Ophthalmic Drug Delivery

Ophthalmic Drug Delivery

Editors

Francisco Javier Otero-Espinar
Anxo Fernández Ferreiro

MDPI

Basel • Beijing • Wuhan • Barcelona • Belgrade • Novi Sad • Cluj • Manchester

Editors
Francisco Javier Otero-Espinar
Department of Pharmacology, Pharmacy and Pharmaceutical Technology
University of Santiago de Compostela (USC)
Santiago de Compostela
Spain

Anxo Fernández Ferreiro
Hospital Pharmacy & Pharmacology Group
SERGAS and Health Research Institute Santiago Compostela
Santiago de Compostela
Spain

Editorial Office
MDPI
St. Alban-Anlage 66
4052 Basel, Switzerland

This is a reprint of articles from the Special Issue published online in the open access journal *Pharmaceutics* (ISSN 1999-4923) (available at: www.mdpi.com/journal/pharmaceutics/special_issues/ophthalmic_drugdelivery).

For citation purposes, cite each article independently as indicated on the article page online and as indicated below:

Lastname, A.A.; Lastname, B.B. Article Title. *Journal Name* **Year**, *Volume Number*, Page Range.

ISBN 978-3-0365-8797-4 (Hbk)
ISBN 978-3-0365-8796-7 (PDF)
doi.org/10.3390/books978-3-0365-8796-7

Contents

Preface . . . . **vii**

Tobias Auel, Linus Großmann, Lukas Schulig, Werner Weitschies and Anne Seidlitz
The EyeFlowCell: Development of a 3D-Printed Dissolution Test Setup for Intravitreal Dosage Forms
Reprinted from: *Pharmaceutics* **2021**, *13*, 1394, doi:10.3390/pharmaceutics13091394 . . . . **1**

Deyanira Barbosa-Alfaro, Vanessa Andrés-Guerrero, Ivan Fernandez-Bueno, María Teresa García-Gutiérrez, Esther Gil-Alegre and Irene Teresa Molina-Martínez et al.
Dexamethasone PLGA Microspheres for Sub-Tenon Administration: Influence of Sterilization and Tolerance Studies
Reprinted from: *Pharmaceutics* **2021**, *13*, 228, doi:10.3390/pharmaceutics13020228 . . . . **15**

Karine Bigot, Pauline Gondouin, Romain Bénard, Pierrick Montagne, Jenny Youale and Marie Piazza et al.
Transferrin Non-Viral Gene Therapy for Treatment of Retinal Degeneration
Reprinted from: *Pharmaceutics* **2020**, *12*, 836, doi:10.3390/pharmaceutics12090836 . . . . **36**

Simon Hauri, Paulina Jakubiak, Matthias Fueth, Stefan Dengl, Sara Belli and Rubén Alvarez-Sánchez et al.
Understanding the Half-Life Extension of Intravitreally Administered Antibodies Binding to Ocular Albumin
Reprinted from: *Pharmaceutics* **2020**, *12*, 810, doi:10.3390/pharmaceutics12090810 . . . . **58**

Pradeep Kumar Bolla, Vrinda Gote, Mahima Singh, Manan Patel, Bradley A. Clark and Jwala Renukuntla
Lutein-Loaded, Biotin-Decorated Polymeric Nanoparticles Enhance Lutein Uptake in Retinal Cells
Reprinted from: *Pharmaceutics* **2020**, *12*, 798, doi:10.3390/pharmaceutics12090798 . . . . **76**

Philip Chennell, Mouloud Yessaad, Florence Abd El Kader, Mireille Jouannet, Mathieu Wasiak and Yassine Bouattour et al.
Do Ophthalmic Solutions of Amphotericin B Solubilised in 2-Hydroxypropyl-γ-Cyclodextrins Possess an Extended Physicochemical Stability?
Reprinted from: *Pharmaceutics* **2020**, *12*, 786, doi:10.3390/pharmaceutics12090786 . . . . **93**

Baptiste Berton, Philip Chennell, Mouloud Yessaad, Yassine Bouattour, Mireille Jouannet and Mathieu Wasiak et al.
Stability of Ophthalmic Atropine Solutions for Child Myopia Control
Reprinted from: *Pharmaceutics* **2020**, *12*, 781, doi:10.3390/pharmaceutics12080781 . . . . **110**

Yoshiyuki Kubo, Miki Yamada, Saki Konakawa, Shin-ichi Akanuma and Ken-ichi Hosoya
Uptake Study in Lysosome-Enriched Fraction: Critical Involvement of Lysosomal Trapping in Quinacrine Uptake But Not Fluorescence-Labeled Verapamil Transport at Blood-Retinal Barrier
Reprinted from: *Pharmaceutics* **2020**, *12*, 747, doi:10.3390/pharmaceutics12080747 . . . . **127**

Roseline Mazet, Xurxo García-Otero, Luc Choisnard, Denis Wouessidjewe, Vincent Verdoot and Frédéric Bossard et al.
Biopharmaceutical Assessment of Dexamethasone Acetate-Based Hydrogels Combining Hydroxypropyl Cyclodextrins and Polysaccharides for Ocular Delivery
Reprinted from: *Pharmaceutics* **2020**, *12*, 717, doi:10.3390/pharmaceutics12080717 . . . . **140**

Raphael Mietzner, Christian Kade, Franziska Froemel, Diana Pauly, W. Daniel Stamer and Andreas Ohlmann et al.
Fasudil Loaded PLGA Microspheres as Potential Intravitreal Depot Formulation for Glaucoma Therapy
Reprinted from: *Pharmaceutics* **2020**, *12*, 706, doi:10.3390/pharmaceutics12080706 . . . . **158**

Claudio Iovino, Rodolfo Mastropasqua, Marco Lupidi, Daniela Bacherini, Marco Pellegrini and Federico Bernabei et al.
Intravitreal Dexamethasone Implant as a Sustained Release Drug Delivery Device for the Treatment of Ocular Diseases: A Comprehensive Review of the Literature
Reprinted from: *Pharmaceutics* **2020**, *12*, 703, doi:10.3390/pharmaceutics12080703 . . . . **180**

Jaakko Itkonen, Ada Annala, Shirin Tavakoli, Blanca Arango-Gonzalez, Marius Ueffing and Elisa Toropainen et al.
Characterization, Stability, and In Vivo Efficacy Studies of Recombinant Human CNTF and Its Permeation into the Neural Retina in Ex Vivo Organotypic Retinal Explant Culture Models
Reprinted from: *Pharmaceutics* **2020**, *12*, 611, doi:10.3390/pharmaceutics12070611 . . . . **206**

Takuya Miyagawa, Zhi-Yu Chen, Che-Yi Chang, Ko-Hua Chen, Yang-Kao Wang and Guei-Sheung Liu et al.
Topical Application of Hyaluronic Acid-RGD Peptide-Coated Gelatin/Epigallocatechin-3 Gallate (EGCG) Nanoparticles Inhibits Corneal Neovascularization via Inhibition of VEGF Production
Reprinted from: *Pharmaceutics* **2020**, *12*, 404, doi:10.3390/pharmaceutics12050404 . . . . **236**

Rubén Varela-Fernández, Victoria Díaz-Tomé, Andrea Luaces-Rodríguez, Andrea Conde-Penedo, Xurxo García-Otero and Asteria Luzardo-Álvarez et al.
Drug Delivery to the Posterior Segment of the Eye: Biopharmaceutic and Pharmacokinetic Considerations
Reprinted from: *Pharmaceutics* **2020**, *12*, 269, doi:10.3390/pharmaceutics12030269 . . . . **253**

Noriaki Nagai, Miyu Ishii, Ryotaro Seiriki, Fumihiko Ogata, Hiroko Otake and Yosuke Nakazawa et al.
Novel Sustained-Release Drug Delivery System for Dry Eye Therapy by Rebamipide Nanoparticles
Reprinted from: *Pharmaceutics* **2020**, *12*, 155, doi:10.3390/pharmaceutics12020155 . . . . **292**

Javier Rodríguez Villanueva, Jorge Martín Esteban and Laura J. Rodríguez Villanueva
Retinal Cell Protection in Ocular Excitotoxicity Diseases. Possible Alternatives Offered by Microparticulate Drug Delivery Systems and Future Prospects
Reprinted from: *Pharmaceutics* **2020**, *12*, 94, doi:10.3390/pharmaceutics12020094 . . . . **303**

Preface

Research in ophthalmic drug delivery has developed significant advances in the last few years, and efforts have been made to develop more effective topical formulations to increase drug bioavailability, efficiency, and safety. Drug delivery to the posterior segment of the eye remains a great challenge in the pharmaceutical industry due to the complexity and particularity of the eye's anatomy and physiology. Some advances have been made with the purpose of maintaining constant drug levels in the site of action. The anatomical ocular barriers have a great impact on drug pharmacokinetics and, subsequently, on the pharmacological effect.

Despite the increasing interest in efficiently reaching the posterior segment of the eye with reduced adverse effects, there is still a need to expand the knowledge of ocular pharmacokinetics that allow the development of safer and more innovative drug delivery systems. These novel approaches may greatly improve the lives of patients with ocular pathologies.

Francisco Javier Otero-Espinar and Anxo Fernández Ferreiro
Editors

pharmaceutics

Article

The EyeFlowCell: Development of a 3D-Printed Dissolution Test Setup for Intravitreal Dosage Forms

Tobias Auel [1], Linus Großmann [1], Lukas Schulig [2], Werner Weitschies [1] and Anne Seidlitz [1,*]

1 Center of Drug Absorption and Transport, Department of Biopharmaceutics and Pharmaceutical Technology, Institute of Pharmacy, University of Greifswald, 17489 Greifswald, Germany; tobias.auel@uni-greifswald.de (T.A.); linus.grossmann@uni-greifswald.de (L.G.); werner.weitschies@uni-greifswald.de (W.W.)

2 Department of Pharmaceutical and Medicinal Chemistry, Institute of Pharmacy, University of Greifswald, 17489 Greifswald, Germany; lukas.schulig@uni-greifswald.de

* Correspondence: anne.seidlitz@uni-greifswald.de; Tel.: +49-3834-420-4898

Abstract: An in vitro dissolution model, the so-called EyeFlowCell (EFC), was developed to test intravitreal dosage forms, simulating parameters such as the gel-like consistency of the vitreous body. The developed model consists of a stereolithography 3D-printed flow-through cell with a polyacrylamide (PAA) gel as its core. This gel needed to be coated with an agarose sheath because of its low viscosity. Drug release from hydroxypropyl methylcellulose-based implants containing either triamcinolone acetonide or fluorescein sodium was studied in the EFC using a schematic eye movement by the EyeMovementSystem (EyeMoS). For comparison, studies were performed in USP apparatus 4 and USP apparatus 7. Significantly slower drug release was observed in the PAA gel for both model drugs compared with the compendial methods. Drug release from fluorescein sodium-containing model implants was completed after 40 min in USP apparatus 4, whereas drug release in the gel-based EFC lasted 72 h. Drug release from triamcinolone acetonide-containing model implants was completed after 35 min in USP apparatus 4 and after 150 min in USP apparatus 7, whereas this was delayed until 96 h in the EFC. These results suggest that compendial release methods may overestimate the drug release rate in the human vitreous body. Using a gel-based in vitro release system such as the EFC may better predict drug release.

Keywords: in vitro model; in vitro drug release; intravitreal implants; SLA 3D-printing; triamcinolone acetonide; USP apparatus 4; USP apparatus 7; vitreous substitute; dissolution

Citation: Auel, T.; Großmann, L.; Schulig, L.; Weitschies, W.; Seidlitz, A. The EyeFlowCell: Development of a 3D-Printed Dissolution Test Setup for Intravitreal Dosage Forms. *Pharmaceutics* **2021**, *13*, 1394. https://doi.org/10.3390/pharmaceutics13091394

Academic Editors: Monica M. Jablonski and Ingunn Tho

Received: 29 July 2021
Accepted: 31 August 2021
Published: 3 September 2021

1. Introduction

The incidence of eye diseases has increased steadily in recent years as a result of demographic change. In particular, diseases of the posterior segment of the eye, such as diabetic retinopathy, macular edema, or age-related macular degeneration, are more and more common [1–3]. Intravitreal therapy as a minimally invasive procedure, in which suspensions, solutions, or implants containing antibodies like bevacizumab (Avastin®) or glucocorticoids like dexamethasone (Ozurdex®) or triamcinolone acetonide (TA) are injected into the human vitreous body, is becoming increasingly crucial for the treatment of such clinical conditions [4]. Implants, in particular, provide better patient compliance because of their sustained release, as the intervals between the individual applications may be extended [5].

For ethical and practical reasons, in vivo studies in humans in preclinical development of new intravitreal dosage forms are complicated. On the one hand, an in vivo determination of the drug in the vitreous body is almost impossible. On the other hand, the human eye is a susceptible organ, where even minor damages can lead to visual impairment. Therefore, the use of animal models plays a significant role in preclinical development. Aside from rats and mini-pigs, rabbits are the most commonly used animal species [6].

Even if animal models provide preliminary conclusions regarding the behavior of dosage forms in the human vitreous, it must be taken into account that the physiological conditions differ to a variable extent; that is, different vitreous volumes, aqueous flows, and vitreous diffusional pathlength between the species may complicate the transferability of results from in vivo studies [7,8]. Another important aspect is the age-related liquefaction of the human vitreous body. Whereas this frequently occurs in humans with increasing age, possibly leading to a different release and distribution behavior of dosage forms, young animals used in in vivo studies have a more gel-like vitreous body that cannot reflect this fact [9–11]. For this reason, the combination of in vivo animal studies with more biorelevant in vitro models is a possible option to reduce the number of animal studies and obtain a better first idea of the behavior of new drug formulations in the human vitreous body.

Compendial release apparatuses of the United States Pharmacopeia (USP) such as the flow-through cell (USP apparatus 4) or the reciprocating holder (USP apparatus 7) are the first approach for dissolution testing of new intravitreal dosage forms. Both are recommended, for example, for in vitro release studies of implants [12]. The so-called shake-flask method, in which implants are incubated with release medium in tubes under agitation, is also commonly found in the literature [13,14]. With these methods, it is possible to represent lower liquid volumes, as they are present at many application sites of implants. Nevertheless, when it comes to simulating the physiological conditions of the human vitreous body, unique characteristics such as the gel-like consistency or the aqueous flow are neglected here. There are only a few in vitro models that try to simulate the behavior of drug formulations in the human vitreous. One of them is the PK-Eye developed by Awwad et al., which attempts to simulate the clearance of drugs via the aqueous flow-through the anterior chamber of the eye [15]. Another model is the EyeMovementSystem (EyeMoS) created by Loch et al. [16] and adjusted by Stein et al. [17], which takes the influence of simulated eye movements on the distribution and release of drugs into account. Both models investigate the influence of individual aspects on the distribution behavior of active ingredients in a simulated human vitreous body. However, they are nevertheless fairly limited regarding the information they provide about the release of the drugs from different dosage forms.

This work aimed to develop a gel-based flow-through system and combine it with the previously developed EyeMoS so that continuous dissolution testing is possible over a more extended time. Until now, it was necessary for dissolution studies in the EyeMoS either to perform multiple studies with different endpoints or to transfer the test objects into fresh gels at defined time points. This transfer meant that the dosage form was subjected to mechanical stress. By adding a flow-through system around the gel, sampling from an external vessel should be possible without affecting the dosage form.

For this purpose, model implants based on hydroxypropyl methylcellulose (HPMC) containing fluorescein sodium (FS) or TA were manufactured by hot-melt extrusion. In the first studies, the model was tested with the analytically accessible, hydrophilic model substance FS, which is used as a dye in fluorescein angiography for staining tissue layers, among other applications [18]. The glucocorticoid TA is used as a vascular endothelial growth factor (VEGF) inhibitor in the therapy of diseases of the posterior segment of the eye [19].

The drug release from the implants was investigated in the newly developed so-called EyeFlowCell (EFC) after injection into a gel-like core. For this purpose, a polyacrylamide (PAA) gel developed by Loch et al. was used, corresponding to the human vitreous body in essential characteristics such as water content, pH, density, and viscosity [16]. As the PAA gel used by Loch et al. has a low viscosity, a setup had to be found to prevent it from being washed away by the flowing media. For this purpose, the PAA gel was coated with a form-stable agarose sheath and the dual gel was placed centrally in a 3D-printed basket so that the release medium could flow around it. By combining it with the EyeMoS, the influence of schematic eye movement on drug release was investigated.

Moreover, for reasons of comparison, dissolution studies were performed in the USP standard apparatuses 4 (flow-through cell) and 7 (reciprocating holder).

2. Materials and Methods

2.1. Materials

Sodium chloride, potassium chloride, disodium hydrogen phosphate, and potassium dihydrogen phosphate as components of phosphate buffered saline (PBS) pH 7.4 were purchased from AppliChem (Darmstadt, Germany). A PAA gel developed by Loch et al. [16] simulating the vitreous body was prepared according to the composition given in Table 1. Rotiphoresis gel 30 (37.5:1), ammonium peroxodisulfate, and tetramethylethylenediamine were purchased from Carl Roth (Karlsruhe, Germany). Agarose for the PAA gel-sheath was purchased from Sigma Aldrich, Germany. Model implants were prepared via hot-melt extrusion of FS (Sigma Aldrich, St. Louis, MO, USA) or TA (Caelo, Hilden, Germany) as active pharmaceutical ingredients, hydroxypropyl methylcellulose (HPMC; Affinisol 100LV/Affinisol 15LV; Dow Chemicals, Midland, TX, USA) and polyethylene glycol (PEG) 6000 (Carl Roth). All chemicals and solvents for the high-performance liquid chromatography (HPLC) were of analytical quality. A standard Formlabs Clear Resin (Formlabs, Somerville, MA, USA) was used for the 3D-printed EFC.

Table 1. Composition of the modified polyacrylamide gel by Loch et al.

Compound	Content (%)
phosphate buffered saline pH 7.4	92.21
rotiphoresis gel 30	6.69
ammonium peroxodisulfate	1
tetramethylethylendiamine	0.1

2.2. Methods

2.2.1. Preparation of the Model Implants

For the preparation of the drug-loaded model implants, the components listed in Table 2 were mixed, dried in an oven for 24 h at 40 °C, and then extruded with a twin-screw extruder (Three-Tec ZE12, Seon, Switzerland) through a 0.5 mm nozzle. The powder inlet was cooled to 15 °C, and the barrel was heated to 180 °C. A Three-Tec conveyor belt was used to stretch the extrudates. The produced filaments were cut to a length of approximately 6 mm with a disposable scalpel, and their mass was determined individually using a Sartorius SE2 ultra-micro balance (Sartorius, Goettingen, Germany).

Table 2. Composition of the powder mixtures for fluorescein sodium and triamcinolone acetonide implants produced via hot-melt extrusion.

Compound	Batch 1 Content (%)	Batch 2 Content (%)
fluorescein sodium	40	-
triamcinolone acetonide	-	20
silicone dioxide	0.5	0.5
polyethylene glycol 6000	10	10
hydroxypropyl methylcellulose	49.5	69.5

2.2.2. Fabrication of the EyeFlowCell

The 3D-printed dissolution chambers, the so-called EyeFlowCell, were designed with FreeCAD (version 0.17), sliced with Preform (version 3.4.5) software, and printed with a Formlabs Form 3 (Formlabs, Somerville, MA, USA) stereolithography printer. A clear resin was used as material for all cells. A schematic view of the intended design is shown in Figure 1. The chamber was developed to consist of a closed bottom side and a top side with an injection channel for injecting the dosage forms to be tested and a basket keeps the vitreous substitute centered in the middle. Sealing is achieved by a self-manufactured sealing ring made of silicone; the injection channel is closed by a plug so no medium can leak out this way. In contrast to conventional flow-through cells, the dissolution chamber is perfused with a release medium from the bottom inlet to the top outlet. Special holders were printed from polylactic acid (Formfutura, Nijmegen, The Netherlands) using an Ultimaker 3 Extended (Ultimaker, Ultrecht, The Netherlands) to mount the EFC on the EyeMoS.

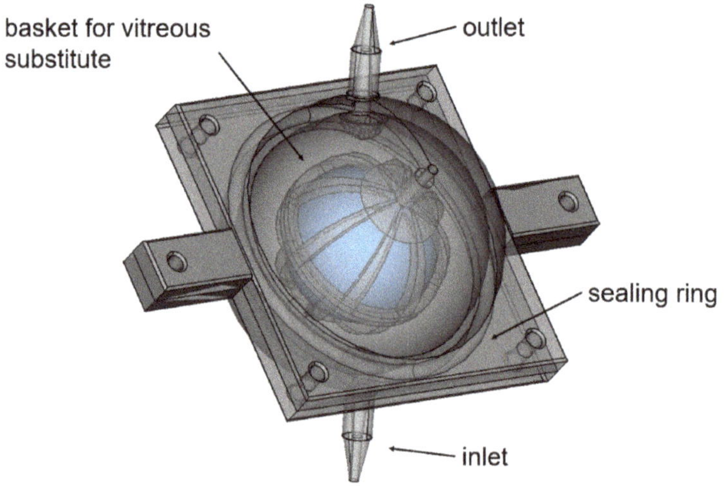

Figure 1. Schematic view of the EyeFlowCell. The vitreous substitute should be placed centrally in the basket allowing the flow to pass through the inlet to the outlet and surround the substitute.

2.2.3. Fabrication of the Vitreous Substitute

In order to prevent the PAA gel from washing out, a method to produce a sheath around it had to be developed. To mimic the volume of the human vitreous body, a spheric 4 mL gel body of the PAA gel was cast in silicone molds (r = 10 mm; Figure 2a) and frozen at −80 °C for at least 2 h (Figure 2b). A 2% agarose solution in PBS 7.4 mixture was heated on a heating plate to 100 °C under agitation until the agarose was completely dissolved and then cooled down to 50–60 °C. Evaporation loss was corrected and the frozen PAA gel was fixed centrally with a metal rod in a larger silicone mold (r = 14 mm; Figure 2c). This mold was used to coat the PAA gel with the hot agarose solution and create a uniform, 4 mm thick sheath. The dual gel was stored at 8 °C for at least 2 h.

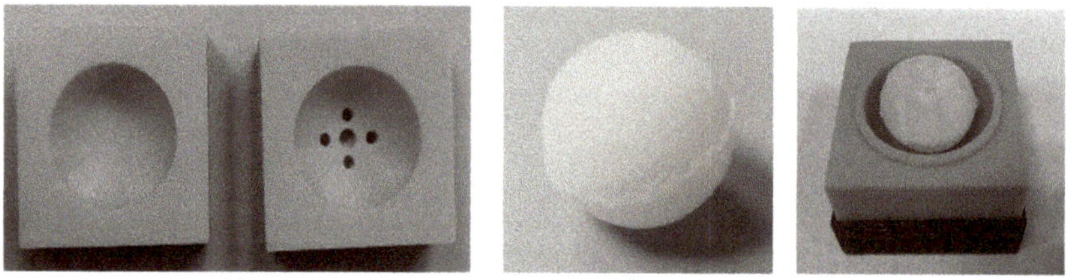

(**a**) (**b**) (**c**)

Figure 2. (**a**) Silicone molds for the production of the polyacrylamide (PAA) gel vitreous body substitutes; (**b**) frozen PAA gel core; (**c**) mounted PAA gel-core before coating with agarose-solution.

2.2.4. In Vitro Drug Release Studies Using Compendial Methods

In vitro release testing of the FS and TA-containing HPMC implants in USP apparatus 4 was performed using flow-through cells under sink conditions at room temperature in a closed system. A magnetic stirrer stirred the test volume of 100 mL PBS in a vessel at 250 rpm. An Ismatec IPC peristaltic pump was used to circulate the release medium at a flow rate of 5 mL/min through the cells. Samples of 1 mL were withdrawn at predetermined time points from the vessel and replaced with fresh PBS after sampling. In vitro release of TA-containing HPMC implants was furthermore studied under sink conditions in a USP 7 apparatus (400-DS Dissolution Apparatus 7, Agilent Technologies, Santa Clara, CA, USA) at room temperature. Cells were filled with a volume of 10 mL of PBS and each cell was loaded with a 12-port mesh basket dipping at 30 dips per minute through an externally controlled magnetic plate. A sample volume of 1 mL was withdrawn at each time point, and the remaining volume was discarded and replaced with 10 mL of fresh PBS.

2.2.5. In Vitro Drug Release Studies in the EyeFlowCell

The release testing of the drug-loaded model implants was performed in the newly developed system combined with or without the EyeMovementSystem (EyeMoS). For both methods, 100 mL PBS 7.4 was used as the release medium. The medium container was stirred at room temperature by a magnetic stirrer at 250 rpm. An Ismatec IPC peristaltic pump was used to circulate the release medium at a flow rate of 5 mL/min through the chambers. A picture of this setup is shown in Figure 3.

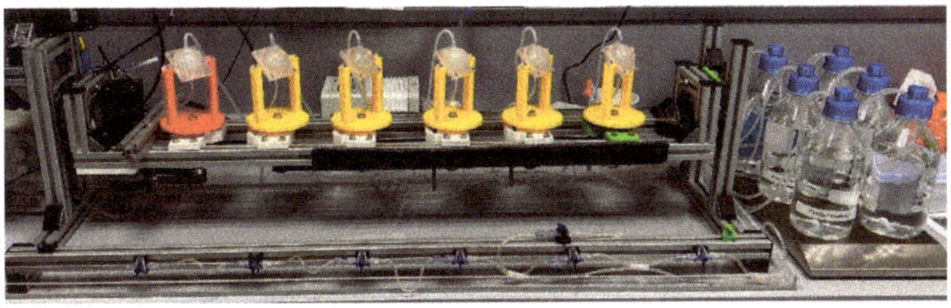

Figure 3. Setup of the EyeFlowCell combined with the EyeMoS.

For the release in the EFC, the gel vitreous bodies were prepared as described above and inserted into the dissolution chambers. The drug-loaded implants were injected into the gel vitreous bodies with a Sterican cannula (0.5 × 16 mm) through the injection channel. The cannula was fitted with a spacer to ensure reproducible injection, placing the implant centrally in the vitreous substitute. For dissolution testing with the simulated eye movement, the repetitive 24 h scheme given in Table 3 was used, which was also used in previous works [16,17]. To determine the residual drug content in the gel, TA or FS was extracted from the gel with 10 mL of acetone. Extraction was carried out in an incubator at room temperature for 24 h and 150 rpm. The PAA gel collapsed upon exposure to the solvent and was removed with the parts of the agarose sheath. The acetone was then evaporated, and the residue was taken up in 10 mL PBS and measured by high-performance liquid chromatography (TA) or fluorescence spectroscopy (FS).

Table 3. Movement pattern of the applied schematic eye movement.

	Movement Pattern (x-Axis)	Angle (°)	Angular Velocity (°/s)
Mode 1	Slow pursuit movement	35	41
Mode 2	Fast pursuit movement	33	83
Mode 3	Saccadic movement	42	165
Mode 4	Pursuit movement with distinct amplitudes	90	330
	Movement pattern y-axis	20	60
	24 h day rhythm Minutes (mode)	290 min (mode 1), 5 min (mode 3) 280 min (mode 4), 5 min (mode 3) 260 min (mode 2), 5 min (mode 3) 300 min (mode 1), 5 min (mode 3) 285 min (mode 4), 5 min (mode 3)	

2.2.6. Quantification

TA was quantified using a Shimadzu Nexera XR Modular high-pressure liquid chromatography system (Shimadzu, Kyoto, Japan) consisting of a SIL-20ACxr autosampler, a CTO-10AC column oven, SPD-M20A diode array detector, DGU-20A3R degasser, CBM-20A system controller, and LC-20AD pumps. A Kinetix Polar C18 column (2.6 μm, 150 × 2.1 mm; Phenomenex, Torrance, CA, USA) was used. The column oven was heated to 40 °C, and the wavelength of the detector was set to 238 nm. The mobile phase consisted of 30% millipore water and 70% methanol, both mixed with 0.5% formic acid. The injection volume was 20 μL, the flow rate was 0.45 mL/min, and the retention time was approximately 1.8 min. The concentration range for the calibration was 0.1–10 μg/mL with a coefficient of determination (R^2) of 0.999. The evaluation was performed with the software LabSolution (Shimadzu).

FS was determined by UV/vis spectrometry using a Cary 60 spectrophotometer (Agilent, San Diego, CA, USA) with a fiber optic-based system (slit width 10 mm). In a two-minute interval, measurements were carried out at a wavelength of 490 nm (λ_{max} of fluorescein) and 600 nm (baseline correction). The calibration range was 0.1–10 μg/mL (coefficient of determination $R^2 = 0.999$). All FS experiments were performed under protection from light.

3. Results

3.1. Preparation of the Vitreous Substitute

The PAA gel used to simulate the vitreous body had to be covered with a form-giving agarose sheath because of its low viscosity. For this purpose, the frozen PAA gel core was coated with a warm agarose solution in a special silicone mold. On contact with the gel, this solution cooled and formed a 4 mm thick agarose sheath. An agarose solution of 2% proved to be practicable in handling. Cracks occurred in the sheath at lower concentrations, so washing out of the gel core could not be avoided entirely. At higher concentrations, the warm agarose solution was too viscous to cast a uniformly thick sheath without defects. Figure 4a shows a schematic view of the dual gel. The coated dual gel is shown in Figure 4b.

Even after the release studies, both the inner PAA gel and the outer agarose sheath were intact. Images of vitreous substitutes that were cut in half after a release experiment are shown in Figure 5. There is a clear separation between the viscous PAA gel and the form-stable agarose sheath.

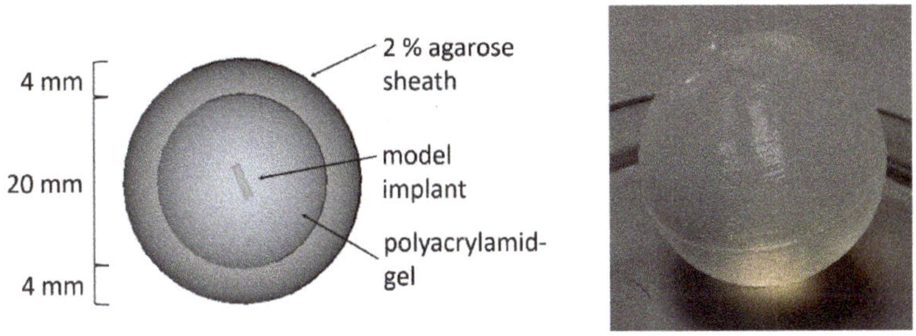

(a) (b)

Figure 4. (**a**) Schematic view of the dual gel: the inner polyacrylamide gel core simulates the human vitreous body. Dosage forms like implants or suspensions can be injected into the polyacrylamide gel. The core is coated with a 4 mm thick 2% agarose sheath to maintain the form. (**b**) Photography of the agarose-coated polyacrylamide gel.

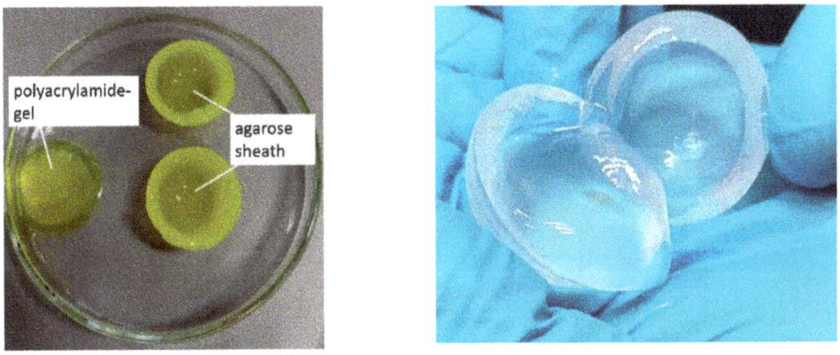

(a) (b)

Figure 5. (**a**) Cut open agarose sheath after the end of a fluorescein sodium dissolution study; (**b**) cut open agarose sheath after the end of a triamcinolone acetonide dissolution study.

3.2. Fabrication of the EyeFlowCell

The 3D-printed dissolution chamber, called EyeFlowCell, is depicted in Figure 6a. Printing was achieved in a suitable resolution and the planned properties were achieved. The dimensions of the EFC are 60 mm × 60 mm × 52 mm (width, length, height). The chamber volume is 51 mL, of which 11.5 mL is occupied by the inner basket for the vitreous substitute. The central basket for holding the vitreous substitute has an inner radius of 14 mm. The basket itself consists of eight bars with a width of 2.8 mm, which are connected at the top in a 1.4 mm thick ring. Leak tightness was achieved with the custom-made sealing ring. The upper side of the model as shown in Figure 6b has an injection channel with a diameter of 3.5 mm, intended for direct injection of the dosage form to be tested into the inner vitreous substitute. The cell is attached to a holder via two cantilevers so that the orientation allows a vertically upward flow through the cell.

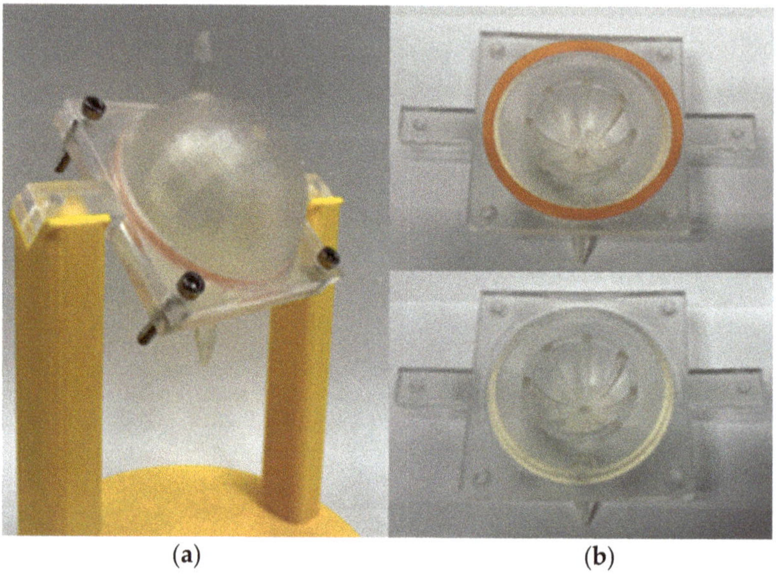

Figure 6. 3D-printed EyeFlowCell; (**a**) complete cell mounted on a 3D-printed holder; (**b**) separate top and bottom side of the EyeFlowCell.

3.3. Drug Loaded Model Implants

TA- and FS-loaded implants based on HPMC were successfully extruded. Microscopic images of the extruded implants are shown in Figure 7. The filaments exhibit a relatively uniform diameter of 0.49 mm with a homogeneous matrix and a slightly rough surface. The length of the cut implants was approximately 6 mm. The actual drug loading of the implants was 29.5 ± 1.4% for the implants with FS and 17.3 ± 0.8% for those with TA. In relation to the powder mixture, the drug content of the FS filaments deviates significantly. On the one hand, thermal stress during extrusion and, on the other hand, photoinstabilities could be responsible for this. Before the dissolution experiments, the mass of the investigated implants was determined and used for calculating the drug content. The average mass of FS implants was 1.627 ± 0.103 mg containing 0.480 ± 0.030 mg FS, and the TA implants weighed 1.421 ± 0.219 mg with an amount of 0.246 ± 0.038 mg TA incorporated.

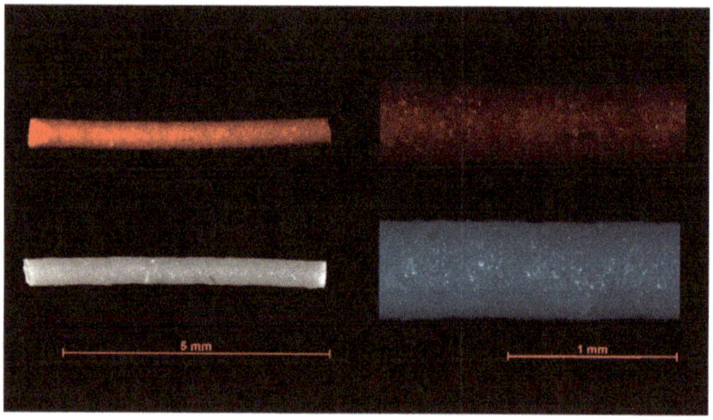

Figure 7. Microscopic images of extruded fluorescein sodium and triamcinolone acetonide HPMC implants.

3.4. Dissolution Studies

The drug release of FS- or TA-containing HPMC implants was tested in the EFC, as shown in Figure 8 (FS) and Figure 9 (TA). For both the hydrophilic FS and the more lipophilic TA, no difference can be seen between the respective profiles in the EFC independent of whether or not the movement was applied. The release of the FS-containing HPMC implants after 72 h was 110.0 ± 4.4% with EyeMoS versus 113.1 ± 7.2% without EyeMoS. In comparison, even minimally less drug is released without the movement by the EyeMovementSystem. However, the slight difference shows that the movement does not seem to have any influence in this experiment. Moreover, there is no difference in the release profiles of the TA-containing HPMC implants. After four days, a plateau was reached for both release profiles in the EFC. At this time, 91.3 ± 1.6% was released when testing with movement, while without movement, 91.3 ± 0.9% of the theoretical drug load was released.

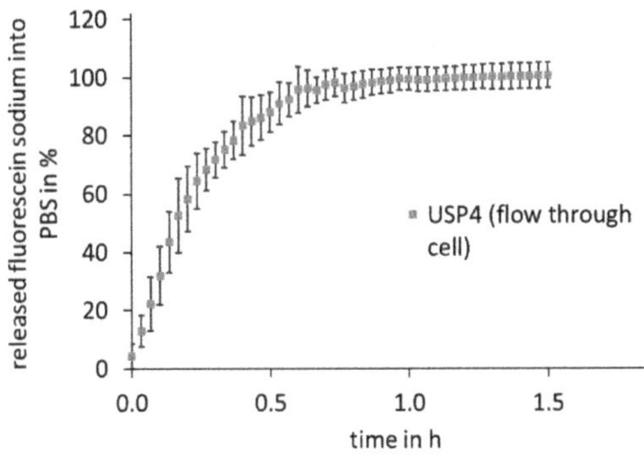

(**a**)

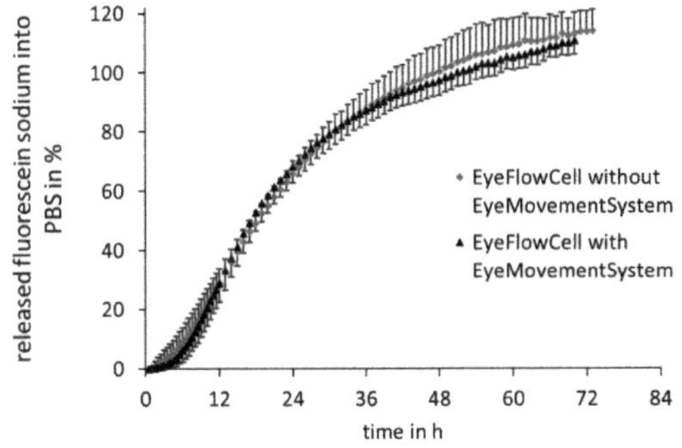

(**b**)

Figure 8. Mean fluorescein sodium release profiles obtained from HPMC model implants in PBS 7.4; (**a**) in the USP apparatus 4 (RT, 250 rpm) $n = 5 \pm$ SD; (**b**) in the EyeFlowCell with and without agitation with EyeMovement System (RT, 250 rpm) $n = 5 \pm$ SD.

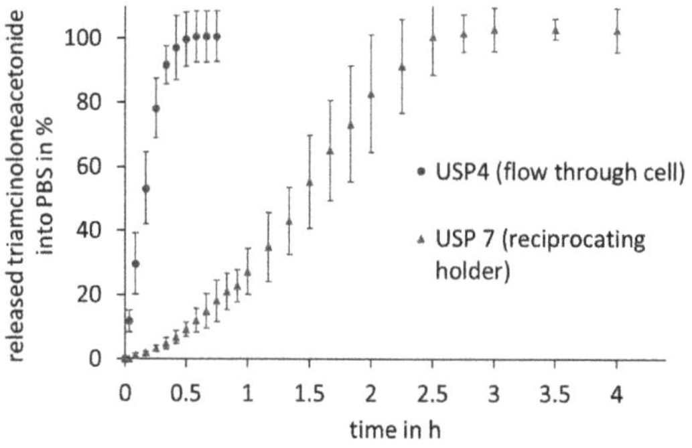

(**a**)

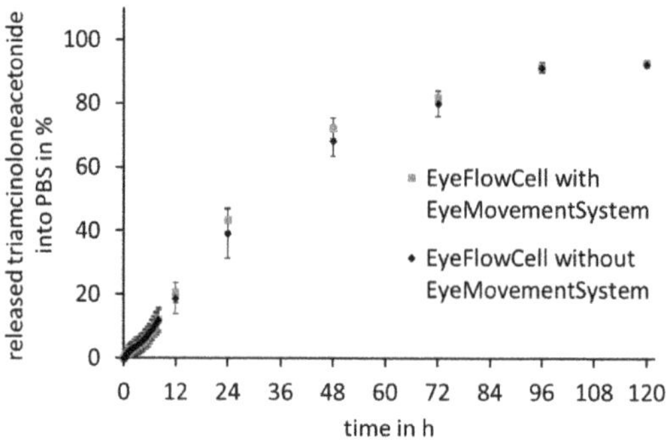

(**b**)

Figure 9. Mean triamcinolone acetonide release profiles obtained from HPMC model implants in PBS 7.4; (**a**) in the USP apparatus 4 (RT, 250 rpm) and USP apparatus 7 (RT, 30 dips/min), $n = 5 \pm$ SD; (**b**) in the EyeFlowCell with and without agitation with EyeMovementSystem, $n = 5 \pm$ SD.

Comparing the profiles with those obtained using compendial methods, a slower release can be seen in the EFC for both drugs. While for the TA-containing implants in the USP apparatus 7, there is a low release at the beginning, in the USP apparatus 4, a rapid increase in the amount released can be seen directly for TA as well as for FS. In USP apparatus 4, the plateau and thus the complete release of TA with 100.5 ± 8.1% is even reached after 35 min, while in USP apparatus 7, the reciprocating holder, 100.6 ± 12.0% is released after 150 min into the surrounding medium. The release from the FS-containing implants reached a plateau of 95.5 ± 4.5% after approximately 40 min in USP apparatus 4.

4. Discussion

Monographed pharmacopeia release systems offer many advantages for the in vitro characterization of dosage forms. They assure defined and reproducible conditions for drug release from different dosage forms. As a result, they provide comparability of collected data. However, these systems usually have little in common with the conditions at the respective application sites. Therefore, they offer great advantages for quality control, but lack predictability of the actual behavior of the dosage form in vivo. The general approach for developing a gel-based flow-through cell is based on the assumption that the degradation, swelling, and thus release behavior of dosage forms like implants depends on the medium surrounding them. In the case of intravitreal application, this is the gel-like vitreous body. This site of application is poorly reflected by compendial release systems, leading to differences in in vitro behavior compared with the situation in vivo.

Suitable systems for continuous dissolution studies, which provide a better preliminary understanding of how the dissolution might occur in vivo, are lacking so far. While there are several approaches for human vitreous body substitution in vivo, in vitro drug release in these has not been studied in detail so far [20,21]. Apart from the PAA gel by Loch et al. used here, which has already been used for release studies, and another vitreous substitute developed by Awwad et al. from hyaluronic acid and agar, which was used to determine the clearance of PLGA microparticles or antibodies, there is little literature on in vitro experiments. One reason for this could be the problems associated with sampling from gels.

The use of 3D-printing is beneficial for dissolution test setup development. The individual options for design and layout allow new dissolution test models to be adapted quickly and easily, depending on requirements. The stereolithography printing used here enables the precise production of fine models. In previous works, it has been used to produce a Franz cell for permeation studies or to print tablets containing drugs, for example, [22,23]. The EFC is intended to simulate the human vitreous body, which is why a gel was used as a dissolution medium to simulate the human vitreous body, resembling the vitreous body in some essential properties [16]. In the human vitreous body, the gel-like structure is formed by an interaction of primary collagen and hyaluronic acid [24,25]. In contrast, in the PAA gel, this is achieved by crosslinking acrylic amide with tetramethylethylenediamine. The negative charge of the glycosaminoglycan hyaluronic acid is not considered here, for which interactions and inhibition of the diffusion of cations have been described [26]. This point should be an approach for future developments to revise the inner gel core, the in vitro vitreous substitute.

In order to maintain sink conditions, the use of a flow-through system around this gel was chosen. Moreover, this offers the advantage of sampling from a liquid medium, as the determination of the release into gels usually requires extraction for sampling, and thus leads to multiple experiments with different endpoints. Compared with USP apparatus 4, however, the EFC requires a larger minimum volume of the release medium. Owing to the chamber volume of 51 mL and the tubing system, at least 100 mL of release medium is required, whereas in USP apparatus 4, 50 mL or even less is sufficient depending on the cell and tubing design. Because the PAA gel used as the vitreous substitute possesses a low viscosity, it had to be enclosed in a 2% agarose coating to prevent it from being liquefied and washed away by the flow. Preliminary tests have shown that a sheath thickness of 4 mm is necessary to produce a uniform reproducible shell. A spherical coating was chosen because it visually reflects the almost spherical vitreous body and ensures simple and reproducible handling. Preliminary experiments with dye solution (data not shown) have indicated that the diffusion of the drug from the inner PAA gel into the dissolution medium is not significantly hindered.

To test this system, simple model implants were produced from HPMC and FS or TA. HPMC is a water-soluble polymer commonly used in hot-melt extrusion, which has excellent properties for processing. FS was chosen as an analytically well-accessible hydrophilic model substance. The glucocorticoid TA belongs to the VEGF inhibitors and is used as an intravitreal suspension for various diseases like macular edema [27], and was thus selected as a model substance. The length and diameter of the fabricated implants were based on the intravitreal implant Ozurdex® (Allergan), which is approved in Europe.

An extreme discrepancy in dissolution times is noticeable when comparing the dissolution profiles between the EFC and the standard apparatuses. Because of the flow of the medium in USP apparatus 4 and the dipping in USP apparatus 7, the release is completed within 35–150 min, whereas this takes several days in the EFC. This time difference can be attributed to the movement of the dosage form in the medium associated with convective transport of the drug after dissolution, which does not occur when gels are used as injection sites. Another reason for the slower drug release in the EFC could be the dissolution of the implants. As these are immobilized in the gel and degradation products also have to diffuse out of the PAA gel core, slower degradation may result in slower drug release. Moreover, no diffusion of the drugs is required in the compendial setups, so that the released drug can be determined without delay. Comparing the two releases in the EFC, it can be seen that the applied movement had no influence on the release rate in these first investigations. All release profiles in the EFC can be divided into three phases: at the beginning, there is a lag-time of 1.5–2 h, during which almost no drug is released into the medium. In this phase, the drug is most likely distributed in the inner gel core, and is thus not yet detectable in the surrounding medium. Subsequently, the release curves increase constantly over several days until they reach a plateau.

Because diffusion processes play a role in the distribution within the gel and between the different media and, according to Fick's law, these are only driven by the concentration gradient, this result was expected. These results demonstrate that the PAA gel, intended to simulate the human vitreous body, can significantly slow down drug release from HPMC implants. Assuming that the dosage form behaves approximately the same in the human vitreous, it can be hypothesized that compendial methods significantly overestimate the rate of drug release for both hydrophilic and lipophilic drugs, at least for the release from HPMC implants tested here. However, to confirm this hypothesis and the suitability of EFC to predict the in vivo behavior of dosage forms, in vivo release data are required. Diffusion, as well as convection, plays an essential role in the human vitreous. The elimination of drugs occurs either via the posterior chamber of the eye or the retina, thus the drug has to be distributed in the vitreous body [28]. The distribution processes that take place in the vitreous body could thus be roughly simulated with the distribution in the gel as a vitreous body substitute. Because of the limited volume of the PAA gel, solubility in it could be a limiting factor. Even if sink conditions exist in the release medium, non-sink conditions in the PAA gel could affect the concentration gradient between the vitreous substitute and the dosage form, thus slowing down release. It may be expected that this effect is more pronounced for drugs with low solubility in the water-based gel.

The use of the EFC is not only limited to implants owing to the PAA gel core. An investigation of suspensions or nanoparticles would also be possible because separation of the particles from the release medium used for sampling is assured when using the EFC. If the results for implants are transferred to nanoparticles, this would probably also be considered with a slower drug release in the EFC compared with compendial methods.

All experiments in this work were performed at room temperature because temperature control of the EFC could not be implemented thus far. This detail is to be seen as a disadvantage compared with the compendial methods, in which the temperature can be easily adjusted. Especially in the dissolution of implants and the disintegration process of polymers, temperature plays a major role. This aspect must be considered in future developments in any case.

Because mainly young animals are used in preclinical in vivo studies, the gel used in this work should take this aspect into account [13,29]. However, using a pure gel body as a vitreous substitute here only represents idealized physiological conditions. With aging, the human vitreous body liquefies [25], so that an applied movement might influence the release behavior because of the addition of convective processes [9]. Because the incidence of many posterior eye diseases (diabetic retinopathy, age-related macular degeneration, and macular edema) increases with age, simulation of a liquefied vitreous should be included in further experiments. A simulation of a vitrectomized vitreous body would also be possible with the EFC. Stein et al. showed that the addition of silicone oil to an in vitro vitreous substitute has an influence on distribution processes [30]. Because of the outer agarose sheath, the inner gel core can be easily adapted to these different conditions.

In conclusion, the EFC, a gel-based flow-through cell, was developed to simulate the human vitreous body in this work. With this, a continuous dissolution study of intravitreal implants is possible without the need for multiple experiments with different endpoints or manual transfer of the implants. In the future, temperature control of the system needs to be considered to take the influence of body temperature into account. Further steps should include the testing of commercially available dosage forms using this setup. However, model evaluation based on the comparison of in vitro and in vivo data is complicated for intravitreal products because in vivo data regarding release into the vitreous are not available owing to the local release of small amounts of drug over time and the inaccessibility of human vitreous for sampling. Nevertheless, the model is a first approach to investigate intravitreal dosage forms under more biorelevant conditions in preclinical development.

5. Conclusions

Models of more biorelevant in vitro release in preclinical development can better predict the dissolution behavior of dosage forms in vivo. Official compendial drug dissolution methods generally represent aqueous systems that often inadequately reflect physiological conditions. The EFC developed here as a modified flow-through cell represents a first approach to study intravitreal dosage forms, in which a gel simulates the human vitreous body. The setup was successfully printed with a 3D printer using stereolithography. It was shown that drug release from FS- or TA-containing HPMC implants was significantly slower when using a gel system compared with two standard compendial methods (USP apparatus 4 and 7). The EFC represents a gel-based release system that allows continuous dissolution testing of intravitreal dosage forms. Further studies, specifically on long-term suitability, need to be conducted to further evaluate the system.

Author Contributions: Conceptualization, T.A., L.G., W.W. and A.S.; methodology, T.A. and L.G.; software, L.S.; validation, T.A. and L.G; investigation, T.A. and L.G.; data curation, T.A.; writing—original draft preparation, T.A. and A.S.; writing—review and editing, T.A., L.G., L.S., W.W. and A.S.; funding acquisition, W.W. and A.S. All authors have read and agreed to the published version of the manuscript.

Funding: This research received no external funding.

Institutional Review Board Statement: Not applicable.

Informed Consent Statement: Not applicable.

Data Availability Statement: The data presented in this study are available on request from the corresponding author.

Acknowledgments: The authors thank Agilent Technologies, Inc., USA, and Sandra Klein for the supply of the 400-DS reciprocating holder apparatus and Katharina Tietz for assistance with the experiments.

Conflicts of Interest: The authors declare no conflict of interest.

References

1. Wong, W.L.; Su, X.; Li, X.; Cheung, C.M.G.; Klein, R.; Cheng, C.Y.; Wong, T.Y. Global prevalence of age-related macular degeneration and disease burden projection for 2020 and 2040: A systematic review and meta-analysis. *Lancet Glob. Health* **2014**, *2*, e106–e116. [CrossRef]
2. Voleti, V.B.; Hubschman, J.P. Age-related eye disease. *Maturitas* **2013**, *75*, 29–33. [CrossRef]
3. Finger, R.P.; Fimmers, R.; Holz, F.G.; Scholl, H.P.N. Incidence of blindness and severe visual impairment in Germany: Projections for 2030. *Investig. Ophthalmol. Vis. Sci.* **2011**, *52*, 4381–4389. [CrossRef] [PubMed]
4. Fogli, S.; Del Re, M.; Rofi, E.; Posarelli, C.; Figus, M.; Danesi, R. Clinical pharmacology of intravitreal anti-VEGF drugs. *Eye* **2018**, *32*, 1010–1020. [CrossRef] [PubMed]
5. Fredenberg, S.; Wahlgren, M.; Reslow, M.; Axelsson, A. The mechanisms of drug release in poly(lactic-co-glycolic acid)-based drug delivery systems—A review. *Int. J. Pharm.* **2011**, *415*, 34–52. [CrossRef]
6. Awwad, S.; Henein, C.; Ibeanu, N.; Khaw, P.T.; Brocchini, S. Preclinical challenges for developing long acting intravitreal medicines. *Eur. J. Pharm. Biopharm.* **2020**, *153*, 130–149. [CrossRef]
7. del Amo, E.M.; Urtti, A. Rabbit as an animal model for intravitreal pharmacokinetics: Clinical predictability and quality of the published data. *Exp. Eye Res.* **2015**, *137*, 111–124. [CrossRef] [PubMed]
8. Rowe-Rendleman, C.L.; Durazo, S.A.; Kompella, U.B.; Rittenhouse, K.D.; Di Polo, A.; Weiner, A.L.; Grossniklaus, H.E.; Naash, M.I.; Lewin, A.S.; Horsager, A.; et al. Drug and gene delivery to the back of the eye: From bench to bedside. *Investig. Ophthalmol. Vis. Sci.* **2014**, *55*, 2714–2730. [CrossRef] [PubMed]

9. Tan, L.E.; Orilla, W.; Hughes, P.M.; Tsai, S.; Burke, J.A.; Wilson, C.G. Effects of vitreous liquefaction on the intravitreal distribution of sodium fluorescein, fluorescein dextran, and fluorescent microparticles. *Investig. Ophthalmol. Vis. Sci.* **2011**, *52*, 1111–1118. [CrossRef]
10. Stein, S.; Hadlich, S.; Langner, S.; Biesenack, A.; Zehm, N.; Kruschke, S.; Oelze, M.; Grimm, M.; Mahnhardt, S.; Weitschies, W.; et al. 7.1 T MRI and T2 mapping of the human and porcine vitreous body post mortem. *Eur. J. Pharm. Biopharm.* **2018**, *131*, 82–91. [CrossRef]
11. Henein, C.; Awwad, S.; Ibeanu, N.; Vlatakis, S.; Brocchini, S.; Tee Khaw, P.; Bouremel, Y. Hydrodynamics of Intravitreal Injections into Liquid Vitreous Substitutes. *Pharmaceutics* **2019**, *11*, 371. [CrossRef]
12. Seidlitz, A.; Weitschies, W. In-vitro dissolution methods for controlled release parenterals and their applicability to drug-eluting stent testing. *J. Pharm. Pharmacol.* **2012**, *64*, 969–985. [CrossRef]
13. Fialho, S.L.; Behar-Cohen, F.; Silva-Cunha, A. Dexamethasone-loaded poly(ε-caprolactone) intravitreal implants: A pilot study. *Eur. J. Pharm. Biopharm.* **2008**, *68*, 637–646. [CrossRef]
14. Matter, B.; Ghaffari, A.; Bourne, D.; Wang, Y.; Choi, S.; Kompella, U.B. Dexamethasone Degradation in Aqueous Medium and Implications for Correction of In Vitro Release from Sustained Release Delivery Systems. *AAPS PharmSciTech* **2019**, *20*. [CrossRef]
15. Awwad, S.; Lockwood, A.; Brocchini, S.; Khaw, P.T. The PK-Eye: A Novel in Vitro Ocular Flow Model for Use in Preclinical Drug Development. *J. Pharm. Sci.* **2015**, *104*, 3330–3342. [CrossRef]
16. Loch, C.; Nagel, S.; Guthoff, R.; Seidlitz, A.; Weitschies, W. The vitreous model—A new in vitro test method simulating the vitreous body. *Biomed. Tech.* **2012**, *57*, 281–284. [CrossRef]
17. Stein, S.; Auel, T.; Kempin, W.; Bogdahn, M.; Weitschies, W.; Seidlitz, A. Influence of the test method on in vitro drug release from intravitreal model implants containing dexamethasone or fluorescein sodium in poly (D,L-lactide-co-glycolide) or polycaprolactone. *Eur. J. Pharm. Biopharm.* **2018**, *127*, 270–278. [CrossRef]
18. Spaide, R.F.; Klancnik, J.M.; Cooney, M.J. Retinal vascular layers imaged by fluorescein angiography and optical coherence tomography angiography. *JAMA Ophthalmol.* **2015**, *133*, 45–50. [CrossRef]
19. German Society of Ophthalmology (DOG); German Retina Society (RG); Professional Association of Ophthalmologists in Germany (BVA). Statement of the German Ophthalmological Society, the German Retina Society, and the Professional Association of Ophthalmologists in Germany on treatment of diabetic macular edema. *Ophthalmologe* **2021**, *118*, 40–67. [CrossRef]
20. Mondelo-García, C.; Bandín-Vilar, E.; García-Quintanilla, L.; Castro-Balado, A.; del Amo, E.M.; Gil-Martínez, M.; Blanco-Teijeiro, M.J.; González-Barcia, M.; Zarra-Ferro, I.; Fernández-Ferreiro, A.; et al. Current Situation and Challenges in Vitreous Substitutes. *Macromol. Biosci.* **2021**, 2100066. [CrossRef]
21. Yu, Z.; Ma, S.; Wu, M.; Cui, H.; Wu, R.; Chen, S.; Xu, C.; Lu, X.; Feng, S. Self-assembling hydrogel loaded with 5-FU PLGA microspheres as a novel vitreous substitute for proliferative vitreoretinopathy. *J. Biomed. Mater. Res. Part A* **2020**, *108*, 2435–2446. [CrossRef] [PubMed]
22. Wang, J.; Goyanes, A.; Gaisford, S.; Basit, A.W. Stereolithographic (SLA) 3D printing of oral modified-release dosage forms. *Int. J. Pharm.* **2016**, *503*, 207–212. [CrossRef]
23. Sil, B.C.; Alvarez, M.P.; Zhang, Y.; Kung, C.P.; Hossain, M.; Iliopoulos, F.; Luo, L.; Crowther, J.M.; Moore, D.J.; Hadgraft, J.; et al. 3D-printed Franz type diffusion cells. *Int. J. Cosmet. Sci.* **2018**, *40*, 604–609. [CrossRef] [PubMed]
24. Käsdorf, B.T.; Arends, F.; Lieleg, O. Diffusion Regulation in the Vitreous Humor. *Biophys. J.* **2015**, *109*, 2171–2181. [CrossRef]
25. Le Goff, M.M.; Bishop, P.N. Adult vitreous structure and postnatal changes. *Eye* **2008**, *22*, 1214–1222. [CrossRef]
26. Kim, H.; Robinson, S.B.; Csaky, K.G. Investigating the movement of intravitreal human serum albumin nanoparticles in the vitreous and retina. *Pharm. Res.* **2009**, *26*, 329–337. [CrossRef] [PubMed]
27. Soheilian, M.; Eskandari, A.; Ramezani, A.; Rabbanikhah, Z.; Soheilian, R. A pilot study of intravitreal diclofenac versus intravitreal triamcinolone for uveitic cystoid macular edema. *Ocul. Immunol. Inflamm.* **2013**, *21*, 124–129. [CrossRef]
28. del Amo, E.M.; Rimpelä, A.K.; Heikkinen, E.; Kari, O.K.; Ramsay, E.; Lajunen, T.; Schmitt, M.; Pelkonen, L.; Bhattacharya, M.; Richardson, D.; et al. Pharmacokinetic aspects of retinal drug delivery. *Prog. Retin. Eye Res.* **2017**, *57*, 134–185. [CrossRef]
29. Rauck, B.M.; Friberg, T.R.; Medina Mendez, C.A.; Park, D.; Shah, V.; Bilonick, R.A.; Wang, Y. Biocompatible reverse thermal gel sustains the release of intravitreal bevacizumab in vivo. *Investig. Ophthalmol. Vis. Sci.* **2013**, *55*, 469–470. [CrossRef]
30. Stein, S.; Bogdahn, M.; Rosenbaum, C.; Weitschies, W.; Seidlitz, A. Distribution of fluorescein sodium and triamcinolone acetonide in the simulated liquefied and vitrectomized Vitreous Model with simulated eye movements. *Eur. J. Pharm. Sci.* **2017**, *109*, 233–243. [CrossRef]

pharmaceutics

MDPI

Article

Dexamethasone PLGA Microspheres for Sub-Tenon Administration: Influence of Sterilization and Tolerance Studies

Deyanira Barbosa-Alfaro [1,2], Vanessa Andrés-Guerrero [1,2,3], Ivan Fernandez-Bueno [3,4], María Teresa García-Gutiérrez [4], Esther Gil-Alegre [1], Irene Teresa Molina-Martínez [1,2,3], José Carlos Pastor-Jimeno [3,4,5], Rocío Herrero-Vanrell [1,2,3,*] and Irene Bravo-Osuna [1,2,3]

[1] Innovation, Therapy and Pharmaceutical Development in Ophthalmology (InnOftal) Research Group, UCM 920415, Complutense University of Madrid, 28040 Madrid, Spain; deyanira.barbosa@hotmail.com (D.B.-A.); vandres@ucm.es (V.A.-G.); megil@ucm.es (E.G.-A.); iremm@ucm.es (I.T.M.-M.); ibravo@ucm.es (I.B.-O.)

[2] Departamento de Farmacia Galénica y Tecnología Alimentaria, Facultad de Farmacia, Universidad Complutense de Madrid (UCM), IdISSC, 28040 Madrid, Spain

[3] Thematic Research Network in Ophthalmology (Oftared) Carlos III National Institute of Health, 28040 Madrid, Spain; ivan.fernandez.bueno@uva.es (I.F.-B.); pastor@ioba.med.uva.es (J.C.P.-J.)

[4] Instituto Universitario de Oftalmobiología Aplicada (IOBA), Universidad de Valladolid, 47011 Valladolid, Spain; tgarcia@ioba.med.uva.es

[5] Department of Ophthalmology, Hospital Clínico Universitario of Valladolid, 47003 Valladolid, Spain

* Correspondence: rociohv@ucm.es

Citation: Barbosa-Alfaro, D.; Andrés-Guerrero, V.; Fernandez-Bueno, I.; García-Gutiérrez, M.T.; Gil-Alegre, E.; Molina-Martínez, I.T.; Pastor-Jimeno, J.C.; Herrero-Vanrell, R.; Bravo-Osuna, I. Dexamethasone PLGA Microspheres for Sub-Tenon Administration: Influence of Sterilization and Tolerance Studies. *Pharmaceutics* **2021**, *13*, 228. https://doi.org/10.3390/pharmaceutics13020228

Academic Editor: Hwa Jeong Lee

Received: 21 December 2020

Accepted: 2 February 2021

Published: 6 February 2021

Abstract: Many diseases affecting the posterior segment of the eye require repeated intravitreal injections with corticosteroids in chronic treatments. The periocular administration is a less invasive route attracting considerable attention for long-term therapies. In the present work, dexamethasone-loaded poly(lactic-*co*-glycolic) acid (PLGA) microspheres (Dx-MS) were prepared using the oil-in-water (O/W) emulsion solvent evaporation technique. MS were characterized in terms of mean particle size and particle size distribution, external morphology, polymer integrity, drug content, and in vitro release profiles. MS were sterilized by gamma irradiation (25 kGy), and dexamethasone release profiles from sterilized and non-sterilized microspheres were compared by means of the similarity factor (f_2). The mechanism of drug release before and after irradiation exposure of Dx-MS was identified using appropriate mathematical models. Dexamethasone release was sustained in vitro for 9 weeks. The evaluation of the in vivo tolerance was carried out in rabbit eyes, which received a sub-Tenon injection of 5 mg of sterilized Dx-MS (20–53 μm size containing 165.6 ± 3.6 μg Dx/mg MS) equivalent to 828 μg of Dx. No detectable increase in intraocular pressure was reported, and clinical and histological analysis of the ocular tissues showed no adverse events up to 6 weeks after the administration. According to the data presented in this work, the sub-Tenon administration of Dx-MS could be a promising alternative to successive intravitreal injections for the treatment of chronic diseases of the back of the eye.

Keywords: dexamethasone; poly(lactic-*co*-glycolic) acid; ophthalmology; microspheres; periocular administration; gamma sterilization; tolerance

1. Introduction

According to the World Health Organization, there are 2.2 billion people globally who have a vision impairment or blindness. Of this, available data suggest a conservative estimate of at least one billion people with moderate or severe distance vision impairment or blindness that could have been prevented or has yet to be addressed. This number includes those with moderate or severe distance vision impairment or blindness due to unaddressed refractive error (123.7 million), cataract (65.2 million), age-related macular degeneration (10.4 million), glaucoma (6.9 million), corneal opacities (4.2 million), diabetic retinopathy (3 million), and trachoma (2 million), as well as near-vision impairment caused by unaddressed presbyopia (826 million). The estimate is based on recently published epidemiological data on the global magnitude of near-vision impairment [1] and the global magnitude and causes of bilateral distance vision impairment and blindness [2]. With such a large number of cases each year, it is critical that an optimal treatment is used in ophthalmic chronic diseases.

Many diseases affecting the posterior segment of the eye, such as macular edema secondary to diabetic retinopathy, to central and branch retinal vein occlusion, after surgery (retinal detachment or epiretinal membrane peeling, Irvine–Gass syndrome (post cataract surgery), or after posterior uveitis, require long-term treatments with corticosteroids. Since it is particularly difficult to achieve effective levels of therapeutics in the vitreous/retina following a topical or systemic administration, intraocular drug delivery devices that are capable of maintaining effective intravitreal levels for long periods, with minimal systemic exposure, have attracted considerable attention [3–6]. Of special interest is the design of intravitreal biodegradable implants that can be placed into the vitreous without the need for surgical procedures and without the need to be removed later on. Their development represents a significant advance because they are able to maintain therapeutic concentrations of drugs in the vitreous for long periods (from days to months) [7,8]. However, they present problems such as the ability to migrate to the anterior segment in pseudophakic patients, or the management of secondary ocular hypertensions. An intravitreal biodegradable implant loaded with dexamethasone (Dx) (0.7 mg) is currently in the clinical practice marketed for the treatment of macular edema due to retinal vein occlusion and noninfectious uveitis (Ozurdex™; Allergan Inc., Irvine, CA, USA) [9–12].

In addition to drug implants, other formulations capable of achieving sustained intraocular therapeutic drug concentrations are being studied, for example, microparticles made up of biodegradable polymers, injected as an aqueous suspension in a periocular or intraocular fashion to achieve sustained drug levels [13,14]. Biodegradable poly(lactic-*co*-glycolic) acid (PLGA) microspheres form a depot after their injection acting as an in situ biodegradable implant [15]. The main advantage of microspheres is that doses and specific combination therapy can be easily tuned for each patient as different doses of active substances could be administered by changing the amount of microspheres.

Considering the administration route, the most effective way to achieve appropriate drug concentrations in the posterior eye segment is via intravitreal injection. However, intravitreal administration has potential severe side-effects such as retinal detachment and endophthalmitis [16]. Furthermore, the risk of secondary adverse events increases with the number of injections. Some treatments, for example antiangiogenic treatments at the retinal level, are based on intravitreal injection of anti-vascular endothelial growth factor (anti-VEGF) active compounds once a month for life; thus, with time, these injection side-effects become another problem to deal with from a clinical point of view, in addition to the disease itself.

A potentially less invasive alternative is periocular administration, such as the retrobulbar, subconjunctival, and posterior sub-Tenon injections. Periocular administrations routes are being explored to avoid the mentioned problem, with the studies performed in the case of corticosteroid administration being especially relevant [17]. Among the periocular routes explored, the sub-Tenon seems suitable to treat the deep zones of the back of the eye and it could be an alternative to intravitreal injections, especially with respect to the administration of polymeric drug delivery systems, able to release the loaded active compound for months in a sustained manner. It is important to remark the advantages of the sub-Tenon administration, which is adjacent to the sclera and delivers the drug directly into the retina and vitreous. The sclera is a highly hypovascular porous fibrous tissue (16 nm effective pore size) [18] with low blood absorption and high permeability, and it offers a large surface and a large volume of injection (up to 5 mL) [19], if compared with the vitreous cavity, whose volume of injection is limited to 20–200 μL. After scleral permeation, the compounds reach the ciliary body anteriorly and the choroid posteriorly. For retinal delivery, drugs also need to be able to permeate across the retinal pigment epithelium, which forms an effective cellular barrier due to tight junctions between the retinal pigment epithelium (RPE) cells. In addition to these barriers, the feasibility of drugs to access the vitreous after periocular administration has been reported. For example, according to experimental studies in rabbit eyes, the administration of dimethyl vancomycin via sub-Tenon administration provided an effective drug concentration in the vitreous [20]. Furthermore, previous studies have shown that, after peribulbar or subconjunctival injection of dexamethasone, significant levels of the active substance can be measured in the vitreous, and these levels are achieved by direct diffusion of the drug through the sclera [21]. For example, in a very interesting approach, Huang et al. [22] evaluated some pharmacokinetic parameters of dexamethasone sodium phosphate (DSP) in the rabbits' posterior segment tissue following, among others, sub-Tenon perfusion showing $t_{\frac{1}{2}}$ values for DSP of 14.32 h, 7.65 h, and 4.89 h for vitreous, choroidal/retinal compound, and sclera, respectively. Three years later, the same group demonstrated the efficacy of the sub-Tenon infusion of DSP in experimental autoimmune uveitis in rabbits [23]. For large molecules, these routes have shown a slower diffusion rate or less sustained effect relative to intravitreal injections. In humans, an anti-inflammatory and anti-infective response was reported in a limited phase II study, in which biodegradable microspheres containing triamcinolone acetonide and ciprofloxacin were administered via sub-Tenon injection, in a small group of patients after cataract extraction and intraocular lens implantation [24]. Considering this, sub-Tenon administration provides new possibilities to evaluate DDS as a new tool that is able to prolong a drug's efficacy in the posterior segment of the eye, considerably reducing the number of interventions by the ophthalmologist and, subsequently, limiting the risks associated, especially in chronic treatments. Moreover, this route can be exploited for long-term treatment without serious side-effects and potential interference with the optical path [25].

From a technological point of view, an essential issue in the development of formulations intended for ophthalmic administration is the sterilization process. The use of gamma-irradiation is the most suitable sterilization method for PLGA-based microparticles [15,26,27]. However, this radiation method can have effects on the biodegradable polyesters, i.e., the formation of reactive radicals, which may compromise the drug substance incorporated into the device. Therefore, drug stability under irradiation conditions and changes in drug release properties need to be carefully evaluated [28,29].

The purpose of this investigation was to develop a sterilized formulation of dexamethasone-loaded PLGA microspheres (Dx-MS) able to control the release of the drug, while being at the same time well tolerated after sub-Tenon administration. To that, microspheres were designed, prepared, and characterized in vitro. Then, microspheres were injected periocularly (sub-Tenon administration) into rabbit eyes to evaluate the tolerance of the formulation in terms of clinical evaluation and histological analysis.

2. Materials and Methods

Poly(D,L-lactide-*co*-glycolide) (PLGA, ratio 50:50; Resomer® RG 502) was purchased from Boehringer Ingelheim (C.H. Boehringer Sohn AG & Ko. KG, Ingelheim am Rhein, Germany). Polyvinyl alcohol (PVA, 67,000 g/mol) was supplied by Merck KGaA (Darmstadt, Germany). Dexamethasone (Dx, M_W 392.5 g/mol; aqueous solubility at 37 °C = 0.12 mg/mL) was obtained from Sigma-Aldrich (Schnelldorf, Darmstadt, Germany). All other chemicals were reagent grade and used as received.

2.1. Preparation of Microspheres

Dx-loaded PLGA microspheres (Dx-MS) were prepared using the oil-in-water (O/W) emulsion solvent evaporation technique as previously described [30]. Briefly, 80 mg of Dx was suspended in 0.8 mL of PLGA/dichloromethane (50% *w*/*v*) by ultrasonication in a water/ice bath for 5 min (Elma. Transsonic 460, Singen, Germany). Then, the suspension was gently sonicated at low temperature (Sonicator KL, Qsonica Llc, Newtown, CT, USA) for 1 min. The so-prepared organic phase was emulsified with 5 mL of PVA MilliQ® water solution (1% w/v). Emulsification was performed in a homogenizer (Polytron® RECO, Kinematica GmbH PT 3000, Lucerna, Switzerland) at different speeds (5500–9500 rpm) for 2 min. Subsequently, 10 mL of a PVA solution (0.1%) was added to the emulsion and kept in the same homogenization conditions for an extra minute. Finally, the emulsion was poured into 90 mL of an aqueous PVA solution (0.1%) and kept under constant stirring for 3 h at room temperature, to allow the extraction and the subsequent evaporation of the organic solvent. Once formed, microspheres were washed with MilliQ® water to eliminate PVA and sieved according to their particle size (106–53 µm, 53–38 µm, 38–20 µm, or 20–2 µm). Particles were then rapidly frozen (methanol/ice mixture) and freeze-dried to obtain a free-flowing microsphere powder. They were kept at −20 °C under dry conditions until use. Three independent batches (same composition) of microspheres were prepared in each experimental condition (four different homogenization speeds). For each experimental condition, microspheres with sizes 53–38 µm and 38–20 µm were selected for further analysis. For the in vitro release profile, 10 different batches of the selected formulation were prepared, and the whole 53–20 fraction was selected.

2.2. Microspheres Characterization

2.2.1. Production Yield

The production yield percentage ($PY\%$) of each size fraction was calculated from the following Equation (1):

$$PY(\%) = \frac{M_T(microspheres)}{M_T(PLGA) + M_T(Dx)} \times 100, \tag{1}$$

where M_T is the mass of each component in the formulation.

2.2.2. Mean Particle Size, Particle Size Distribution, and Morphology of Microspheres

Mean particle size and particle size distribution were measured by static light scattering (Microtrac S3500, Montgomeryville, PA, USA). Samples were prepared by suspending microspheres in distilled water. Microsphere morphology was evaluated by scanning electron microscopy (SEM; Jeol, JSM-6335F, Tokyo, Japan). Prior to that, each powder sample was spread on a double-sided carbon tape mounted on an aluminum stub to be gold-coated under vacuum (K550X ion sputter, Emitech, UK) for 3 min at 25 mA. SEM images were recorded at an acceleration voltage of 5.0 kV and 2500× magnification.

2.2.3. Polymer Integrity

The molar mass of the polymers was evaluated by high-performance gel permeation chromatography (GPC). The assay was performed with a blank column of PLgel (PLgel 3 µm MIXED-E and PLgel 5 µm MIXED-D, both 7.8 mm × 300 mm), preceded by a PLgel 5 µm guard, 50 mm × 7.5 mm from Varian (Polymer Laboratories, Church Stretton, Shropshire, UK). The equipment included a Waters 1525 binary HPLC pump and a Waters 2414 Refractive Index Detector (Waters, Saint-Quentin en Yvelines, France). The column was maintained at 33 °C using a Waters heating column system. Tetrahydrofuran (THF) was filtered (Sartolon Polyamid, 0.45 µm, Göttingen, Germany) and degassed before use. The flow rate was 1 mL/min of THF. Before injection, samples were filtered using a polytetrafluoroethylene (PTFE) membrane (0.22 µm, 0.2 mm × 13 mm, Teknokroma, Barcelona, Spain). The injection volume was 20 µL (Hamilton syringe, Reno, NV, USA).

The column was calibrated using polystyrene standards of different molar masses: 381, 1100, 2950, 6520, 18,600, and 43,700 g/mol (Waters, Mainz, Germany), prepared by their dissolution in THF at a concentration ranging from 0.4 to 1.6 mg/mL, depending on the molar mass needed. Experimental samples were dissolved in THF at concentrations ranging from 1 to 2 mg/mL.

2.2.4. Drug Quantification by HPLC

Dexamethasone was quantified by HPLC, according to the method described in the Spanish Royal Pharmacopoeia, with minor modifications. The method was validated with respect to linearity, accuracy, and reliability in the range of concentrations of 2–20 μg/mL.

The HPLC system consisted of two Waters Millipore 510 pumps, an autosampler Waters 712DWSP, and a Waters 490E ultraviolet/visible light (UV/Vis) detector. Analyses were performed on a 15 cm × 5 mm reverse-phase C18 5-μm column (Tracer Excel 120 ODSA, Teknokroma, Barcelona, Spain) preceded by a guard cartridge SEA 18, 100 mm × 4.0 mm (Teknokroma, Barcelona, Spain). The column was maintained at 45 °C using a heating column system (Waters TCM/CMM). The mobile phase consisted on a gradient of acetonitrile–water 35:65 *v*/*v* (phase A) and acetonitrile (phase B) delivered at a flow rate of 1.0 mL/min. The initial mobile phase condition A 100%-B 0% was progressively changed to A 0%-B 100% from t = 10 min to t = 25 min. Subsequently, initial conditions were recovered in the subsequent 5 min, which ran until the end of the assay (t = 35 min). The injection volume was 20 μL. UV detection of analytes was carried out at 254 nm.

2.2.5. Encapsulation Efficiency of Dexamethasone-Loaded Microspheres (Dx-MS)

Sterilized and non-sterilized microspheres (5 mg) were dissolved in 5 mL of dichloromethane. Then, 12 mL of ethanol was added to promote polymer precipitation. Samples were further centrifuged (5000 rpm, 10 min) and the supernatant was recovered and filtered (0.45 μm). Dexamethasone in the supernatant was quantified by HPLC as described in Section 2.2.4.

The encapsulation efficiency (EE%) was calculated as follows (Equation (2)):

$$\mathrm{EE\%} = \frac{Actual\ drug\ content}{Theorical\ drug\ content} \times 100. \quad (2)$$

2.2.6. In Vitro Release Studies

Duplicates of 5 mg of microspheres of each batch (sterilized and non-sterilized) were suspended in 2 mL of phosphate-buffered saline (PBS, pH 7.4) isotonized with NaCl. Samples (protected from light) were placed in a shaker bath with a constant agitation speed of 100 rpm (Clifton Shaking Bath NE5, Nikel Electro Ltd., Weston-super-Mare, UK; Avon, London, UK) at 37 °C. At preset times (1 h, 24 h, 48 h, and once every 3 days until the end of the study), the microparticle suspensions were gently centrifuged (3000 rpm, 3 min), and 2 mL of the supernatant was recovered and replaced with the same volume of fresh PBS, to continue the release study and assure sink conditions. The remaining microparticles and the fresh release media were gently mixed in a vortex before being replaced again in the shaker bath. The concentration of dexamethasone in the supernatant samples was analyzed using the HPLC method described in Section 2.2.4. Both the cumulative release (% vs. t) plot and the release rate (%/day) plot, calculated as the amount of drug released at each time point divided by the number of days between sample point, are presented.

2.2.7. Analysis of Drug Release Mechanism

Two model-dependent approaches were selected to characterize the dissolution profiles: the Korsmeyer–Peppas equation (Equation (3)) [31,32] and the Heller and Baker equation (Equation (4)) [33].

$$\frac{Q_t}{Q_\infty} = K \cdot t^n, \quad (3)$$

$$\frac{dQ}{dt} = \frac{A}{2}\frac{\sqrt{2 \cdot P_0 \cdot e^{K_c \cdot t} \cdot C_0}}{t}, \quad (4)$$

where, in Equation (3), Q_t/Q_∞ represents the fraction of drug released at time t, K, is the kinetic constant of the release process, characteristic of the drug/polymer system, t is the release time, and n is the release exponent that describes the drug release mechanism. In Equation (4), A is the contact area, P_0 is the initial drug permeability, K_c is the first-order kinetic polymeric alteration rate constant, C_0 is the initial drug concentration, and t is the time. In both cases, only the data points with less than 60% release were used.

Considering microspheres as a matrix, i.e., heterogeneous and porous systems that hydrate when in contact with the aqueous medium, the release profile of the drug will depend on both the diffusion rate of the active principle in the matrix and the rate of hydration of the polymer. If the erosion phenomena described within the mechanisms that affect this type of release are also considered, the kinetics that can be manifested in these studies can be complex. That is why, in this work, two models were selected that have proven to be useful to describe these complex systems. One of these treatments is that proposed by Korsmeyer et al. (Korsmeyer equation). According to this model, when polymeric materials in contact with a solvent are hardly modified or adapt quickly to the new situation, the predominant mechanism is Fick diffusion, with the transfer rate (dQ/dt) being inversely proportional to the square root of time, i.e., the value of n in the above equation is equal to 0.5. This situation is also known as case I transport. If the transfer rate is influenced both by the diffusion of the solute and by modifications in the reticular structure of the polymer (coupling of the solvent molecules or hydration, relaxation, or breakage of the polymer chains), then this value of n is greater than 0.5, and the below situations can be established.

Anomalous transport is where the release of the solute is controlled both by its diffusion and by the structural modification of the lattice. The value of n is then between 0.5 and 1. Transport case II and super-case II occur when the transfer rate is not controlled by diffusion mechanisms, but by the alterations that take place in the polymer structure (coupling, rupture, or adjustment), manifesting a kinetic that is good; it depends linearly on time (zero-order, n equal to 1), being called case II transport, and it can be of higher degree ($n > 1$), which in this case is called super-case II transport. Later, Ritger and Peppas described different values of n depending on the geometry of the devices. For spherical matrices, the corresponding extreme values of n are 0.43 and 0.85 [34,35].

Another of the equations proposed for those cases in which homogeneous polymer erosion processes are developed is that described by Heller and Baker, where the transfer rate corresponds to Higuchi's basic approach, but introduces a variable permeability coefficient throughout time, which depends on the alteration in the polymer structure (internal erosion process), admitting that this last process responds to a kinetics of order one. This treatment can only be applied when the transfer rate increases with time (since an increase in the diffusion coefficient is admitted), and the results close to or after the time in which the maximum transfer rate is manifested should not be considered.

2.3. Sterilization of Microspheres

Dx-MS were subjected to ^{60}Cobalt radiation at 25 kGy. Samples were placed into 2 mL glass vials before closing with rubber and an overseal closure. Vials were sterilized in dry ice to assure a low temperature (−78.5 °C) during the irradiation process [36].

After sterilization, microspheres were further characterized in terms of mean particle size and particle size distribution, morphological evaluation, polymer integrity, drug content, and in vitro release profiles using the protocols described above. The drug release kinetics was evaluated according to the model-dependent approaches already mentioned. Furthermore, the dexamethasone release profiles from sterilized and non-sterilized microspheres were further compared using a model-independent approach, by calculating the similarity factor (f_2) (Equation (5)).

$$f_2 = 50 \times Log\left\{\left[1 + (1/n)\sum_{t=1}^{n}|R_t - T_t|^2\right]^{-0.5} \times 100\right\}, \quad (5)$$

where Log is the logarithm base 10, n is the number of observations, R_t is the average percentage drug dissolved from the reference formulation, and T_t is average percentage drug dissolved from the test formulation.

2.4. *In Vivo Studies*

A total of 22 female pigmented rabbits weighing 2.5–3.5 kg were used. The procedure assured animal welfare, and it was approved by the University of Valladolid Ethics Committee on animal experimentation and welfare. Furthermore, the protocols herein comply with the ARVO Statement for the Use of Animals in Ophthalmology and Vision Research and are in accordance with the European Communities Council Directive (86/609/EEC).

Before administration, animals were anesthetized by applying an intramuscular injection of 30 mg/kg of ketamine (Imalgene® 1000, 100 mg, Merial Laboratorios S.A., Barcelona, Spain) and 6 mg/kg of xylazine (Rompun® 2%, 2 g, Bayer AG, Barcelona, Spain). Pinna and pedal reflexes were used to monitor the level of anesthesia. Topical anesthesia was applied on the eye prior to the procedure via topical instillation of tetracaine chlorhydrate (Colircusí Anestésico Doble® 0.05%, Alcon Cusí, Barcelona, Spain).

Microspheres were injected at the posterior superotemporal juxtascleral area (sub-Tenon). Briefly, the upper eyelid was retracted, and the superior rectus muscle was rotated nasally to expose the superior temporal quadrant of the eye. The conjunctiva was held with toothed forceps, and a buttonhole was cut with Westcott scissors. Afterward, a blunt dissection was conducted in order to introduce a metal cannula, 19G (model Stevens, Magnolia, NJ, USA), under the Tenon's capsule. The cannula was fixed to a syringe preloaded with the microparticle suspension, and the formulation was slowly delivered into the sub-Tenon's space. Finally, the cannula was carefully removed. In order to avoid any post-injection leakage, a sterile cotton-tipped applicator was used to gently press over the insertion area. Tobramycin ointment (Tobrex® 3 mg/g, Alcon Cusí, Barcelona, Spain) was applied at the site of injection. On day 0, a sub-Tenon injection of 5 mg of Dx-PLGA microspheres (dose: 828 µg of dexamethasone) in PBS (100 µL) was applied to the left eye of each animal. The right eye was used as the control and received 100 µL of PBS. A clinical evaluation was performed in all eyes until the end of the study.

A physical examination and scored ophthalmic evaluation of the animals were performed at the time of injection and 1, 7, 14, 28, and 42 days later. Anterior pole evaluation was performed by slit-lamp biomicroscopy (Kowa SL-15; Kowa Optimed Inc., Torrance, CA, USA) following the scored method described by Hackett and McDonald [23]. Posterior pole evaluation was performed by inverted image ophthalmoscopy (Keeler Ltd., Windsor, UK) with non-contact lenses and pharmacological midriasis with Tropicamide® (Colircusí Tropicamida® colirio; Alcon Cusí S.A.). Intraocular pressure (IOP) was scored by contact tonometry (Tono-Pen VetTM Tonometer; Reichert Inc., Depew, NY, USA). The following clinical signs were evaluated: conjunctival congestion, swelling and discharge, aqueous flare, light reflex, iris involvement, pannus, vitreous opacity, vascular congestion, vitreous and retinal hemorrhage, retinal detachment, and intraocular pressure (Table 1).

Table 1. Ophthalmic evaluation using scored method.

	Anterior Pole Evaluation [23]	
Conjunctival congestion	0	Normal, blanched to reddish pink conjunctiva
	1 to 3	From reddish color confined to the palpebral conjunctiva to dark red color of both palpebral and bulbar conjunctiva
Conjunctival swelling	0	Normal, no swelling
	1 to 4	From swelling above normal without eversion of the lids to swelling with pronounced eversion of the lids
Conjunctival discharge	0	Normal, no discharge
	1 to 3	From discharge above normal and restricted to the inner portion of the eye to discharge flowing over the eyelids

Table 1. *Cont.*

	Anterior Pole Evaluation [23]	
Aqueous flare	0	Absence of visible light beam in the anterior chamber
	1 to 3	From Tyndall effect barely discernible to Tyndall beam easily discernible
Light reflex	0	Normal pupillary response
	1 or 2	From sluggish to fixed pupillary response
Iris involvement	0	Normal iris without hyperemia
	1 to 4	From minimal injection of secondary vessels to marked injection of secondary and tertiary vessels with marked swelling of the iris stroma
Cornea	0	Normal
	1 to 4	From some loss of transparency to marked loss of transparency of the entire thickness of the corneal stroma
Surface of cornea cloudiness	0	Normal
	1 to 4	From 1–25% to 76–100% area of stromal cloudiness
Pannus	0	Absence
	1 or 2	From vascularization without vessels invading the cornea to vessels invading 2 mm or more of the cornea
Fluorescein staining	0	Absence
	1 to 4	From slight and confined to a small focus to extreme fluorescein staining
Lens	Normal/abnormal	
	Posterior Pole Evaluation	
Vitreous opacity	Yes/No	
Vascular congestion	Yes/No	
Vitreous and/or retinal hemorrhage	Yes/No	
Retinal detachment	Yes/No	

Two animals were euthanized at day 42 post injection, and the eyes were submitted for histological processing and microscopic evaluation by hematoxylin and eosin staining. The tissue response in the areas of the injection site was evaluated for quantity of inflammation (− absence; + mild; ++ moderated; +++ severe; +/− does not fall into one of the defined categories), predominant cell type of the inflammatory infiltrate, presence of foreign body giant cell reaction (+ present; − absent), and presence of residual microspheres (+ present; +/− focal, occasional; − absent).

2.5. Statistical Analysis

The data were represented as means ± SD for n values. Statistically significant differences were calculated by one-way analysis of variance (ANOVA). The differences were considered significant at $p < 0.05$.

3. Results

3.1. Microsphere Preparation and Characterization

Data concerning the preparation parameters and the characteristics of the formulations are compiled in Table 2. As can be observed, the production yield was independent of the emulsification speed ($p = 0.9905$) with values around 60% in all cases.

Table 2. Production yield (Y) and particle size distribution of formulations elaborated at different homogenization speeds (HS) ($n = 3$).

Formulation	HS (rpm)	Y (%)	Size Distribution (%)				
			>106 μm	106–53 μm	53–38 μm	38–20 μm	20–2 μm
1	5500	59.4 ± 1.4	9.8 ± 2.8	48.1 ± 2.2	16.9 ± 0.8	16.8 ± 0.2	8.4 ± 0.6
2	8500	60.4 ± 3.0	-	19.5 ± 5.2	32.0 ± 1.3	32.7 ± 2.9	15.8 ± 1.1
3	9500	60.2 ± 2.8	-	18.1 ± 1.7	28.8 ± 2.6	33.3 ± 1.2	19.8 ± 3.7
4	10,500	59.9 ± 1.2	-	16.0 ± 3.7	26.7 ± 0.6	34.1 ± 2.3	23.3 ± 1.1

As expected, this parameter did clearly influence the particle size distribution, showing a shift to smaller particle sizes, especially when using emulsification speeds higher or equal to 9500 rpm. In all cases, particles exhibited a spherical shape with only some small pores and no crystals on the surface, as shown by SEM (Figure 1).

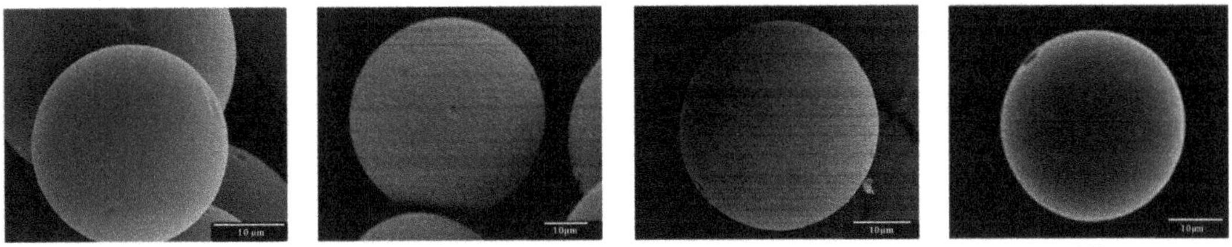

(a) (b) (c) (d)

Figure 1. Dexamethasone (Dx)-loaded poly(lactic-*co*-glycolic) acid (PLGA) microspheres (MS, 20–53 μm) prepared using the oil-in-water (O/W) emulsion solvent evaporation technique at (**a**) 5500 rpm, (**b**) 8500 rpm, (**c**) 9500 rpm, and (**d**) 10,500 rpm.

In Table 3, Dx loading of the two fractions of interest (53–38 μm and 38–20 μm) is presented, as well as the percentage encapsulation efficiency (EE%). Considering the fraction with the biggest particle size (53–38 μm), the highest encapsulation efficiency was achieved by formulation 4 with values of 103.2% ± 0.4%. The values of the two granulometric fractions in the case of formulation 3 resulted in nonsignificant differences ($p = 0.896$), and the complete 53–20 μm fraction was selected for the in vivo studies.

Table 3. Drug loading (μg Dx/mg MS) and percentage encapsulation efficiency (EE%) for the fractions of interest of each formulation ($n = 3$).

Formulation	μg Dx/mg MS		EE (%)	
	53–38 μm	38–20 μm	53–38 μm	38–20 μm
1	154.3 ± 4.7	131.1 ± 4.7	92.5 ± 3.0	78.6 ± 2.7
2	161.4 ± 2.5	150.1 ± 4.9	86.7 ± 1.4	89.9 ± 2.9
3	164.0 ± 6.0	162.7 ± 7.2	98.1 ± 3.6	97.3 ± 4.3
4	172.0 ± 0.9	146.7 ± 1.8	103.2 ± 0.4	94.0 ± 1.1

3.2. Sterilization of Dx PLGA Microspheres

The size and morphology of the Dx-MS was not influenced by the sterilization procedure ($p = 0.540$), as shown in Figures 2 and 3. The product retained its physical characteristics, and particles were free-flowing without showing clumping and/or aggregation behavior.

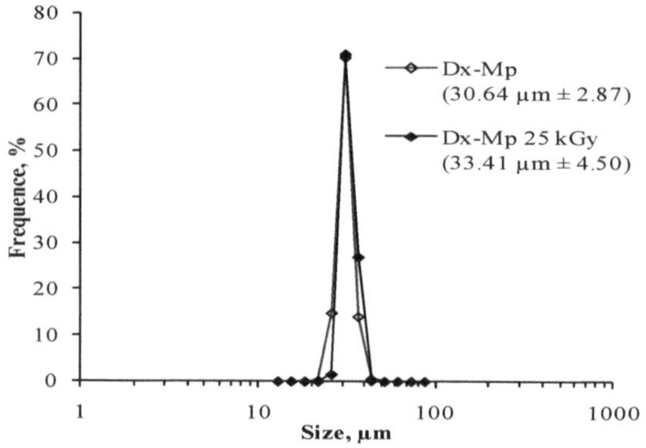

Figure 2. Particle size distribution of dexamethasone-loaded microspheres (53–20 μm): ◊ before and ♦ after sterilization.

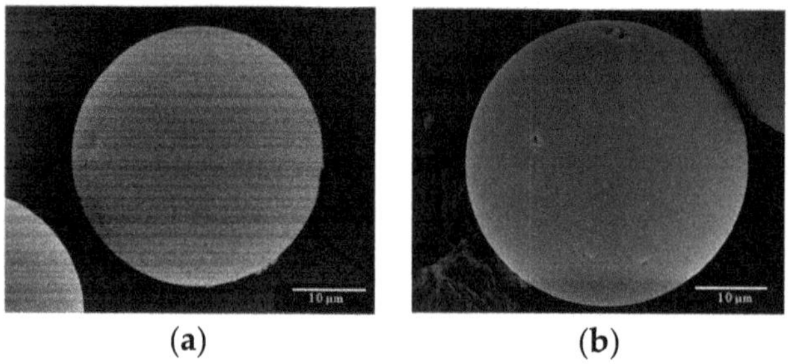

Figure 3. SEM pictures of dexamethasone-loaded PLGA microspheres: (**a**) before and (**b**) after γ-irradiation (applied dose: 25 kGy).

The drug content and release characteristics of 10 independent batches of sterilized microspheres were also analyzed. According to the results, dexamethasone content remained unaltered with a mean value of 165.6 ± 3.6 μg Dx/mg MS (Figure 4). These systems also provided a controlled release of the drug for 9 weeks (Figure 5a,b).

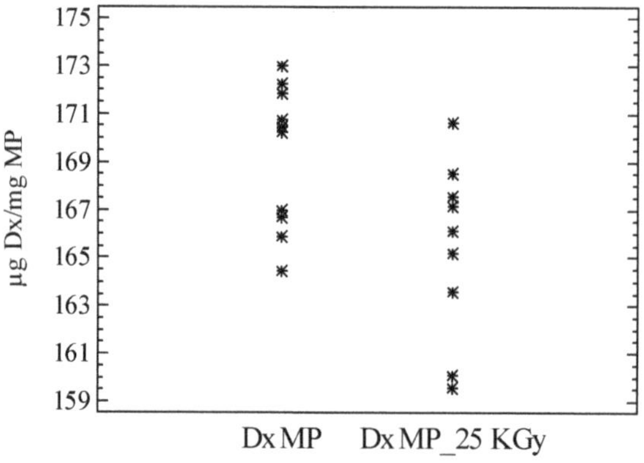

Figure 4. Dexamethasone loading in the microparticles (μg Dx/mg MS) before (Dx MS) and after sterilization (Dx-MS 25 kGy) (n = 10).

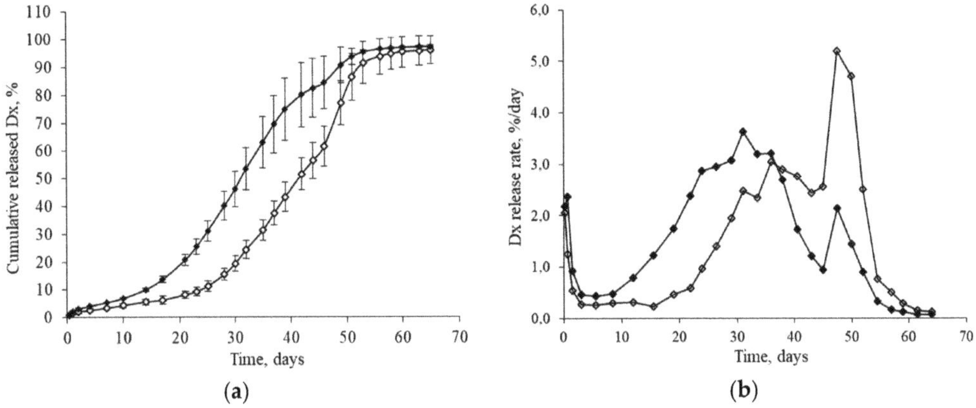

Figure 5. Release profile of dexamethasone from non-sterilized (◇) and sterilized (♦) PLGA microspheres (53–20 μm, prepared at 9500 rpm). (**a**) Cumulative release (%) and (**b**) release rate (%/day). Data points (± standard deviations) (n = 10).

The release profile of Dx from the PLGA MS exhibited sensible changes after sterilization (Figure 5a,b). For example, the time necessary to release 50% of loaded dexamethasone was reduced to 12 days for gamma-irradiated samples as compared with non-sterilized particles. The similarity factor f_2 was selected as a model-independent method to compare the two release profiles, obtaining an f_2 value of 35.5, lower than the similarity limit (f_2 = 50), confirming that the changes in the release profile were due to the sterilization process. These changes in the Dx release profile after gamma-irradiation were attributed to the induction of ester bond cleavage and the resulting decrease in the polymer molecular weight [26,37,38].

As can be observed in Figure 6a,c, experimental data fit the Korsmeyer–Peppas equation showing a biphasic behavior. Determination coefficient and "n" values are compiled in Table 4. In accordance with this model, the first phase of the release (0–17 days) was characterized by an anomalous transport (n = 0.51), indicating that not only drug diffusion, but also polymeric matrix changes controlled the release of dexamethasone [39]. In the second phase (17 days until the end), the strong alterations produced on the polymeric matrix structure might control the drug release (n > 0.85), according to a Super Case II transport.

Table 4. Values of kinetic parameters of drug release profiles before and after sterilization. The value of "n" of Korsmeyer–Peppas model (95% confidence level, CL), "K_c" of Heller and Baker model, and coefficients of determination (r^2).

Drug Release	**Korsmeyer-Peppas Model**			**Heller and Baker Model**		
	Phase	r^2	**n (CL)**	**Phase**	r^2	**K_c (days^{-1})**
Dx-MS	1	0.987	0.51 (0.46–0.56)	1	0.977	0.16
	2	0.995	2.79 (2.66–2.91)	2	0.991	0.34
Dx-MS, 25 kGy	1	0.993	0.46 (0.41–0.51)	1	0.995	0.30
	2	0.996	2.06 (1.96–2.16)			

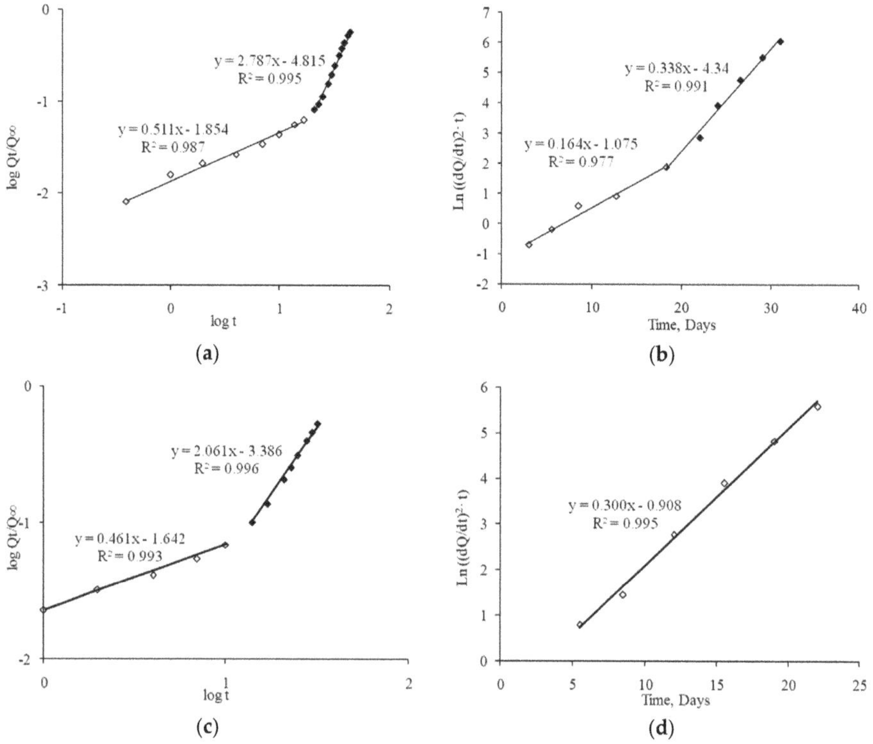

Figure 6. Kinetic fitting of dexamethasone release data: (**a**) Korsmeyer—Peppas model before sterilization; (**b**) Heller and Baker model before sterilization; (**c**) Korsmeyer—Peppas model after sterilization; (**d**) Heller and Baker model after sterilization.

Figure 6b,d show the fitting of experimental data for the first 32 days of the release assay to the Heller and Baker model, considering that a homogeneous polymer erosion occurs during the drug release. According to this model, two polymeric change rates occurred (data shown in Table 4). The first phase (approximately the first 17 days of the study) was characterized by a slow polymer alteration (K_c = 0.16 day^{-1}). In the second phase, an increase in the polymeric alteration rate was achieved (K_c = 0.34 day^{-1}).

In order to complete and integrate the information obtained from the kinetic evaluation of the drug release profiles, both the polymer molecular weight (M_W) and the morphological aspects of microspheres were monitored during the release study (Figure 7). Effectively, during the first 15–17 days, microspheres did not appreciably change their external morphology and, therefore, exhibited a spherical shape over this time period. At the same time, only a moderate reduction in PLGA M_W (15%) was observed. This behavior should be in concordance with the anomalous transport proposed after Korsmeyer–Peppas fitting and with the low polymer erosion rate observed after Heller and Baker treatment. During weeks 3 and 4, microspheres maintained their spherical structure; however, their surfaces started to deteriorate more. This may be explained by the higher polymer erosion rate observed (Table 4), which was confirmed by the reduction in the polymer M_W (45% of the initial value). No further M_W reduction was observed until the end of the study. However, according to the SEM pictures, in the fifth week of the release, the inner microsphere structure appeared to be so weak that particles disintegrated, which may be the origin of the Super Case II transport observed according to Korsmeyer–Peppas fitting in the second phase of the study.

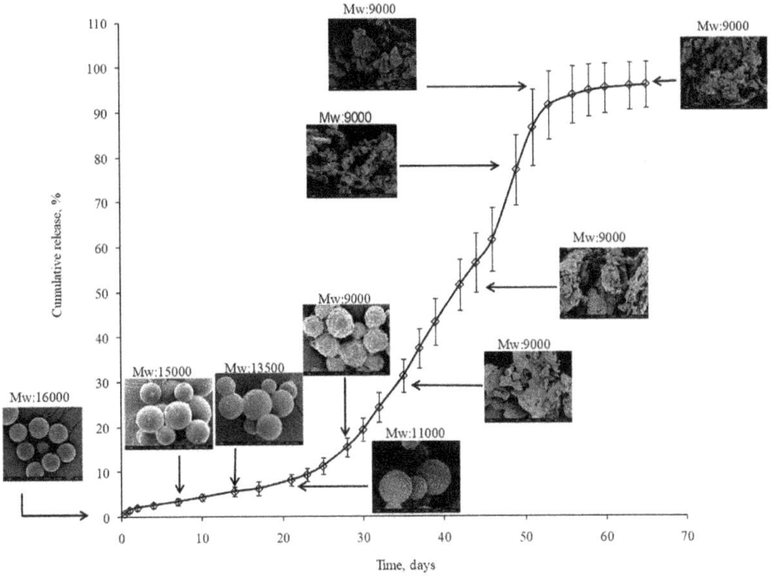

(**a**)

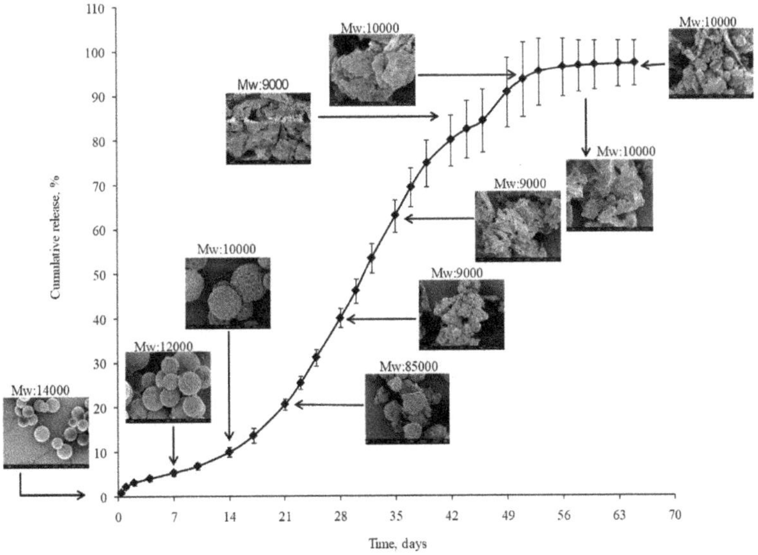

(**b**)

Figure 7. PLGA molecular weight (gel permeation chromatography (GPC) data) and microsphere morphology (SEM pictures) during the in vitro release assay of non-sterilized (**a**) and sterilized (**b**) microspheres.

The kinetic analysis of drug release data following both Korsmeyer–Peppas and Heller and Baker models showed changes related to the polymer matrix modifications due to sterilization. On one hand, the Korsmeyer·Peppas studies (Table 4, Figure 6c) showed a more extended Super Case II transport kinetic starting 1 week before (at day

10 instead of day 17) for sterilized MS. Furthermore, the Heller and Baker fitting (Table 4, Figure 6d) behaved in a monophasic manner, with a high polymer alteration rate constant (0.30 day^{-1}). Additionally, both the PLGA molecular weight measurement and the SEM pictures of sterilized microspheres during the release process confirmed the kinetic results, showing a higher erosion of the polymer both on the surface (surfaces began to deteriorate after 2 weeks of study) and in the inner structure; therefore, particles disintegrated after 3 weeks (Figure 7b).

3.3. In Vivo Evaluation

Table 5 shows the results of the ophthalmic clinical signs evaluated after sub-Tenon injection. Among the clinical signs evaluated, only conjunctival congestion was observed.

Table 5. Summary of ophthalmic clinical observations (anterior and posterior segment). Rabbits received a single sub-Tenon injection of Dx-loaded microspheres in the left eye (LE). The right eye (RE) was used as the control.

Sign	Prescreen		1 day		7 days		14 days		28 days		42 days	
	RE	LE	RE	LE	RE	LE	RE	LE	RE	LE	RE	LE
Conjunctival congestion	1/20	2/20	5/20	19/20 *	0/15	7/15 **	0/11	0/11	0/7	0/7	0/6	0/6
Conjunctival discharge	0/20	0/20	0/20	0/20	0/15	0/15	0/11	0/11	0/7	0/7	0/6	0/6
Conjunctival swelling	0/20	0/20	0/20	0/20	0/15	0/15	0/11	0/11	0/7	0/7	0/6	0/6
Aqueous flare	0/20	0/20	0/20	0/20	0/15	0/15	0/11	0/11	0/7	0/7	0/6	0/6
Light reflex	0/20	0/20	0/20	0/20	0/15	0/15	0/11	0/11	0/7	0/7	0/6	0/6
Iris involvement	0/20	0/20	0/20	0/20	0/15	0/15	0/11	0/11	0/7	0/7	0/6	0/6
Surface of cornea cloudiness	0/20	0/20	0/20	0/20	0/15	0/15	0/11	0/11	0/7	0/7	0/6	0/6
Pannus	0/20	0/20	0/20	0/20	0/15	0/15	0/11	0/11	0/7	0/7	0/6	0/6
Fluorescein staining	0/20	0/20	0/20	0/20	0/15	0/15	0/11	0/11	0/7	0/7	0/6	0/6
Lens	0/20	0/20	0/20	0/20	0/15	0/15	0/11	0/11	0/7	0/7	0/6	0/6
Vitreous opacity	0/20	0/20	0/20	0/20	0/15	0/15	0/11	0/11	0/7	0/7	0/6	0/6
Vascular congestion	0/20	0/20	0/20	0/20	0/15	0/15	0/11	0/11	0/7	0/7	0/6	0/6
Vitreous and retinal hemorrhage	0/20	0/20	0/20	0/20	0/15	0/15	0/11	0/11	0/7	0/7	0/6	0/6
Retinal detachment	0/20	0/20	0/20	0/20	0/15	0/15	0/11	0/11	0/7	0/7	0/6	0/6

* Animals showed minimal conjunctival congestion, except two animals that presented mild congestion. ** Animals showed minimal conjunctival congestion, except one animal that presented mild congestion.

Experimental eyes presented different degrees (minimal or mild) of conjunctival congestion at 1 day (19/20) and at 7 days (7/15); however, in all cases, conjunctival congestion disappeared at 14 days post injection. In addition, conjunctival congestion was present in the control eye of 25% of animals at 1 day (5/20). As hypothesized by other authors, the conjunctival congestion observed in both eyes (treated and untreated) could be due to the sub-Tenon injection itself [40].

No other clinical changes were observed in terms of conjunctival discharge, conjunctival swelling, aqueous flare, light reflex modification, iris involvement, surface of cornea cloudiness, pannus, fluorescein staining, loss of lens transparency, vitreous opacity, vascular congestion, vitreous and/or retinal hemorrhage, and/or retinal detachment. According to these results, microspheres were well tolerated in the short term after periocular injection.

In the present study, intraocular pressure (IOP) remained unchanged with mean values of 19.4 ± 1.8 mmHg (control eyes) and 18.8 ± 2.8 mmHg (experimental eyes) during the 45 days of follow-up. The statistical analysis of IOP values showed no significant differences ($p > 0.05$) between groups (Figure 8).

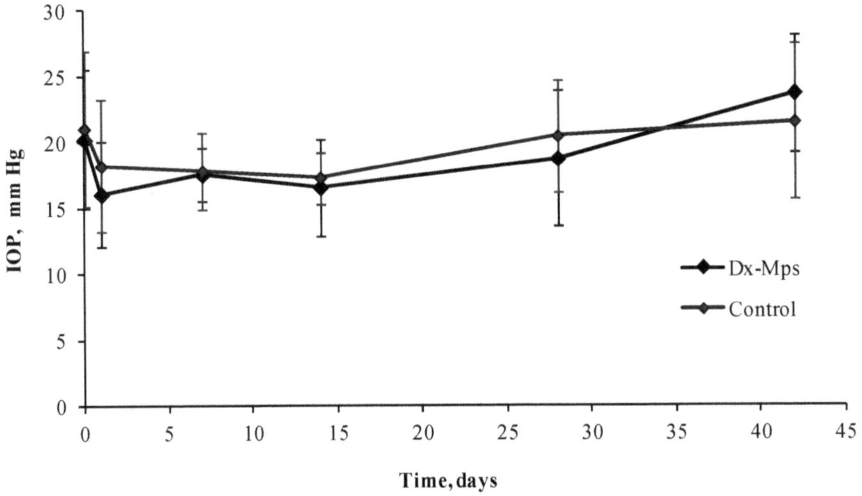

Figure 8. Intraocular pressure (IOP) mean values (± standard error of the mean (SEM)) obtained at different times of the study: before injection, and 1, 7, 14, 28, and 42 days after injection, for control and eyes that received a sub-Tenon injection of Dx-MS. No significant differences were found between groups ($p > 0.05$).

3.4. Histological Analysis

Four eyes (two experimental and two control eyes) were subjected to histopathology studies at 42 days after injection (Figure 9, Table 6). After dosing with Dx-MS, ocular tissues close to the injection site showed occasional macrophages. As no inflammatory signs were noted in the eyes belonging to the control group, the immunological reaction observed in experimental eyes might be related to the presence of microspheres at the administration site. Additionally, scattered occasional residues of microspheres were observed in one experimental eye.

Table 6. Scored histopathological evaluation at 42 days after sub-Tenon injection of Dx-microspheres in PBS (left eye, LE) and control eye (right eye, RE).

Eyes Evaluated	Inflammation at the Injection Site	Presence of Foreign Body Giant Cell Reaction	Presence of Microparticles Residues
Rabbit 1 and 2 RE (control)	− (Absent)	− (Absent)	− (Absent)
Rabbit 1 LE (Dx-MS)	− (Absent)	− (Absent)	− (Absent) No significant residues; occasional foamy macrophages
Rabbit 2 LE (Dx-MS)	− (Absent)	− (Absent)	+/− (focal) Scattered occasional residues; single foamy macrophage

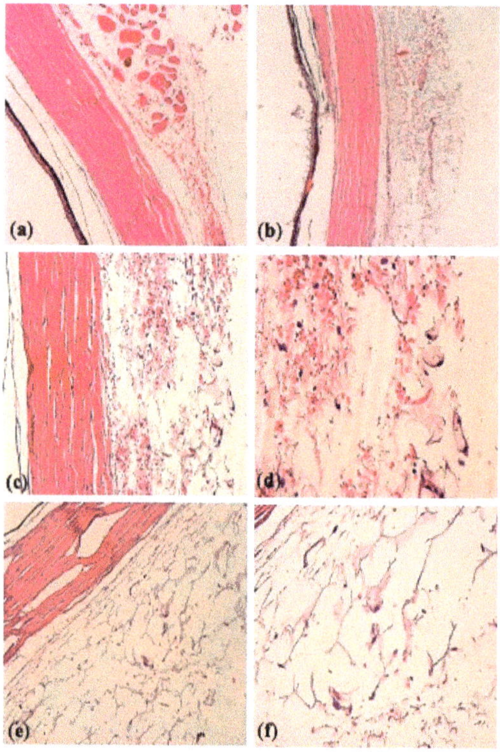

Figure 9. Histopathologic analysis of episcleral tissue injection site, after sub-Tenon injection of Dx-microspheres in phosphate-buffered saline (PBS) (left eye, **a**,**b**) and control eye (right eye, **c**–**f**). (**a**,**b**) Untreated eyes of two different rabbits, showing absence of tissue reaction; (**c**,**d**) Dx-microparticle-treated eye (rabbit 1), showing presence of occasional foamy macrophages and no microsphere residues; (**e**,**f**) Dx-microsphere-treated eye (rabbit 2), showing presence of single foamy macrophages and scattered occasional microspheres residues. Magnification: 10× (**a**,**b**); 20× (**c**,**e**); 40× (**d**,**f**).

4. Discussion

Current developments in the therapy of ophthalmic chronic diseases are directed toward the use of new drug delivery systems, with the objective to allow sustained therapeutic levels of drugs at ocular target sites. In this sense, biodegradable microspheres have been demonstrated to provide long-term delivery of drugs, and their utility in ophthalmology has been previously reported [3,15,41–44]. One of the main advantages of these systems is that they can be administered as a conventional injection using a small=gauge needle. Furthermore, depending on the patients' needs, a proper dose of the active substance can be adjusted by administering a specific amount of microspheres, allowing a personalized therapy. The most effective route of administration to achieve appropriate drug levels in the posterior segment of the eye is intravitreal injection. However, the use of this route in chronic therapies has potential side-effects, such as retinal detachment or endophthalmitis, and other alternatives are under study. In this experimental work, biodegradable PLGA microspheres loaded with the anti-inflammatory dexamethasone were designed to allow a long-term release of the drug by periocular administration, in line with previous studies in which authors demonstrated that this drug can diffuse through the sclera and can be detected in the retina and vitreous [21–23].

Even though PLGA is a Food and Drug Administration (FDA)-approved polymer to be used in devices, it is desirable to minimize the amount of PLGA administered to the eye. This can be achieved by fabricating PLGA microparticles that exhibit a high drug-loading capacity. In this sense, all formulations and size fractions presented in this work showed excellent encapsulation characteristics, with high drug loadings in all the assayed conditions). These results are in accordance with those reported by other authors [45]. Another desirable attribute of microparticles is that they should exhibit a particle size that is small enough to pass through a cannula, needed to inject these formulations in the form of aqueous suspensions. As formulation 3 did not show significant differences between the two granulometric fractions assayed (53–38 μm and 38–20 μm), the complete 20–53 μm fraction, with a mean particle size of 31 ± 3 μm, was chosen as the most suitable for injection.

Many authors have proposed a gamma-irradiation sterilization process as one of the least aggressive and more suitable sterilization approaches for PLGA microspheres with no significant changes in MS properties [15,26,28,29]. In the present work, the surface morphology and particle size distribution of microspheres remained unaltered after the sterilization process under the described conditions. However, changes in the release profile of dexamethasone were observed in sterilized batches, which might be attributed to the induction of ester-bond cleavage and the resulting decrease in polymer molecular weight [26,37,38]. It is well known that a decrease in M_W may have an important effect on the mobility of the polymer chain and, hence, on the free volume available for water and drug diffusion [28]. Effectively, in this study, a reduction in the PLGA molecular weight by 11% was quantified after irradiation. These results are in agreement with other works, wherein a loss in M_W was documented for PLGA MS after gamma sterilization [30,37,46].

Ideally, drug delivery devices will maintain therapeutic concentrations locally for months. Poly(lactic acid), poly(glycolic acid), and their copolymers degrade safely via hydrolysis into natural products of lactic and glycolic acids, which are metabolized into CO_2 and water [47]. PLGA is preferred for microparticle preparation in part because of its slow and reproducible degradation rate. PLGA has been used in several FDA-approved parenteral drug applications that are currently on the market, with one of them being used in ophthalmology, for intravitreal administration [7]. Although several authors have demonstrated that the in vitro/in vivo correlation is not optimal for ocular tissues [47], in vitro release studies remain a preliminary step necessary to determine the potential suitability of developed formulations. In the present work, changes in the release profile were detected and attributed to the induction of ester-bond cleavage and the resulting decrease in polymer molecular weight after the gamma irradiation [26,37,38]. However, the results shown in this work demonstrate that the developed microspheres were able to control the release of dexamethasone until even 9 weeks after their sterilization, a requirement needed for the use of these systems in vivo.

Microspheres were well tolerated after periocular injection. Among the clinical signs evaluated, only conjunctival congestion was observed. As hypothesized by other authors, the conjunctival congestion observed in both eyes (treated and untreated) could be due to the sub-Tenon injection itself [40]. In fact, Saishin et al. (2003) observed that, 20 days after periocular administration of unloaded PLGA–glucose microspheres and PKC412 microspheres (25% or 50%) in pigs, mild conjunctival congestion was similarly observed among the three groups, and there were no discernible signs of inflammation or irritation. In addition, Amrite et al. [48] did not find any signs of inflammation, including redness or edema, after a single subconjunctival injection of PLGA microspheres loaded with celecoxib in rats.

Concerning the nature of the administered drug, different adverse events can occur after corticosteroid therapy. The most common adverse reactions are cataract formation and elevated intraocular pressure [10,49], as well as the promotion of ocular herpes simplex virus reactivation [50]. In the present work, no clinical signs of cataract formation were denoted during the 6 weeks of observation. However, it is important to remark that the treatment-related cataract formation may take longer periods to become apparent [10]. The increase in IOP after administration of corticosteroids is of particular concern [10,51]. Whereas this increment reverts to normal values when the treatment is finished, the glaucomatous damage of the optic nerve head is irreversible, and patients need an ocular hypotensive treatment for the duration of the corticosteroid treatment in order to avoid permanent damage. This fact is of special importance in chronic treatment with steroids. Effectively, some authors showed glaucomatous symptoms associated with the ocular administration of corticosteroids due to the increment of IOP, typically after systemic and topical administration [52]. In the present study, IOP remained unchanged during the assay (42 days) with a mean after injection of 19.4 $\pm$ 1.8 mmHg (control eye) and 18.8 $\pm$ 2.8 mmHg (experimental eye). The statistical analysis of IOP values showed no significant differences ($p > 0.05$) between groups.

Scattered occasional residues of microspheres were observed in one experimental eye. According to the previous extensive in vitro evaluation of microspheres presented in this work, once administered, PLGA microspheres might undergo progressive polymer hydrolysis while remaining visible for at least 6 weeks. It is, thus, not uncommon to find small portions of polymeric material in histological samples. These small portions might suffer progressive degradation until disappearance, with no observable tissue damage, according to previous tolerance studies where PLGA microspheres were intravitreally [15] or periocularly [24] administered, and this was even noted with the use of the more hydrophobic PLGA (85:15), which presents a lower degradation rate [53].

A total of 42 days after periocular injection, Dx-MS were still detected in the sub-Tenon space by histopathology studies, indicating that they were able to properly reach the injection site. No clinical signs of inflammation were observed during the study, although it is true that particles were loaded with an anti-inflammatory drug that could mask this symptom. On the contrary, an immunological reaction was observed at the site of administration. This "foreign body reaction" resulted analogous to that observed after the previously described intravitreal injection of 10 mg of PLGA microspheres into rabbits [54], and similar to that described for microspheres injected intramuscularly in rabbits, which gradually decreased with time [55].

The findings presented in this work are promising since, to date, research has shown limited data on creating a proficient system for delivering small-particle-size drugs (such as dexamethasone) periocularly over a prolonged period of time. By encapsulating dexamethasone in PLGA microspheres with the method optimized here, it has been demonstrated that a slow and sustained drug delivery can be achieved in a local environment, resulting in long-term delivery of the drug for over 9 weeks.

5. Conclusions

The periocular administration of microparticulate systems can be considered as a good alternative to overcome the limitation of the frequent intravitreal administration of drugs. Dx-MS developed in this work represent a suitable formulation for sub-Tenon administration. Particles exhibited a high encapsulation efficiency, as well as prolonged and sustained release rates, and they were resistant to gamma sterilization. Microspheres were well tolerated after in vivo administration with no increase in IOP for at least 42 days. Although prolonged efficacy and tolerance studies are needed to study the effect of these systems in more depth, this formulation is presented as a potential alternative for the long-term delivery of ophthalmic drugs to the back of the eye.

Author Contributions: Conceptualization, R.H.-V., I.B.-O., and J.C.P.-J.; methodology, R.H.-V., I.B.-O., and I.T.M.-M.; software, D.B.-A. and V.A.-G.; validation, D.B.-A. and E.G.-A.; formal analysis, D.B.-A. and V.A.-G.; investigation, D.B.-A.; resources, R.H.-V. and I.T.M.-M.; data curation, D.B.-A., I.F.-B., M.T.G.-G., E.G.-A., and V.A.-G.; writing—original draft preparation, D.B.-A.; writing—review and editing, D.B.-A., V.A.-G., R.H.-V., and I.B.-O.; visualization, R.H.-V., I.B.-O., and I.T.M.-M.; supervision, R.H.-V. and I.T.M.-M.; project administration, R.H.-V. and I.T.M.-M.; funding acquisition, R.H.-V., I.B.-O., and I.T.M.-M. All authors read and agreed to the published version of the manuscript.

Funding: This research was funded by the Spanish Ministry of Education and Ministry of Science and Technology (MAT 2017-83858-C2-1-R), RETICS RD16/0008/0001, RD16/0008/0004, RD16/0008/0009, UCM Research Group 920415, CONACYT (Mexico), and Junta de Castilla y León (Spain).

Institutional Review Board Statement: The use of animals in this study was in accordance with the recommendations of the Association for Research in Vision and Ophthalmology (ARVO) for the Use of Animals in Ophthalmic and Vision Research. It was approved by the Animal Research and Welfare Ethics Committee of the University of Valladolid (Spain) in agreement with European (Council Directive 2010/63/UE) and Spanish regulations (RD 53/2013).

Informed Consent Statement: Not applicable

Acknowledgments: The authors are grateful to Alfonso Rodríguez, Centro de Microscopía Electrónica Luis Bru (CAI, UCM), for technical SEM assistance.

Conflicts of Interest: The authors declare no conflict of interest.

References

1. Fricke, T.R.; Tahhan, N.; Resnikoff, S.; Papas, E.; Burnett, A.; Ho, S.M.; Naduvilath, T.; Naidoo, K.S. Global Prevalence of Presbyopia and Vision Impairment from Uncorrected Presbyopia: Systematic Review, Meta-analysis, and Modelling. *Ophthalmology* **2018**, *125*, 1492–1499. [CrossRef] [PubMed]
2. Bourne, R.R.A.; Flaxman, S.R.; Braithwaite, T.; Cicinelli, M.V.; Das, A.; Jonas, J.B.; Keeffe, J.; Kempen, J.H.; Leasher, J.; Limburg, H.; et al. Magnitude, temporal trends, and projections of the global prevalence of blindness and distance and near vision impairment: A systematic review and meta-analysis. *Lancet Glob. Health* **2017**, *5*, e888–e897. [CrossRef]
3. Bravo-Osuna, I.; Andrés-Guerrero, V.; Abal, P.P.; Molina-Martinez, I.T.; Herrero-Vanrell, R. Pharmaceutical microscale and nanoscale approaches for efficient treatment of ocular diseases. *Drug Deliv. Transl. Res.* **2016**, *6*, 686–707. [CrossRef] [PubMed]
4. Herrero-Vanrell, R.; De La Torre, M.V.; Andrés-Guerrero, V.; Barbosa-Alfaro, D.; Molina-Martínez, I.; Bravo-Osuna, I. Nano and microtechnologies for ophthalmic administration, an overview. *J. Drug Deliv. Sci. Technol.* **2013**, *23*, 75–102. [CrossRef]
5. Ribeiro, A.M.; Figueiras, A.; Veiga, F. Improvements in Topical Ocular Drug Delivery Systems: Hydrogels and Contact Lenses. *J. Pharm. Pharm. Sci.* **2015**, *18*, 683–695. [CrossRef] [PubMed]
6. Cao, Y.; Samy, K.E.; Bernards, D.A.; Desai, T.A. Recent advances in intraocular sustained-release drug delivery devices. *Drug Discov. Today* **2019**, *24*, 1694–1700. [CrossRef] [PubMed]
7. Hickey, T.; Kreutzer, D.; Burgess, D.; Moussy, F. Dexamethasone/PLGA microspheres for continuous delivery of an anti-inflammatory drug for implantable medical devices. *Biomaterials* **2002**, *23*, 1649–1656. [CrossRef]
8. Short, B.G. Safety Evaluation of Ocular Drug Delivery Formulations: Techniques and Practical Considerations. *Toxicol. Pathol.* **2008**, *36*, 49–62. [CrossRef]
9. Chang-Lin, J.-E.; Burke, J.A.; Peng, Q.; Lin, T.; Orilla, W.C.; Ghosn, C.R.; Zhang, K.-M.; Kuppermann, B.D.; Robinson, M.R.; Whitcup, S.M.; et al. Pharmacokinetics of a Sustained-Release Dexamethasone Intravitreal Implant in Vitrectomized and Nonvitrectomized Eyes. *Investig. Opthalmol. Vis. Sci.* **2011**, *52*, 4605–4609. [CrossRef]
10. Kuppermann, B.D.; Blumenkranz, M.S.; Haller, J.A.; Williams, G.A.; Weinberg, D.V.; Chou, C.; Whitcup, S.M. Randomized Controlled Study of an Intravitreous Dexamethasone Drug Delivery System in Patients With Persistent Macular Edema. *Arch. Ophthalmol.* **2007**, *125*, 309–317. [CrossRef]
11. Haller, J.A.; Kuppermann, B.D.; Blumenkranz, M.S.; Williams, G.A.; Weinberg, D.V.; Chou, C.; Whitcup, S.M. Randomized Controlled Trial of an Intravitreous Dexamethasone Drug Delivery System in Patients With Diabetic Macular Edema. *Arch. Ophthalmol.* **2010**, *128*, 289–296. [CrossRef] [PubMed]
12. Haller, J.A.; Bandello, F.; Belfort, R.; Blumenkranz, M.S.; Gillies, M.; Heier, J.; Loewenstein, A.; Yoon, Y.-H.; Jacques, M.-L.; Jiao, J.; et al. Randomized, Sham-Controlled Trial of Dexamethasone Intravitreal Implant in Patients with Macular Edema Due to Retinal Vein Occlusion. *Ophthalmology* **2010**, *117*, 1134–1146. [CrossRef]
13. Hsu, J. Drug delivery methods for posterior segment disease. *Curr. Opin. Ophthalmol.* **2007**, *18*, 235–239. [CrossRef] [PubMed]
14. Silva-Cunha, A.; Fialho, S.L.; Naud, M.-C.; Behar-Cohen, F. Poly-epsilon-caprolactone intravitreous devices: An in vivo study. *Invest Ophthalmol. Vis. Sci.* **2009**, *50*, 2312–2318. [CrossRef] [PubMed]
15. Herrero-Vanrell, R.; Refojo, M.F. Biodegradable microspheres for vitreoretinal drug delivery. *Adv. Drug Deliv. Rev.* **2001**, *52*, 5–16. [CrossRef]
16. Jager, R.D.; Aiello, L.P.; Patel, S.C.; Cunningham, E.T. Risks of Intravitreous Injection: A Comprehensive Review. *Retina* **2004**, *24*, 676–698. [CrossRef] [PubMed]
17. Fung, A.T.; Tran, T.; Lim, L.L.; Samarawickrama, C.; Arnold, J.; Gillies, M.; Catt, C.; Mitchell, L.; Symons, A.; Buttery, R.; et al. Local delivery of corticosteroids in clinical ophthalmology: A review. *Clin. Exp. Ophthalmol.* **2020**, *48*, 366–401. [CrossRef] [PubMed]
18. Wen, H.; Hao, J.; Li, S.K. Characterization of Human Sclera Barrier Properties for Transscleral Delivery of Bevacizumab and Ranibizumab. *J. Pharm. Sci.* **2013**, *102*, 892–903. [CrossRef]
19. Guise, P. Sub-Tenon's anesthesia: An update. *Local Reg. Anesth.* **2012**, *5*, 35–46. [CrossRef]

20. Duan, Y.; Yang, Y.; Huang, X.; Lin, D. Preliminary study of a controllable device for subtenon drug infusion in a rabbit model. *Acta Ophthalmol.* **2017**, *95*, 595–601. [CrossRef] [PubMed]
21. Geroski, D.H.; Edelhauser, H.F. Drug delivery for posterior segment eye disease. *Investig. Ophthalmol. Vis. Sci.* **2000**, *41*, 961–964.
22. Huang, X.; Liu, S.; Yang, Y.; Duan, Y.; Lin, D. Controllable continuous sub-tenon drug delivery of dexamethasone disodium phosphate to ocular posterior segment in rabbit. *Drug Deliv.* **2017**, *24*, 452–458. [CrossRef] [PubMed]
23. Huang, X.; Duan, Y.; Zhao, L.; Liu, S.; Qin, D.; Zhang, F.; Lin, D. Dexamethasone pharmacokinetics characteristics via sub-tenon microfluidic system in uveitis rabbits. *J. Drug Deliv. Sci. Technol.* **2020**, *57*, 101639. [CrossRef]
24. Paganelli, F.; Cardillo, J.A.; Melo, L.A.S.; Lucena, D.R.; Silva, A.A.; De Oliveira, A.G.; Höfling-Lima, A.L.; Nguyen, Q.D.; Kuppermann, B.D.; Belfort, R. A Single Intraoperative Sub-Tenon's Capsule Injection of Triamcinolone and Ciprofloxacin in a Controlled-Release System for Cataract Surgery. *Investig. Opthalmol. Vis. Sci.* **2009**, *50*, 3041–3047. [CrossRef] [PubMed]
25. Nayak, K.; Misra, M. A review on recent drug delivery systems for posterior segment of eye. *Biomed. Pharmacother.* **2018**, *107*, 1564–1582. [CrossRef]
26. Friess, W.; Schlapp, M. Sterilization of gentamicin containing collagen/PLGA microparticle composites. *Eur. J. Pharm. Biopharm.* **2006**, *63*, 176–187. [CrossRef] [PubMed]
27. Puthli, S.; Vavia, P. Formulation and Performance Characterization of Radio-Sterilized "Progestin-Only" Microparticles Intended for Contraception. *AAPS PharmSciTech* **2009**, *10*, 443–452. [CrossRef]
28. Faisant, N.; Siepmann, J.; Richard, J.; Benoit, J. Mathematical modeling of drug release from bioerodible microparticles: Effect of gamma-irradiation. *Eur. J. Pharm. Biopharm.* **2003**, *56*, 271–279. [CrossRef]
29. Mohr, D.; Wolff, M.; Kissel, T. Gamma irradiation for terminal sterilization of 17beta-estradiol loaded poly-(D,L-lactide-co-glycolide) microparticles. *J. Control. Release* **1999**, *61*, 203–217. [CrossRef]
30. Martínez-Sancho, C.; Herrero-Vanrell, R.; Negro, S. Study of gamma-irradiation effects on aciclovir poly(D,L-lactic-co-glycolic) acid microspheres for intravitreal administration. *J. Control. Release* **2004**, *99*, 41–52. [CrossRef]
31. Korsmeyer, R.W.; Von Meerwall, E.; Peppas, N.A. Solute and penetrant diffusion in swellable polymers. II. Verification of theoretical models. *J. Polym. Sci. Part B Polym. Phys.* **1986**, *24*, 409–434. [CrossRef]
32. Korsmeyer, R.W.; Lustig, S.R.; Peppas, N.A. Solute and penetrant diffusion in swellable polymers. I. Mathematical modeling. *J. Polym. Sci. Part B Polym. Phys.* **1986**, *24*, 395–408. [CrossRef]
33. Hellen, J.; Baker, R. *Theory and Practice of Controlled Drug Delivery from Bioerodible Polymers*; Controlled Release of Bioactive Materials; Academic Press: New York, NY, USA, 1980.
34. Ritger, P.L.; Peppas, N.A. A simple equation for description of solute release II. Fickian and anomalous release from swellable devices. *J. Control. Release* **1987**, *5*, 37–42. [CrossRef]
35. Ritger, P.L.; Peppas, N.A. A simple equation for description of solute release I. Fickian and non-fickian release from non-swellable devices in the form of slabs, spheres, cylinders or discs. *J. Control. Release* **1987**, *5*, 23–36. [CrossRef]
36. Herrero-Vanrell, R.; Ramirez, L. Biodegradable PLGA Microspheres Loaded with Ganciclovir for Intraocular Administration. Encapsulation Technique, in Vitro Release Profiles, and Sterilization Process. *Pharm. Res.* **2000**, *17*, 1323–1328. [CrossRef] [PubMed]
37. Schwach, G.; Oudry, N.; Delhomme, S.; Lück, M.; Lindner, H.; Gurny, R. Biodegradable microparticles for sustained release of a new GnRH antagonist–part I: Screening commercial PLGA and formulation technologies. *Eur. J. Pharm. Biopharm.* **2003**, *56*, 327–336. [CrossRef]
38. Yip, E.Y.; Wang, J.; Wang, C.-H. Sustained release system for highly water-soluble radiosensitizer drug etanidazole: Irradiation and degradation studies. *Biomaterials* **2003**, *24*, 1977–1987. [CrossRef]
39. Peppas, N.A. *1.* Commentary on an exponential model for the analysis of drug delivery: Original research article: A simple equation for description of solute release: I II. Fickian and non-Fickian release from non-swellable devices in the form of slabs, spheres, cylinders or discs, 1987. *J. Control. Release Off. J. Control. Release Soc.* **2014**, *190*, 31–32.
40. Saishin, Y.; Takahashi, K.; Melia, M.; Vinores, S.A.; Campochiaro, P.A. Inhibition of protein kinase C decreases prostaglandin-induced breakdown of the blood-retinal barrier. *J. Cell Physiol.* **2003**, *195*, 210–219. [CrossRef]
41. Andrés-Guerrero, V.; Zong, M.; Ramsay, E.; Rojas, B.; Sarkhel, S.; Gallego, B.; De Hoz, R.; Ramírez, A.I.; Salazar, J.J.; Triviño, A.; et al. Novel biodegradable polyesteramide microspheres for controlled drug delivery in Ophthalmology. *J. Control. Release* **2015**, *211*, 105–117. [CrossRef]
42. Gómez-Ballesteros, M.; Andrés-Guerrero, V.; Parra, F.; Marinich, J.; De-las-Heras, B.; Molina-Martínez, I.T.; Vazquez, B.; San Román, F.; Herrero-Vanrell, R. HEMA/Bayfit-MA nanoparticles improve the hypotensive effect of acetazolamide in rabbit eyes. In Proceedings of the International Forum on Advances in Pharmaceutical Technology, Santiago de Compostela, Spain, 5 November 2015.
43. Herrero-Vanrell, R.; Bravo-Osuna, I.; Andrés-Guerrero, V.; Vicario-De-La-Torre, M.; Molina-Martínez, I.T. The potential of using biodegradable microspheres in retinal diseases and other intraocular pathologies. *Prog. Retin. Eye Res.* **2014**, *42*, 27–43. [CrossRef] [PubMed]
44. Peters, T.; Kim, S.-W.; Castro, V.; Stingl, K.; Strasser, T.; Bolz, S.; Schraermeyer, U.; Mihov, G.; Zong, M.; Andres-Guerrero, V.; et al. Evaluation of polyesteramide (PEA) and polyester (PLGA) microspheres as intravitreal drug delivery systems in albino rats. *Biomaterials* **2017**, *124*, 157–168. [CrossRef] [PubMed]

45. Siepmann, J.; Faisant, N.; Akiki, J.; Richard, J.; Benoit, J.P. Effect of the size of biodegradable microparticles on drug release: Experiment and theory. *J. Control. Release* **2004**, *96*, 123–134. [CrossRef] [PubMed]
46. Bittner, B.; Mäder, K.; Kroll, C.; Borchert, H.H.; Kissel, T. Tetracycline-HCl-loaded poly(DL-lactide-co-glycolide) microspheres prepared by a spray drying technique: Influence of gamma-irradiation on radical formation and polymer degradation. *J. Control. Release* **1999**, *59*, 23–32. [CrossRef]
47. Fialho, S.; Rêgo, M.B.; Siqueira, R.C.; Jorge, R.; Haddad, A.; Rodrigues, A.L.; Maia-Filho, A.; Silva-Cunha, A. Safety and Pharmacokinetics of an Intravitreal Biodegradable Implant of Dexamethasone Acetate in Rabbit Eyes. *Curr. Eye Res.* **2006**, *31*, 525–534. [CrossRef] [PubMed]
48. Amrite, A.C.; Ayalasomayajula, S.P.; Cheruvu, N.P.S.; Kompella, U.B. Single Periocular Injection of Celecoxib-PLGA Microparticles Inhibits Diabetes-Induced Elevations in Retinal PGE2, VEGF, and Vascular Leakage. *Investig. Opthalmol. Vis. Sci.* **2006**, *47*, 1149–1160. [CrossRef] [PubMed]
49. Kuppermann, B.D.; Herrero-Vanrell, R.; Cardillo, J.A. Clinical applications of the sustained-release dexamethasone implant for treatment of macular edema. *Clin. Ophthalmol.* **2011**, *5*, 139–146. [CrossRef] [PubMed]
50. Al-Dujaili, L.J.; Clerkin, P.P.; Clement, C.; E McFerrin, H.; Bhattacharjee, P.S.; Varnell, E.D.; E Kaufman, H.; Hill, J.M. Ocular herpes simplex virus: How are latency, reactivation, recurrent disease and therapy interrelated? *Futur. Microbiol.* **2011**, *6*, 877–907. [CrossRef]
51. Herschler, J. Increased Intraocular Pressure Induced by Repository Corticosteroids. *Am. J. Ophthalmol.* **1976**, *82*, 90–93. [CrossRef]
52. Mohan, R.; Muralidharan, A.R. Steroid induced glaucoma and cataract. *Indian J. Ophthalmol.* **1989**, *37*, 13–16. [PubMed]
53. Ayalasomayajula, S.; Kompella, U.B. Subconjunctivally administered celecoxib-PLGA microparticles sustain retinal drug levels and alleviate diabetes-induced oxidative stress in a rat model. *Eur. J. Pharmacol.* **2005**, *511*, 191–198. [CrossRef] [PubMed]
54. Veloso, A.A.; Zhu, Q.; Herrero-Vanrell, R.; Refojo, M.F. Ganciclovir-loaded polymer microspheres in rabbit eyes inoculated with human cytomegalovirus. *Investig. Ophthalmol. Vis. Sci.* **1997**, *38*, 665–675.
55. Visscher, G.E.; Robison, R.L.; Maulding, H.V.; Fong, J.W.; Pearson, J.E.; Argentieri, G.J. Biodegradation of and tissue reaction to 50:50 poly(DL-lactide-co-glycolide) microcapsules. *J. Biomed. Mater. Res.* **1985**, *19*, 349–365. [CrossRef] [PubMed]

pharmaceutics

MDPI

Article

Transferrin Non-Viral Gene Therapy for Treatment of Retinal Degeneration

Karine Bigot [1], Pauline Gondouin [1], Romain Bénard [1], Pierrick Montagne [1], Jenny Youale [1,2], Marie Piazza [1], Emilie Picard [2], Thierry Bordet [1,*] and Francine Behar-Cohen [2,3,*]

1 Eyevensys, Biopark, 11 rue Watt, 75013 Paris, France; karine.bigot@eyevensys.com (K.B.); pauline.gondouin@eyevensys.com (P.G.); romain.benard@eyevensys.com (R.B.); pierrick.montagne@eyevensys.com (P.M.); jenny.youale@eyevensys.com (J.Y.); marie.piazza@eyevensys.com (M.P.)

2 Centre de Recherche des Cordeliers, INSERM, Sorbonne Université, USPC, Université Paris Descartes, Team 17, 75006 Paris, France; emilie.picard@crc.jussieu.fr

3 Ophtalmopole, Cochin Hospital, AP-HP, Assistance Publique Hôpitaux de Paris, 24 rue du Faubourg Saint-Jacques, 75014 Paris, France

* Correspondence: thierry.bordet@eyevensys.com (T.B.); francine.behar-cohen@parisdescartes.fr (F.B.-C.)

Received: 7 August 2020; Accepted: 28 August 2020; Published: 1 September 2020

Abstract: Dysregulation of iron metabolism is observed in animal models of retinitis pigmentosa (RP) and in patients with age-related macular degeneration (AMD), possibly contributing to oxidative damage of the retina. Transferrin (TF), an endogenous iron chelator, was proposed as a therapeutic candidate. Here, the efficacy of TF non-viral gene therapy based on the electrotransfection of pEYS611, a plasmid encoding human TF, into the ciliary muscle was evaluated in several rat models of retinal degeneration. pEYS611 administration allowed for the sustained intraocular production of TF for at least 3 and 6 months in rats and rabbits, respectively. In the photo-oxidative damage model, pEYS611 protected both retinal structure and function more efficiently than carnosic acid, a natural antioxidant, reduced microglial infiltration in the outer retina and preserved the integrity of the outer retinal barrier. pEYS611 also protected photoreceptors from N-methyl-N-nitrosourea-induced apoptosis. Finally, pEYS611 delayed structural and functional degeneration in the RCS rat model of RP while malondialdehyde (MDA) ocular content, a biomarker of oxidative stress, was decreased. The neuroprotective benefits of TF non-viral gene delivery in retinal degenerative disease models further validates iron overload as a therapeutic target and supports the continued development of pEY611 for treatment of RP and dry AMD.

Keywords: iron; retinal degeneration; age-related macular degeneration; retinitis pigmentosa; transferrin; gene therapy; plasmid electrotransfection

1. Introduction

Iron is essential for retinal metabolism and visual cycle, but excessive ferrous iron (Fe^{2+}) can generate reactive oxygen species (ROS) and consecutive oxidative damage to the cellular environment (reviewed in [1,2]). Iron particles cause oxidative damage to rat photoreceptors, with greater damage to cones than rods [3] and iron-induced photoreceptor cell death was associated with lipid peroxidation [4], activation of the nucleotide-binding oligomerization domain (NOD)-like receptor family pyrin domain-containing 3 (NLRP3) inflammasome signaling pathway, and induction of necrotic and apoptotic markers [3,5,6]. In addition, the phagocytosis of Fe^{2+}-oxidized photoreceptor outer segments further damage the retinal pigment epithelium (RPE) [7], markedly decreasing phagocytosis activity and lysosomal function [8], and possibly inducing RPE de-differentiation [9]. To tightly control the intracellular iron level, several proteins regulate iron import, storage, and export. Transferrin (TF) binds ferric iron (Fe^{3+}) with a very high affinity (association constant is 10^{20} M^{-1} at pH 7.4) and is then internalized by transferrin receptors (TFRs), allowing iron to enter into the cell. Inside cells, iron dissociates from TF and enters in the labile iron pool while TF is recycled at the cell membrane. Intracellular iron is supplied to cytosolic proteins for storage (ferritins), taken up by the mitochondria or released from the cell by ferroportin, a membrane transporter requiring ferroxidases, such as ceruloplasmin or hephaestin, to convert the ferrous Fe^{2+} to ferric Fe^{3+} form. In addition, iron-sensitive intracellular proteins, such as iron-regulatory proteins (IRP1 and IRP2), hepcidin or hypoxia-inducing factor (HIF), serve as check points to control the intracellular iron concentration (recently reviewed in [2]).

Iron-mediated retinal cell death has been shown to occur in various models of retinal degeneration and suspected to occur in age-related macular degeneration (AMD) and retinitis pigmentosa (RP). Indeed, iron deposits (including labile iron) were observed in postmortem AMD macula at the RPE–choroid interface within metal-storing melanosomes, in drusens, in the central layer of the calcified Bruch's membrane but also in the neurosensory retina [10–12]. The level of iron in the aqueous humor of dry AMD patients undergoing cataract surgery was two-fold higher than in age-matched controls [13] and the expression of proteins involved in iron homeostasis, such as ferritin and ferroportin, was increased in the macula of AMD patients with geographic atrophy [11]. Similarly, increased expression of TF was shown in the retinas of AMD patients relative to those of healthy control patients, which suggests that iron regulation is impaired [14]. Finally, several polymorphisms in iron homeostasis genes have been identified as risk factors for AMD, such as the TF receptors (TFR1 and TFR2) genes [15], IRP1 and IRP2 genes [16], and the heme oxygenase-1 and -2 (HMOX1/2) genes [17]. We and others have characterized the role of iron homeostasis dysregulation and associated oxidative injury in the pathogenesis of RP. In the Royal College of Surgeons (RCS) rat [18] and in the rd10 mouse [19,20], two models of RP, degeneration of the retina was associated with altered iron homeostasis and its progression correlated with iron overload. Furthermore, mutation in the feline leukemia virus subgroup C cellular receptor 1 (FLVCR1), a gene encoding a heme-transporter protein involved in iron homeostasis, is also causing syndromic autosomal-recessive RP [21].

Whether loss of iron homeostasis is a cause or a consequence of various retinal diseases remains unknown, but it is undeniable that an excess of free iron is pathogenic, and that its neutralization with chemical chelators protects the retina not only in rodent models with impaired mechanisms of iron homeostasis [22,23] but also in models of inherited retinal dystrophies [24–26]. Chemical iron chelators failed so far to reach clinical stage because of limited ocular bioavailability and/or ocular side-effects (cataract, retinopathy optic neuritis) probably due to chelation of intracellular iron store necessary for retina cells' function [2,27]. Conversely, the natural iron transporter TF was proven to be safe in the eye when overexpressed in transgenic mouse or when delivered intraperitoneally or intravitreally in the rat even after repeated administration of high doses (up to 240 μg per eye) [19,28–30]. Thus, we proposed to use TF as a therapeutic candidate for safe iron chelation in ocular diseases. Although vitreous humor contains a high amount of TF in physiologic conditions both as the free form (apo-TF) and the iron-bound form (holo-TF) [31], the expression of TF and of its receptor is upregulated in retinal degeneration or inflammation [14,20,29] suggesting that TF levels could be a limiting factor in disease conditions. We recently reported that both the TF saturation rate and levels of free iron were increased in the vitreous and in the subretinal fluid of patients with retinal detachment, together correlated with reduced postoperative visual recovery [6], identifying TF as a good candidate to buffer free iron in the eye. When injected into the vitreous, TF distributes throughout the neural retina and the RPE via its receptors and is rapidly eliminated from the retina by a transretinal elimination route [30], suggesting that local delivery of the protein itself would require repeated administration in the context of chronic retinal diseases. Importantly, TF was highly potent to preserve photoreceptors in animal models of retinal degeneration induced by iron overload, light exposure, inherited genetic mutations, or retinal detachment [6,19,30]. In these models, TF restored iron homeostasis, reduced oxidative stress, inflammation, and cell death, preserving photoreceptor cells and visual function [6,30].

In the present study, we evaluated a non-viral gene therapy strategy that combines a plasmid coding for human TF (pEYS611), and an electrotransfection system to deliver DNA plasmids into the ciliary muscle, in order to sustainably produce apo-TF into the eye. Such a technology was previously shown to efficiently allow the production of a variety of secreted proteins, including trophic factors, anti-TNF, or anti-VEGF [32–36]. We investigated the therapeutic potential of pEYS611 in several rat models of induced retinal degeneration, including the RCS rat model of RP and the photo-oxidative damage model, evaluating both retinal histology and function. These findings further validate iron overload as a therapeutic target for the treatment of retinal degeneration and pEYS611 as a valuable product to neutralize ocular iron excess.

2. Materials and Methods

2.1. *pEYS611 Plasmid Construct*

pEYS611 is a 5201-base pair plasmid DNA coding for the human transferrin (TF). The codon-optimized cDNA sequence of TF was de novo synthesized by GeneArt (ThermoFisher Scientific, Waltham, MA, USA), subcloned into the NTC8685 plasmid backbone (Nature Technology Corporation, Lincoln, NE, USA) [37] by enzymatic restriction and verified by sequencing. Transgene expression was placed under the control of an optimized chimeric CMV-HTLV-1R ubiquitous promoter and the ß-globin intron. pEYS611 plasmid was amplified through an antibiotic-free selection procedure in modified *E. coli* cells [38] and formulated in sterile Tris-EDTA buffered saline at a final concentration of 5 mg/mL.

2.2. *Animals*

Male Wistar and Sprague Dawley rats were obtained from Janvier Labs (Le Genest-Saint-Isle, France) to conduct the light-induced damage and the N-methyl-N-nitrosourea (MNU)-induced retinal degeneration models, respectively, as previously reported (see below). New Zealand rabbits were provided by CEGAV (Saint Mars d'Egrenne, France). Pigmented dystrophic RCS and pigmented control non-dystrophic RDY rats were a gift from Dr Emeline Nandrot (Institut de la Vision, Paris, France).

Rats were group-housed (maximum 3 rats per cage) and rabbits were individually housed. Each cage contained an environmental enrichment. Animals were fed ad libitum with a diet for maintenance; they were maintained in a temperature-controlled room at 21–23 °C with the light-environment consisting of 12- or 18-h light per day for rabbits and rats, respectively.

Animals were acclimated for at least one week in the animal facility prior any experiments. All experimental methods and protocols were carried out according to standard operating procedures with approval by the Institutional Ethic Committees of Sorbonne university and National veterinary school of Alfort and French Ministry of Higher Education, Research and Innovation (certificates APAFIS#7001-2015100815363248, APAFIS#11019-2017082415542346, APAFIS#7411-2016102710489557 and APAFIS#15364-20180531109399950). In addition, experiments complied with the ARVO statement for animal experimentation and followed European guidelines for animal welfare.

2.3. *Plasmid Electrotransfection Procedure in Rat and Rabbit Ciliary Muscle*

Animals were anesthetized by intramuscular injection of a mixture of ketamine (8% Imalgen 1000, Merial, France) and xylazine (2% Rompun, Bayer AG, Leverkusen, Germany). Electrotransfection of pEYS611 in the rat ciliary muscle was performed as previously described [34]. Briefly, following protrusion of the eye with an operating field, injection of the plasmid solution (10 µL) was performed transclerally using a 30G needle parallel to the limbus. An iridium/platinum wire electrode (cathode, Good Fellow, Lille, France) was then inserted into the transscleral tunnel, and a semi-annular stainless-steel sheet electrode (anode, Good Fellow, Lille, France) was placed on the sclera, facing the wire electrode. The eye was humidified by instillation of an additional drop of 0.9% NaCl solution to facilitate conductance. Square-wave electrical pulses (200 V/cm, 5 Hz, 10 ms, 8 pulses) were generated with Eyevensys proprietary Pulse Generator.

Plasmid electrotransfection in rabbits was performed using a dedicated ocular device similar to a device previously described for human application [35]. When placed on the nasal scleral surface and adjusted with the limbus, such a device allows for precise and consistent guiding of the plasmid injection into the posterior longitudinal ciliary muscle fibers using a 29G-needle (30 µL). A tracer dye insuring proper ciliary muscle injection was used for training of operators and demonstration purpose as described in Figure 1. Following instillation of two to three drops of physiological solution (0.9% NaCl) on the eye, a square-wave electrical pulse sequence was delivered in between the surface electrode and the needle electrodes inserted in the anterior vitreous just beneath the ciliary muscle. Electric pulses (high voltage = 500 V/cm, 1 Hz, 100 µs, 1 pulse duration, 10 s break; low voltage = 200 V/cm, 1 Hz, 100 ms, 4 pulses) were delivered with an Eyevensys Pulse Generator. All animals received post-operative ophthalmic gel of carbomer onto the cornea (Lacrigel, Laboratoire Europhta, Monaco).

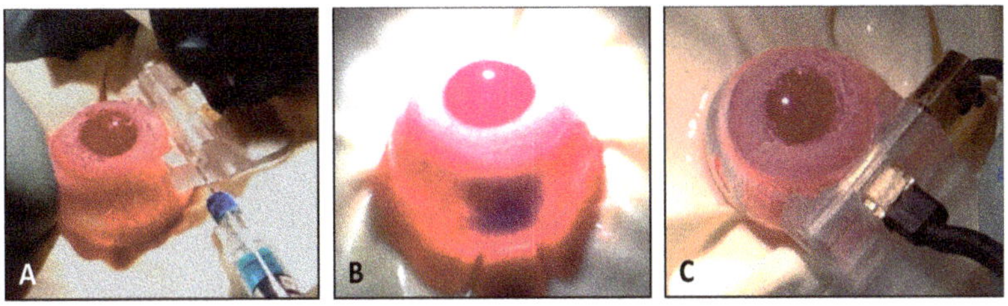

Figure 1. Ciliary muscle electrotransfection procedure in rabbit. (**A**) Plasmid injection in the rabbit ciliary muscle was performed using a dedicated ocular device placed on the nasal scleral surface. (**B**) Tracer dye (blue) was used for the demonstration purpose only and was not used during administration of pEYS611. (**C**) Following adjusted placement of the ocular device so that its superior part fits with the limbus, the comb electrode was inserted into ocular tissues until its stop position.

2.4. *Quantification of Human Transferrin (TF) in Ocular Fluids and Tissues*

Quantification of TF in ocular fluids and in retinal tissues was performed using a specific enzyme-linked immunosorbent assay (ELISA). Briefly, goat anti-human TF polyclonal antibodies (Bio-Rad, Hercules, CA, USA) were coated on a 96-well high-binding affinity plate. Captured human TF was detected using a biotinylated goat polyclonal antibody raised against the human TF (Bio-Rad, Hercules, CA, USA) and revealed with streptavidin-horse radish peroxidase (HRP, Sigma-Aldrich, St. Louis, MI, USA) enzyme and tetramethylbenzidine (TMB) substrate (Sigma-Aldrich, St. Louis, MI, USA). The 450-nm absorbance was measured using the Infinite F200 plate reader (Tecan, Männedorf, Switzerland). Recombinant human TF (Bio-Rad, Hercules, CA, USA) was used as a standard. The lower limit of quantification (LLoQ) in rat ocular fluids (aqueous humor and vitreous pooled together) and in rabbit aqueous humor, vitreous and retina/RPE/choroid complex was defined as 195.3 and 39 pg/mL, respectively. Concentrations of human TF were calculated using a four-parameter logistic curve fit (4-PL, MyAssays software) from the standard curve. Values were expressed as mean ± standard error of the mean (sem) in ng/mL of fluids or ng/g of tissues.

2.5. *Light-Induced Damage Rat Model*

Male Wistar rats (4-week-old at arrival) were maintained for 3 weeks prior to light exposure in a dimly lit environment (maximum 200 lux) by placing the ventilated cages at the bottom of the rack to reduce variation in the photoreceptor sensibility between animals, as previously described [30]. Dark adaptation was performed during at least 15 h before light exposure. Animals were then placed in individual transparent cages with access to food and water (Hydrogel, Janvier Labs, Saint Berthevin,

France), and retina light-induced damage (LID) was induced by exposition under a cold white LED of 6500 lux mounted on a lamp board (slightly raised to allow airflow) during 24 h. After light exposure, animals returned to normal cyclic light conditions as described above. Control animals underwent dark adaptation but then returned to rearing cyclic light conditions without being exposed to the cold white LED (no LID group). Retinal functionality was assessed by electroretinography (ERG) eight days after LID. Animals were then sacrificed for histopathological evaluations and quantification of human TF in ocular fluids.

2.6. N-Methyl-N-Nitrosourea (MNU)-Induced Retinal Degeneration Model in Rat

N-methyl-N-nitrosourea-induced retinopathy was induced as previously reported [39]. Briefly, eight-week-old male Sprague Dawley rats received a single intraperitoneal injection (i.p.) of N-methyl-N-nitrosourea (MNU) dissolved in 0.9% NaCl (Sigma-Aldrich, St. Louis, MI, USA) at the dose of 60 mg/kg body weight, while age-matched control animals received a single i.p. injection of vehicle (no MNU). Animals were sacrificed 3 or 7 days following the injections for histopathological evaluation of the retina (n = up to 5 rats/group/timepoint).

2.7. Electroretinogram (ERG) Recordings

Animals were dark-adapted for at least 15 h prior to ERG and all manipulations were performed under dim red light. Rats were anesthetized by intramuscular injection of a mixture of ketamine and xylazine. Pupils were dilated with topical 0.5% tropicamide. ERGs were recorded simultaneously in both eyes using a rodent full-integrated ERG system (Celeris, Diagnosys, Cambridge, UK). Saline lubricant eye drops were added to the end of the electrode and on the cornea to ensure optimal contact between the eye and the electrode. Electrode stimulators were placed directly onto the surface of the eye from the front and down, ensuring the whole eye was covered and there was good contact to the eye. For scotopic ERG in the dark-adapted state, flash intensities ranged from 0.01 to 3 cd·s/m^2. For photopic ERG in the light-adapted state, flash intensities ranged from 3 to 10 cd·s/m^2. Amplitudes of a-waves (negative waves) were measured from the baseline to the bottom of the a-wave trough, and b-wave amplitudes (positive waves) were measured from the bottom of the a-wave trough to the peak of the b-wave. Implicit times of the a-and b-waves were measured from the time of stimulus to peaks. Results were expressed in microvolts (µV) for amplitudes and milliseconds (ms) for implicit times. The values obtained for all eyes from the same experimental group were average and values are expressed as mean ± sem.

2.8. Histology

Oriented ocular globes were fixed for at least 24 h in Hartman's fixative solution (Sigma-Aldrich, St. Louis, MI, USA) and embedded in paraffin. Five-µm sagittal sections containing optic nerve (ON) were performed and stained with hematoxylin and eosin (HE). HE sections from 3 consecutive slides were examined by light microscopy at a magnification of 20× and color images were obtained using a NanoZoomer-XR Digital slide scanner (Hamamatsu Photonics, Hamamatsu city, Japan). Images were analyzed using NDP View software. The outer nuclear layer (ONL thickness) in the LID model or the total retinal thickness (from the internal limiting membrane to the retinal pigment epithelium) and the outer retinal thickness (from the outer plexiform layer to the retinal pigment epithelium) in the MNU rat model were measured every 500 µm from the ON to the inferior and the superior ciliary processes. Thickness profiles along the retina were generated by averaging, for each distance, the values obtained for all eyes, as previously described [30] and values are expressed as mean ± sem. The photoreceptor ratio was calculated as the percentage of outer retinal thickness/total retinal thickness, as previously described [40].

2.9. Immunochemistry and TUNEL Assay

Immunofluorescent staining was performed on 5-µm-thick paraffin sections. Dewaxed slides were incubated with different primary antibodies: mouse anti-Glial fibrillary acid protein (GFAP, Sigma-Aldrich, St. Louis, MI, USA), rabbit anti-anti-ionized calcium-binding adapter molecule 1 (Iba1, Wako, Richmond, VA, USA), mouse anti-CD68 (Bio-Rad, Hercules, CA, USA), rabbit anti-cone arrestin (Sigma-Aldrich, St. Louis, MI, USA), and anti-serum albumin (MyBiosource, San Diego, CA, USA). Control sections were incubated without primary antibodies. The corresponding Alexa-conjugated secondary antibody (Thermo Fisher Scientific, Carlsbad, CA, USA) was used to reveal the primary antibodies. Final counterstaining with 4.6-diamidino-2-phenylindole (DAPI, Sigma-Aldrich, St. Louis, MI, USA) was performed to locate retinal structures. Slices were mounted with a Fluoromount mounting medium (Sigma Aldrich, St. Louis, MI, USA) under a lamella for microscopic examination using a fluorescence microscope with apotome module (Zeiss, Oberkochen, Germany), a fluorescence microscope with Spinning Disk (CSU-Xi, Intelligent Imaging Innovations, Denver, CO, USA), or a NanoZoomer-XR Digital slide scanner (Hamamatsu, Japan). Cone photoreceptors' quantification was done by masked counting for each retinal section of the number of cone-arrestin-positive cells in the outer nuclear layer.

The TUNEL assay was performed on 5-µm-thick paraffin sections using a commercial apoptosis detection kit (Promega, Madison, WI, USA) and following the manufacturer's instructions. Images were recorded with a NanoZoomer-XR Digital slide scanner (Hamamatsu, Japan) at 20-fold magnification and the fluorescent staining level in the whole retina was quantified using Image J software.

2.10. Retina/RPE/Choroid Flat Mounts

Following transversal sectioning of the globe, the anterior segments, lens, and vitreous were removed, and five radial cuts were made in the remaining eyecups containing retina, RPE, choroid, and sclera. Immunofluorescent staining was performed using a rabbit anti-zonula occludens-1 antibody (ZO-1, Thermo Fisher, Waltham, MA, USA) and corresponding Alexa-conjugated secondary antibody (Life Technologies, Carlsbad, CA, USA). Retina/RPE/choroid complexes were flat-mounted with a Fluoromount mounting medium (Sigma Aldrich, St. Louis, MI, USA) for microscopic examination using a Spinning Disk (CSU-Xi).

2.11. MDA Content Assay in Ocular Fluids

Quantification of malondialdehyde (MDA) in rat ocular fluids was performed using a method adapted from Giera and colleagues' publication [41]. Diluted samples underwent alkaline hydrolysis and were then neutralized in the presence of perchloric acid. Derivatization was performed using the 2-amonoacridone, as the derivative agent, in a citrate buffer solution at 40 °C. Following cooling, the MDA level was determined by HPLC. Methyl-MDA was used as standard and the lower limit of quantification was defined as 25 nM. Values were expressed as mean ± sem.

2.12. Statistical Analysis

To take into account the correlation between the 2 eyes of the same rat, a mixed linear model was used to define a treatment effect on ONL thickness and ERG parameters in the LID rat model. Statistical analyses were performed using SAS 9.4 software and differences between groups and interactions were declared significant at the 5% level of significance.

For the other parameters, statistical analyses were performed using Prism 8 software (GraphPad). Tests for normality for each group were performed using the Shapiro–Wilk test. For normal distribution, one-way ANOVA followed by Tukey's multiple comparisons test were used to define differences between groups. For non-normal distribution, the Kruskal–Wallis test followed by Dunn's multiple comparisons test were used to define differences between groups. Differences were declared significant at a 5% level of significance.

3. Results

3.1. pEYS611 Administration Allows Sustained Intraocular Production of Human Transferrin in Rats and Rabbits

Electrotransfection of pEYS611 plasmid (Figure 2A; 30 μg/eye) in the rat ciliary muscle allowed for the expression and secretion of human transferrin (TF) in ocular fluids (vitreous and aqueous humor), with an average maximal concentration of 141 ± 47 ng/mL reached within three days after the administration (Figure 2B). The protein was still measured 90 days following plasmid electrotransfection.

In rabbits, the maximal concentration of human TF in both vitreous and aqueous humor was reached within five days following pEYS611 administration at the dose of 45 μg/eye with the concentration being 5-fold higher in the vitreous than in the aqueous humor 28 days following the administration (Figure 2C; 1.6 ± 0.7 ng/mL in vitreous vs. 0.31 ± 0.2 ng/mL in aqueous humor). Six months after plasmid administration, human TF was still quantified in the vitreous of 75% of the treated eyes, allowing for a sustained expression of the protein, with an exposure and mean residence time of 184,061 pg.d.ml-1 and 58 days, respectively. Human TF was also quantified within two days in retina/RPE/choroid complex (data not shown), demonstrating that human TF produced and secreted by the ciliary muscle cells rapidly penetrated into the retina. A high TF protein concentration was observed in the retina/RPE/choroid complex 28 days following plasmid administration (Figure 2D; 3.4 ± 1.9 ng/g of tissue) and was still high at 6 months in this compartment (2.5 ± 1.3 ng/g of tissue vs. 0.7 ± 0.4 and 0.1 ± 0.1 ng/mL in vitreous and aqueous humor, respectively), demonstrating a high exposure (336,061 pg·d·g^{-1}) and long residence time (73 days) of human TF in the posterior segment of the eye.

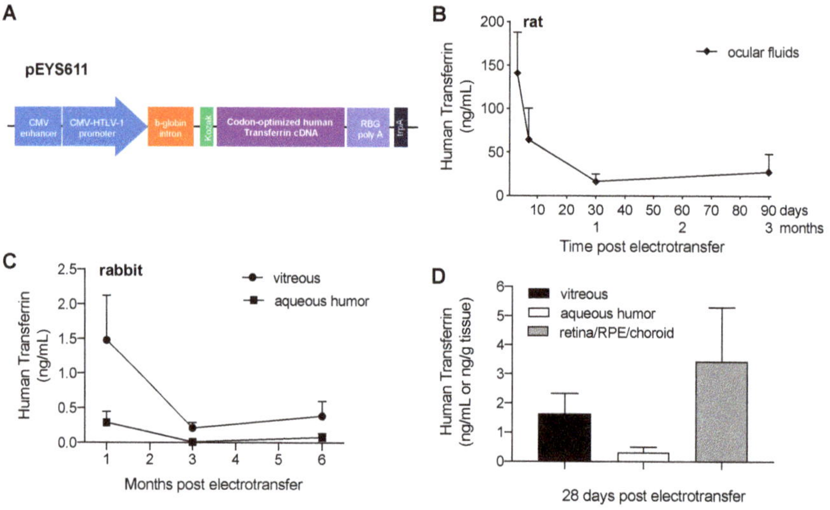

Figure 2. pEYS611-driven sustained human transferrin (TF) intraocular production in rats and rabbits. (**A**) The human TF expression cassette is composed of a human cytomegalovirus (CMV) enhancer, a chimeric CMV-HTLV (human T-cell leukemia virus)-I ubiquitous promoter, the ß-globin intron, and a Kozak sequence driving the expression of the human TF. (**B**,**C**) Human TF expression profiles in rat ocular fluids (**B**, *n* = 5–7 animals per timepoint) and rabbit aqueous humor and vitreous (**C**, *n* = 3–9 animals per timepoint) after bilateral ciliary muscle administration of pEYS611 at the doses of 30 and 45 μg/eye, respectively, demonstrated sustained expression of human TF for at least 3 and 6 months, in rat and rabbits, respectively. (**D**) Human TF distribution in rabbit eyes 28 days following pEYS611 administration demonstrated that the expressed protein reaches the back of the eye. Values are presented as mean ± sem.

3.2. *pEYS611 Preserves Photoreceptor Cells from Photo-Oxidative Damage*

We previously reported the protective effect of intravitreal injection of recombinant TF in the light-induced retinal damage (LID) rat model, a well-established model of oxidative stress-induced retinal degeneration [30]. Here, we wished to confirm the protective effect of pEYS611-driven TF delivery in this model. pEYS611 was electrotransfered at doses of 0.3, 3, or 30 µg/eye in the rat ciliary muscle three days prior the LID induction performed on day 0 (D0) to achieve maximum TF expression at the time of disease initiation. ERG and ONL thickness were measured 8 days following light exposure. As expected, light exposure resulted in an extended loss of photoreceptor cells as evidenced by a reduction of 77% to 88% of the ONL thickness in the inferior and superior poles of the retina, respectively (Figure 3A,B). Notifiable changes in the morphology of cone photoreceptors were also observed following light exposure (Figure 3D). Almost all cones had no inner and outer segments, axon, and terminal pedicle. The remaining inner and outer segments were highly shortened and disorganized. Similarly, the remaining terminal pedicles were smaller and flatter, directly abutting cone cell bodies. The number of cone photoreceptors appeared dramatically reduced in response to light compared to the non-exposed control group as demonstrated with the cone arrestin-positive cells counting (18.9 ± 7.0 vs. 179.5 ± 11.8 cone arrestin-positive cells per whole retinal section, $p = 0.0003$, Figure 3E). In accordance with morphological modifications of the photoreceptor cell layer, a dramatic deterioration of scotopic and photopic b-wave amplitudes was observed when compared to unexposed control animals (Figure 4, $p < 0.0001$). These results confirmed the induction of severe retinal degeneration after light exposure in these experimental conditions.

pEYS611 treatment at the three doses tested led to the preservation of the ONL (Figure 3A). On the inferior part of the retina, the ONL thickness of all pEYS611-treated animals was significantly thicker than that of exposed untreated control animals ($p < 0.0001$), with the average ONL thickness corresponding to about 80–90% of the average ONL thickness of unexposed control animals regardless of the tested dose (Figure 3B). A significant preservation of the ONL on the superior pole of the retina was also observed, with protective effects correlating with the pEYS611 dose and TF intraocular levels (Figure 3C). Indeed, the average ONL thickness in pEYS611-treated animals at the dose of 0.3, 3, and 30 µg/eye corresponded to 30%, 49%, and 63%, respectively, of the average ONL thickness of the unexposed control animals ($p < 0.0001$). A significant increase of the cone photoreceptor density was also observed in comparison to untreated exposed animals (90.6 ± 14.3 cone arrestin-positive cells per whole section, $p = 0.0498$; Figure 3E). Despite the shorter axon length and flatter terminal pedicle, the surviving cone photoreceptors displayed a similar morphology to those observed in the control unexposed animals, with preserved cell body sizes and preserved inner and outer segment morphologies (Figure 3D). pEYS611 treatments also led to the preservation of both the mixed rod-cone and cone-mediated ERG responses, confirming a functional beneficial effect in treated animals (Figure 4). In scotopic conditions, a- and b-wave amplitudes were significantly increased in all pEYS611-treated animals in comparison to untreated LID animals ($p < 0.05$). Thus, pEYS611 administration significantly rescued from 24% to 26% of the photoreceptor response and from 23% to 32% of the internal retinal response of a normal nonexposed retinal light response. Similarly, the photopic b-wave amplitude was significantly increased by pEYS611 treatments in comparison to untreated exposed animals ($p < 0.05$), with a preservation of 22% to 29% of a normal unexposed retinal light response. In both scotopic and photopic conditions, no functional dose–response was evidenced.

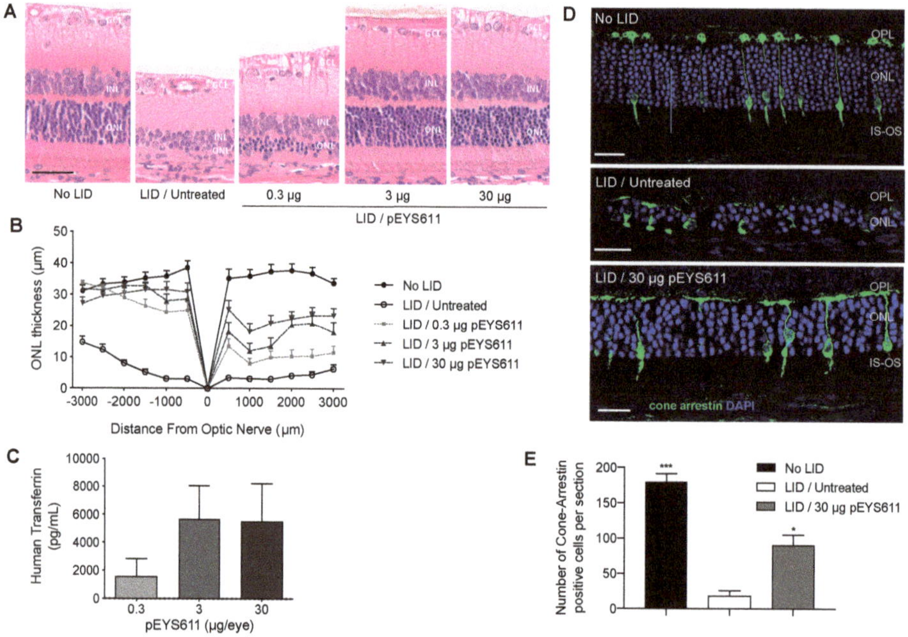

Figure 3. Dose-dependent effects of pEYS611 administration in the rat light-induced damage (LID) model. Rats received a single ciliary muscle electrotransfection of pEYS611 at the dose of 0.3, 3, or 30 µg/eye on day (-) 3 (D-3) or left untreated (n = 8 animals/group). Except for the unexposed animals (no LID), retinal degeneration was induced on D0 by 24 h of bright light exposure (6500 lux). Dark- and light-adapted electroretinography (ERG) responses were recorded simultaneously from both eyes on D8. Following ERG recordings, animals were sacrificed for analysis of human TF levels in ocular fluids and histological evaluations. (**A**) Representative images of retina section (superior pole) stained with hematoxylin eosin. Scale bar, 50 µm. (**B**) ONL thickness was measured every 500 µm from the optic nerve (0) to the inferior (−) and superior (+) poles of the retina. Compared with no LID control animals, the ONL of LID/untreated animals was thinner. Treatment with pEYS611 resulted in a dose-dependent preservation of the ONL, correlating with human TF levels measured in ocular fluids (**C**). (**D**) Representative images of cone-arrestin staining at a distance of 1500–2000 µm from the optic nerve in the superior part of the retina (4.6-diamidino-2-phenylindole (DAPI) in blue/cone arrestin in green). Scale bar, 25 µm. (**E**) The number of cone-arrestin-positive cells per retinal section was significantly higher in LID/pEYS611-treated animals compared to LID/untreated rats. All values are presented as mean ± sem. * $p < 0.05$; *** $p < 0.001$ using Dunn's multiple comparisons test versus LID/untreated group. IS, inner segment; ONL, outer nuclear layer; OPL, outer plexiform layer; OS, outer segment.

In response to light exposure, intense GFAP immunoreactive profiles were observed in astrocytes (located in the GCL) and in Müller cell processes extended through the inner nuclear layer (INL), demonstrating macroglia activation representative of the extent of retinal damage (Figure 5A, middle). In addition, light exposure led to microglial activation and migration in the outer retina and positive-CD68 macrophages' infiltration in the sub-retinal space, representative of an intense inflammatory response (Figure 5B, middle). In contrast, pEYS611 treatment reduced macroglial activation, as shown by a lower GFAP staining in treated animals (Figure 5A, right). Microglial cells' migration into the outer retina was also reduced following pEYS611 administration, and most of the IBA/CD68 labelled cells remaining properly localized in the inner retina, while infiltrated macrophages were no longer observed in the subretinal space (Figure 5B, right).

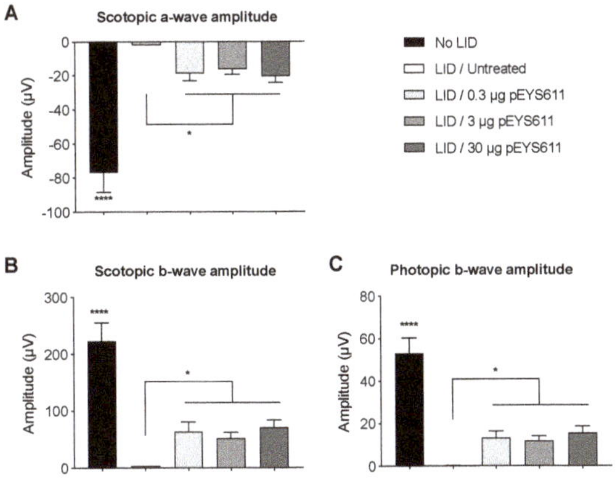

Figure 4. pEYS611 maintains retinal function in the rat LID model. Rats received a single ciliary muscle electrotransfection of pEYS611 at the dose of 0.3, 3, or 30 µg/eye on D-3 or left untreated (n = 8 animals/group). Except for unexposed animals (no LID), retinal degeneration was induced on D0 by 24 h of bright light exposure (6500 lux). Dark- and light-adapted ERG responses were recorded simultaneously from both eyes on D8. (**A**,**B**) Average amplitude (µV) of scotopic a-and b-waves from ERG responses elicited by a stimulus intensity of 3 cd·s/m^2 and (**C**) amplitude of photopic b-wave from ERG responses elicited by a stimulus intensity of 10 cd·s/m^2 are presented as mean ± sem. * $p < 0.05$; **** $p < 0.0001$ using a repeated measure mixed model and determination of confidence intervals versus LID/untreated group.

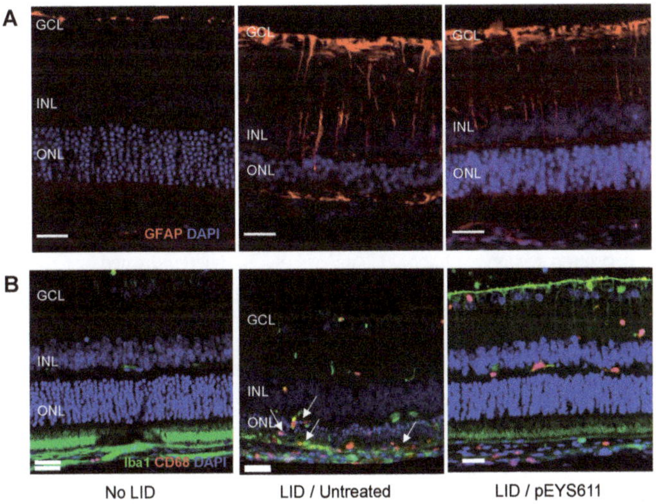

Figure 5. pEYS611 diminishes light-induced macroglia activation and microglia/macrophage retinal migration. Rat received a single ciliary muscle electrotransfection of pEYS611 (30 µg/eye) on D-3 or left untreated (n = 8 animals/group). Except for unexposed animals (no LID), retinal degeneration was induced on D0 by 24 h of bright light exposure (6500 lux). anti-Glial fibrillary acid protein (GFAP) and Iba1/CD68 staining was performed on D8. (**A**) Representative images of GFAP staining (red) in the inferior central part of the retina. (**B**) Representative images of Iba1 (green) and CD68 (red) immunostaining in the inferior central part of the retina. Arrows indicate microglial cells and macrophages accumulating in the outer retina of LID/untreated animals. Scale bar, 25 µm. GCL, ganglion cell layer; INL, inner nuclear layer; ONL, outer nuclear layer.

3.3. pEYS611 Preserves RPE Cells from Photo-Oxidative Damage

The RPE tight junctions were examined 8 days following light exposure on flat-mounted retina/RPE/choroid complexes immunostained for zonula occludens-1 (ZO-1), a tight-junction-associated protein. In untreated LID animals (Figure 6A, middle), the integrity of RPE tight junctions was lost, with a high degree of disruption in comparison to nonexposed animals (Figure 6A, left). In contrast, pEYS611 treatment preserved the RPE border structures. Almost the totality of the middle area of the RPE monolayer showed RPE with normal morphology (Figure 6A, right). Breakdown of the retinal epithelial barrier was then evaluated by albumin diffusion into the retina 8 days following light-induced retinal degeneration. Albumin diffusion in both the inferior and superior parts of the retina was significantly increased in untreated LID animals in comparison to no LID animals ($p < 0.0001$; Figure 6B,C). This result confirmed that, in our experimental conditions, light exposure alters the outer blood retinal barrier formed by tight junctions between RPE cells and allows the passage of albumin from the choroid to the retina, as previously described [42]. pEYS611 administration reduced by about 60–70% albumin diffusion into both the inferior and superior poles of the retina compared to untreated LID animals ($p < 0.0001$; Figure 6B,C).

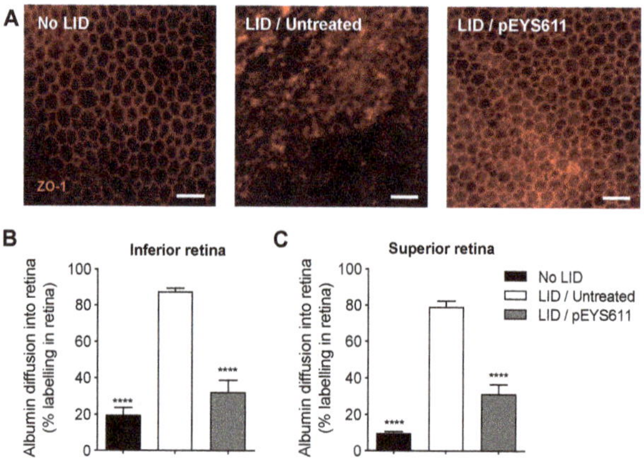

Figure 6. pEYS611 preserves the integrity of the outer BRB following light damage. Rat received a single ciliary muscle electrotransfection of pEYS611 (30 µg/eye) on D-3 or left untreated ($n = 8$ animals/group). Except for unexposed animals (no LID), retinal degeneration was induced on D0 by 24 h of bright light exposure (6500 lux). ZO-1 and albumin staining were performed on D8. (**A**) Representative images of flat-mounted retina/RPE/choroid ZO-1 staining at a distance of 1500–2000 µm from the ON. Scale bar, 50 µm. (**B**,**C**) Albumin into the retina was quantified in the inferior (**B**) and superior (**C**) poles of the retina. Percentage of albumin diffusion per retina section is presented as mean ± sem. **** $p < 0.0001$ using Tukey's multiple comparisons test versus LID/untreated group.

3.4. pEYS611 Provides Benefits over Antioxidant

The efficacy of EYS611 gene therapy was compared to the efficacy of carnosic acid (CA), an antioxidant that previously demonstrated efficacy on both retinal structure and function in the LID rat model [43]. CA (BOC Sciences, Shirley, NY, USA) was daily administered by intraperitoneal injection at the dose of 25 mg/kg/day for five days prior to light exposure as previously described [43] while pEYS611 (30 µg/eye) was electrotransfered once in the rat ciliary muscle three days prior to the light exposure. In our experimental conditions, a systemic repeated administration of CA prior to the light exposure led to significantly thicker ONL in comparison to untreated exposed animals (average ONL thickness of 9.61 ± 1.93 µm and 14.29 ± 1.89 µm, respectively; $p = 0.0012$) (Figure 7A). Nevertheless, this effect was restricted to the inferior pole of the retina. In this experiment, protective effects of pEYS611 were confirmed, with the average ONL thickness in both the inferior and superior poles of the retina being significantly higher than in CA-treated LID animals (30.66 ± 1.71 μm and 14.29 ± 1.89 μm and 21.02 ± 2.41 μm vs. 3.22 ± 0.83, respectively; $p = 0.0002$ and $p < 0.0001$), corresponding to a preservation of, respectively, 73% and 52% of the total ONL as compared to unexposed animals. In addition, about 50% of the cone photoreceptor cells were preserved in pEYS611-treated animals while preservation of cone photoreceptor cells was not observed in CA-treated animals (data not shown). In accordance with the histological results, CA treatment did not preserve ERG function while pEYS611 treatment led to a significant preservation of both scotopic and photopic b-wave amplitudes in comparison to untreated LID animals (Figure 7B).

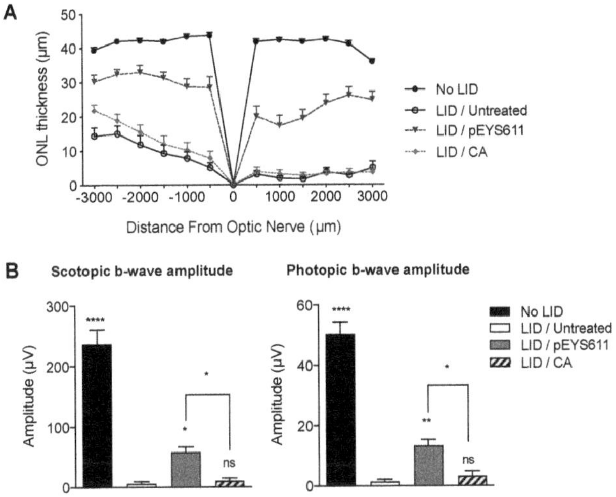

Figure 7. pEYS611 shows benefit over the antioxidant in the rat LID model. Rats received a single ciliary muscle electrotransfection of pEYS611 (30 μg/eye) on D-3 or daily administration of CA (25 mg/kg/day) from D-5 to D0 ($n = 8$ animals/group). Except for unexposed animals (no LID), retinal degeneration was induced on D0 by 24 h of bright light exposure (6500 lux). Dark- and light-adapted ERG responses were recorded simultaneously from both eyes on D8. Following ERG recordings, animals were sacrificed for histological examinations. (**A**) ONL thickness was measured every 500 μm from the optic nerve (0) to the inferior (−) and superior (+) poles of the retina, values are presented as mean ± sem. (**B**) Amplitude (μV) of b-waves from ERG responses elicited by a stimulus intensity of 3 cd·s/m^2 (left) and of 10 cd·s/m^2 (right) are presented as mean ± sem. * $p < 0.05$; ** $p < 0.01$; **** $p < 0.0001$ using repeated measure mixed model versus LID/untreated group.

3.5. *pEYS611 Preserves Photoreceptors Cell in the MNU-Induced Retinal Degeneration Rat Model*

To further confirm the effect of TF on oxidative stress-induced photoreceptor cell death, we tested the efficacy of pEYS611 treatment in the N-methyl-N-nitrosourea (MNU) intoxication model, an alkylating agent causing oxidative radical generation [44] and a rapid and specific apoptosis of photoreceptors in rats [45–47].

One week after MNU injection, retinas from untreated rats showed thinning with selective loss of the photoreceptor cells as demonstrated by the noticeable reduction of the photoreceptor ratio in comparison to non-intoxicated control animals (average photoreceptor ration 17.9 ± 0.6% vs. 44.9 ± 0.4%, respectively; Figure 8A,B). In contrast, pEYS611 (30 μg/eye) gene delivery 3 days prior to the MNU intoxication significantly inhibited MNU-induced ONL thinning and loss of photoreceptors, especially in the mid-peripheral superior retina (31.8 ± 2.0% vs. 20.5 ± 1.1%, respectively; Figure 8B). TUNEL staining indicated the presence of 15% apoptotic cells in the whole retina in MNU untreated rats compared to nonexposed animals. pEYS611 administration reduced by about 90% the TUNEL staining in the outer nuclear layer (Figure 8C,D), demonstrating that TF could protect photoreceptors from different types of oxidative stress.

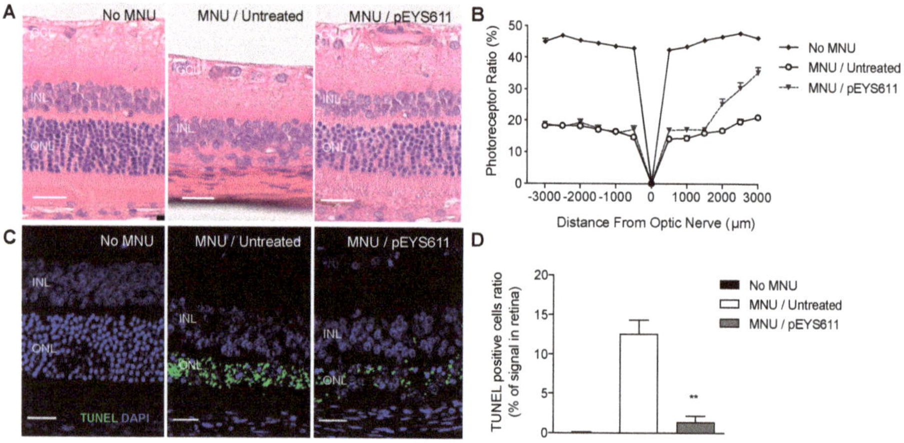

Figure 8. pEYS611 prevents photoreceptors from N-methyl-N-nitrosourea (MNU)-induced cell death in rats. Rats received bilateral ciliary muscle electrotransfection of pEYS611 at the dose 30 µg/eye on D-3 or left untreated ($n = 8$ animals/group). Except for not intoxicated rats (no MNU; $n = 3$ animals), retinal degeneration was induced by intraperitoneal injection of MNU (60 mg/kg) on D0. Histological analyses were performed on D3 and D8. (**A**) Representative images of the hematoxylin eosin-stained retinal sagittal section at D8. Images were performed at a distance of 2000–2500 µm from the optic nerve. (**B**) Outer retinal thickness and total retinal thickness were measured every 500 µm from the optic nerve (0) to the inferior (−) and superior (+) poles of the retina. The photoreceptor ratio was calculated as (outer retinal thickness/total retinal thickness) × 100. (**C**) Representative images of TUNEL staining on the retinal section (superior pole) performed on D3. (**D**) TUNEL immunostaining is presented as a percentage of the stained surface area over the entire retina. All values are presented as mean ± sem. ** $p < 0.01$ using Dunn's multiple comparisons test versus MNU/untreated group. Scale bar, 25 µm. INL, inner nuclear layer; GCL, ganglion cell layer; ONL: outer nuclear layer.

3.6. *pEYS611 Slows down Retinal Degeneration in the RCS Rat*

Finally, the efficacy of EYS611 gene therapy was evaluated on the Royal College of Surgeons (RCS) rat, a well-known model of inherited retinitis pigmentosa. In this model, mutation in the receptor tyrosine kinase gene (Mertk-/-) causes a defect in photoreceptor outer segment phagocytosis by RPE cells. The resulting accumulation of debris in the subretinal space leads to a progressive loss of photoreceptor, evidenced as early as postnatal day 18 (PND18) onward, with complete degeneration within 2 to 3 months [48–50].

pEYS611 at the dose of 25 µg/g per eye was administered to RCS rats at PND18 and its effects monitored at PND45 and PND60 in comparison to untreated RCS rats and to untreated non-dystrophic age-matched RDY control rats. As expected, an extended loss of photoreceptor cells was observed in untreated RCS animals at PND45 and PND60 as evidenced by a significant reduction of the ONL thickness as compared to RDY control animals (Figure 9A,B). At PND45, the average ONL thickness was reduced in both inferior (−47%, $p < 0.0001$) and superior (−34%, $p < 0.0001$) parts of the retina in comparison to age-matched RDY rats. At PND60, ONL degeneration progressed, with a reduction of about 70% of the average ONL thickness ($p < 0.0001$, Figure 9A,B). In contrast, pEYS611 significantly slowed the progression of the disease, compared to untreated RCS rats (Figure 9A,B). As early as 27 days post-administration (PND45), the average ONL was significantly thicker in pEYS611-treated animals than in the untreated RCS animals, both in the inferior (+30%, $p < 0.0001$) and in the superior retina (+33.7%, $p < 0.0001$). Despite the progression of the disease, the ONL thickness remained significantly thicker at PND60 in pEYS611-treated RCS animals in comparison to untreated RCS rats ($p < 0.0001$).

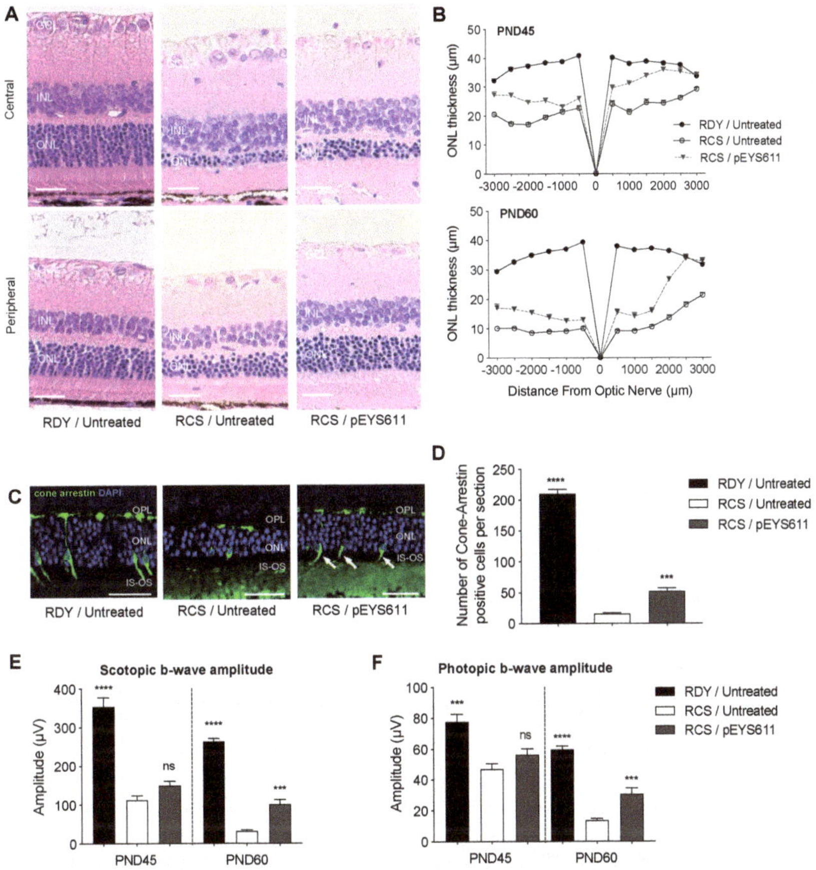

Figure 9. pEYS611 preserves retinal structure and function in RCS rats. At PND18, RCS rat received a bilateral injection and electrotransfection of pEYS611 in the ciliary muscle at the dose 25 µg/eye. Non-dystrophic RDY rats were used as the control and were left untreated. On PND45 and PND60, animals were sacrificed for histological examinations. (**A**) Representative images of hematoxylin/eosin-stained central (top) and peripheral (bottom) superior retina at PND60. (**B**) ONL thickness was measured every 500 µm from the optic nerve (0) to the inferior (−) and superior (+) poles of the retina. (**C**) Representative images of cone-arrestin staining in peripheral superior poles of the retina at PND60 (cone arrestin in green/DAPI in blue). (**D**) Number of cone-arrestin-positive cells per section in the whole retina was drastically reduced in RCS/untreated rats compared to RDY normal rats at PND60. pEYS611 treatment significantly preserved cones. *** $p < 0.001$; **** $p < 0.0001$ using Tukey's multiple comparisons test versus RCS/untreated group. (**E**,**F**) Light- and dark-adapted ERG responses were recorded simultaneously from both eyes at PND45 and PND60. Amplitude (µV) of scotopic and photopic b-waves from ERG responses elicited by a stimulus intensity of 3 cd·s/m^2 (**E**) and 10 cd·s/m^2 (**F**), respectively, are presented. *** $p < 0.001$; **** $p < 0.0001$ using the repeated measure mixed model versus RCS/untreated group. All values are presented as mean ± sem. Scale bar, 25 µm. GCL, ganglion cell layer; INL, inner nuclear layer; IS: inner segment, ONL: outer nuclear layer, OPL: outer plexiform layer, OS: outer segment.

Cone arrestin staining and positive cells quantification were performed at PND60, i.e., 42 days following pEYS611 ciliary muscle administration. Noticeable changes in the morphology of the remaining cone photoreceptors were observed in untreated RCS rats (Figure 9C). Most of the outer segments (OSs) were lost and the remaining inner segments (ISs) were swollen. Similarly, the remaining terminal pedicles were smaller and flatter, with most of them directly abutting cone cell bodies, especially in the central retina (data not shown). In addition, the total number of cone photoreceptors appeared dramatically reduced compared to non-dystrophic RDY animals (16.1 ± 1.1 vs. 210.6 ± 6.9 cone arrestin-positive cells per retinal section, $p < 0.0001$, Figure 9D). Morphological ONL preservation in the inferior and superior parts of the retina was associated with significant preservation of cone photoreceptor cells in pEYS611-treated animals (Figure 9C, right panel), with more than 3 times as many cells than in the untreated RCS group (52 1 ± 5.1 vs. 16.1 ± 1.1 cone arrestin-positive cells per retinal section, $p = 0.0002$, Figure 9D). In addition, preservation of the cell body was associated with the preservation of axons (despite shorter length) and outer segments (especially in the peripheral retina).

The extended loss of photoreceptor cells in untreated RCS animals was related to a significant progressive decrease of a-wave (data not shown) and b-wave amplitudes (Figure 9E,F) from both dark- and light-adapted ERG as compared to non-dystrophic age-matched RDY rats ($p < 0.0001$). Scotopic and photopic implicit times (regardless of the waves) were also increased by disease progression (data not shown), confirming the alteration of rod- and cone-mediated retinal function in RCS rats. pEYS611 treatment led to the preservation of both the mixed rod-cone response and cone-mediated response as demonstrated by significant higher scotopic and photopic ERG b-wave amplitudes at PND60 in comparison to untreated RCS animals ($p < 0.001$).

Finally, we looked for surrogate markers of pEYS611 biological activity in ocular fluids of RCS rats and measured the content in malondialdehyde (MDA), a common marker of lipid peroxidation that accumulates in many pathological conditions [51,52]. Ocular fluids from untreated RCS rats had a significant elevation in the mean MDA content compared to ocular fluids from RDY control animals at PND45 (62.7 ± 8.3 μM vs. 34.0 ± 3.4 μM, $p = 0.0093$). Interestingly pEYS611-treated RCS rats demonstrated a reduction in MDA content in ocular fluids when compared to untreated RCS rats (40.7 ± 11.3 μM), corresponding to a 35% reduction.

4. Discussion and Conclusions

Non-viral gene delivery of TF using ciliary muscle electrotransfection allows for the sustained intraocular production of human TF in both rats and rabbits. Though the produced protein is not 100% homologous to the animal species (73% and 79% for rat and rabbit TF, respectively), no sign of immune response or inflammation was observed, confirming the good safety profile of human TF as previously reported after repeated IVT injections in rat [30]. Not only human TF was measured in the vitreous for at least 3 and 6 months in rats and rabbits after one single electrotransfection, but pEYS611 showed protective effects in the long term in the RCS rat (up to 42 days after electrotransfection), demonstrating that human TF remains biologically active. In addition, the expressed TF protein widely distributed in all compartments of the eye and concentrated in the outer retina, allowing significant preservation of the retina in different models of retinal degeneration. Similar observations have been made following ciliary muscle electrotransfection of plasmids coding for other proteins, such as anti-TNF in animal models of uveitis [34,53], anti-VEGF in a rat model of choroidal neovascularization [54], and neurotrophic factors in rat models of retinal dystrophies [55], confirming that plasmid electrotransfection into the ciliary muscle is a valuable approach to deliver any therapeutic proteins to the retina.

To gain confidence in the therapeutic potential of TF non-viral gene therapy for the treatment of retinal degeneration and because no animal models fully replicate human conditions, the effect of pEYS611 treatment has been evaluated in several induced and inherited models of retinal degeneration. The light damage in rats is a well-established model of retinal degeneration inducing photoreceptor-specific cell death, breakdown of the blood–retina barrier, oxidative stress, inflammation, and subsequent loss of functional vision [56,57], recapitulating some of the hallmarks of dry AMD and

RP [58–60]. We and others also reported modification of iron metabolism and iron overload in the injured outer retina following light damage [29,30,61], making this model a relevant model to evaluate the pharmacodynamics effects of pEYS611. Indeed, we previously showed that intravitreal injection of a high dose of human TF was efficient to rescue photoreceptors from light-induced cell death, with morphological and functional preservation being associated with reduced iron overload and decreased oxidative stress-induced heme oxygenase expression [30]. Here, TF non-viral gene therapy similarly and very consistently protected the inferior outer retina from LID even when delivered at a very low dose while higher TF protein concentrations were required to fully preserve the superior retina. This regional effect of pEYS611 is in agreement with a previous observation reporting higher susceptibility of the superior retina to light damage [62]. Increasing the plasmid dose from 0.3 to 3 or 30 μg/eye induced an increase in human TF vitreous levels, with no statistically significant difference between 3 or 30 μg, suggesting that in the rat eye, other strategies could be used to reach higher protein levels, such as repeated administrations in other muscle quadrants [33,36]. Although a clear morphologic dose–response effect was observed between 0.3 and 3 μg of pEYS611, with a higher number of cones protected, no significant change was noted with increasing the dose from 3 to 30 μg/eye, which correlates with TF levels. Interestingly, at a functional level, a similar improvement in the retinal light response was measured with either the lowest or the highest dose of plasmid, suggesting that even a very low dose of TF might be sufficient to neutralize iron excess and subsequent cell death. Although cones were better preserved with the high dose of pEYS611, some cones still presented morphological abnormalities and might be not functional, possibly explaining the apparent discrepancy between the morphological and functional results. Interestingly, at the highest dose of plasmid used, TF not only protected photoreceptors from cell death but also prevented the RPE barrier breakdown, as witnessed by reduced albumin leakage, preserved RPE structure, and reduced retinal inflammation. The anti-inflammatory properties of TF have already been shown in the ischemic brain [63], but the protective role of TF on the RPE barrier had not been evidenced previously, confirming that TF might have additional non-iron-mediated effects as shown by transcriptomic analysis of TF effects in a retinal detachment model [6]. The superiority of TF over CA, a well-known antioxidant, is in line with this observation. In our hands, the protection achieved with CA was less prominent compared to previously published results [43]. This discrepancy might be explained by the more drastic light damage conditions used in our study, i.e., 24-h exposure at 6500 lux versus 5-h exposure at 5000 lux in Rezaie and colleagues' study [43]. In line with the neuroprotective properties of TF, pEYS611 at 30μg/eye significantly reduced photoreceptor apoptosis induced by MNU with an efficacy comparable to that reported following administration of caspase 3 or calpain inhibitors [40,64]. Here again, a regional protective effect of pEYS611 was observed in line with the less pronounced toxicity of MNU in both the peripheral and superior retina [39]. Taken together, our results and others support broader neuroprotective functions of TF beyond its iron chelation activity.

These results are of great therapeutic importance for the treatment of retinal degenerative disorders with still unmet needs. Beyond gene mutation, accumulating evidence suggests that oxidative stress is a key contributor to cone degeneration in RP [65–67]. Gene replacement using viral gene therapy is only possible for a very limited number of genotyped RP patients, leaving most patients without any therapeutic options. Here, we first report the benefit of TF in the RCS rat model of RP, which presents spontaneous retinal degeneration due to a mutation in the Mertk gene [49,68], and sharing many similarities with autosomal recessive RP (arRP) caused by mutations in MERTK in humans. When administered at disease onset, pEYS611 significantly delayed retinal degeneration and vision loss. Interestingly, the benefit observed following pEYS611 treatment was in the same range to that reported following subretinal injection of viral vectors aiming at correcting the Mertk gene and administered at much earlier timepoints [69,70], reinforcing the neuroprotective potential of such a non-viral gene therapy approach for RP patients. The benefit of TF is also not specific of a particular RP mutation or gene. Indeed, we previously reported the benefit of TF in rd10 mice, a murine model of inherited RP due to the mutation of the Pde6b gene [19] and in P23H rats, carrying a mutation of the Rho gene [30]. Taken together, these results strongly support further development of pEYS611 gene therapy to slow down photoreceptor degeneration and to preserve visual performances in all RP patients regardless of their underlying genetic defect. While RP is most often characterized by a slowly degenerative process complicating the clinical evaluation of a new drug candidate, we identified the aqueous humor MDA level as a potential surrogate biomarker of the activity of TF. Whether the MDA content in aqueous humor of RP patients is increased remains to be demonstrated. In a very limited cohort of RP patients, Campochiaro and colleagues did not observe any changes in the MDA content both in aqueous humor and in serum [67] while they showed a significant reduction in the reduced to oxidized glutathione (GSH/GSSG) ratio in aqueous humor and a significant increase in the aqueous protein carbonyl content. The authors suggested that most lipids are too hydrophobic to enter into the aqueous humor, but our results in RCS rats, using another method to detect MDA, suggest otherwise. Indeed, whilst most MDA assays are based on its derivatization with thiobarbituric (TBA) [71], a more accurate and sensitive method based on selective derivatization with 2-aminoacridone (2-AA) combined with HPLC detection was used herein (Daruich et al., 2020, Molecular Vision In press). This method, initially optimized for the measurement of free and protein-bound MDA in human tears, might be a valuable tool to (re)investigate the MDA content in aqueous humor and/or vitreous of RP patients.

Beyond RP, pEYS611 gene therapy approach targeting iron-mediated ocular oxidative stress has a strong upside potential for the treatment of more frequent invalidating retinal degenerative diseases, such as dry AMD, a leading cause of blindness for which there is still no treatment option. The causal link between AMD pathogenicity and iron overload remains to be established, but some evidence is provided supporting that iron homeostasis dysregulation is associated with AMD [72]. Retinal iron levels increase with age [73], AMD-affected maculae have increased iron especially in the RPE and Bruch's membrane compared to healthy age-matched controls [10,12], and iron levels in aqueous humor were increased by more than two-fold in patients with dry AMD [13]. An upregulation by about 2-fold of both TF transcript and protein is also described in AMD patients [14]. Melanin usually buffers the iron content and preserves the RPE and the choroid from a pro-oxidant environment. However, its content in RPE decreases with age while iron accumulates in melanosomes, leading to the formation of free radicals in aging retinas [74]. In addition to the obvious potential of iron chelation to protect photoreceptors cells, prevention of the deleterious effects of iron-induced damages on the blood–retina barrier is another interest of TF non-viral gene therapy to treat AMD since the degeneration of the RPE cells is closely related to the pathogenesis of non-exudative AMD. Aforementioned, pEYS611 administration preserves the integrity of the outer blood retinal barrier formed by tight junctions between RPE cells, reducing the diffusion of albumin from the choroid to the retina.

In conclusion, pEYS611 appears as a promising approach for the treatment of retinal degeneration. By combining a non-viral gene therapy and a safe delivery approach, electrotransfection of plasmids into the ciliary muscle provides huge advantages over current viral vectors in development for RP or other retinal degeneration: (i) The administration procedure is minimally invasive and does not require subretinal surgery, thus allowing intervention at an earlier stage of the disease with no risk of retinal injury; (ii) the lack of immunogenicity of plasmid DNA allows for re-dosing; and (iii) this delivery approach allows for a fine-tuning of the expressed therapeutic protein by modulating the plasmid dose and/or the surface of transfected muscle [36], offering the possibility to adapt the treatment to the patient's disease progression. Finally, plasmid DNA have no limited cargo capacity, offering the possibility to deliver almost any therapeutic proteins or even to combine therapeutic proteins on the same plasmid to address multiple pathogenic pathways.

Author Contributions: Conceptualization, E.P. and F.B.-C.; Methodology, K.B. and E.P.; Validation, K.B.; Formal Analysis, K.B.; Investigation, P.G., R.B., P.M., J.Y. and M.P.; Data Curation, P.G. and R.B.; Writing—Original Draft Preparation, K.B. and T.B.; Writing—Review and Editing, K.B., T.B., E.P., and F.B.-C.; Visualization, K.B.; Supervision, K.B., T.B., and F.B.-C.; Project Administration, K.B., P.G., and R.B. All authors have read and agreed to the published version of the manuscript.

Funding: This research received no external funding.

Acknowledgments: Authors sincerely thank Eyevensys's team for support and helpful discussions, Thomas Hohman for critical review of the program, Maëva Dupuis-Deniaud (MDSAT consulting) for statistical analysis, Firas Bassissi for pharmacokintetics analysis, Jean-Jacques Sauvain (Unisanté, Centre universitaire de médecine générale et santé publique, Lausanne, Switzerland) for the development of the MDA method, and Aurélien Thomas and Gregory Plateel (Unité de Toxicologie et Chimie Forensiques, Lausanne, Switzerland) for assistance with MDA quantification in ocular fluids.

Conflicts of Interest: K.B., P.G., R.B., P.M., M.P., J.Y., and T.B. are employees of Eyevensys. K.B., P.G., R.B., and T.B. hold grants of Eyevensys stock. F.B.-C. is founder and shareholder of Eyevensys. E.P. and F.B.-C. have issued and pending patents claiming for the use of transferrin for the treatment of retinal disorders. The other co-authors have no conflict.

References

1. Song, D.; Dunaief, J.L. Retinal iron homeostasis in health and disease. *Front. Aging Neurosci.* **2013**, *5*, 1–13. [CrossRef]
2. Picard, E.; Daruich, A.; Youale, J.; Courtois, Y.; Behar-Cohen, F. From Rust to Quantum Biology: The Role of Iron in Retina Physiopathology. *Cells* **2020**, *9*, 705. [CrossRef]
3. Rogers, B.S.; Symons, R.C.A.; Komeima, K.; Shen, J.K.; Xiao, W.; Swaim, M.E.; Yuan, Y.G.; Kachi, S.; Campochiaro, P.A. Differential sensitivity of cones to iron-mediated oxidative damage. *Investig. Opthalmol. Vis. Sci.* **2007**, *48*, 438–445. [CrossRef]
4. Dixon, S.J.; Lemberg, K.M.; Lamprecht, M.R.; Skouta, R.; Zaitsev, E.M.; Gleason, C.E.; Patel, D.N.; Bauer, A.J.; Cantley, A.M.; Yang, W.S.; et al. Ferroptosis: An iron-dependent form of nonapoptotic cell death. *Cell* **2012**, *149*, 1060–1072. [CrossRef]
5. Chaudhary, K.; Promsote, W.; Ananth, S.; Veeranan-Karmegam, R.; Tawfik, A.; Arjunan, P.; Martin, P.; Smith, S.B.; Thangaraju, M.; Kisselev, O.; et al. Iron Overload Accelerates the Progression of Diabetic Retinopathy in Association with Increased Retinal Renin Expression. *Sci. Rep.* **2018**, *8*, 1–12. [CrossRef]
6. Daruich, A.; Le Rouzic, Q.; Jonet, L.; Naud, M.C.; Kowalczuk, L.; Pournaras, J.A.; Boatright, J.H.; Thomas, A.; Turck, N.; Moulin, A.; et al. Iron is neurotoxic in retinal detachment and transferrin confers neuroprotection. *Sci. Adv.* **2019**, *5*, eaau9940. [CrossRef]
7. Akeo, K.; Hiramitsu, T.; Yorifuji, H.; Okisaka, S. Membranes of retinal pigment epithelial cells in vitro are damaged in the phagocytotic process of the photoreceptor outer segment discs peroxidized by ferrous ions. *Pigment Cell Res.* **2002**, *15*, 341–347. [CrossRef]
8. Chen, H.; Lukas, T.J.; Du, N.; Suyeoka, G.; Neufeld, A.H. Dysfunction of the retinal pigment epithelium with age: Increased iron decreases phagocytosis and lysosomal activity. *Investig. Opthalmol. Vis. Sci.* **2009**, *50*, 1895–1902. [CrossRef]
9. Shu, W.; Baumann, B.H.; Song, Y.; Liu, Y.; Wu, X.; Dunaief, J.L. Ferrous but not ferric iron sulfate kills photoreceptors and induces photoreceptor-dependent RPE autofluorescence. *Redox Biol.* **2020**, *34*, 101469. [CrossRef]
10. Hahn, P.; Milam, A.H.; Dunaief, J.L. Maculas Affected by Age-Related Macular Degeneration Contain Increased Chelatable Iron in the Retinal Pigment Epithelium and Bruch's Membrane. *Arch. Opthalmol.* **2003**, *121*, 1099–1105. [CrossRef]
11. Dentchev, T.; Hahn, P.; Dunaief, J.L. Strong labeling for iron and the iron-handling proteins ferritin and ferroportin in the photoreceptor layer in age-related macular degenerationNo Title. *Arch. Opthalmol.* **2005**, *123*, 1745–1746. [CrossRef]
12. Biesemeier, A.; Yoeruek, E.; Eibl, O.; Schraermeyer, U. Iron accumulation in Bruch's membrane and melanosomes of donor eyes with age-related macular degeneration. *Exp. Eye Res.* **2015**, *137*, 39–49. [CrossRef]
13. Jünemann, A.; Stopa, P.; Michalke, B.; Chaudhri, A.; Reulbach, U.; Huchzermeyer, C.; Schlötzer-Schrehardt, U.; Kruse, F.E.; Zrenner, E.; Rejdak, R. Levels of Aqueous Humor Trace Elements in Patients with Non-Exsudative Age-related Macular Degeneration: A Case-control Study. *PLoS ONE* **2013**, *8*, e56734. [CrossRef]
14. Chowers, I.; Wong, R.; Dentchev, T.; Farkas, R.H.; Iacovelli, J.; Gunatilaka, T.L.; Medeiros, N.E.; Presley, J.B.; Campochiaro, P.A.; Curcio, C.A.; et al. The iron carrier transferrin is upregulated in retinas from patients with age-related macular degeneration. *Investig. Opthalmol. Vis. Sci.* **2006**, *47*, 2135–2140. [CrossRef]

15. Wysokinski, D.; Danisz, K.; Pawlowska, E.; Dorecka, M.; Romaniuk, D.; Robaszkiewicz, J.; Szaflik, M.; Szaflik, J.; Blasiak, J.; Szaflik, J.P. Transferrin receptor levels and polymorphism of its gene in age-related macular degeneration. *Acta Biochim. Pol.* **2015**, *62*, 177–184. [CrossRef]
16. Synowiec, E.; Pogorzelska, M.; Blasiak, J.; Szaflik, J.; Szaflik, J.P. Genetic polymorphism of the iron-regulatory protein-1 and-2 genes in age-related macular degeneration. *Mol. Biol. Rep.* **2012**, *39*, 7077–7087. [CrossRef]
17. Synowiec, E.; Szaflik, J.; Chmielewska, M.; Wozniak, K.; Sklodowska, A.; Waszczyk, M.; Dorecka, M.; Blasiak, J.; Szaflik, J.P. An association between polymorphism of the heme oxygenase-1 and-2 genes and age-related macular degeneration. *Mol. Biol. Rep.* **2012**, *39*, 2081–2087. [CrossRef]
18. Yefimova, M.G.; Jeanny, J.C.; Keller, N.; Sergeant, C.; Guillonneau, X.; Beaumont, C.; Courtois, Y. Impaired retinal iron homeostasis associated with defective phagocytosis in Royal College of surgeons rats. *Investig. Opthalmol. Vis. Sci.* **2002**, *43*, 537–545.
19. Picard, E.; Jonet, L.; Sergeant, C.; Vesvres, M.H.; Behar-Cohen, F.; Courtois, Y.; Jeanny, J.C. Overexpressed or intraperitoneally injected human transferrin prevents photoreceptor degeneration in rd10 mice. *Mol. Vis.* **2010**, *16*, 2612–2625.
20. Deleon, E.; Lederman, M.; Berenstein, E.; Meir, T.; Chevion, M.; Chowers, I. Alteration in iron metabolism during retinal degeneration in rd10 mouse. *Investig. Opthalmol. Vis. Sci.* **2009**, *50*, 1360–1365. [CrossRef]
21. Rajadhyaksha, A.M.; Elemento, O.; Puffenberger, E.G.; Schierberl, K.C.; Xiang, J.Z.; Putorti, M.L.; Berciano, J.; Poulin, C.; Brais, B.; Michaelides, M.; et al. Mutations in FLVCR1 cause posterior column ataxia and retinitis pigmentosa. *Am. J. Hum. Genet.* **2010**, *87*, 643–654. [CrossRef]
22. Hadziahmetovic, M.; Song, Y.; Wolkow, N.; Iacovelli, J.; Grieco, S.; Lee, J.; Lyubarsky, A.; Pratico, D.; Connelly, J.; Spino, M.; et al. The oral iron chelator deferiprone protects against iron overload-induced retinal degeneration. *Investig. Opthalmol. Vis. Sci.* **2011**, *52*, 959–968. [CrossRef]
23. Zhao, L.; Wang, C.; Song, D.; Li, Y.; Song, Y.; Su, G.; Dunaief, J.L. Systemic administration of the antioxidant/iron chelator α-lipoic acid protects against light-induced photoreceptor degeneration in the mouse retina. *Investig. Opthalmol. Vis. Sci.* **2014**, *55*, 5979–5988. [CrossRef]
24. Obolensky, A.; Berenshtein, E.; Lederman, M.; Bulvik, B.; Alper-Pinus, R.; Yaul, R.; Deleon, E.; Chowers, I.; Chevion, M.; Banin, E. Zinc-desferrioxamine attenuates retinal degeneration in the rd10 mouse model of retinitis pigmentosa. *Free Radic. Biol. Med.* **2011**, *51*, 1482–1491. [CrossRef]
25. Hadziahmetovic, M.; Pajic, M.; Grieco, S.; Song, Y.; Song, D.; Li, Y.; Cwanger, A.; Iacovelli, J.; Chu, S.; Ying, G.; et al. The Oral Iron Chelator Deferiprone Protects Against Retinal Degeneration Induced through Diverse Mechanisms. *Transl. Vis. Sci. Technol.* **2012**, *1*, 2. [CrossRef]
26. Wang, K.; Peng, B.; Xiao, J.; Weinreb, O.; Youdim, M.B.H.; Lin, B. Iron-chelating drugs enhance cone photoreceptor survival in a mouse model of retinitis pigmentosa. *Investig. Opthalmol. Vis. Sci.* **2017**, *58*, 5287–5297. [CrossRef]
27. Lakhanpal, V.; Schocket, S.; Jiji, R. Deferoxamine (Desferal)-induced toxic retinal pigmentary degeneration and presumed optic neuropathyitle. *Opthalmology* **1984**, *91*, 443–452. [CrossRef]
28. Picard, E.; Fontaine, I.; Jonet, L.; Guillou, F.; Behar-Cohen, F.; Courtois, Y.; Jeanny, J.C. The protective role of transferrin in Müller glial cells after iron-induced toxicity. *Mol. Vis.* **2008**, *14*, 928–941.
29. Picard, E.; Ranchon-Cole, I.; Jonet, L.; Beaumont, C.; Behar-Cohen, F.; Courtois, Y.; Jeanny, J.C. Light-induced retinal degeneration correlates with changes in iron metabolism gene expression, ferritin level, and aging. *Investig. Opthalmol. Vis. Sci.* **2011**, *52*, 1261–1274. [CrossRef]
30. Picard, E.; Le Rouzic, Q.; Oudar, A.; Berdugo, M.; El Sanharawi, M.; Andrieu-Soler, C.; Naud, M.-C.; Jonet, L.; Latour, C.; Klein, C.; et al. Targeting iron-mediated retinal degeneration by local delivery of transferrin. *Free Radic. Biol. Med.* **2015**, *89*, 1105–1121. [CrossRef]
31. Hawkins, K.N. Contribution of plasma proteins to the vitreous of the rat. *Curr. Eye Res.* **1986**, *5*, 655–663. [CrossRef]
32. Bloquel, C.; Bejjani, R.A.; Bigey, P.; Bedioui, F.; Doat, M.; BenEzra, D.; Scherman, D.; Behar-Cohen, F. Plasmid electrotransfer of eye ciliary muscle: Principles and therapeutic efficacy using hTNF-α soluble receptor in uveitis. *FASEB J.* **2006**, *20*, 389–391. [CrossRef]
33. El Sanharawi, M.; Kowalczuk, L.; Touchard, E.; Omri, S.; de Kozak, Y.; Behar-Cohen, F. Protein delivery for retinal diseases: From basic considerations to clinical applications. *Prog. Retin. Eye Res.* **2010**, *29*, 443–465. [CrossRef]

34. Touchard, E.; Benard, R.; Bigot, K.; Laffitte, J.-D.; Buggage, R.; Bordet, T.; Behar-Cohen, F. Non-viral ocular gene therapy, pEYS606, for the treatment of non-infectious uveitis: Preclinical evaluation of the medicinal product. *J. Control. Release* **2018**, *285*, 244–251. [CrossRef]
35. Bordet, T.; Behar-Cohen, F. Ocular gene therapies in clinical practice: Viral vectors and nonviral alternatives. *Drug Discov. Today* **2019**, *24*, 1685–1693. [CrossRef]
36. Touchard, E.; Kowalczuk, L.; Bloquel, C.; Naud, M.-C.; Bigey, P.; Behar-Cohen, F. The ciliary smooth muscle electrotransfer: Basic principles and potential for sustained intraocular production of therapeutic proteins. *J. Gene Med.* **2010**, *12*, 904–919. [CrossRef]
37. Luke, J.M.; Vincent, J.M.; Du, S.X.; Gerdemann, U.; Leen, A.M.; Whalen, R.G.; Hodgson, C.P.; Williams, J.A. Improved antibiotic-free plasmid vector design by incorporation of transient expression enhancers. *Gene Ther.* **2011**, *18*, 334–343. [CrossRef]
38. Luke, J.M.; Carnes, A.E.; Williams, J.A. Development of Antibiotic-Free Selection System for Safer DNA Vaccination. *DNA Vaccines* **2014**, *1143*, 91–111.
39. Tao, Y.; Chen, T.; Fang, W.; Peng, G.; Wang, L.; Qin, L.; Liu, B.; Huang, Y.F. The temporal topography of the N-Methyl- N-nitrosourea induced photoreceptor degeneration in mouse retina. *Sci. Rep.* **2015**, *5*, 1–14. [CrossRef]
40. Yoshizawa, K.; Yang, J.; Senzaki, H.; Uemura, Y.; Kiyozuka, Y.; Shikata, N.; Oishi, Y.; Miki, H.; Tsubura, A. Caspase-3 inhibitor rescues *N*-methyl-*N*-nitrosourea-induced retinal degeneration in Sprague-Dawley rats. *Exp. Eye Res.* **2000**, *71*, 629–635. [CrossRef]
41. Giera, M.; Kloos, D.-P.; Raaphhorst, A.; Mayboroda, O.A.; Deelder, A.M.; Lingerman, H.; Niessen, W.M. Mild and selective labeling of malondialdehyde with 2-aminoacridone: Assessment of urinary malondialdehyde levels. *Analyst* **2011**, *136*, 2763–2769. [CrossRef]
42. Krigel, A.; Berdugo, M.; Picard, E.; Levy-Boukris, R.; Jaadane, I.; Jonet, L.; Dernigoghossian, M.; Andrieu-Soler, C.; Torriglia, A.; Behar-Cohen, F. Light-induced retinal damage using different light sources, protocols and rat strains reveals LED phototoxicity. *Neuroscience* **2016**, *339*, 296–307. [CrossRef]
43. Rezaie, T.; McKercher, S.R.; Kosaka, K.; Seki, M.; Wheeler, L.; Viswanath, V.; Chun, T.; Joshi, R.; Valencia, M.; Sasaki, S.; et al. Protective effect of carnosic acid, a pro-electrophilic compound, in models of oxidative stress and light-induced retinal degeneration. *Investig. Opthalmol. Vis. Sci.* **2012**, *53*, 7847–7854. [CrossRef]
44. Tsuruma, K.; Yamauchi, M.; Inokuchi, Y.; Sugitani, S.; Shimazawa, M.; Hara, H. Role of oxidative stress in retinal photoreceptor cell death in N-methyl-N-nitrosourea-treated mice. *J. Pharmacol. Sci.* **2012**, *118*, 351–362. [CrossRef]
45. Nakajima, M.; Yuge, K.; Senzaki, H.; Shikata, N.; Miki, H.; Uyama, M.; Tsubura, A. Photoreceptor apoptosis induced by a single systemic administration of N-methyl-N-nitrosourea in the rat retina. *Am. J. Pathol.* **1996**, *148*, 631–641.
46. Nakajima, M.; Nambu, H.; Shikata, N.; Senzaki, H.; Miki, H.; Tsubura, A. Pigmentary degeneration induced by N-met hyl-N-nitrosourea and the fate of pigment epithelial cells in the rat retina. *Pathol. Int.* **1996**, *46*, 874–882. [CrossRef]
47. Yoshizawa, K.; Nambu, H.; Yang, J.; Oishi, Y.; Senzaki, H.; Shikata, N.; Miki, H.; Tsubura, A. Mechanisms of photoreceptor cell apoptosis induced by N-methyl-N-nitrosourea in Sprague-Dawley rats. *Lab. Investig.* **1999**, *79*, 1359–1367.
48. Mullen, R.J.; LaVail, M.M. Inherited retinal dystrophy: Primary defect in pigment epithelium determined with experimental rat chimeras. *Science* **1976**, *192*, 799–801. [CrossRef]
49. Nandrot, E.; Dufour, E.M.; Provost, A.C.; Péquignot, M.O.; Bonnel, S.; Gogat, K.; Marchant, D.; Rouillac, C.; De Condé, B.S.; Bihoreau, M.T.; et al. Homozygous deletion in the coding sequence of the c-mer gene in RCS rats unravels general mechanisms of physiological cell adhesion and apoptosis. *Neurobiol. Dis.* **2000**, *7*, 586–599. [CrossRef]
50. Di Pierdomenico, J.; García-Ayuso, D.; Pinilla, I.; Cuenca, N.; Vidal-Sanz, M.; Agudo-Barriuso, M.; Villegas-Pérez, M.P. Early events in retinal degeneration caused by rhodopsin mutation or pigment epithelium malfunction: Differences and similarities. *Front. Neuroanat.* **2017**, *11*, 14. [CrossRef]
51. Barrera, G.; Pizzimenti, S.; Daga, M.; Dianzani, C.; Arcaro, A.; Cetrangolo, G.P.; Giordano, G.; Cucci, M.A.; Graf, M.; Gentile, F. Lipid peroxidation-derived aldehydes, 4-hydroxynonenal and malondialdehyde in aging-related disorders. *Antioxidants* **2018**, *7*, 102. [CrossRef]

52. Del Rio, D.; Stewart, A.J.; Pellegrini, N. A review of recent studies on malondialdehyde as toxic molecule and biological marker of oxidative stress. *Nutr. Metab. Cardiovasc. Dis.* **2005**, *15*, 316–328. [CrossRef]
53. Kowalczuk, L.; Touchard, E.; Camelo, S.; Naud, M.C.; Castaneda, B.; Brunel, N.; Besson-Lescure, B.; Thillaye-Goldenberg, B.; Bigey, P.; BenEzra, D.; et al. Local ocular immunomodulation resulting from electrotransfer of plasmid encoding soluble TNF receptors in the ciliary muscle. *Investig. Opthalmol. Vis. Sci.* **2009**, *50*, 1761–1768. [CrossRef]
54. El Sanharawi, M.; Touchard, E.; Benard, R.; Bigey, P.; Escriou, V.; Mehanna, C.; Naud, M.C.; Berdugo, M.; Jeanny, J.C.; Behar-Cohen, F. Long-term efficacy of ciliary muscle gene transfer of three sFlt-1 variants in a rat model of laser-induced choroidal neovascularization. *Gene Ther.* **2013**, *20*, 1093–1103. [CrossRef]
55. Touchard, E.; Heiduschka, P.; Berdugo, M.; Kowalczuk, L.; Bigey, P.; Chahory, S.; Gandolphe, C.; Jeanny, J.C.; Behar-Cohen, F. Non-viral gene therapy for GDNF production in RCS rat: The crucial role of the plasmid dose. *Gene Ther.* **2012**, *19*, 886–898. [CrossRef]
56. Noell, W.K.; Walker, V.S.; Kang, B.S.; Berman, S. Retinal damage by light in rats. *Investig. Opthalmol.* **1966**, *5*, 450–473.
57. Chen, L.; Wu, W.; Dentchev, T.; Zeng, Y.; Wang, J.; Tsui, I.; Tobias, J.W.; Bennett, J.; Baldwin, D.; Dunaief, J.L. Light damage induced changes in mouse retinal gene expression. *Exp. Eye Res.* **2004**, *79*, 239–247. [CrossRef]
58. Wenzel, A.; Grimm, C.; Samardzija, M.; Remé, C.E. Molecular mechanisms of light-induced photoreceptor apoptosis and neuroprotection for retinal degeneration. *Prog. Retin. Eye Res.* **2005**, *24*, 275–306. [CrossRef]
59. Shen, J.; Yang, X.; Dong, A.; Petters, R.M.; Peng, Y.W.; Wong, F.; Campochiaro, P.A. Oxidative damage is a potential cause of cone cell death in retinitis pigmentosa. *J. Cell. Physiol.* **2005**, *203*, 457–464. [CrossRef]
60. Marc, R.E.; Jones, B.W.; Watt, C.B.; Vazquez-Chona, F.; Vaughan, D.K.; Organisciak, D.T. Extreme retinal remodeling triggered by light damage: Implications for age related macular degeneration. *Mol. Vis.* **2008**, *14*, 782–806.
61. Hadziahmetovic, M.; Kumar, U.; Song, Y.; Grieco, S.; Song, D.; Li, Y.; Tobias, J.W.; Dunaief, J.L. Microarray analysis of murine retinal light damage reveals changes in iron regulatory, complement, and antioxidant genes in the neurosensory retina and isolated RPE. *Investig. Opthalmol. Vis. Sci.* **2012**, *53*, 5231–5241. [CrossRef]
62. Tanito, M.; Kaidzu, S.; Ohira, A.; Anderson, R.E. Topography of retinal damage in light-exposed albino rats. *Exp. Eye Res.* **2008**, *87*, 292–295. [CrossRef]
63. Guardia Clausi, M.; Paez, P.M.; Pasquini, L.A.; Pasquini, J.M. Inhalation of growth factors and apo-transferrin to protect and repair the hypoxic-ischemic brain. *Pharmacol. Res.* **2016**, *109*, 81–85. [CrossRef]
64. Kuro, M.; Yoshizawa, K.; Uehara, N. Calpain Inhibition Restores Basal Autophagy and Suppresses MNU-induced Photoreceptor Cell Death in Mice. *In Vivo* **2011**, *25*, 617–624.
65. Komeima, K.; Rogers, B.S.; Lu, L.; Campochiaro, P.A. Antioxidants reduce cone cell death in a model of retinitis pigmentosa. *Proc. Natl. Acad. Sci. USA* **2006**, *103*, 11300–11305. [CrossRef]
66. Usui, S.; Oveson, B.C.; Lee, S.Y.; Jo, Y.-J.; Yoshida, T.; Miki, A.; Miki, K.; Iwase, T.; Lu, L.; Campochiaro, P.A. NADPH oxidase plays a central role in cone cell death in retinitis pigmentosa. *J. Neurochem.* **2009**, *110*, 1028–1037. [CrossRef]
67. Campochiaro, P.A.; Strauss, R.W.; Lu, L.; Hafiz, G.; Wolfson, Y.; Shah, S.M.; Sophie, R.; Mir, T.A.; Scholl, H.P. Is There Excess Oxidative Stress and Damage in Eyes of Patients with Retinitis Pigmentosa? *Antioxid. Redox Signal.* **2015**, *23*, 643–648. [CrossRef]
68. D'Cruz, P.M.; Yasumura, D.; Weir, J.; Matthes, M.T.; Abderrahim, H.; LaVail, M.M.; Vollrath, D. Mutation of the receptor tyrosine kinase gene Mertk in the retinal dystrophic RCS rat. *Hum. Mol. Genet.* **2000**, *9*, 645–651. [CrossRef]
69. Smith, A.J.; Schlichtenbrede, F.C.; Tschernutter, M.; Bainbridge, J.W.; Thrasher, A.J.; Ali, R.R. AAV-mediated gene transfer slows photoreceptor loss in the RCS rat model of retinitis pigmentosa. *Mol. Ther.* **2003**, *8*, 188–195. [CrossRef]
70. Tschernutter, M.; Schlichtenbrede, F.C.; Howe, S.; Balaggan, K.S.; Munro, P.M.; Bainbridge, J.W.; Thrasher, A.J.; Smith, A.J.; Ali, R.R. Long-term preservation of retinal function in the RCS rat model of retinitis pigmentosa following lentivirus-mediated gene therapy. *Gene Ther.* **2005**, *12*, 694–701. [CrossRef]
71. Yagi, K. A simple fluorometric assay for lipoperoxide in blood plasma. *Biochem. Med.* **1976**, *15*, 212–216. [CrossRef]

72. Shu, W.; Dunaief, J.L. Potential treatment of retinal diseases with iron chelators. *Pharmaceuticals* **2018**, *11*, 112. [CrossRef]
73. Hahn, P.; Ying, G.-S.; Beard, J.; Dunaief, J.L. Iron levels in human retina: Sex difference and increase with age. *Neuroreport* **2006**, *17*, 1803–1806. [CrossRef]
74. Rózanowski, B.; Burke, J.M.; Boulton, M.E.; Sarna, T.; Rózanowska, M. Human RPE melanosomes protect from photosensitized and iron-mediated oxidation but become pro-oxidant in the presence of iron upon photodegradation. *Investig. Opthalmol. Vis. Sci.* **2008**, *49*, 2838–2847. [CrossRef]

pharmaceutics

MDPI

Article

Understanding the Half-Life Extension of Intravitreally Administered Antibodies Binding to Ocular Albumin

Simon Hauri [1,*], Paulina Jakubiak [1,†], Matthias Fueth [1], Stefan Dengl [2], Sara Belli [1], Rubén Alvarez-Sánchez [1] and Antonello Caruso [1]

1 Roche Pharma Research and Early Development, Pharmaceutical Sciences, Roche Innovation Center Basel, F. Hoffmann-La Roche Ltd., Grenzacherstrasse 124, CH-4070 Basel, Switzerland; jakubiak.paulina@gene.com (P.J.); matthias.fueth@roche.com (M.F.); sara.belli@roche.com (S.B.); ruben.alvarez_sanchez@roche.com (R.A.-S.); antonello.caruso@roche.com (A.C.)

2 Roche Pharma Research and Early Development, Large Molecule Research, Roche Innovation Center Munich, F. Hoffmann-La Roche Ltd., Nonnenwald 2, D-82377 Penzberg, Germany; stefan.dengl@roche.com

* Correspondence: simon.hauri@roche.com

† Current address: Preclinical and Translational Pharmacokinetics and Pharmacodynamics, Genentech, 1 DNA Way, South San Francisco, CA 94080-4990, USA.

Received: 10 July 2020; Accepted: 20 August 2020; Published: 26 August 2020

Abstract: The burden associated with frequent injections of current intravitreal (IVT) therapeutics may be reduced by long-acting delivery strategies. Binding to serum albumin has been shown to extend the ocular half-life in rabbits, however, the underlying molecular mechanisms and translational relevance remain unclear. The aim of this work was to characterize the in vitro and in vivo formation of complexes between human serum albumin (HSA) and an antigen-binding fragment of a rabbit antibody linked to an anti-HSA nanobody (FabA). The ocular and systemic pharmacokinetics of ^{3}H-labeled FabA (0.05 mg/eye IVT) co-formulated with HSA (1 and 15 nmol/eye) were assessed in Dutch belted rabbits. Next, FabA was incubated in vitreous samples from cynomolgus monkeys and human donors (healthy and diseased) supplemented with species-specific serum albumin. Finally, the FabA-albumin complexes formed in vitro and in vivo were analyzed by radio-size exclusion chromatography. A 3-fold increase in FabA vitreal exposure and half-life was observed in rabbits co-administered with 15 nmol HSA compared to 1 nmol and a control arm. The different pharmacokinetic behavior was explained with the formation of higher molecular weight FabA–albumin complexes. The analysis of vitreous samples revealed the existence of predominantly 1:1 complexes at endogenous or low concentrations of supplemented albumin. A shift towards 1:2 complexes was observed with increasing albumin concentrations. Overall, these results suggest that endogenous vitreal albumin concentrations are insufficient for half-life extension and warrant supplementation in the dosing formulation.

Keywords: ocular drug delivery; ocular pharmacokinetics; half-life extension; albumin; therapeutic proteins; size exclusion chromatography

1. Introduction

As the number of patients with vision-threatening conditions has been steadily increasing in recent years, largely driven by the growth and ageing of the world's population [1], so have the efforts directed at finding novel treatments. As a notable example, the development of anti-vascular endothelial growth factor (VEGF) therapeutics has transformed the management of neovascular age-related macular degeneration (nAMD), diabetic retinopathy (DR) and diabetic macular edema (DME) [2,3]. The antibodies ranibizumab (Lucentis®) and aflibercept (Eylea®) are the current standard of care to treat these retinal diseases [4,5], with off-label use of bevacizumab (Avastin®) being common [4]. Recently, a novel fusion protein, brolucizumab (Beovu®), was also approved for the treatment of nAMD [6,7]. All anti-VEGF biologics are administered through intravitreal (IVT) injections every 4–12 weeks [8,9]. The dosing frequency can be reduced in clinical practice, leading in some cases to suboptimal treatment [10]. In addition, IVT injections are invasive and can pose a significant medical, psychological, and financial burden on patients and healthcare systems alike. For these reasons, treatment options with less frequent dosing regimens are desirable, potentially improving outcomes and compliance [11].

To address such needs, a common approach in protein drug discovery is to optimize the molecular properties influencing the target suppression and maximum feasible dose, such as the binding affinity, stability and aggregation. In addition, durability can be enhanced by reducing the rate of ocular elimination, which is driven by diffusion from the vitreous body to the anterior chamber and by aqueous humor (AH) turnover [12]. Diffusivity decreases inversely with macromolecular size, so larger antibody formats, PEGylation or conjugation to biopolymers result in prolonged ocular retention [13–18]. This may also be achieved with binding to constituents of the vitreous matrix, such as collagen (type II) and hyaluronic acid [19,20], or association with soluble proteins, like albumin [21]. Parallel to the development of novel therapeutic agents, continuous effort is being put into designing long-acting delivery strategies applicable to existing and new drugs [22–24]. For instance, the Port Delivery System, an implantable intraocular device, is currently undergoing clinical investigation for sustained delivery of ranibizumab on a 6-month refill regimen [25].

Among these approaches, binding to albumin may be considered appealing because of its undetermined biological function [26] and relatively high abundance in ocular fluids. In the human vitreous, albumin was shown to be approximately equimolar to the standard-of-care doses of IVT antibodies [20]. However, its small size (66.4 kDa) and correspondingly short ocular half-life (reported as 2–4 days in rabbit [27,28]) may limit the prolongation of ocular half-life and therefore its suitability as a retention target.

The effects of albumin binding on antibody pharmacokinetics (PK) were recently investigated in rat and rabbit eyes by Fuchs and Igney [21]. To this end, a nanobody molecule (BI-X, 40 kDa) was used containing one high affinity binding site to human serum albumin (HSA) and showing no specific binding to rat or rabbit albumin. In rabbits, co-administration with albumin led to a 3-fold increase in the vitreal half-life of BI-X (10.1 days with HSA vs. 3.2 days without). Association of one BI-X and one albumin molecule would result in a 106 kDa complex, however, the observed half-life exceeded that of macromolecules with similar molecular weight (MW) (40–150 kDa, 2–6 days [29,30]). Fuchs and Igney [21] hypothesized complexation with multiple HSA molecules, since commercially available human and bovine serum albumins are known to form oligomers after reconstitution from powders [31,32]. While oligomeric complexes could theoretically explain the long retention observed in vivo, their nature and stoichiometry were not investigated experimentally in the original study [21]. It also remains unclear whether the endogenous albumin concentration in the human vitreous is conducive to a meaningful half-life extension.

In this work, we investigated the molecular mechanisms underlying the binding of macromolecules to vitreal albumin by means of in vitro and in vivo experiments. We aimed to determine the vitreal albumin concentration leading to the formation of high MW complexes and understand the potential impact on ocular drug retention. To this end, we assessed the IVT PK in rabbits of a radiolabeled antigen-binding mAb fragment (Fab) linked to an anti-albumin nanobody and co-formulated with different amounts of albumin. We incubated the Fab in cynomolgus monkey and human vitreous humor (VH), supplemented with different amounts of species-specific serum albumin. Finally, we characterized the nature of Fab–albumin complexes formed in vitro and in vivo with radio-size exclusion chromatography (radio-SEC). Herein, we present the results of these investigations and assess the scope and translatability of albumin binding as a long-acting drug delivery approach.

2. Materials and Methods

2.1. Materials

A HSA binding immunoglobulin single variable domain (nanobody, VHH) sequence (ALB8 from WO 2012/131078 A1 [33]) was recombinantly fused via a 3× GGGGS-linker to the C-terminus of the heavy chain of a species-matched rabbit Fab (rabFab) [17]. The C-terminus of the nanobody was modified by a His6-tag (FabA). In addition, rabFab with a 3× GGGGS-linker-His6-tag at the C-terminus of the heavy chain (without the nanobody sequence) was produced as the non-albumin binding control molecule (FabB). The MW of the antibodies was 59.5 and 47.4 kDa for FabA and FabB, respectively.

The DNA sequences were cloned into mammalian expression vectors that were used for transfection of HEK293F cells (Invitrogen, Waltham, MA, USA). After expression of the proteins, cleared supernatants were subjected to affinity chromatography (cOmpleteTM His-Tag purification resin, Sigma-Aldrich, St Louis, MO, USA). Bound protein was eluted in 50 mM Na_2HPO_4 (Sigma-Aldrich, St Louis, MO, USA), 300 mM NaCl (Sigma-Aldrich, St Louis, MO, USA), 500 mM imidazole (Sigma-Aldrich, St Louis, MO, USA), pH 8.0. Eluted protein was subjected to preparative size exclusion chromatography (SEC) (HiLoad 26/60 Superdex 200 prep grade, GE Healthcare Life Sciences, Marlborough, MA, USA) in 1× PBS, pH 7.0. The biochemical quality of the final product was high with a 100% monomer peak on analytical high-performance liquid chromatography (HPLC) SEC (BioSuite, Waters Corporation, Milford, MA, USA) for both proteins. Identity of the proteins was verified by mass spectrometry.

Human, rabbit (RSA) and porcine serum albumin (PSA) were purchased from Sigma-Aldrich (St Louis, MO, USA). Cynomolgus serum albumin (CSA) was purchased from antibodies-online GmbH (Aachen, Germany) and Abcam (Cambridge, UK). Frozen cynomolgus monkey and human (diabetic with and without retinopathy) VH samples were provided by Anawa Trading SA (Kloten, Switzerland).

2.2. Albumin Binding Kinetics and Cross-Reactivity

In order to determine the affinity of the Fabs to serum albumin from different species, interaction of the compounds with HSA, CSA, RSA, and PSA was tested by surface plasmon resonance. The selected albumin concentration range was based on the binding affinity of the nanobody for HSA reported in the original patent [33].

In brief, an anti-His capturing antibody (28995056, GE Healthcare Life Sciences, Marlborough, MA, USA) was immobilized to a Series S Sensor Chip CM3 (29104990, GE Healthcare Life Sciences, Marlborough, MA, USA) using standard amine coupling chemistry, resulting in a surface density of approximately 5000 resonance units. As the running and dilution buffer, HBS-P+ (10 mM HEPES (Sigma-Aldrich, St Louis, MO, USA), 150 mM NaCl pH 7.4, 0.05% surfactant P20 (Sigma-Aldrich, St Louis, MO, USA)) was used. The measurement temperature was set to 25 °C. The antibodies were captured to the surface with resulting capture levels of approximately 15 resonance units. Dilution series of HSA, CSA, RSA, and PSA in the range 22.2–1800 nM were injected for 180 s, dissociation was monitored for 300 s at a flow rate of 30 µL/min. Subsequently, the surface was regenerated by injecting 10 mM glycine pH 1.5 for 60 s. Bulk refractive index differences were corrected by subtracting blank injections and by subtracting the response obtained from the control flow cell without captured antibody. Rate constants were calculated using the Langmuir 1:1 binding model within the Biacore Evaluation software (GE Healthcare Life Sciences, Marlborough, MA, USA).

2.3. Native Intact Mass Spectrometry of Protein Complexes

FabA–HSA complex composition was characterized by high-resolution intact mass spectrometry. Protein separation was carried out by SEC on an Ultimate 3000 UHPLC system (Thermo Fisher Scientific, Waltham, MA, USA) using an Acquity BEH SEC column (200 Å, 1.7 × 100 mm; Waters Corporation, Milford, MA, USA) with 100 mM ammonium acetate pH 6.8 as mobile phase. The method run time was 10 min at 250 µL/min isocratic flow. Intact mass analysis was performed on a maXis II qToF instrument (Bruker Corporation, Billerica, MA, USA). The ion polarity was set to positive mode, covering the mass range of 800–10,000 *m/z*. Spectra were recorded at 0.5 Hz. Capillary voltage was 4500 V at a nebulizer pressure of 2 bar and a dry gas flow rate of 10 L/min at 280 °C. In-source fragmentation was enabled at 30 eV. The raw files were analyzed using Compass DataAnalysis 4.4 SR1 (Bruker Corporation, Billerica, MA, USA) and PMI-Intact v3.8-11 x64 (Protein Metrics Inc., San Carlos, CA, USA).

2.4. Radiolabeling

FabA and FabB were chemically labeled with ^{3}H-propionic acid esterification activated by N-hydroxysuccinimide [34]. The specific activity of FabA was 1.5 mCi/mg (90 Ci/mmol) and yielded a protein concentration of 2.15 mg/mL. The specific activity of FabB was 2.3 mCi/mg (110 Ci/mmol) and yielded a protein concentration of 2.23 mg/mL. The endotoxin levels measured after sterile filtration using 0.20 μm syringe filter-discs were 0.832 EU/mL and 0.641 EU/mL for FabA and FabB, respectively.

2.5. Ocular Pharmacokinetics Study in Rabbits

An in vivo study was performed with the goal of investigating the effects of albumin binding on ocular pharmacokinetics. The animal experimentation was approved by the local veterinary authorities and was conducted in strict accordance with the Swiss federal regulations on animal care and laboratory use and in adherence to the rules of the Association for Assessment and Accreditation of Laboratory Animal Care International. The husbandry license number is 1009H F. Hoffmann-La Roche Ltd. and animal permission number 2764 (valid since 01.07.2018).

^{3}H-labeled FabA and FabB were administered to female Dutch belted rabbits allocated to three study groups (n = 4/group). Each group received 0.05 mg Fab premixed with HSA. Group 1 was dosed FabA with 1 nmol HSA, group 2 FabA with 15 nmol HSA, and group 3 FabB with 1 nmol HSA. Molar quantities of HSA were selected based on serum albumin concentration values reported in healthy humans and cynomolgus monkeys (group 1 and 3) as well as patients with different types of retinopathies (group 2). Table 1 summarizes all values available in the literature to date, to the best of our knowledge. A volume of 50 μL of the filtered (0.22 μm) formulation was injected intravitreally with a syringe (BD Micro-Fine, 30 G × 8 mm) to both eyes. Blood was withdrawn from the ear vein into K3-EDTA tubes and plasma produced by centrifugation (10 min at 2000× g at 4 °C) at 0, 1, 2, 5, 7, 24, 48, 72, 168, and 336 h post-dose. AH and VH samples were collected in-life from anesthetized rabbits at 24, 74, 168, and 336 h post-dose in a composite design. For AH sampling, a 30 G needle was inserted through the cornea into the anterior chamber and a maximum of 20 μL of aqueous was sampled. For VH sampling, a 22 G butterfly needle was inserted through the sclera and pars plana for 5–10 mm, and a maximum of 20 μL of vitreous was gently aspirated from the center of the vitreal cavity. Safety of the method and possible effects on the eye were evaluated by frequent ophthalmic examinations (biomicroscopy and indirect ophthalmoscopy) over the study period. Radioactivity in the VH, AH and plasma samples was counted with a TopCount NXT HTS Microplate Counter (Perkin Elmer, Waltham, MA, USA). A non-compartmental analysis of the composite concentration-time profiles was performed in Phoenix WinNonlin version 6.4 (Certara USA Inc., Princeton, NJ, USA, 2015).

2.6. In Vitro Sample Preparation

To test the contribution of albumin to multimeric complex formation, FabA was incubated in vitro with different concentrations of HSA and CSA in PBS, human and cynomolgus monkey vitreous humor (VH) at 37 °C for 18 h, as summarized in Table 2. Low (0.57 μM) and high (5.7 μM) dose levels of radiolabeled FabA were tested. For the high dose, the specific activity of FabA was kept constant and supplemented with unlabeled FabA. The samples were stored at −20 °C prior to further analysis. Cynomolgus monkey and human VH samples collected post mortem were obtained from a commercial provider. Upon receipt of the samples, albumin concentration was determined using the Millipore Human ALB/Serum albumin ELISA kit (Sigma-Aldrich Chemie GmbH, Buchs, Switzerland) according to manufacturer's instructions. Absorbance at 450 nm was measured on an EnSpire Multimode Plate Reader (Perkin Elmer, Waltham, MA, USA).

Table 1. Summary of literature values of albumin concentration in the VH of healthy humans and cynomolgus monkeys, as well as patients undergoing vitrectomy.

Species	Disease	Reported Albumin Concentration (mg/L)	Measure [1]	Calculated Albumin Concentration (μM) [2]	Reference
Human	Healthy [3]	293 ± 18	Mean ± S.E.M. (95% confidence interval: 155.8–429.4)	4.41 ± 0.27	[35,36]
		249 ± 150	Mean ± S.E.M.	3.75 ± 2.26	[35–37]
	Non-diabetic patients	300	Median (range: 83–1900)	4.52	[38]
	Diabetic patients without retinopathy or proliferative diabetic retinopathy (PDR)	280 ± 10	Mean ± S.D.	4.22 ± 016	Current study [3]
		700	Median (range: 80–1200)	10.5	[38]
	Non-PDR patients	1160 ± 360	Mean ± S.E.M.	17.47 ± 5.42	[39]
	PDR	699 ± 77	Mean ± S.D.	10.5 ± 1.16	Current study [3]
		536 ± 212	Mean ± S.E.M. (95% confidence interval: 81.3–991.1)	8.07 ± 3.19	[35,36]
		1600	Median (range: 700–3000)	24.10	[38]
		2564 ± 665	Mean ± S.E.M.	38.61 ± 10.0	[39]
	Traumatic proliferative vitreoretinopathy	743 ± 232	Mean ± S.E.M. (95% confidence interval: 217.9–1267)	11.2 ± 3.49	[35,36]
	Idiopathic proliferative vitreoretinopathy	2215 ± 867	Mean ± S.E.M. (95% confidence interval: 254.6–4176.4)	33.36 ± 13.1	[35,36]
Cynomolgus monkey	Healthy	35 ± 4	Mean ± S.D.	0.53 ± 0.05	Current study [3]
		86.8 ± 4.0	Mean ± S.E.M. (calculated from reported 40% of total protein content: 217 μg/mL ± 4.6%)	1.31 ± 0.060	[40]

[1] S.E.M.: standard error of the mean; S.D.: standard deviation.[2] Calculated using albumin MW of 66.4 kDa.[3] Vitreous samples collected post mortem.

Table 2. List of amounts, volumes and concentrations used in all experiments.

Experiment	FabA Dose	^{3}H-FabA Concentration [1]		Albumin Concentration [2]	
		μM	mg/L	μM	mg/L
Formulation of in vivo rabbit study		16.8	1000	20.0	1328
		16.8	1000	300	19,920
In vivo rabbit VH	Low dose [3]	0.57	33	0.67	44
		0.57	33	10.0	664
In vitro cynomolgus monkey VH	Low dose	0.57	33	0.53	35
		0.57	33	50.0	3320
		0.57	33	100	6640
		0.57	33	250	16,600
	High dose [4]	5.7	330	0.53	35
		5.7	330	50.0	3320
		5.7	330	100	6640
		5.7	330	250	16,600
In vitro human VH (no eye disease)	Low dose	0.57	33	4.22	280
		0.57	33	50.0	3320
		0.57	33	100	6640
		0.57	33	250	16,600
	High dose [4]	5.7	330	4.22	280
		5.7	330	50.0	3320
		5.7	330	100	6640
		5.7	330	250	16,600
In vitro human VH (PDR)	Low dose	0.57	33	10.53	699
		0.57	33	50.0	3320

[1] Calculated using FabA MW of 59.5 kDa. [2] Calculated using albumin MW of 66.4 kDa. [3] Calculated assuming a rabbit vitreous humor volume of 1.5 mL [13]. [4] 10-fold of low dose (0.57 μM ^{3}H-FabA complemented with 5.13 μM unlabeled FabA).

2.7. *Radio Size Exclusion Chromatography*

To characterize the nature of Fab–albumin complex formation in vivo, SEC studies were performed with the vitreous humor samples obtained in the rabbit study. As outlined in Table 2, FabA and FabB were also incubated with HSA and CSA in PBS, as well as in human and cynomolgus monkey VH at 37 °C for 18 h. The samples were stored at −20 °C prior to SEC analysis.

Protein separation was carried out by SEC on an Agilent 1290 Infinity II UHPLC system (Agilent Technologies Inc, Santa Clara, CA, USA) using an Acquity BEH SEC column (200 Å, 1.7 × 100 mm, Waters Corporation, Milford, MA, USA) with 100 mM sodium phosphate buffer at pH 7.4 containing 10% ethanol as mobile phase. The method run time was 10 min at 250 μL/min isocratic flow. Fractions were collected between 4 and 10 min for 0.05 min (12.5 μL) in a Deepwell LumaPlate384 (Perkin Elmer, Waltham, MA, USA) and radioactivity was measured on a TopCount NXT HTS Microplate Counter (Perkin Elmer, Waltham, MA, USA).

3. Results

3.1. Albumin Binding Kinetics Experiments

FabA and FabB binding kinetics to the serum albumin of different species are summarized in Table 3. FabA showed a high affinity interaction with HSA in a two-digit nanomolar range. The molecule was fully cross-reactive to CSA with comparable on- and off-rates, but did not interact with RSA or PSA. For FabB, no interaction with serum albumin from the different species was detected.

Table 3. Binding kinetics of FabA and FabB to albumin of different species.

Compound	HSA			CSA			RSA			PSA		
	ka (1/Ms)	kd (1/s)	KD (nM)	ka (1/Ms)	kd (1/s)	KD (nM)	ka (1/Ms)	kd (1/s)	KD (nM)	ka (1/Ms)	kd (1/s)	KD (nM)
FabA	110,000 ± 10,000	0.0061 ± 0.0001	55 ± 6	99,000 ± 4000	0.0065 ± 0.0004	66 ± 6	n.d.	n.d.	n.d.	n.d.	n.d.	n.d.
FabB	n.d.	n.d.	n.d.	n.d.	n.d.	n.d.	n.d.	n.d.	n.d.	n.d.	n.d.	n.d.

n.d.: no detectable interaction.

Verification of HSA binding after radiolabeling of the compounds for use in vivo confirmed that the labeling procedure did not have an impact on their binding properties (Table 4).

Table 4. Binding kinetics of FabA (unlabeled and radiolabeled) and FabB to HSA.

Compound	HSA		
	ka (1/Ms)	kd (1/s)	KD (nM)
FabA	64,400	0.00640	99
Radiolabeled FabA	64,700	0.00626	97
FabB	n.d.	n.d.	n.d.

n.d.: no detectable interaction.

3.2. Native LC-MS

To investigate the composition of the protein complexes, unlabeled FabA was incubated with HSA and analyzed by size exclusion chromatography coupled to mass spectrometry (SEC-MS). The experiment was performed under non-denaturing conditions at neutral pH to prevent protein complex dissociation during the chromatographic separation. By measuring the intact mass of FabA, albumin and the FabA–albumin complexes, the composition of the different molecular weight species was investigated (Figure 1). The UV chromatogram shows four distinct peaks at 280 nm absorption (Figure 1A). Fifteen µM of FabA and HSA were measured separately, to define migration times and reference mass spectra (Figure 1A, peak 1 and 2). To favor 1:1 complex formation, 15 µM of FabA was incubated with 15 µM of HSA, resulting in a 126 kDa complex at a migration time of 4.8 min (Figure 1A, peak 3). For the formation of the 1:2 complexes, 15 µM FabA and 75 µM HSA were incubated and detected at a migration of time 4.2 min with masses for FabA and multimeric albumin (Figure 1A, peak 4). The underlying mass spectra in all four peaks were deconvoluted to intact protein masses. Peak 1 consisted of a protein with the mass of 59 kDa, corresponding to FabA (Figure 1B). It is also in good alignment with the molecular weight standard with a faster migration time than the 66 kDa marker. Peak 2 contained a single mass of 67 kDa, which is the mass of HSA (Figure 1C). Migration time of peak 3 was just before the 150 kDa marker and when deconvoluted, several masses were identified: The 59 kDa mass of FabA, the 67 kDa of HSA and a 126 kDa mass corresponding to the 1:1 FabA–HSA complex (Figure 1D). The slowest migrating peak 4 contained again FabA, but no 67 kDa HSA. Instead, HSA was found in its dimeric form at 133 kDa. The 126 kDa complex was still present and additionally two large masses were found at 186 and 193 kDa (Figure 1E). These high molecular weight complexes could consist of two FabA and one HSA or vice versa.

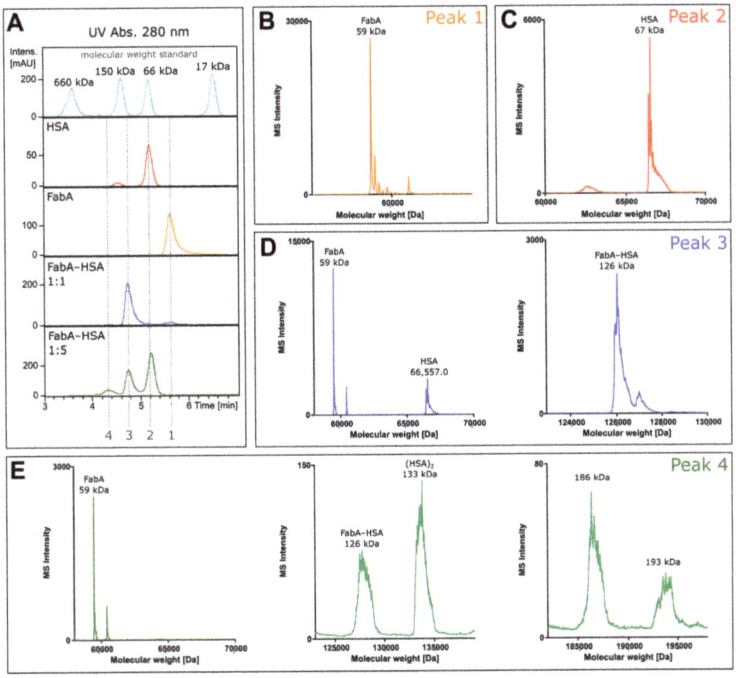

Figure 1. Native mass spectrometry of intact proteins. (**A**) UV size exclusion chromatograms FabA, HSA and FabA–HSA complexes formed after 4 h incubation with human VH supplemented with albumin (at 1:1 and 1:5 ratio). (**B**) Deconvoluted intact mass spectrum of chromatographic peak 1 corresponding to a molecular weight of FabA and (**C**) HSA. (**D**) Deconvoluted spectra of two mass ranges. The lower mass range contains FabA and HSA, while the higher mass range covers the equimolar FabA–HSA complex of 126 kDa. (**E**) Deconvoluted intact mass spectra of three mass ranges, with FabA in the lowest, FabA–HSA and dimeric $(HSA)_2$ in the middle, and two high molecular mass complexes of 186 and 193 kDa in the highest.

3.3. Ocular Pharmacokinetics Study

Ocular and plasma PK were studied in rabbits after an IVT injection of human albumin-binding FabA (0.05 mg; 0.84 nmol; 50 μL) co-formulated with HSA at molar quantities of 1 (group 1) and 15 nmol (group 2). An equal dose of FabB lacking the albumin-binding moiety was co-administered with 1 nmol HSA and served as negative control (group 3). At each time point, VH, AH and plasma concentrations of the test molecules were calculated as mean ± standard deviation (S.D.) from four individual samples. The composite concentration-time profiles in rabbit ocular fluids and plasma are depicted in Figure 2, and the individual data is reported in the Supplementary Information (Table S1). The pharmacokinetic parameters calculated by non-compartmental analysis are summarized in Table 5.

The VH PK data demonstrated that approximately a 3-fold extension of vitreous half-life was achieved in the group that received FabA with the excess of 15 nmol HSA ($t_{1/2}$ = 149 h) when compared to FabB dosed with 1 nmol HSA ($t_{1/2}$ = 52 h) or FabA co-administered with an equimolar amount of HSA ($t_{1/2}$ = 58 h). The observed prolongation of the vitreous half-life, related to a decrease in the ocular clearance, resulted in an increased overall exposure to FabA in the VH in low and high HSA concentration groups (AUCinf = 104 and 230 h·nmol/mL, respectively) compared to the FabB group (AUCinf = 72.8 h·nmol/mL). Similarly, longer residence times were observed for HSA-binding FabA (MRTinf = 79.1 h for group 1 and 129 h for group 2) than for FabB (MRTinf = 68.6 h). The volume of distribution based on nominal dose was calculated as 0.68, 0.79 and 0.87 mL for groups 1, 2 and 3, respectively.

The concentration measurements in AH indicated a later t_{max} for FabA (168 h for 1 nmol HSA and 74 h for 15 nmol HSA) than FabB (24 h). Minimal differences were observed in the AH exposure across groups, with the AUCinf calculated to be 5.32, 6.68 and 4.70 h·nmol/mL for group 1, 2 and 3, respectively. These comparable AUC values could be explained by a complete transfer of the compounds from the vitreous into the anterior chamber and a comparable anterior clearance across molecules, dictated by the AH flow. The respective $t_{1/2}$ values in the aqueous humor were calculated to 50.9, 87.0 and 50.4 h.

Both FabA and FabB were found circulating in plasma at very low levels with similar exposures across study groups, in line with the lack of cross-reactivity with rabbit serum albumin. Nonetheless, the average plasma concentration of FabA in both low and high HSA concentration groups showed a bi-phasic behavior in the systemic absorption phase, with a first lower concentration peak and a second absorption peak appearing later than the FabB t_{max}. This effect was more prominent and consistently observed in all individuals of the 15 nmol HSA group, possibly reflecting differences in ocular kinetics and systemic absorption rates between the free and complexed FabA.

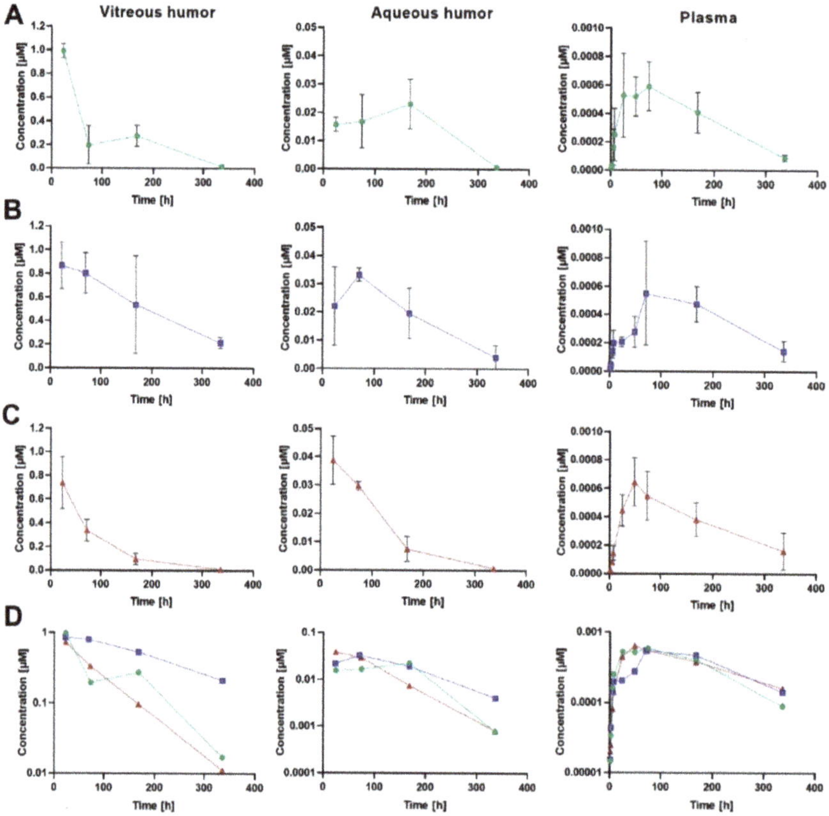

Figure 2. Concentration-time profiles of FabA and FabB in rabbit VH, AH and plasma after a single IVT injection of 0.05 mg per eye of the respective molecule co-formulated with HSA. Panel (**A–C**) represent the concentrations obtained in each matrix for group 1 (FabA and 1 nmol HSA), group 2 (FabA and 15 nmol HSA) and group 3 (FabB and 1 nmol HSA), respectively. Composite data are plotted as mean ± S.D. Panel (**D**) depicts overlaid semi-log profiles of group 1, 2 and 3 without error bars for greater readability.

Table 5. Pharmacokinetic parameters calculated for FabA and FabB in rabbit VH, AH and plasma after a single IVT injection of 0.05 mg of the respective molecule co-administered with 1 nmol (FabA and FabB) and 15 nmol HSA (FabA). The parameters were computed by non-compartmental analysis of composite profiles, assuming extravascular (plasma and AH) or intravenous (VH) dosing.

Parameter	Unit	Vitreous Humor			Aqueous Humor			Plasma		
		FabA 1 nmol HSA	FabA 15 nmol HSA	FabB 1 nmol HSA	FabA 1 nmol HSA	FabA 15 nmol HSA	FabB 1 nmol HSA	FabA 1 nmol HSA	FabA 15 nmol HSA	FabB 1 nmol HSA
C_{max}	nmol/mL	0.99	0.87	0.74	0.023	0.033	0.039	0.0006	0.0006	0.0007
t_{max}	h	24	24	24	168	74	24	72	72	48
$t_{1/2}$	h	58.0	149	52.1	50.9	87.0	50.4	94.6	130	147
MRT_{inf}	h	83.8	213	72.5	129	149	86.5	154	213	224
AUC_{inf}	h·nmol/mL	104	230	72.8	5.32	6.68	4.70	0.14	0.15	0.16
V_{ss}/F	mL	0.68	0.79	0.87	11.6	15.8	13.0	840	1051	1128
CL/F	mL/h	0.008	0.004	0.012	0.16	0.13	0.18	6.15	5.60	5.31

3.4. Radio Size Exclusion Chromatography Studies on Rabbit Vitreous Samples and Dosing Formulations

To investigate the underlying molecular mechanism of half-life extension in vivo, the rabbit VH samples were analyzed by SEC and radiometric detection. SEC allows to determine the stoichiometry of the FabA–albumin complexes by separating them by their hydrodynamic radius. For the VH samples from the group dosed at 1:1 ratio of FabA and HSA, the radio-signal for FabA was observed at a retention time corresponding to a MW between 66 and 150 kDa. This was in good agreement with the theoretical MW of the expected 1:1 complex, namely 126 kDa (Figure 3A). For the VH samples of the 15:1 molar ratio group, the radio signal shifted to the higher MW species greater than 150 kDa, consistent with the MW of a 1:2 complex of about 180 kDa (Figure 3B).

These findings suggest the formation of higher stoichiometry complexes because of the higher albumin concentration that could be responsible for the ocular half-life extension observed in vivo.

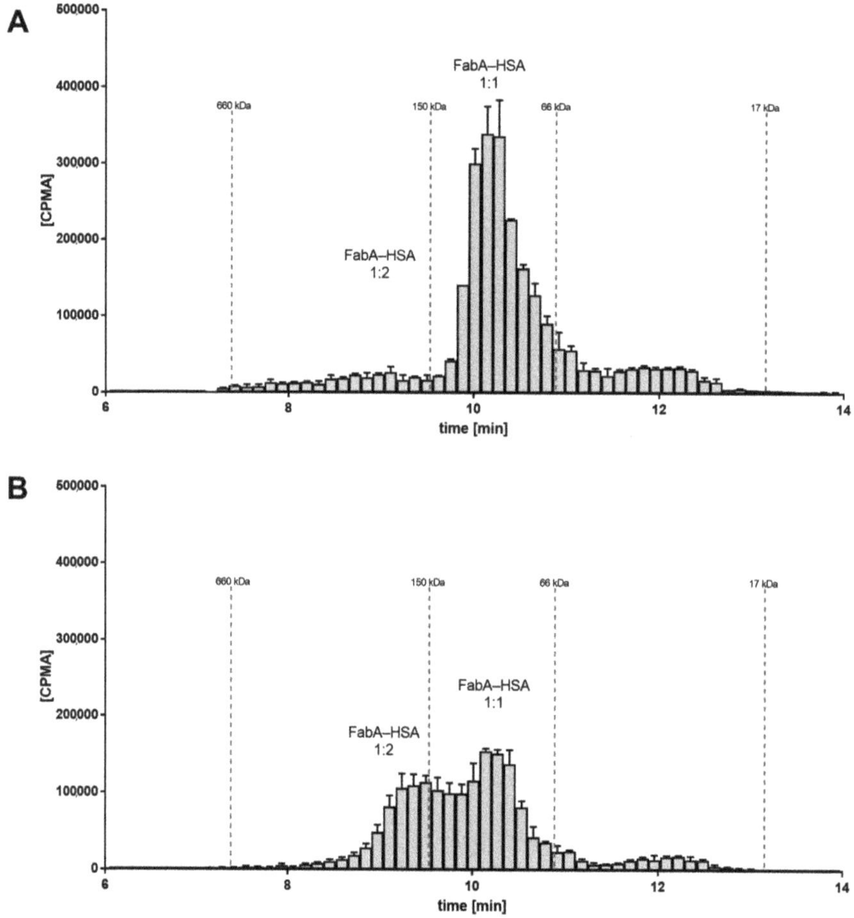

Figure 3. Radio-size exclusion chromatograms of FabA–HSA complexes in rabbit VH samples from the PK study (24 h time point). Error bars are min/max values of the right and left eye. Dotted lines represent the UV absorbance maxima of the MW standard. At low albumin levels (0.67 μM), the majority of the FabA–HSA complexes occur in 1:1 stoichiometry, corresponding to a MW of 126 kDa (**A**). At 15:1 HSA to FabA ratio, higher MW complexes (>150 kDa) were observed (**B**).

SEC analysis of the dosing formulations was also performed in order to verify whether the multimeric complex is formed prior to ocular administration (Figure 4). A concentration range of HSA was tested with FabA to determine a stoichiometric dependency. Additionally, FabA was tested for complex formation with CSA. In the absence of albumin, FabA migrated slightly faster than the 66 kDa marker, as expected from its MW of 59.5 kDa (Figure 4A). Under equimolar conditions, both HSA and CSA predominantly formed the 126 kDa 1:1 complex (Figure 4B,C). In the presence of a 15-fold molar excess of albumin, higher MW complexes were formed by both albumin species variants.

These data indicate that the half-life extending 1:2 stoichiometry can be induced already by co-formulation prior to administration.

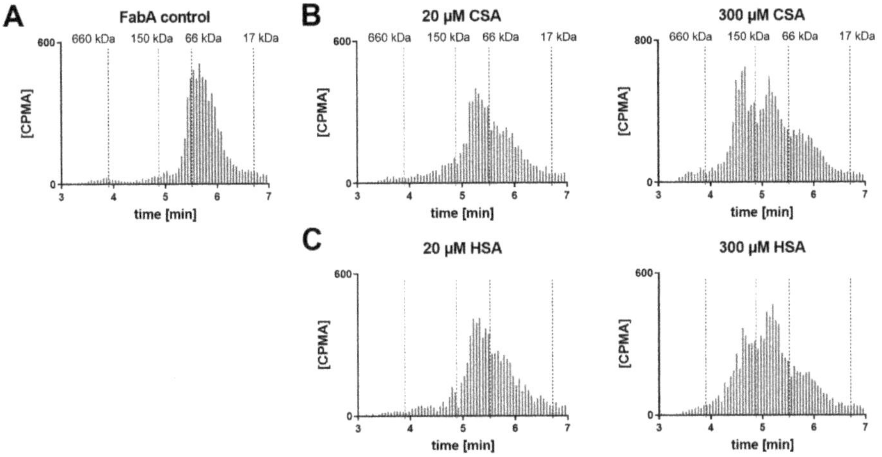

Figure 4. Radio-size exclusion chromatograms of dosing formulations with (**A**) FabA alone and increasing concentrations of (**B**) CSA or (**C**) HSA.

3.5. *FabA–Albumin Complex Formation in Monkey and Human Vitreous Humor*

Given the lack of rabbit cross-reactivity, co-administration of HSA was necessary in the PK study. To assess the complexation profile under more physiological conditions and build the rationale for a potential in vivo study in non-human primates, cynomolgus monkey and human VH samples were tested in vitro for Fab–albumin complex formation.

A VH sample from a cynomolgus monkey was incubated with FabA and supplemented with increasing concentrations of CSA to saturate FabA binding (Figure 5). At endogenous albumin levels, a 1:1 stoichiometry complex could be observed. Upon supplementation with 50, 100 and 250 µM CSA, a shift towards higher MW species was apparent. Increasing the concentration of FabA by 10-fold had a limited effect on the MW of the complexes. The endogenous cynomolgus monkey albumin concentration was determined by ELISA to be 35 mg/L (0.53 µM) (Table 1). This low basal albumin concentration relative to FabA explains why, in the absence of CSA supplementation, only a mixture of non-complexed FabA and 1:1 complexes was detected by SEC.

In a human post mortem vitreous sample from a single donor without eye disease, the endogenous albumin was not conducive to the formation of the 1:2 complex (Figure 6). When exogenous HSA was added, a shift towards the 1:2 stoichiometry could be clearly observed at 50 µM HSA. Increasing the FabA concentration by 10-fold, most FabA remained unbound at endogenous albumin concentrations and a progressive shift to the 1:1 and 1:2 complex was observed with HSA supplementation. The endogenous albumin concentration was determined to be 280 mg/L, or 4.22 µM (Table 1), a level that appears insufficient to form higher MW complexes.

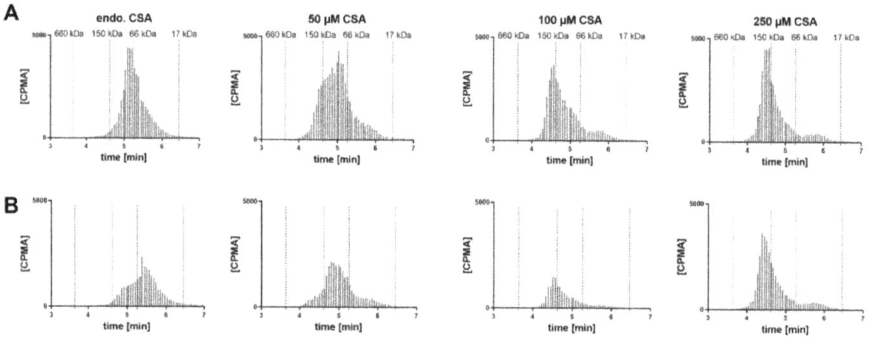

Figure 5. Radio-size exclusion chromatograms of FabA–CSA complexes formed after 4 h incubation in cynomolgus monkey VH supplemented with albumin. Two different concentrations of FabA were tested, namely (**A**) 0.6 and (**B**) 6 µM. Endogenous albumin concentrations were supplemented with 50, 100 and 250 µM of CSA.

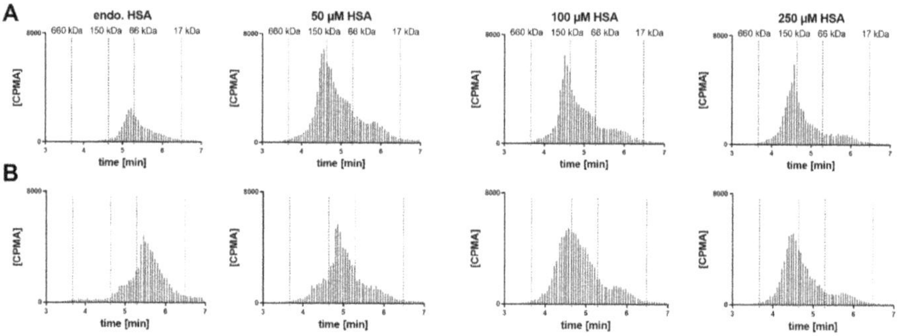

Figure 6. Radio-size exclusion chromatograms of FabA–HSA complexes formed after 4 h incubation in human VH and supplemented with increasing amounts of albumin. Two different concentrations of FabA were tested, namely (**A**) 0.6 and (**B**) 6 µM. Endogenous albumin concentrations were supplemented with 50, 100 and 250 µM of HSA.

A human post mortem VH sample from a single donor with diabetic retinopathy was tested in similar conditions (Figure 7). In the absence of albumin supplementation, mostly 1:1 complexed FabA was detected. Increasing the albumin concentration by supplementation of 50 µM resulted in the formation of the 1:2 complex. The albumin concentration was measured as 699 mg/L (10.5 µM), consistent with previous reports [35,36,38,39] (Table 1).

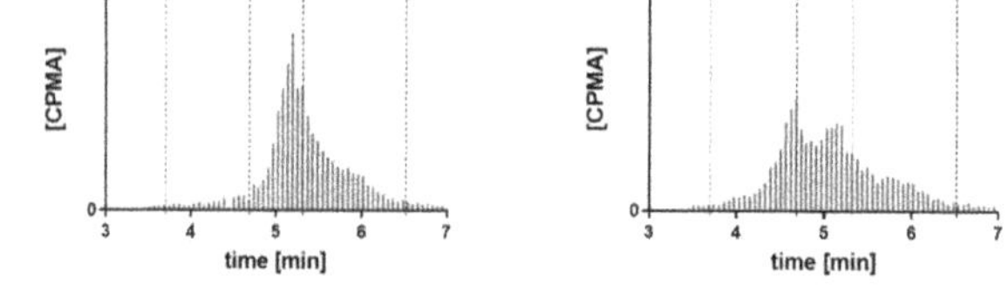

Figure 7. Radio-size exclusion chromatograms of FabA–HSA complexes formed after 4 h incubation with human VH (donor with eye disease) supplemented with albumin. The FabA concentration was 0.57 µM and the HSA concentration was (**A**) at endogenous levels or (**B**) at 50 µM.

4. Discussion

Prolonging the duration of ocular exposure and target engagement is one of the main goals in the optimization of intravitreal antibodies. Most approaches currently pursued for ocular half-life extension aim to reduce the drug's diffusivity. This may be accomplished by binding to a vitreous matrix constituent, such as hyaluronic acid or collagen [19,20], by designing a bulky format of large hydrodynamic radius [14–17] or by enabling it to associate with soluble endogenous macromolecules, such as albumin, and form high MW complexes.

Previously, Fuchs and Igney [21] demonstrated in rats and rabbits that binding to vitreal albumin produces a meaningful increase in ocular retention using an experimental antibody. In this work, we assessed the scope and translatability of this approach by means of a series of in vitro and in vivo investigations with a rabbit Fab linked to an anti-HSA nanobody, FabA (Table 2).

By means of SEC coupled to UV and MS detection, we first confirmed the identity of both HSA and FabA (Figure 1B,C). Next, we showed that following incubation at equimolar concentrations, a new entity was formed with a retention time and mass consistent with a 1:1 complex (Figure 1D). Last, in conditions of excess of albumin, an additional chromatographic peak consistent with a 1:2 stoichiometry was observed. Given the similar MW of the two possible 1:2 complexes (185 and 192 kDa) and the limited resolution of the SEC, the actual identity of this complex, or the possible coexistence of both species, could not be elucidated. However, an albumin dimer was observed exclusively in the 1:2 peak, hinting towards a one FabA to two albumin stoichiometry (Figure 1E).

Next, we assessed the pharmacokinetic profile in rabbits after IVT injection of FabA (Figure 2). Considering the lack of rabbit cross-reactivity of the anti-HSA nanobody (Table 3), we co-formulated FabA with HSA at HSA:FabA molar ratios of approximately 1.2 and 17.9. The study showed small differences in the ocular PK of the low albumin concentration group when compared to the group that received FabB, not bearing the anti-HSA nanobody (Table 5). Approximately a 3-fold increase in vitreal exposure and half-life was instead observed for the high albumin concentration group. These observations suggest the requirement for a certain minimum albumin concentration to allow the formation of FabA–albumin complex(es) with distinct pharmacokinetic behavior.

To characterize the nature of the complexes present in vivo, we conducted additional SEC studies with radiometric detection (Figures 3 and 4). Analysis of VH samples from the rabbit study collected at 24 h post-dose showed a qualitative difference between low and high albumin concentration groups, with the former exhibiting predominantly the 1:1 complex and the latter revealing the coexistence of 1:1 and 1:2 complexes. Similarly, the formulations used in the study revealed the presence of mostly free FabA and 1:1 complex in the low albumin concentration formulation and 1:1 and 1:2 complexes for the high albumin concentration group. Overall, these findings indicate that different FabA–HSA complex profiles were injected and present in the vitreous for the two groups, resulting in differentiated vitreal PK. Furthermore, there seems to be a prerequisite for formation of the 1:2 complex to significantly reduce the clearance of FabA, consistent with the well-established principle that the hydrodynamic radius is a key determinant of ocular retention [13,16,30].

Hypothesizing that the observed half-life extension is the result of pre-formed high MW complexes, rather than their in vivo formation, we investigated the implications under physiological conditions (Figures 5 and 6). We studied the formation of complexes in the human vitreous at endogenous concentrations and with supplementation of albumin. Cynomolgus monkey VH samples were also tested with the goal of identifying a more relevant animal model for potential in vivo studies. These mechanistic investigations showed very similar results in both species. Without albumin supplementation, FabA was mostly present in the free form or 1:1 complex. The amount of free FabA increased with that of FabA, suggesting that the endogenous albumin is insufficient for adequate complexation. When albumin was added to the vitreous samples, a shift towards 1:1 and eventually 1:2 complex forms was observed, with the 1:2 stoichiometry becoming predominant at concentrations of 50 μM or above. By comparison, the albumin concentrations found in the vitreous of healthy human donors (249–293 mg/mL) and cynomolgus monkeys (35–87 mg/mL) (Table 1) are one to two orders of magnitude lower. These results indicate that significantly higher than physiological concentrations of albumin are required for sufficient complexation with FabA, warranting supplementation of albumin in a potential application to cynomolgus monkeys and humans.

Additionally, we performed studies in a human vitreous sample obtained from a diabetic retinopathy patient to assess how the disease state may alter the FabA–albumin complexation profile (Figure 7). In fact, previous studies have shown that patients with retinopathies exhibit increased levels of vitreous albumin, possibly as a result of the vascular leakage associated with the disease (Table 1). In the in vivo rabbit study, the expected albumin concentration for the high albumin dose was between 10 and 15 μM, assuming a VH volume of 1.0–1.6 mL. Therefore, the albumin levels in the human diseased VH should be sufficient to form the 1:2 complex. This was, however, not reflected in the in vitro experiment where the FabA–albumin complex was found predominantly in its 1:1 conformation (Figure 7A). Our results, therefore, suggest similar complexation profiles in patients with and without eye disease and again underline the need for exogenous albumin supplementation to achieve higher order complexes.

In the dynamic in vivo setting, where the concentrations of all entities (FabA, HSA and their complexes) decrease with time after dosing, it is relevant to take into account the kinetics of formation and dissociation of the complexes. If the 1:2 complex forms and dissociates rapidly, as time passes and the concentrations of precursors decrease, it would be expected that the clearance of total FabA accelerates. In contrast, if the 1:2 complex form is irreversible or quasi-irreversible, it would determine the ocular half-life of the binder, being the lowest clearance species. The results of the in vivo rabbit study suggest that the 1:2 complex is rather stable since it was found in significant amounts in both early and late vitreous samples, without an apparent acceleration of clearance at the later time points. We tested this hypothesis by diluting pre-formed complexes in PBS and vitreous humor. However, in both conditions a dissociation of the complex was observed (data not shown). There seems to be a more elaborate underlying mechanism of complex stability than we could reproduce in vitro. Although the nature of the 1:2 complex could not be determined, it is known that albumin has a propensity to aggregate in vitro at concentrations lower than those used for the PK study formulations [31,41]. The aggregation process has been suggested to involve intermolecular disulfide bridging [31,42]. The formation of covalent bonds between two albumin molecules would be consistent with the high stability of the complex, which may be further reinforced by additional interactions with the FabA molecule.

Despite the extension of ocular half-life, a number of caveats arise when considering the potential use of albumin binding as an IVT drug delivery strategy. Co-formulation with albumin seems necessary to induce the formation of longer-residence complexes. This requirement adds on to the technical complexity of the formulation with regard to stability and other manufacturing aspects. Although the vitreal concentrations of albumin are higher in disease, the levels remain insufficient and may be expected to decrease as disease resolves by therapeutic intervention, making the approach self-limiting. Further, it is disadvantageous that binding to serum albumin has been shown to result in decreased systemic clearance and prolonged plasma half-life, after the drug diffuses out of the eye into circulation [20,43].

In this context, designing a larger molecule may be a more practical strategy to achieve the desired increase in hydrodynamic radius than introducing an albumin-binding motif. In addition, albumin is a soluble, mobile species of relatively small size and short ocular half-life. A greater reduction in diffusivity could be achieved by binding to a static retention target, such as collagen type II or hyaluronic acid, which are constituents of the vitreous matrix [20]. Whilst the compact 3D structure of collagen limits its carrying capacity to about 0.1 mg of a Fab [20], hyaluronic acid displays interesting features in terms of its vitreal abundance (34–700 μg/mL) that increases with age [44] and low turnover [45]. These characteristics yield an estimated carrying capacity of approximately 2 mg of a Fab [20], which seems suitable for ocular drug delivery.

In conclusion, we have studied the formation of complexes between albumin and a Fab fragment linked to an albumin binding nanobody and the conditions under which the ocular retention in rabbits is extended. In addition, we have addressed the human relevance of these findings, with the aim of assessing the viability as an ocular drug delivery strategy for the treatment of retinopathies. The need for supplementation of exogenous albumin in a co-formulation and the associated development hurdles led us to conclude that the approach is of limited potential relative to other delivery strategies.

Supplementary Materials: The following are available online at http://www.mdpi.com/1999-4923/12/9/810/s1, Table S1: Summary of individual concentration-time data measured in rabbit plasma, vitreous (VH) and aqueous humor (AH).

Author Contributions: Conceptualization, P.J., S.B. and A.C.; methodology, P.J. and S.H.; software, R.A.-S., P.J. and S.H. validation, S.D., S.H., and P.J.; formal analysis, S.H.; investigation P.J., A.C., R.A.-S., S.D., and S.H.; writing—original draft preparation, P.J., A.C., R.A.-S., S.D., and S.H.; writing—review and editing, S.B.; M.F., visualization, S.H., P.J.; supervision, A.C. All authors have read and agreed to the published version of the manuscript.

Funding: This research was funded by F. Hoffmann-La Roche Ltd.

Acknowledgments: The authors wish to thank Bob Kelley for sharing the sequence of the species-matched rabbit Fab as well as Christian Gassner, Martin Edelmann, Claudia Senn, Anthony Vandjour, Theresa Hartmann and Nora Denk for their technical assistance.

Conflicts of Interest: The authors declare no conflict of interest. The authors are employees of F. Hoffmann-La Roche Ltd. Roche had no role in the design of the experiments; in the collection, analysis, or interpretation of data; in the writing of the manuscript, or in the decision to publish the results.

References

1. Bourne, R.R.A.; Flaxman, S.R.; Braithwaite, T.; Cicinelli, M.V.; Das, A.; Jonas, J.B.; Keeffe, J.; Kempen, J.H.; Leasher, J.; Limburg, H.; et al. Magnitude, temporal trends, and projections of the global prevalence of blindness and distance and near vision impairment: A systematic review and meta-analysis. *Lancet Glob. Health* **2017**, *5*, e888–e897. [CrossRef]
2. Kovach, J.L.; Schwartz, S.G.; Flynn, H.W.; Scott, I.U. Anti-VEGF Treatment Strategies for Wet AMD. *J. Ophthalmol.* **2012**, *2012*, 1–7. [CrossRef] [PubMed]
3. Gower, N.J.D.; Barry, R.; Edmunds, M.R.; Titcomb, L.C.; Denniston, A.K. Drug discovery in ophthalmology: Past success, present challenges, and future opportunities. *BMC Ophthalmol.* **2016**, *16*, 11. [CrossRef]
4. Meyer, C.H.; Holz, F.G. Preclinical aspects of anti-VEGF agents for the treatment of wet AMD: Ranibizumab and bevacizumab. *Eye* **2011**, *25*, 661–672. [CrossRef] [PubMed]
5. Semeraro, F.; Morescalchi, F.; Duse, S.; Parmeggiani, F.; Gambicorti, E.; Costagliola, C. Aflibercept in wet AMD: Specific role and optimal use. *Drug Des. Dev. Ther.* **2013**, *7*, 711–722. [CrossRef] [PubMed]
6. Markham, A. Brolucizumab: First Approval. *Drugs* **2019**, *79*, 1997–2000. [CrossRef]
7. Dugel, P.U.; Koh, A.; Ogura, Y.; Jaffe, G.J.; Schmidt-Erfurth, U.; Brown, D.M.; Gomes, A.V.; Warburton, J.; Weichselberger, A.; Holz, F.G.; et al. HAWK and HARRIER: Phase 3, Multicenter, Randomized, Double-Masked Trials of Brolucizumab for Neovascular Age-Related Macular Degeneration. *Ophthalmology* **2020**, *127*, 72–84. [CrossRef] [PubMed]
8. Li, J.; Zhang, H.; Sun, P.; Gu, F.; Liu, Z.-L. Bevacizumab vs ranibizumab for neovascular age-related macular degeneration in Chinese patients. *Int. J. Ophthalmol.* **2013**, *6*, 169–173.
9. Dans, K.C.; Freeman, S.R.; Lin, T.; Meshi, A.; Olivas, S.; Cheng, L.; Amador-Patarroyo, M.J.; Freeman, W.R. Durability of every-8-week aflibercept maintenance therapy in treatment-experienced neovascular age-related macular degeneration. *Graefe's Arch. Clin. Exp. Ophthalmol.* **2019**, *257*, 741–748. [CrossRef]
10. Ciulla, T.A.; Huang, F.; Westby, K.; Williams, D.F.; Zaveri, S.; Patel, S.C. Real-world Outcomes of Anti–Vascular Endothelial Growth Factor Therapy in Neovascular Age-Related Macular Degeneration in the United States. *Ophthalmol. Retin.* **2018**, *2*, 645–653. [CrossRef]
11. Shah, S.S.; Denham, L.V.; Elison, J.R.; Bhattacharjee, P.S.; Clement, C.; Huq, T.; Hill, J.M. Drug delivery to the posterior segment of the eye for pharmacologic therapy. *Expert Rev. Ophthalmol.* **2010**, *5*, 75–93. [CrossRef] [PubMed]

12. Del Amo, E.M.; Vellonen, K.-S.; Kidron, H.; Urtti, A. Intravitreal clearance and volume of distribution of compounds in rabbits: In silico prediction and pharmacokinetic simulations for drug development. *Eur. J. Pharm. Biopharm.* **2015**, *95*, 215–226. [CrossRef] [PubMed]
13. Caruso, A.; Futh, M.; Alvarez-Sanchez, R.; Belli, S.; Diack, C.; Maass, K.F.; Schwab, D.; Kettenberger, H.; Mazer, N.A. Ocular Half-Life of Intravitreal Biologics in Humans and Other Species: Meta-Analysis and Model-Based Prediction. *Mol. Pharm.* **2020**, *17*, 695–709. [CrossRef]
14. Shatz, W.; Hass, P.E.; Mathieu, M.; Kim, H.S.; Leach, K.; Zhou, M.; Crawford, Y.G.; Shen, A.; Wang, K.; Chang, D.P.; et al. Contribution of Antibody Hydrodynamic Size to Vitreal Clearance Revealed through Rabbit Studies Using a Species-Matched Fab. *Mol. Pharm.* **2016**, *13*, 2996–3003. [CrossRef]
15. Shatz, W.; Hass, P.E.; Peer, N.; Paluch, M.T.; Blanchette, C.; Han, G.; Sandoval, W.; Morando, A.; Loyet, K.M.; Bantseev, V.; et al. Identification and characterization of an octameric PEG-protein conjugate system for intravitreal long-acting delivery to the back of the eye. *PLoS ONE* **2019**, *14*, e0218613. [CrossRef]
16. Crowell, S.; Wang, K.; Famili, A.; Shatz, W.; Loyet, K.M.; Chang, V.; Liu, Y.; Prabhu, S.; Kamath, A.V.; Kelley, R.F. Influence of Charge, Hydrophobicity, and Size on Vitreous Pharmacokinetics of Large Molecules. *Transl. Vis. Sci. Technol.* **2019**, *8*, 1. [CrossRef] [PubMed]
17. Famili, A.; Crowell, S.R.; Loyet, K.M.; Mandikian, D.; Boswell, C.A.; Cain, D.; Chan, J.; Comps-Agrar, L.; Kamath, A.; Rajagopal, K. Hyaluronic Acid–Antibody Fragment Bioconjugates for Extended Ocular Pharmacokinetics. *Bioconjugate Chem.* **2019**, *30*, 2782–2789. [CrossRef] [PubMed]
18. Perlroth, D.V.; Charles, S.A.; Aggen, J.; Benoit, D.; To, W.; Mosyak, L.; Lin, L.; Cohen, J.; Ishino, T.; Somers, W. Dual PDGF/VEGF Antagonists. U.S. Patent 9,840,553 B2, 12 December 2017.
19. Oh, E.J.; Park, K.; Kim, K.S.; Kim, J.; Yang, J.-A.; Kong, J.-H.; Lee, M.Y.; Hoffman, A.S.; Hahn, S.K. Target specific and long-acting delivery of protein, peptide, and nucleotide therapeutics using hyaluronic acid derivatives. *J. Control. Release* **2010**, *141*, 2–12. [CrossRef] [PubMed]
20. Ghosh, J.G.; Nguyen, A.A.; Bigelow, C.E.; Poor, S.; Qiu, Y.; Rangaswamy, N.; Ornberg, R.; Jackson, B.; Mak, H.; Ezell, T.; et al. Long-acting protein drugs for the treatment of ocular diseases. *Nat. Commun.* **2017**, *8*, 14837. [CrossRef]
21. Fuchs, H.; Igney, F. Binding to Ocular Albumin as a Half-Life Extension Principle for Intravitreally Injected Drugs: Evidence from Mechanistic Rat and Rabbit Studies. *J. Ocul. Pharmacol. Ther.* **2017**, *33*, 115–122. [CrossRef]
22. Geroski, D.H.; Edelhauser, H.F. Drug delivery for posterior segment eye disease. *Investig. Ophthalmol. Vis. Sci.* **2000**, *41*, 961–964.
23. Yavuz, B.; Kompella, U.B. Ocular Drug Delivery. In *Pharmacologic Therapy of Ocular Disease*; Whitcup, S.M., Azar, D.T., Eds.; Springer International Publishing: Cham, Switzerland, 2017; Volume 242, pp. 57–93.
24. Iyer, S.; Radwan, A.E.; Hafezi-Moghadam, A.; Malyala, P.; Amiji, M. Long-acting intraocular Delivery strategies for biological therapy of age-related macular degeneration. *J. Control. Release* **2019**, *296*, 140–149. [CrossRef] [PubMed]
25. Campochiaro, P.A.; Marcus, D.M.; Awh, C.C.; Regillo, C.; Adamis, A.P.; Bantseev, V.; Chiang, Y.; Ehrlich, J.S.; Erickson, S.; Hanley, W.D.; et al. The Port Delivery System with Ranibizumab for Neovascular Age-Related Macular Degeneration. *Ophthalmology* **2019**, *126*, 1141–1154. [CrossRef] [PubMed]
26. Nickerson, C.S. Engineering the Mechanical Properties of Ocular Tissues. Ph.D. Thesis, California Institute of Technology, Pasadena, CA, USA, November 2005. [CrossRef]
27. Maurice, D.M. Protein Dynamics in the Eye Studied with Labelled Proteins. *Am. J. Ophthalmol.* **1959**, *47*, 361–368. [CrossRef]
28. Molokhia, S.A.; Jeong, E.-K.; Higuchi, W.I.; Li, S.K. Transscleral iontophoretic and intravitreal delivery of a macromolecule: Study of ocular distribution in vivo and postmortem with MRI. *Exp. Eye Res.* **2009**, *88*, 418–425. [CrossRef]
29. Del Amo, E.M.; Urtti, A. Rabbit as an animal model for intravitreal pharmacokinetics: Clinical predictability and quality of the published data. *Exp. Eye Res.* **2015**, *137*, 111–124. [CrossRef]
30. Gadkar, K.; Pastuskovas, C.V.; Le Couter, J.E.; Elliott, J.M.; Zhang, J.; Lee, C.V.; Sanowar, S.; Fuh, G.; Kim, H.S.; Lombana, T.N.; et al. Design and Pharmacokinetic Characterization of Novel Antibody Formats for Ocular Therapeutics. *Investig. Opthalmology Vis. Sci.* **2015**, *56*, 5390. [CrossRef]
31. Jordan, G.M.; Yoshioka, S.; Terao, T. The Aggregation of Bovine Serum Albumin in Solution and in the Solid State. *J. Pharm. Pharmacol.* **1994**, *46*, 182–185. [CrossRef]

32. Atmeh, R.F.; Arafa, I.M.; Al-Khateeb, M. Albumin aggregates: Hydrodynamic shape and physico-chemical properties. *Jordan J. Chem.* **2007**, *2*, 169–182.
33. Gschwind, A.; Ott, R.G.; Boucneau, J.; Buyse, M.-A.; Depla, E. Bispecific Binding Molecules Binding to VEGF and Ang2. WIPO Patent No. WO 2012/131078 Al, 30 March 2012.
34. Müller, G.H. Protein labelling with 3H-NSP (N-succinimidyl-[2,3-3H]propionate). *J. Cell Sci.* **1980**, *43*, 319–328.
35. Clausen, R.; Weller, M.; Hilgers, R.D.; Heimann, K.; Wiedemann, P. Quantitative determination of 5 vitreal proteins in the normal vitreous body and proliferative retinal diseases. *Fortschr. Ophthalmol. Z. Dtsch. Ophthalmol. Ges.* **1990**, *87*, 283–286. (In German)
36. Clausen, R.; Weller, M.; Wiedemann, P.; Heimann, K.; Hilgers, R.-D.; Zilles, K. An immunochemical quantitative analysis of the protein pattern in physiologic and pathologic vitreous. *Graefe's Arch. Clin. Exp. Ophthalmol.* **1991**, *229*, 186–190. [CrossRef] [PubMed]
37. Ishizaki, T. Immunochemical quantitative study of soluble proteins in the human vitreous. *Nippon. Ganka Gakkai Zasshi* **1984**, *88*, 1487–1491. (In Japanese) [PubMed]
38. Fosmark, D.S.; Bragadóttir, R.; Berg, J.P.; Berg, T.J.; Lund, T.; Sandvik, L.; Hanssen, K.F.; Stene-Johansen, I. Increased vitreous levels of hydroimidazolone in type 2 diabetes patients are associated with retinopathy: A case-control study. *Acta Ophthalmol. Scand.* **2007**, *85*, 618–622. [CrossRef] [PubMed]
39. Spranger, J.; Möhlig, M.; Osterhoff, M.; Bühnen, J.; Blum, W.F.; Pfeiffer, A. Retinal Photocoagulation Does Not Influence Intraocular Levels of IGF-I, IGF-II and IGF-BP3 in Proliferative Diabetic Retinopathy—Evidence for Combined Treatment of PDR with Somatostatin Analogues and Retinal Photocoagulation? *Horm. Metab. Res.* **2001**, *33*, 312–316. [CrossRef] [PubMed]
40. Van Bockxmeer, F.M.; Martin, C.E.; Constable, I.J. Iron-binding proteins with vitreous humour. *Biochim. Biophys. Acta Gen. Subj.* **1983**, *758*, 17–23. [CrossRef]
41. White, J.; Heß, D.; Raynes, J.K.; Laux, V.; Haertlein, M.; Forsyth, T.; Jeyasingham, A. The aggregation of "native" human serum albumin. *Eur. Biophys. J.* **2015**, *44*, 367–371. [CrossRef]
42. Maruyama, T.; Katoh, S.; Nakajima, M.; Nabetani, H. Mechanism of bovine serum albumin aggregation during ultrafiltration. *Biotechnol. Bioeng.* **2001**, *75*, 233–238. [CrossRef]
43. Sleep, D.; Cameron, J.; Evans, L.R. Albumin as a versatile platform for drug half-life extension. *Biochim. Biophys. Acta Gen. Subj.* **2013**, *1830*, 5526–5534. [CrossRef] [PubMed]
44. Balazs, E.A.; Denlinger, J.L. Aging changes in the vitreus. In *Aging and Human Visual Function*; Modern Aging Research Series Vol. 2; Sekuler, R., Kline, D., Dismukes, K., Eds.; Alan R. Liss, Inc.: New York, NY, USA, 1982; Volume 2, pp. 45–57.
45. Laurent, U.B.; Fraser, J. Turnover of hyaluronate in the aqueous humour and vitreous body of the rabbit. *Exp. Eye Res.* **1983**, *36*, 493–503. [CrossRef]

pharmaceutics

Article

Lutein-Loaded, Biotin-Decorated Polymeric Nanoparticles Enhance Lutein Uptake in Retinal Cells

Pradeep Kumar Bolla [1], Vrinda Gote [2], Mahima Singh [3], Manan Patel [3], Bradley A. Clark [1] and Jwala Renukuntla [1,*]

1 Department of Basic Pharmaceutical Sciences, Fred Wilson School of Pharmacy, High Point University, High Point, NC 27262, USA; bollaniper@gmail.com (P.K.B.); bclark@highpoint.edu (B.A.C.)
2 Division of Pharmacology and Pharmaceutical Sciences, School of Pharmacy, University of Missouri, 2464 Charlotte Street, Kansas City, MO 64108, USA; vrindagote@mail.umkc.edu
3 Department of Pharmaceutical Sciences, University of the Sciences in Philadelphia, Philadelphia, PA 19104, USA; msingh@mail.usciences.edu (M.S.); mpatel@biolinkonline.com (M.P.)
* Correspondence: jrenukun@highpoint.edu; Tel.: +1-336-841-9729

Received: 28 July 2020; Accepted: 21 August 2020; Published: 24 August 2020

Abstract: Age related macular degeneration (AMD) is one of the leading causes of visual loss and is responsible for approximately 9% of global blindness. It is a progressive eye disorder seen in elderly people (>65 years) mainly affecting the macula. Lutein, a carotenoid, is an antioxidant, and has shown neuroprotective properties in the retina. However, lutein has poor bioavailability owing to poor aqueous solubility. Drug delivery to the posterior segment of the eye is challenging due to the blood–retina barrier. Retinal pigment epithelium (RPE) expresses the sodium-dependent multivitamin transporter (SMVT) transport system which selectively uptakes biotin by active transport. In this study, we aimed to enhance lutein uptake into retinal cells using PLGA–PEG–biotin nanoparticles. Lutein loaded polymeric nanoparticles were prepared using O/W solvent-evaporation method. Particle size and zeta potential (ZP) were determined using Malvern Zetasizer. Other characterizations included differential scanning calorimetry, FTIR, and in-vitro release studies. In-vitro uptake and cytotoxicity studies were conducted in ARPE-19 cells using flow cytometry and confocal microscopy. Lutein was successfully encapsulated into PLGA and PLGA–PEG–biotin nanoparticles (<250 nm) with uniform size distribution and high ZP. The entrapment efficiency of lutein was ≈56% and ≈75% for lutein-loaded PLGA and PLGA–PEG–biotin nanoparticles, respectively. FTIR and DSC confirmed encapsulation of lutein into nanoparticles. Cellular uptake studies in ARPE-19 cells confirmed a higher uptake of lutein with PLGA–PEG–biotin nanoparticles compared to PLGA nanoparticles and lutein alone. In vitro cytotoxicity results confirmed that the nanoparticles were safe, effective, and non-toxic. Findings from this study suggest that lutein-loaded PLGA–PEG–biotin nanoparticles can be potentially used for treatment of AMD for higher lutein uptake.

Keywords: lutein; PLGA; PLGA–PEG–biotin; ARPE-19; retina; macular edema; age-related macular degeneration; biotin-decorated nanoparticles; polymeric nanoparticles; targeted therapy

---

1. Introduction

The eye is considered as one of the most sophisticated sensory organs of the human body due to its intricate anatomical structure. Anatomically, the eye can be broadly classified into two segments; i.e., (a) the anterior segment comprising cornea, aqueous humor, conjunctiva, ciliary body, iris, and lens, and (b) the posterior segment consisting of sclera, choroid, Bruch's membrane, retinal pigment epithelium, retina, optic nerve, and vitreous humor [1,2]. All the components of the anterior and posterior segments co-ordinate functionally and enable vision formation [3]. Alterations in the arrangement of these structures due to several factors such as aging, infection, inflammation, exposure to UV light, injury, air pollution, and over/under secretion of ocular fluids result in ocular diseases. Based on the localization, the diseases can be categorized into diseases affecting the anterior segment (ocular pain and inflammation, allergic conjunctivitis, blepharitis, keratitis, sty, anterior uveitis, and glaucoma) [4] and posterior segment (macular edema (cystic and diabetic macular edema), retinitis, age-related macular degeneration (AMD), proliferative vitreoretinopathy, diabetic retinopathy, choroidal neovascularization, and others) [3]. AMD is one of the leading causes of visual loss and is responsible for approximately 9% of global blindness [5]. It is a progressive eye disorder common in the elderly population (>65 years) mainly affecting the macula (central region of the retina) which is responsible for vision [6]. In 2012, it was estimated that 50 million people worldwide and 10 million people in the US suffered from AMD [6]. Till now, there was no clear understanding of the pathophysiology of AMD; however, it is a complicated disorder involving several risk factors which include smoking, UV light exposure, inflammation, and genetic factors [6–8]. The early stage of AMD is characterized by the deposition of yellowish deposits, known as soft drusen accumulations, in the retinal pigment epithelium and Bruch's membrane. The later stage of the disease is associated with loss of vision due to atrophy of photoreceptors and retinal pigment epithelium, retinal scarring, and detachment of retina [6,8]. If untreated, AMD is the leading cause of vision loss in 45% of all visual disability cases in the US alone [7]. Currently, there is no cure for AMD, and very few treatments such as anti-vascular endothelial growth factor (VEGF) have been proven to slow the progression of AMD. In addition, it is hypothesized that antioxidants and anti-inflammatory agents such as carotenoids (lutein, zeaxanthin, α-carotene, β-carotene, lycopene, and β-cryptoxanthin) protect against AMD by absorbing UV light, reducing oxidative stress, and stabilizing cell membranes [9].

Lutein is a dihydroxy xanthophyll carotenoid (β,ε-carotene-3,3′-diol) and is ubiquitously available from a variety of green leafy vegetables, fruits, flowers, egg yolk, etc. [10,11]. Since humans/animals cannot synthesize lutein, it must be obtained from the diet. It has been reported in the literature that lutein intake has improved the visual acuity and prevented the progression on AMD [12]. In 2016, Allison et al. showed that lutein was selectively taken up by the retinal pigment epithelial cells and showed protection against oxidative stress induced damage [13,14]. In addition, a recently completed clinical study has also demonstrated the protective effects of lutein in early stage AMD. Thus, it is hypothesized that lutein supplementation could halt the progression of AMD by reducing the oxidative stress in the retina caused by hypoxia and intense exposure to UV light [6]. Unfortunately, lutein has poor bioavailability due to high lipophilicity (log P 7.9) and poor aqueous solubility. [15,16].

Management of ocular/ophthalmic diseases is mainly achieved by using conventional topical products such as ophthalmic solutions, suspensions, and ointments [17]. However, the bioavailability of drugs administered by these conventional drug delivery systems is very low, ranging from 1% to 5% for hydrophobic drugs and <0.5% for hydrophilic drugs [17]. Drug delivery to the posterior part of the eye is challenging as the diseases affecting posterior segment require long-term delivery at a higher dose to the targeted tissues such as retina, choroid and Bruch's membrane. Moreover, treatment strategies such as oral, intraocular, and periocular routes have limited success due to the presence of static barriers such as sclera, retinal pigment epithelium (RPE), and multidrug resistance efflux pumps [3,18]. Various approaches have been explored in improving the ocular bioavailability, which include traditional formulation improvements, use of prodrugs, and carrier mediated drug transport. Formulation improvements include development of novel formulations such as suspensions, ointments, gels, nanoparticles, solutions, microemulsions, niosomes, liposomes, micelles, and others [1,2,17]. Transport of drugs, ions, and nutrients into and out of the ocular cell occurs mainly through transporters, receptors, and transmembrane proteins [19–21]. Transmembrane transporters/receptors are also involved in cellular processes such as absorption, distribution, and elimination of xenobiotics and nutrients [21,22]. Several transporters/receptors have been identified in the eye, which include glucose transporters, peptide transporters, amino acid transporters, nucleoside/nucleobase transporters, vitamin transporters, and nutrient receptors [21,22]. Various vitamin transporters have been characterized on the retinal epithelium which include folate, biotin, and ascorbic acid [20,22]. Transporter-mediated drug delivery can be achieved by conjugation of drug to a specific substrate/nutrient such as folic acid or biotin. The nutrient will be recognized by the transporter proteins and conjugated drug is translocated across the cell membrane thus increasing permeability [22].

Biotin (vitamin B7) is an essential water-soluble vitamin useful for cell growth, function, and development. It is a co-factor for several carboxylase enzymes which catalyze multiple metabolic reactions and acts as a regulator in cell signaling pathways and gene expression. Biotin cannot be synthesized in mammalian cells and therefore must be obtained from exogenous sources. Biotin transport in cells is mediated through sodium-dependent multivitamin transporter (SMVT) or biotin transporter. Biotin transporter is a high-affinity transporter involved in transport of biotin, whereas SMVT is a low-affinity transporter involved in the transport of biotin, pantothenic acid, and lipoic acid. It has been reported in the literature that SMVT is abundantly expressed in the blood–retina barrier and retinal cells (D407 cells). Thus, it is known that biotinylated prodrugs and polymeric nanoparticles utilize the SMVT and biotin transporters for enhanced permeability of drugs [19,23]. Moreover, scientists have reported that biotin-decorated polymeric nanoparticles have enhanced the uptake of poorly soluble drugs such as doxorubicin [24], SN-38 [25], and 15,16-dihydrotanshinone [26]. Therefore, we hypothesize that lutein-loaded PLGA–PEG–biotin polymeric nanoparticles can enhance the uptake of lutein into the retinal cells through SMVT transport system.

Polymeric nanoparticles are known to improve the bioavailability of drugs with poor biopharmaceutical properties [27,28]. Furthermore, polymeric nanoparticles have advantages, including biocompatibility, enhanced stability, sustained release, and improved efficacy [28–32]. Polymeric nanoparticles are prepared using biodegradable polymers such as poly(lactide co-glycolide) (PLGA), gelatin, chitosan, albumin, alginate polycaprolactone, polyglycolides, poly (methyl methacrylate), and polyethylene glycol (PEG) [28,33]. Previously, lutein was encapsulated into several nanocarriers, such as PLGA nanoparticles, liposomes, nanoemulsions, nanocrystals, lipid nanocapsules, and nanodispersions [34–40]. In the present study we aimed to prepare and characterize lutein-loaded polymeric nanoparticles (PLGA and PLGA–PEG–biotin) and evaluate their enhanced uptake in retinal cells.

2. Materials and Methods

2.1. Materials

Lutein (90%) was purchased from Acros Organics (Fair Lawn, NJ, USA). Dimethyl sulfoxide (DMSO), methanol (HPLC grade), tetrahydrofuran (HPLC grade), dichloromethane, sodium chloride, disodium hydrogen phosphate, potassium dihydrogen phosphate, MTT (3-(4,5-dimethylthiazol-2-yl)-2,5-diphenyltetrazolium bromide), and ammonium chloride (NH_4Cl) were purchased from Fisher Scientific (Fair Lawn, NJ, USA). Sodium dodecyl sulphate (SDS) and polyvinyl alcohol (PVA: MW: 30,000–70,000) were procured from Sigma Aldrich (St. Louis, MO, USA). PLGA (50:50; Mw: 10,000 Da) and PLGA–PEG–biotin (50:50; Mw: 10,000 Da–2000 Da) were purchased from Akina PolySciTech, Inc, West Lafayette, IN, USA. Dulbecco's modified Eagle medium (DMEM, Gibco's), Dulbecco's phosphate-buffered saline (DPBS), Triton-X, and trypsin (TrypLE, Gibco) were purchased from Thermo Fisher Scientific (Fair Lawn, NJ, USA). Cellulose ester dialysis tubing (Biotech grade; Mw: 300 kDa) was procured from Spectrum Laboratories, Inc (Gardena, CA, USA). Fluorescein isothiocyanate (FITC) and 4′,6-diamidino-2-Phenylindole (DAPI) were purchased from Invitrogen, Labelling and Detection, Molecular Probes, ThermoFisher Scientific, (Fair Lawn, NJ, USA). Human retinal pigment epithelial cell line (ARPE-19) was purchased from American Type Culture Collection (ATCC, Manassas, VA, USA).

2.2. Methods

2.2.1. Preparation of Lutein-Loaded Polymeric Nanoparticles

Lutein-loaded polymeric nanoparticles were prepared using the oil-in-water (O/W) emulsion solvent evaporation method reported earlier with slight modifications (Figure 1) [41,42]. In brief, 100 mg of polymer (PLGA or PLGA–PEG–biotin) was dissolved in 5 mL of dichloromethane and lutein (20 mg) was dissolved in 2 mL dichloromethane separately. The polymer and lutein solutions were mixed to form a homogenous organic phase. The organic phase was sonicated in a bath sonicator for 5 min followed by slow addition to an aqueous solution of 2% PVA (20 mL) under continuous stirring on a magnetic stirrer. The resultant mixture was sonicated at 30% amplitude for 5 min using a probe sonicator (Fisher Scientific™ Model 505 Sonic Dismembrator) to obtain an emulsion. The sonication step was performed in an icebath to prevent overheating of the emulsion. After sonication, the emulsion was stirred gently at room temperature overnight until complete evaporation of dichloromethane. Un-entrapped lutein and PVA residue were removed from the emulsion by washing three times with deionized water using Hitachi ultracentrifuge at 22,000× *g* for 1 h. Finally, the nanoparticles formed were lyophilized using laboratory freeze dryer (Harvestright, Salt Lake City, UT, USA) for 24 h.

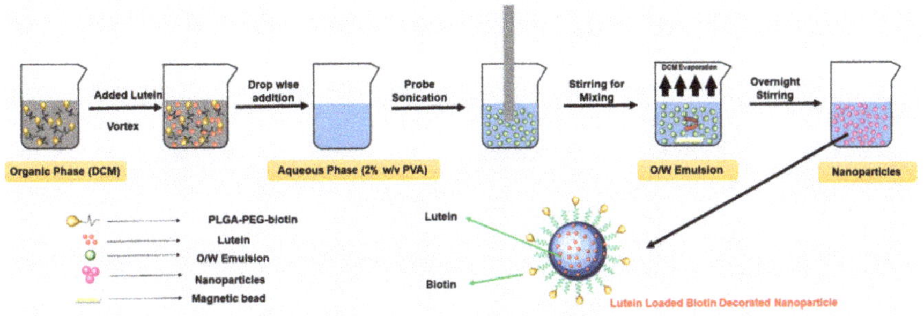

Figure 1. Schematic representation of oil in water emulsion-solvent evaporation method for preparation of lutein loaded PLGA-PEG-biotin nanoparticles.

2.2.2. Determination of Size, Polydispersity Index, and Zeta Potential

The particle size, polydispersity index (PDI), and zeta-potential (ZP) of lutein-loaded PLGA and PLGA–PEG–biotin nanoparticles were measured using the dynamic light scattering (DLS) technique. The nanoparticles (200 µL) were dispersed in 10 mL of double distilled de-ionized water and measurements were determined using Malvern Zetasizer Nano ZS90 (Malvern Instruments, Malvern, UK) at 25 °C. All the measurements were performed in triplicate (n = 3).

2.2.3. Lutein Quantification Using HPLC

The amount of lutein in the samples was quantified using Waters Alliance e2695 HPLC (Waters Corporation, Milford, MA, USA) equipped with 2996 photodiode array (PDA) detector and Empower 2.0 software. The analysis was performed using reverse-phase Waters® C-18 column (5 µm; 250 mm × 4.6 mm) under isocratic conditions (flow rate of 1 mL/min at 25 °C). Mobile phase was a mixture (90:10) of methanol and tetrahydrofuran. The analyte was monitored at 450 nm. Sample injection volume was 20 µL and the run time was 10 min. Retention time of lutein was 3.85 min [43]. All the samples injected were filtered through 0.45 µm membrane filter. Stock solution (1 mg/mL) of lutein was prepared in the mobile phase, and calibration standards (n = 3) ranging from (1 µg/mL to 100 µg/mL) were serially diluted in the mobile phase. Similar standard curve was also prepared by dissolving lutein in DMSO. Calibration curves were obtained by plotting peak area against the concentration of lutein. The lutein content in the samples was determined quantitatively using the linear regression equations from the calibration curves ($R^2 > 0.99$). The HPLC method provided rapid and reproducible results without a significant difference in intra and inter-day analysis.

2.2.4. Determination of Lutein Encapsulation Efficiency (%EE) and Drug Loading (%DL)

The encapsulation and loading of lutein into nanoparticles were determined by quantifying the lutein content in freeze dried nanoparticles using HPLC. In brief, the freeze-dried nanoparticles (10 mg) were dissolved in 10 mL DMSO and the amount of lutein was determined using HPLC. The %EE and %DL of lutein in the nanoparticles were determined using the following formulae (Equations (1) and (2)). All the measurements were performed on three different samples (n = 3).

$$\%EE = (\text{Amount of lutein remained in nanoparticles})/(\text{Initial amount of lutein}) \times 100 \quad (1)$$

$$\%DL = (\text{Weight of lutein in nanoparticles})/(\text{Weight of polymer used}) \times 100 \quad (2)$$

2.2.5. Differential Scanning Calorimetry (DSC)

Interaction of lutein with PLGA and PLGA–PEG–biotin was confirmed using DSC technique. Calorimetric analysis was performed for lutein, PVA, polymers (PLGA and PLGA–PEG–biotin), and lutein-loaded polymeric nanoparticles using a DSC822e (Mettler Toledo, Columbus, OH, USA) instrument. Samples (3–11 mg) were accurately weighed in aluminum pans (40 µL capacity) and were hermetically sealed using a crimping device. The reference standard was an empty aluminum pan. Nitrogen was purged at a rate of 20 mL/min during the analysis. Samples were held isothermally at 25 °C for 5 min and then heated at 10 °C/min to 280 °C. All the thermograms recorded were analyzed using STARe software.

2.2.6. Fourier Transform Infrared Spectroscopy (FTIR)

A JASCO-FT/IR 4600 instrument (Jasco instruments, Easton, MD, USA) using the attenuated total reflection (ATR) technique was used to record the FTIR spectra of lutein, PVA, polymers (PLGA and PLGA–PEG–biotin), and lutein-loaded polymeric nanoparticles. The sample compartment was flushed with argon prior to each run. Each sample was ground to fine powder with a KBr pellet. The scanning range was from 500–4000 cm^{-1}. After measurement of the spectrum, data were analyzed and plotted. Carbon dioxide (CO_2) and water (H_2O) peaks were subtracted from the original spectrum to obtain the final IR spectrum.

2.2.7. In-Vitro Release Studies

Drug release behavior from lutein-loaded polymeric nanoparticles was determined using the dialysis bag method (MWCO: 300 kDa) [27]. Initially, several release media were screened to determine the solubility of lutein. Phosphate-buffered saline (pH 7.4) with 0.2% *w*/*v* sodium dodecyl sulphate was chosen as the suitable release medium for release studies to maintain sink conditions (saturation solubility: 40.1 ± 8.47 µg/mL) [10]. After selecting the release medium, 1 mL lutein-loaded polymeric nanoparticles (≈1 mg lutein) were transferred to individual dialysis tubing and release medium (1 mL) was added to each tubing. Leakage was prevented by sealing the tubing tightly at both ends. Sealed dialysis tubings loaded with nanoparticles were transferred to 250 mL beakers containing 100 mL of release medium in a shaking water bath (100 rpm) (maintained at 37 ± 0.5 °C). To prevent any evaporation of release medium, beakers were tightly sealed with parafilm. At a pre-determined time-intervals (0.5, 1, 2, 3, 4, 5, 6, 7, 8, and 24 h), samples (10 mL) were collected from each beaker and replaced with 10 mL of fresh release medium. The cumulative amount of drug released from the formulations was quantified using UV spectrophotometer (6405 UV/Vis Spectrophotometer, Jenway, Staffordshire, UK) by measuring the absorbance at λ_{max} of 440 nm at different timepoints. All experiments were performed on three different samples (n = 3).

2.2.8. Cell Culture Studies

Cell Culture

ARPE-19 cells were used to determine the in-vitro cellular uptake and cytotoxicity of lutein and lutein-loaded polymeric nanoparticles (PLGA and PLGA–PEG–biotin). ARPE-19 cells were purchased from American Type Culture Collection and stored in liquid nitrogen. The cells were cultured in DMEM/ F-12 (1:1 ratio) media containing 10% (*v*/*v*) heat-inactivated fetal bovine serum (FBS), 100 U/mL penicillin, 100 μg/mL streptomycin, 1% (*v*/*v*) MEM non-essential amino acids, and 1% sodium bicarbonate. The cells were grown in T-75 Corning flasks and incubated at 37 °C, 5% CO_2, and 95% relative humidity and harvested at 80–90% confluency.

FITC Labelling

The in-vitro cellular uptake levels of lutein-loaded PLGA and PLGA–PEG–biotin nanoparticles, and lutein alone were determined by labeling (surface adsorption) the samples with FITC, which is widely used to label proteins [44], drugs [45], and polymers [46]. FITC labelling was performed according to a previously reported protocol with slight modifications [47]. In brief, 10 μg of lyophilized nanoparticles (PLGA or PLGA–PEG–biotin) were suspended in 50 mM phosphate buffered saline (1 mL) to make a 10 μg/mL of nanoparticle suspension. Separately, FITC was powdered and dissolved in DMSO (1 mg/mL) since FITC was not soluble in water. The FITC solution was added to nanoparticle suspension and incubated in the dark for 12 h at 4 °C. After incubation, 1 mL of 50 mM NH_4Cl was added to the mixture to inactivate unreacted FITC. Further, the FITC labelled polymeric nanoparticles were subjected to dialysis to remove any unreacted FITC and NH_4Cl. Finally, the FITC-labelled nanoparticles were filtered through a 0.22 μm nylon filter to ensure sterility. The samples were aliquoted and stored at −20 °C until further use. The sample for FITC-labelled lutein was prepared in a similar way as described above, except lutein was dissolved in DMSO (5 mg/mL) and then mixed with FITC solution.

In Vitro Cellular Uptake Studies Using Flow Cytometry (Fluorescence-Activated Cell Sorting (FACS))

Intracellular uptake of FITC-labelled nanoparticles and lutein alone in ARPE-19 cells was determined by incubating the cells and then evaluating time-dependent uptake using flow cytometry (FACS). ARPE-19 cells were seeded in a 12-well plate at a density of 0.5×10^6 cells/ well with 1 mL of complete DMEM/F-12 media. The cells were treated with 10 μL of each sample which included control (DMSO), FITC–lutein, FITC–lutein PLGA nanoparticles, and FITC–lutein PLGA–PEG–biotin nanoparticles. Then, the treated cells were incubated for various times (3, 6, 9, and 12 h). At each time point, the media was removed from the wells and the cells were harvested by using 200 μL of trypsin (TrypLE, Gibco). This was followed by 5 min incubation and addition of serum containing DMEM/F-12 media. Further, the cells were collected in FACS tubes and centrifuged at 20,000 rpm for 5 min to obtain a cell pellet. The media was then discarded, and the cells were washed twice using 1 mL of (DPBS). The final sample was prepared in DPBS and acquired by flow cytometry to determine the mean FITC fluorescence intensity of the cells at an excitation wavelength of 490 nm. The mean FITC fluorescence intensity values obtained for all the samples ($n = 3$) were plotted using bar-graphs in GraphPad Prism (version 5.0) and the differences were observed.

In Vitro Cellular Uptake Studies Using Confocal Laser Scanning Microscopy

Intracellular distribution of FITC-labelled polymeric nanoparticles (PLGA and PLGA–PEG–biotin) in ARPE-19 cells was determined using confocal laser scanning microscopy (CLSM). FITC–lutein–PLGA–PEG–biotin nanoparticles, FITC–lutein PLGA nanoparticles and FITC–lutein were prepared using the same method described in earlier sections. The cells were seeded in an 8-chamber confocal microscopy slide precoated with collagen (Nunc Lab-Tek, Thermo Fisher Scientific, Waltham, MA, USA) with 200 μL of complete DMEM/F-12 media. This was followed by 10 μL additions of various treatment samples which included control (DMSO), FITC–lutein, FITC–lutein PLGA nanoparticles, and FITC–lutein PLGA-Peg-biotin nanoparticles into each chamber of the 8-chamber plate. Further, the treatment groups were incubated for 6 and 12 h. At each time point, the culture media was removed, and the cells were washed two times on a shaker with 300 µL of DPBS for 5 min. This was followed by fixing the cells with freshly prepared cold 4% buffered paraformaldehyde solution (200 µL) and incubating at 37 °C for 20 min. After incubation, the fixing solution was removed, and the cells were washed again using 300 µL DPBS (3 times × 5 min each). Further, the nuclei of the cells were stained with 100 µL of DAPI (working solution of 10 µg/mL) for 15 min in dark. The cells were then mounted and sealed with cover slip to prevent any evaporation of mounting media and dehydration of the cells. The ARPE-19 cell slides were stored at 4 °C before the actual analysis. A Leica Confocal Laser Scanning Microscope (Leica TCS SP5, Wetzlar, Germany) was used to analyze the cells for green fluorescence-FITC and blue fluorescence-DAPI.

In Vitro Cell Viability Studies (MTT Assay)

Cellular cytotoxicity of lutein PLGA–PEG–biotin nanoparticles, lutein PLGA nanoparticles and lutein alone were determined in ARPE-19 cells by using MTT (3-(4,5-dimethylthiazol-2-yl)-2,5-diphenyltetrazolium bromide) assay. MTT is a yellow tetrazole dye which is reduced to purple formazan crystals by viable or living cells. The cell viability is determined by measuring the absorbance. ARPE-19 cells were seeded at a density of 1×10^4 cells in a 96-well plate. The cells were supplemented with 200 µL of DMEM/ F-12 culture media (1:1 ratio) containing 10% fetal bovine serum. The samples (lutein–PLGA–PEG–biotin nanoparticles, lutein–PLGA nanoparticles. and lutein) were prepared in serum free DMEM: F-12 media and filtered through a 0.22 µm nylon filter. A small quantity of dichloromethane (200 uL) was added to dissolve lutein in the media. Complete DMEM/F-12 from the cell lines was replaced with 100 µL solution of treatment samples prepared in serum free media. All the three treatment groups were analyzed at four concentrations which included 10, 20, and 50 µg/mL of equivalent lutein. The cells were incubated with each sample for 24 h at 5% CO_2 and 37 °C. After incubation, the cells were washed twice with PBS. Separately, MTT reagent A and MTT reagent B were mixed in the ratio 100:1 to make a stock solution of the dye. Further, 20 µL of MTT stock solution was added to each well and incubated for 3.5 h. Finally, the absorbance of formazan solution was measured using a microplate reader (BioRad, Hercules, CA, USA) at an excitation wavelength of 485 nm. Five percent Triton-X prepared in serum free media served as the positive control and serum free media lacking any samples served as the negative control. Cell viability was calculated according to the formula (Equation (3)).

$$\begin{aligned}\% \text{ Cell Viability} = &(\text{Absorbance of sample-absorbance of negative control})/\\&(\text{Absorbance of positive control-absorbance of negative control}) \times 100\end{aligned} \quad (3)$$

2.2.9. Statistical Analysis

Statistical analysis was performed using GraphPad Prism® software (Version 5.0, San Diego, CA, USA). A non-parametric *t*-test followed by Bonferroni's multiple comparison post-test was used to compare cellular uptake of nano-formulations.

3. Results and Discussion

3.1. Determination of Particle Size, PDI, and ZP

The size, PDI, and ZP of lutein-loaded polymeric nanoparticles are provided in Table 1. Results show that all the lutein-loaded nanoparticles had sizes of <250 nm. The sizes of lutein-loaded PLGA and PLGA–PEG–biotin nanoparticles were 196.4 ± 20.04 nm and 208.0 ± 3.38 nm, respectively. Figure 2 confirms the monodisperse distribution of nanoparticles for both formulations. Zeta potential results revealed that lutein-loaded PLGA–PEG–biotin nanoparticles had higher

ZP values (−27.2 ± 2.04 mV) compared to lutein-loaded PLGA nanoparticles (−11.2 ± 2.12 mV). The shift of ZP values towards higher negativity could be due to the presence of terminal carboxylic groups in the PEG–biotin portion of block polymer. In addition, negative ZP values result in higher stability of nanoparticles due to prevention of non-specific interaction with proteins in biological proteins. PLGA-based polymers were chosen for this study due to unique properties which include biocompatibility, targetability, biodegradability, and versatile biodegradation kinetics. Peroxisomal degradation of PLGA-based polymers will result in the formation of safe degradation products such as lactic acid and glycolic acid, which are removed by the Kreb's cycle [48]. However, due to the hydrophobic nature of PLGA, the nanoparticles are rapidly cleared by the mononuclear phagocyte system using opsonization process. Therefore, coating with hydrophilic polymers such as PEG could bypass the opsonization process due to steric repulsion forces. This results in enhancing the bioavailability and half-lives of the drugs by increasing the circulation time of nanoparticles in the plasma [48,49]. Moreover, all the polymers (PLGA, PLGA–PEG–biotin, PVA) are approved by USFDA as inactive ingredients in various formulations [50].

Table 1. Size, polydispersity index (PDI), zeta-potential (ZP), and encapsulation efficiency (%EE) of lutein-loaded PLGA and PLGA–PEG–biotin nanoparticles (n = 3). Data are represented as means ± standard deviations (SDs).

S.no	Particle Type	Size (nm)	PDI	ZP (mV)	EE (%)
1	Lutein PLGA	196.4 ± 20.04	0.087 ± 0.016	−11.12 ± 2.12	56.05 ± 7.28
2	Lutein PLGA–PEG–biotin	208.0 ± 3.38	0.206 ± 0.016	−27.2 ± 2.04	74.56 ± 10.25

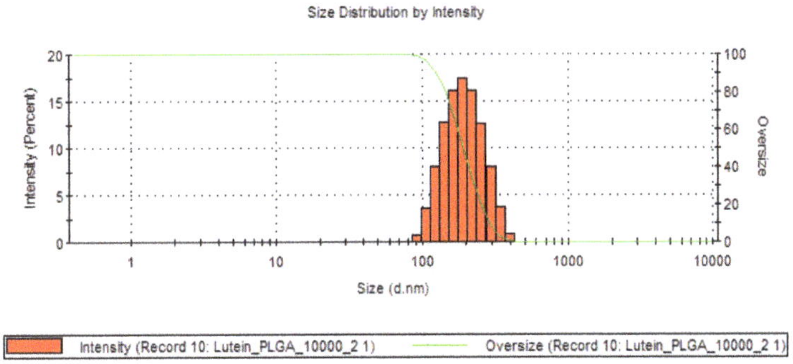

(a)

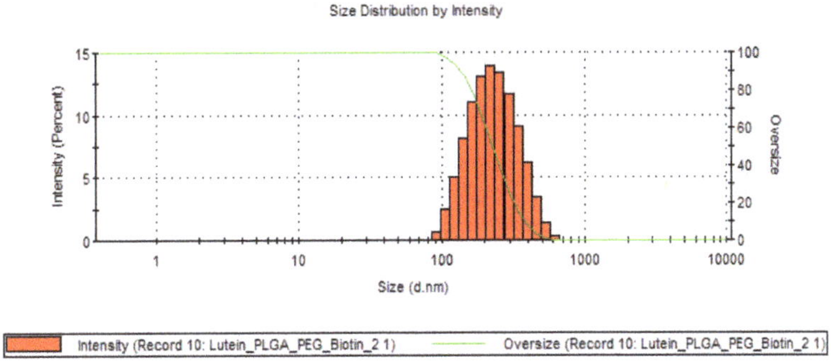

(b)

Figure 2. Size distribution curves of (**a**) lutein–PLGA nanoparticles and (**b**) lutein PLGA–PEG–biotin nanoparticles.

3.2. Determination of Encapsulation Efficiency (%EE) and Drug Loading (%DL)

Results showed that PLGA–PEG–biotin polymer had greater lutein encapsulation compared with the PLGA polymer. The entrapment of lutein values were 56.05% ± 7.28% and 74.56% ± 10.25% for lutein PLGA and PLGA–PEG–biotin nanoparticles, respectively. The lutein loading values in PLGA and PLGA–PEG–biotin nanoparticles were ≈11.2% and ≈14.9%, respectively (Table 1).

3.3. DSC

DSC is a widely used technique to confirm the polymorphic changes of drugs and polymers in formulation research. Thermograms of lutein, polymers, PVA, and lutein-loaded nanoparticles are provided in Figure 3. Results show that lutein has sharp characteristic endothermic peaks at 64.07 °C and 58.15 °C. In addition, PLGA had a small endothermic peak at 45.28 °C. There was no specific peak/melting point observed for PLGA–PEG–biotin and PVA, suggesting their amorphous nature. The characteristic endothermic peak of lutein disappeared in thermograms of lutein-loaded polymeric nanoparticles, suggesting that lutein was rendered amorphous by its interaction with the polymer. The transformation of lutein from crystalline to amorphous form is important, as amorphous forms are characterized by higher solubilities and increased bioavailability [51–54]. Similar results (loss of characteristic peak) were observed in other studies where crystalline drugs such as SN-38, doxorubicin oxcarbazepine, prilocaine, and adefovir were encapsulated into PLGA-based micro- and nanoparticles [24,25,55–57].

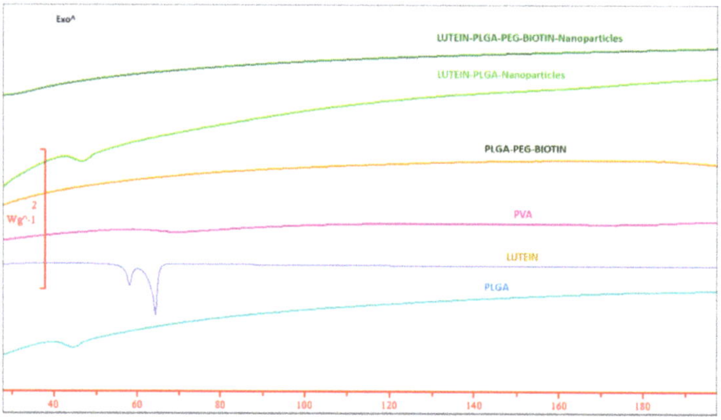

Figure 3. DSC thermograms of lutein-loaded PLGA–PEG–biotin nanoparticles, lutein-loaded PLGA nanoparticles, PLGA–PEG–biotin, PVA, lutein, and PLGA.

3.4. FTIR

FTIR spectroscopy was used to evaluate the surface chemistries of lutein, PVA, PLGA, PLGA–PEG–biotin, lutein-loaded PLGA, and PLGA–PEG–biotin nanoparticles (Figure 4). The broad transmittance band of lutein between 3588.88 and 3073.01 cm^{-1} corresponds to the OH stretching vibrations; it was absent in lutein-loaded PLGA and PLGA–PEG–biotin nanoparticles. In addition, characteristic C–H stretching bands were observed for lutein at 2958 and 2912 cm^{-1}. A strong transmittance of lutein was also observed at 1620.15 cm^{-1} which was absent in the spectra of the lutein-loaded PLGA–PEG–biotin and PLGA nanoparticles. There was no obvious difference in the spectra of the polymers (PLGA and PLGA–PEG–biotin) and lutein-loaded polymeric nanoparticles. Results from FTIR confirm that the characteristic peaks of lutein were absent in the FTIR spectra of lutein-loaded polymeric nanoparticles. This could have been due to the strong interaction of lutein with the polymers which resulted in the absence of characteristic peaks. Similar results were observed for other nanoparticle systems [58]. Moreover, it is evident that the encapsulation of lutein did not result in any structural changes of polymers which might be attributed to either the small concentration of the drug or due to its bonding and non-bonding interactions with the surrounding matrix.

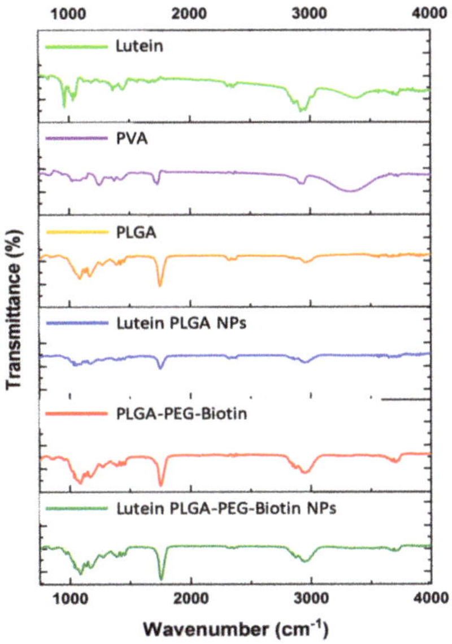

Figure 4. Fourier-transform infrared spectroscopy (FTIR) spectra of freeze-dried lutein-loaded polymeric nanoparticles, PLGA, PLGA–PEG–biotin, PVA, and lutein.

3.5. In-Vitro Release Studies

The in vitro release profile of lutein from PLGA and PLGA–PEG–biotin nanoparticles is provided in Figure 5. Release profiles revealed that the both the nano-formulations showed similar sustained release patterns with 100% of lutein released within 24 h. Higher encapsulation of lutein in the polymers could have resulted in less space for polymer hydration and led to the slower release of lutein [59]. Overall, release studies validate the sustained/controlled release of drugs from polymeric nanoparticles.

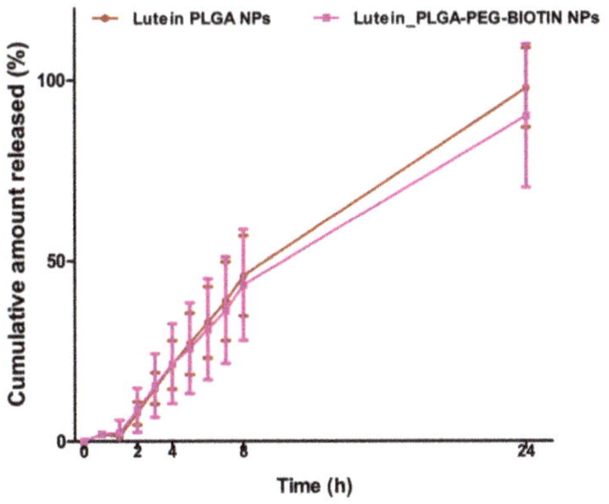

Figure 5. In-vitro release of lutein from lutein-loaded PLGA and PLGA–PEG–biotin NPs. Data are expressed as means ± SDs (n = 3).

3.6. *In-Vitro Cellular Uptake Studies*

In-vitro cellular uptake of lutein was determined in the ARPE-19 cell line to understand the intracellular localization and uptake of the biotin-decorated PLGA-PEG nanoparticles loaded with lutein compared to lutein–PLGA nanoparticles and lutein alone. These studies also helped to compare the uptake of the lutein nanoparticles within the cytoplasm of ARPE-19 cells. FACS and confocal microscopy were used as quantitative and qualitative analysis methods, respectively, to determine the cellular uptake.

3.6.1. FACS Analysis

FITC-labelled, lutein-loaded, biotin-decorated PLGA nanoparticles; PLGA nanoparticles; and lutein alone were incubated with ARPE-19 cells to determine in-vitro uptake at predetermined time points by using flow cytometry (mean FITC florescence intensity). Figure 6 depicts the time- dependent uptakes of FITC-labelled nanoparticles and lutein alone in ARPE-19 cells. Results show that at all time points, there was a significantly higher ($p < 0.05$) mean FITC florescence intensity with lutein-loaded, biotin-decorated nanoparticles and PLGA nanoparticles compared to lutein alone. In addition, it was also observed that at all time points intra cellular uptake of lutein-loaded biotin nanoparticles was numerically higher compared to lutein-loaded PLGA nanoparticles. However, the difference was not statistically significant ($p > 0.05$). Higher uptake with biotin-decorated nanoparticles could be attributed to the presence of a SMVT transporter on the surface of ARPE-19 cells. Results obtained in the study are consistent with other studies evaluating time-dependent uptake of biotinylated nanoparticles for targeted drug delivery [27,56].

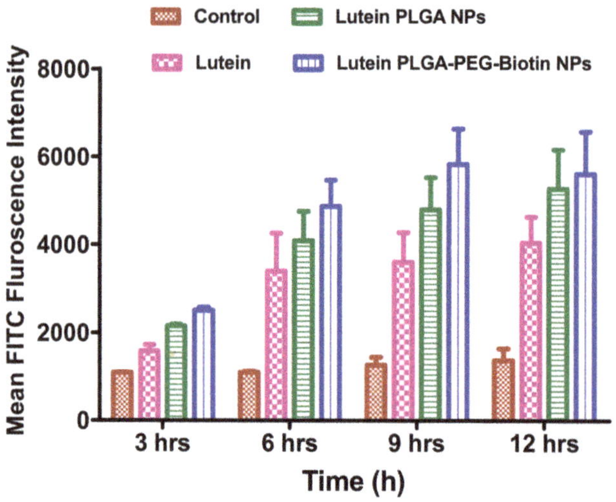

Figure 6. FACS analysis of control, lutein, and lutein-loaded polymeric nanoparticles (PLGA and PLGA–PEG–biotin) for 3, 6, 9, and 12 h in ARPE-19 cells. Data are expressed as means ± SEMs (n = 3).

3.6.2. Confocal Microscopy

In-vitro cellular uptake of FITC labelled lutein nanoparticles (PLGA and PLGA–PEG–biotin) and FITC-labelled lutein was performed using confocal laser scanning microscopy for qualitative analysis of lutein uptake by ARPE-19 cells. At the end of each time point the cells were washed, fixed, stained with DAPI, and mounted on a slide for visual observation for confocal microscopy. Figures 7 and 8 depict the in-vitro uptake of FITC-labelled lutein nanoparticles and FITC-labelled lutein at 6 h and 12 h, respectively. It can be observed clearly that the green fluorescence for FITC increased in all the treatment groups with time. It is also interesting to note that at all timepoints, the fluorescence in the cells treated with FITC-labelled, lutein-loaded polymeric nanoparticles (PLGA and PLGA–PEG–biotin) was higher compared to FITC-labelled lutein. These results are well corroborated with the flow cytometry results. This could mean that biotin-decorated lutein nanoparticles and lutein PLGA nanoparticles are well absorbed via the lipid bilayer of ARPE-19 cells as compared to the lutein alone. Thus, the rate of internalization for lutein nanoparticles (PLGA and PLGA–PEG–biotin) into the cytoplasm and nuclei was higher compared to lutein alone. In addition, at 6 and 12 h timepoints, stronger fluorescence was observed with lutein-loaded PLGA–PEG–biotin nanoparticles compared to lutein-loaded PLGA nanoparticles. The higher uptake with biotin-decorated nanoparticles could be attributed to the SMVT transporter mediated uptake in ARPE-19 cells. Higher expression of biotin transporters on the surface of ARPE-19 cells resulted in higher uptake of lutein compared to other treatment groups.

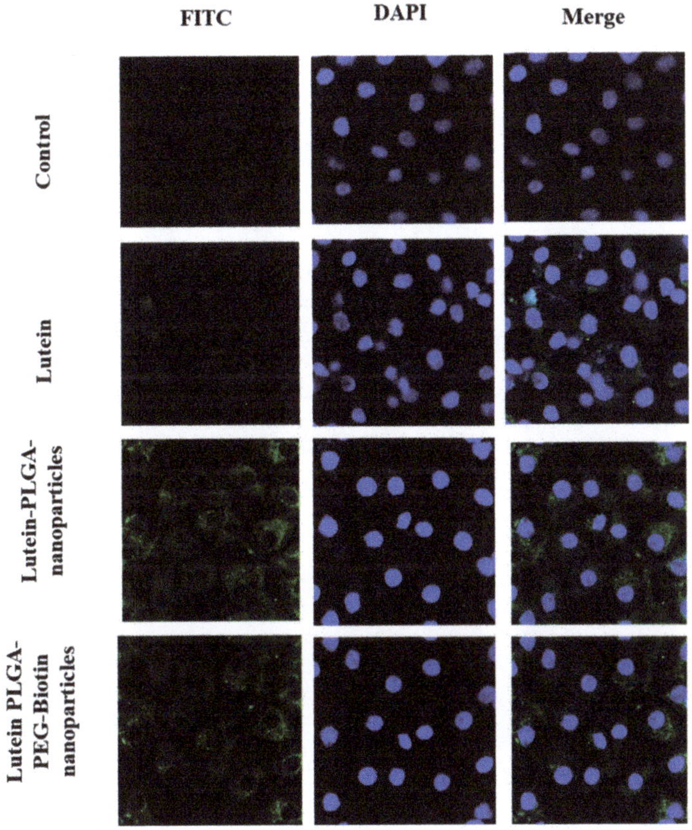

Figure 7. Confocal laser scanning microscopy images of FITC-labelled lutein and FITC-labelled lutein polymeric nanoparticles (PLGA and PLGA–PEG–biotin) at 6 h in ARPE-19 cells.

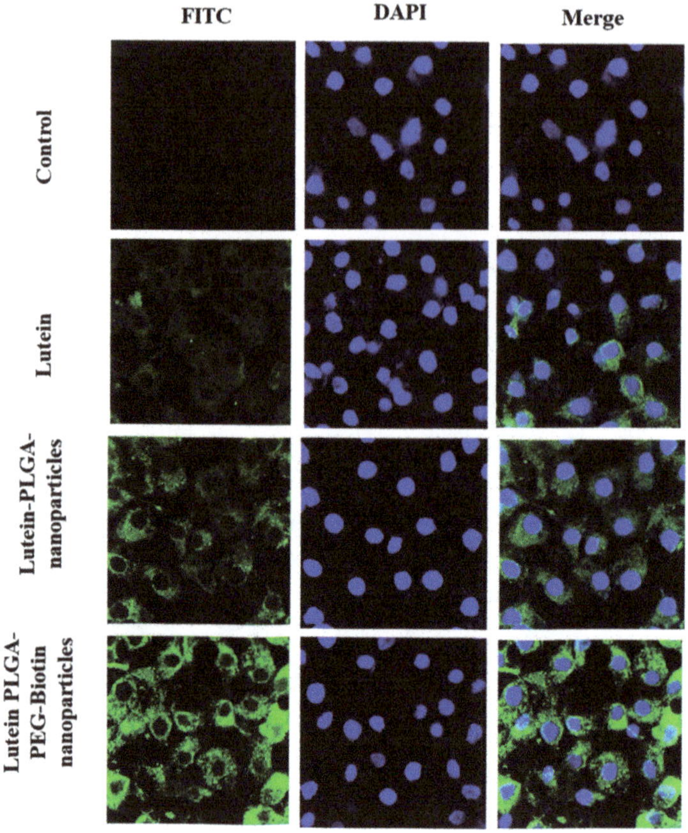

Figure 8. Confocal laser scanning microscopy images of FITC-labelled lutein and FITC-labelled lutein polymeric nanoparticles (PLGA and PLGA–PEG–biotin) at 12 h in ARPE-19 cells.

3.7. *In-Vitro Cytotoxicity Studies*

Figure 9 shows the cell viability (%) of ARPE-19 cells when treated with increasing concentrations of lutein-loaded polymeric nanoparticles and lutein alone. Lutein and lutein-loaded polymeric nanoparticles did not exhibit any significant cytotoxicity at 10, 20, and 50 μg/mL concentrations, proving that these nano-formulations are safe, effective, and non-toxic. Conjugates of biotin to PLGA nanoparticles did not result in any signs of toxicity and they were equivalent to lutein alone.

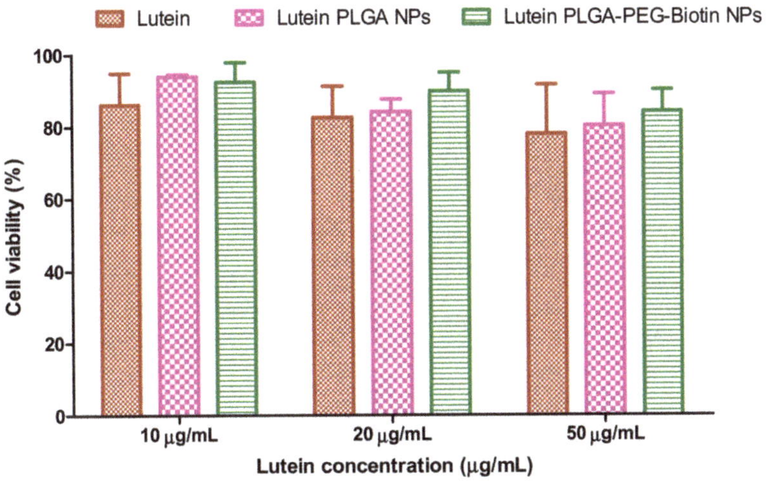

Figure 9. Cell viability (%) of ARPE-19 cells when treated with increasing concentrations of lutein and lutein-loaded polymeric nanoparticles.

4. Conclusions

In conclusion, we have successfully developed and characterized lutein-loaded, biotin-decorated polymeric nanoparticles. The obtained nanoparticles possessed particle sizes of <250 nm with narrow size distributions. Moreover, the biotin targeted nanoparticles showed higher encapsulation efficiency and drug loading. In-vitro cellular uptake studies revealed that biotin-decorated nanoparticles exhibited higher uptake of lutein compared to PLGA nanoparticles and lutein alone. In vitro cytotoxicity results confirmed that the nanoparticles showed higher cell viability compared to lutein alone. Collectively, we have found that the biotin-conjugated nanoparticles may be an appropriate formulation for targeted drug delivery in the treatment of AMD and other retinal diseases. However, these results are preliminary and should be confirmed by evaluating the efficacy, safety, and pharmacokinetics in pre-clinical models.

Author Contributions: Conceptualization, J.R. and P.K.B.; methodology, P.K.B., M.S., M.P., and V.G.; software, P.K.B. and V.G.; formal analysis, P.K.B.; investigation, J.R.; resources, J.R.; data curation, P.K.B. and V.G.; writing—original draft preparation, P.K.B.; writing—review and editing, J.R. and B.A.C.; supervision, J.R. and B.A.C.; funding acquisition, J.R. All authors have read and agreed to the published version of the manuscript.

Funding: This research received no external funding.

Acknowledgments: The authors would like to thank Joint School of Nanoscience and Nanoengineering (Greensboro, NC, USA) for providing access to Malvern Zetasizer.

Conflicts of Interest: All authors declare no conflict of interest.

References

1. Gaudana, R.; Jwala, J.; Boddu, S.H.; Mitra, A.K. Recent perspectives in ocular drug delivery. *Pharm. Res.* **2008**, *26*, 1197. [CrossRef] [PubMed]
2. Gaudana, R.; Ananthula, H.K.; Parenky, A.; Mitra, A.K. Ocular Drug Delivery. *AAPS J.* **2010**, *12*, 348–360. [CrossRef] [PubMed]
3. Nayak, K.; Misra, M. A review on recent drug delivery systems for posterior segment of eye. *Biomed. Pharm.* **2018**, *107*, 1564–1582. [CrossRef] [PubMed]
4. Chen, H. Recent developments in ocular drug delivery. *J. Drug Target.* **2015**, *23*, 597–604. [CrossRef] [PubMed]

5. Keenan, T.D.; Vitale, S.; Agrón, E.; Domalpally, A.; Antoszyk, A.N.; Elman, M.J.; Clemons, T.E.; Chew, E.Y.; Age-Related Eye Disease Study 2 Research Group. AREDS2 Research Group Visual Acuity Outcomes after Anti–Vascular Endothelial Growth Factor Treatment for Neovascular Age-Related Macular Degeneration. *Ophthalmol. Retin.* **2020**, *4*, 3–12. [CrossRef] [PubMed]
6. Ma, L.; Yan, S.-F.; Huang, Y.-M.; Lu, X.-R.; Qian, F.; Pang, H.-L.; Xu, X.-R.; Zou, Z.; Dong, P.-C.; Xiao, X.; et al. Effect of Lutein and Zeaxanthin on Macular Pigment and Visual Function in Patients with Early Age-related Macular Degeneration. *Ophthalmology* **2012**, *119*, 2290–2297. [CrossRef] [PubMed]
7. Richer, S.; Stiles, W.; Statkute, L.; Pulido, J.; Frankowski, J.; Rudy, D.; Pei, K.; Tsipursky, M.; Nyland, J. Double-masked, placebo-controlled, randomized trial of lutein and antioxidant supplementation in the intervention of atrophic age-related macular degeneration: The Veterans LAST study (Lutein Antioxidant Supplementation Trial). *Optom. J. Am. Optom. Assoc.* **2004**, *75*, 216–229. [CrossRef]
8. De Jong, P.T. Age-Related Macular Degeneration. *N. Engl. J. Med.* **2006**, *355*, 1474–1485. [CrossRef]
9. Wu, J.; Cho, E.; Willett, W.C.; Sastry, S.M.; Schaumberg, D.A. Intakes of Lutein, Zeaxanthin, and Other Carotenoids and Age-Related Macular Degeneration During 2 Decades of Prospective Follow-up. *JAMA Ophthalmol.* **2015**, *133*, 1415–1424. [CrossRef]
10. Hu, D.; Lin, C.; Liu, L.; Li, S.; Zhao, Y. Preparation, characterization, and in vitro release investigation of lutein/zein nanoparticles via solution enhanced dispersion by supercritical fluids. *J. Food Eng.* **2012**, *109*, 545–552. [CrossRef]
11. Li, S.-Y.; Fu, Z.; Ma, H.; Jang, W.-C.; So, K.-F.; Wong, D.; Lo, A.C.Y. Effect of Lutein on Retinal Neurons and Oxidative Stress in a Model of Acute Retinal Ischemia/Reperfusion. *Investig. Opthalmol. Vis. Sci.* **2009**, *50*, 836–843. [CrossRef] [PubMed]
12. Moschos, M.M.; Dettoraki, M.; Tsatsos, M.; Kitsos, G.; Kalogeropoulos, C. Effect of carotenoids dietary supplementation on macular function in diabetic patients. *Eye Vis.* **2017**, *4*, 23. [CrossRef] [PubMed]
13. Allison, G.S.; Draper, C.S.; Soekamto, C.; Gong, X.M.; Rubin, L.P. Lutein Protects the Retinal Pigment Epithelium Against Hypoxic and Oxidative Stress: In Vitro Studies. *FASEB J.* **2016**, *30*, 2–5.
14. Gong, X.; Draper, C.S.; Allison, G.S.; Marisiddaiah, R.; Rubin, L.P. Effects of the Macular Carotenoid Lutein in Human Retinal Pigment Epithelial Cells. *Antioxidants* **2017**, *6*, 100. [CrossRef] [PubMed]
15. Ozawa, Y.; Sasaki, M.; Takahashi, N.; Kamoshita, M.; Miyake, S.; Tsubota, K. Neuroprotective Effects of Lutein in the Retina. *Curr. Pharm. Des.* **2012**, *18*, 51–56. [CrossRef]
16. Lutein. 2020. Available online: https://www.drugbank.ca/drugs/DB00137 (accessed on 31 May 2020).
17. Bachu, R.D.; Chowdhury, P.; Al-Saedi, Z.H.F.; Karla, P.K.; Boddu, S.H. Ocular Drug Delivery Barriers—Role of Nanocarriers in the Treatment of Anterior Segment Ocular Diseases. *Pharmaceutics* **2018**, *10*, 28. [CrossRef]
18. Kiernan, D.F.; Lim, J.I. Topical Drug Delivery for Posterior Segment Disease, Retin. Available online: https://retinatoday.com/pdfs/0510RT_Feature_Lim_Mosh.pdf (accessed on 24 July 2020).
19. Cholkar, K.; Ray, A.; Agrahari, V.; Pal, D.; Mitra, A.K. Transporters and receptors in the anterior segment of the eye. In *Ocular Transporters and Receptors*; Elsevier: Amsterdam, The Netherlands, 2013; pp. 115–168.
20. Patel, A.; Gokulgandhi, M.; Khurana, V.; Mitra, A.K. *5-Transporters and Receptors in the Posterior Segment of the Eye*; Woodhead Publishing: Cambridge, UK, 2013; pp. 169–205.
21. Dey, S.; Mitra, A.K. Transporters and receptors in ocular drug delivery: Opportunities and challenges. *Expert Opin. Drug Deliv.* **2005**, *2*, 201–204. [CrossRef]
22. Boddu, S.H.; Nesamony, J. Utility of transporter/receptor(s) in drug delivery to the eye. *World J. Pharmacol.* **2013**, *2*, 1–17. [CrossRef]
23. Vadlapudi, A.D.; Vadlapatla, R.K.; Pal, D.; Mitra, A.K. Functional and Molecular Aspects of Biotin Uptake via SMVT in Human Corneal Epithelial (HCEC) and Retinal Pigment Epithelial (D407) Cells. *AAPS J.* **2012**, *14*, 832–842. [CrossRef]
24. Singh, Y.; Viswanadham, K.D.R.; Jajoriya, A.K.; Meher, J.G.; Raval, K.; Jaiswal, S.; Dewangan, J.; Bora, H.K.; Rath, S.K.; Lal, J.; et al. Click Biotinylation of PLGA Template for Biotin Receptor Oriented Delivery of Doxorubicin Hydrochloride in 4T1 Cell-Induced Breast Cancer. *Mol. Pharm.* **2017**, *14*, 2749–2765. [CrossRef]
25. Mehdizadeh, M.; Rouhani, H.; Sepehri, N.; Varshochian, R.; Ghahremani, M.H.; Amini, M.; Gharghabi, M.; Ostad, S.N.; Atyabi, F.; Baharian, A.; et al. Biotin decorated PLGA nanoparticles containing SN-38 designed for cancer therapy. *Artif. Cells Nanomed. Biotechnol.* **2016**, *45*, 1–10. [CrossRef] [PubMed]

26. Luo, J.; Meng, X.; Su, J.; Ma, H.; Wang, W.; Fang, L.; Zheng, H.; Qin, Y.; Chen, T. Biotin-Modified Polylactic-co-Glycolic Acid Nanoparticles with Improved Antiproliferative Activity of 15,16-Dihydrotanshinone I in Human Cervical Cancer Cells. *J. Agric. Food Chem.* **2018**, *66*, 9219–9230. [CrossRef] [PubMed]
27. Joseph, A.; Wood, T.; Chen, C.-C.; Corry, K.; Snyder, J.M.; Juul, S.E.; Parikh, P.; Nance, E. Curcumin-loaded polymeric nanoparticles for neuroprotection in neonatal rats with hypoxic-ischemic encephalopathy. *Nano Res.* **2018**, *11*, 5670–5688. [CrossRef]
28. El-Say, K.M.; El-Sawy, H. Polymeric nanoparticles: Promising platform for drug delivery. *Int. J. Pharm.* **2017**, *528*, 675–691. [CrossRef]
29. Crucho, C.I.C.; Barros, M.T. Polymeric nanoparticles: A study on the preparation variables and characterization methods. *Mater. Sci. Eng. C* **2017**, *80*, 771–784. [CrossRef]
30. Kumari, A.; Yadav, S.K.; Yadav, S.C. Biodegradable polymeric nanoparticles based drug delivery systems. *Colloids Surf. B Biointerfaces* **2010**, *75*, 1–18. [CrossRef]
31. Khan, I.; Saeed, K.; Khan, I. Nanoparticles: Properties, applications and toxicities. *Arab. J. Chem.* **2019**, *12*, 908–931. [CrossRef]
32. Bahrami, B.; Hojjat-Farsangi, M.; Mohammadi, H.; Anvari, E.; Ghalamfarsa, G.; Yousefi, M.; Jadidi-Niaragh, F. Nanoparticles and targeted drug delivery in cancer therapy. *Immunol. Lett.* **2017**, *190*, 64–83. [CrossRef]
33. Banik, B.L.; Fattahi, P.; Brown, J.L. Polymeric nanoparticles: The future of nanomedicine. *Wiley Interdiscip. Rev. Nanomed. Nanobiotechnol.* **2015**, *8*, 271–299. [CrossRef]
34. Lim, C.; Kim, D.-W.; Sim, T.; Hoang, N.H.; Lee, J.W.; Lee, E.S.; Youn, Y.S.; Oh, K.T. Preparation and characterization of a lutein loading nanoemulsion system for ophthalmic eye drops. *J. Drug Deliv. Sci. Technol.* **2016**, *36*, 168–174. [CrossRef]
35. Tan, T.B.; Yussof, N.S.; Abas, F.; Mirhosseini, H.; Nehdi, I.A.; Tan, C.P. Stability evaluation of lutein nanodispersions prepared via solvent displacement method: The effect of emulsifiers with different stabilizing mechanisms. *Food Chem.* **2016**, *205*, 155–162. [CrossRef] [PubMed]
36. Muhoza, B.; Zhang, Y.; Xia, S.; Cai, J.; Zhang, X.; Su, J. Improved stability and controlled release of lutein-loaded micelles based on glycosylated casein via Maillard reaction. *J. Funct. Foods* **2018**, *45*, 1–9. [CrossRef]
37. Mitri, K.; Shegokar, R.; Gohla, S.; Anselmi, C.; Müller, R.H. Lutein nanocrystals as antioxidant formulation for oral and dermal delivery. *Int. J. Pharm.* **2011**, *420*, 141–146. [CrossRef] [PubMed]
38. Steiner, B.; McClements, D.J.; Davidov-Pardo, G. Encapsulation systems for lutein: A review. *Trends Food Sci. Technol.* **2018**, *82*, 71–81. [CrossRef]
39. Silva, J.; Geiss, J.M.T.; Oliveira, S.M.; Brum, E.D.S.; Sagae, S.C.; Becker, D.; Leimann, F.V.; Ineu, R.P.; Guerra, G.P.; Gonçalves, O.H. Nanoencapsulation of lutein and its effect on mice's declarative memory. *Mater. Sci. Eng. C* **2017**, *76*, 1005–1011. [CrossRef] [PubMed]
40. Brum, A.A.S.; Dos Santos, P.P.; Da Silva, M.M.; Paese, K.; Guterres, S.S.; Costa, T.M.; Pohlmann, A.R.; Jablonski, A.; Flôres, S.H.; Rios, A.D.O. Lutein-loaded lipid-core nanocapsules: Physicochemical characterization and stability evaluation. *Colloids Surf. A Physicochem. Eng. Asp.* **2017**, *522*, 477–484. [CrossRef]
41. Jwala, J.; Boddu, S.H.; Shah, S.; Sirimulla, S.; Pal, D.; Mitra, A.K. Ocular Sustained Release Nanoparticles Containing Stereoisomeric Dipeptide Prodrugs of Acyclovir. *J. Ocul. Pharmacol. Ther.* **2011**, *27*, 163–172. [CrossRef]
42. Boddu, S.H.; Vaishya, R.; Jwala, J.; Vadlapudi, A.; Pal, D.; Mitra, A.K. Preparation and Characterization of Folate Conjugated Nanoparticles of Doxorubicin using Plga-Peg-Fol Polymer. *Med. Chem.* **2012**, *2*, 068–075. [CrossRef]
43. Liu, R.; Sun, M.; Liu, X.; Fan, A.; Wang, Z.; Zhao, Y. Interplay of stimuli-responsiveness, drug loading and release for a surface-engineered dendrimer delivery system. *Int. J. Pharm.* **2014**, *462*, 103–107. [CrossRef]
44. Chaganti, L.K.; Venkatakrishnan, N.; Bose, K. An efficient method for FITC labelling of proteins using tandem affinity purification. *Biosci. Rep.* **2018**, *38*. [CrossRef]
45. Michlewska, S.; Kubczak, M.; Maroto-Díaz, M.; Del Olmo, N.S.; Ortega, P.; Shcharbin, D.; Gómez, R.; De La Mata, F.J.; Ionov, M.; Bryszewska, M. Synthesis and Characterization of FITC Labelled Ruthenium Dendrimer as a Prospective Anticancer Drug. *Biomolecules* **2019**, *9*, 411. [CrossRef] [PubMed]

46. Damgé, C.; Maincent, P.; Ubrich, N. Oral delivery of insulin associated to polymeric nanoparticles in diabetic rats. *J. Control. Release* **2007**, *117*, 163–170. [CrossRef] [PubMed]
47. Mandal, A.; Cholkar, K.; Khurana, V.; Shah, A.; Agrahari, V.; Bisht, R.; Pal, D.; Mitra, A.K. Topical Formulation of Self-Assembled Antiviral Prodrug Nanomicelles for Targeted Retinal Delivery. *Mol. Pharm.* **2017**, *14*, 2056–2069. [CrossRef] [PubMed]
48. Javidfar, S.; Pilehvar-Soltanahmadi, Y.; Farajzadeh, R.; Lotfi-Attari, J.; Shafiei-Irannejad, V.; Hashemi, M.; Zarghami, N. The inhibitory effects of nano-encapsulated metformin on growth and hTERT expression in breast cancer cells. *J. Drug Deliv. Sci. Technol.* **2018**, *43*, 19–26. [CrossRef]
49. Firouzi-Amandi, A.; Dadashpour, M.; Nouri, M.; Zarghami, N.; Serati-Nouri, H.; Jafari-Gharabaghlou, D.; Karzar, B.H.; Mellatyar, H.; Aghebati-Maleki, L.; Babaloo, Z.; et al. Chrysin-nanoencapsulated PLGA-PEG for macrophage repolarization: Possible application in tissue regeneration. *Biomed. Pharm.* **2018**, *105*, 773–780. [CrossRef]
50. USFDA, Inactive Ingredient Search for Approved Drug Products, (n.d.). Available online: https://www.accessdata.fda.gov/scripts/cder/iig/index.cfm (accessed on 28 July 2019).
51. Bolla, P.K.; Kalhapure, R.S.; Rodriguez, V.A.; Ramos, D.V.; Dahl, A.; Renukuntla, J. Preparation of solid lipid nanoparticles of furosemide-silver complex and evaluation of antibacterial activity. *J. Drug Deliv. Sci. Technol.* **2019**, *49*, 6–13. [CrossRef]
52. Bolla, P.K.; Meraz, C.A.; Rodriguez, V.A.; Deaguero, I.G.; Singh, M.; Yellepeddi, V.K.; Renukuntla, J. Clotrimazole Loaded Ufosomes for Topical Delivery: Formulation Development and In-Vitro Studies. *Molecules* **2019**, *24*, 3139. [CrossRef]
53. Rodriguez, V.A.; Bolla, P.K.; Kalhapure, R.S.; Boddu, S.H.; Neupane, R.; Franco, J.; Renukuntla, J. Preparation and Characterization of Furosemide-Silver Complex Loaded Chitosan Nanoparticles. *Processes* **2019**, *7*, 206. [CrossRef]
54. Morissette, S.L. High-throughput crystallization: Polymorphs, salts, co-crystals and solvates of pharmaceutical solids. *Adv. Drug Deliv. Rev.* **2004**, *56*, 275–300. [CrossRef]
55. Musumeci, T.; Serapide, M.; Pellitteri, R.; Dalpiaz, A.; Ferraro, L.; Magro, R.D.; Bonaccorso, A.; Carbone, C.; Veiga, F.; Sancini, G.; et al. Oxcarbazepine free or loaded PLGA nanoparticles as effective intranasal approach to control epileptic seizures in rodents. *Eur. J. Pharm. Biopharm.* **2018**, *133*, 309–320. [CrossRef]
56. Bragagni, M.; Gil-Alegre, M.E.; Mura, P.; Cirri, M.; Ghelardini, C.; Mannelli, L.D.C. Improving the therapeutic efficacy of prilocaine by PLGA microparticles: Preparation, characterization and in vivo evaluation. *Int. J. Pharm.* **2018**, *547*, 24–30. [CrossRef] [PubMed]
57. Ayoub, M.M.; Elantouny, N.G.; Elnahas, H.; Ghazy, F.E.-D.S. Injectable PLGA Adefovir microspheres; the way for long term therapy of chronic hepatitis-B. *Eur. J. Pharm. Sci.* **2018**, *118*, 24–31. [CrossRef] [PubMed]
58. Ahlawat, J.; Deemer, E.M.; Narayan, M. Chitosan Nanoparticles Rescue Rotenone-Mediated Cell Death. *Materials* **2019**, *12*, 1176. [CrossRef] [PubMed]
59. Kamaly, N.; Yameen, B.; Wu, J.; Farokhzad, O.C. Degradable Controlled-Release Polymers and Polymeric Nanoparticles: Mechanisms of Controlling Drug Release. *Chem. Rev.* **2016**, *116*, 2602–2663. [CrossRef] [PubMed]

pharmaceutics

MDPI

Article

Do Ophthalmic Solutions of Amphotericin B Solubilised in 2-Hydroxypropyl-γ-Cyclodextrins Possess an Extended Physicochemical Stability?

Philip Chennell [1,*], Mouloud Yessaad [2], Florence Abd El Kader [2], Mireille Jouannet [2], Mathieu Wasiak [2], Yassine Bouattour [1] and Valérie Sautou [1]

[1] Université Clermont Auvergne, CHU Clermont-Ferrand, CNRS, SIGMA Clermont-Ferrand, ICCF, 63000 Clermont-Ferrand, France; ybouattour@chu-clermontferrand.fr (Y.B.); vsautou@chu-clermontferrand.fr (V.S.)

[2] CHU Clermont-Ferrand, Pôle Pharmacie, 63000 Clermont-Ferrand, France; myessaad@chu-clermontferrand.fr (M.Y.); florence.abdelkader@ch-lepuy.fr (F.A.E.K.); mjouannet@chu-clermontferrand.fr (M.J.); mwasiak@chu-clermontferrand.fr (M.W.)

* Correspondence: pchennell@chu-clermontferrand.fr

Received: 15 July 2020; Accepted: 17 August 2020; Published: 19 August 2020

Abstract: Fungal keratitis is a sight-threatening disease for which amphotericin B eye drops is one of the front-line treatments. Unfortunately, there are currently no commercial forms available, and there is little data concerning the long-term stability of compounded formulations based on intravenous dosages forms. New formulations of amphotericin B ophthalmic solutions solubilised with γ-cyclodextrins have shown promising in-vitro results, but stability data is also lacking. The objective of this study was therefore to investigate the stability of a formulation of ready-to-use amphotericin B solubilised in 2-hydroxypropyl-γ-cyclodextrins (AB-HP-γ-CD), for 350 days. An amphotericin B deoxycholate (ABDC) formulation was used as a comparator. Analyses used were the following: visual inspection, turbidity, osmolality and pH measurements, amphotericin B quantification by a stability-indicating liquid chromatography method, breakdown product research, and sterility assay. AB-HP-γ-CD formulation showed signs of chemical instability (loss of amphotericin B) after 28 and 56 days at 25 °C and 5 °C. Adding an antioxidant (ascorbic acid) to the formulation did not improve stability. ABDC formulation showed signs of physical instability (increased turbidy and amphotericin B precipitation) after 28 days and 168 days at 25 °C and 5 °C. As such, AB-HP-γ-CD formulation does not provide long-term stability for ophthalmic amphotericin B solutions.

Keywords: amphotericin B; γ-cyclodextrins; stability; fungal keratitis

1. Introduction

Fungal (or mycotic) keratitis is a purulent, ulcerative infection of the cornea that can cause corneal opacification and irreversible blindness if left untreated [1,2]. It has been estimated that 1,000,000 cases occur annually in the world, but as it is often under-suspected, it is also underdiagnosed and real numbers might be a lot higher [3]. Risk factors for developing such an affection have been documented as living in a tropical or subtropical environment [4,5], underlying corneal and ocular surface diseases, ocular trauma, and wearing contact lenses [6–8]. Among the fungal germs isolated, the most common are Fusarium species, Aspergillus species, and Candida species [4,7,9–11]. For the treatment of such infections, clinicians have the choice between drugs from two main typical classes of antifungal agents that are azoles (voriconazole, fluconazole, ketoconazole, posaconazole, itraconazole) and polyenes (natamycin and amphotericin B) [12]. Of these drugs, amphotericin B is broad-spectrum agent and is active against most of fungi, especially Candida spp [13], but also possesses very low minimal inhibitory concentrations against Fusarium and Aspergillus [14], allowing it to be also one of the first line treatments of fungal keratitis caused by those germs, at dosages ranging from 0.1% to 0.5% [7,15–17]. Another advantage of amphotericin B is that it seems to be less likely to induce resistances as opposed to azole antifungals [18].

Amphotericin B is a heptaene possessing a heavily hydroxylated region on the ring opposite to the multiple conjugated double bonds, a mycosamine moiety and a carboxylic group (Figure 1A). These latter groups impart a polar character to the molecule (which contributes to the relative insolubility in organic solvents), whereas the opposite unsaturated terminal imparts a nonpolar character (which contributes to its poor aqueous solubility) [18]. Such properties make it hard to create an optimum formulation for ophthalmic delivery. As amphotericin B eye drops are not currently commercially available in the world, the most used formulation consists of diluting a marketed intravenous dosage form of amphotericin B deoxycholate (ABDC) in 5% glucose to reach the desired concentration. Other preparations of lipid-based formulations of amphotericin B can also be used [13,18] but they are far more expensive and not readily available in all countries. Unfortunately, ABDC is known to possess very short (less than two weeks) stability at ambient temperature, and even if longer stabilities of 60 to 120 days have been reported (often at the end point of the studies), not all physicochemical parameters were studied, making it difficult to conclude [19,20]. Overall, these shortfalls make it difficult for compounding pharmacies to adequately manage amphotericin B preparations, and short shelf life at ambient temperature means complexifying transport and storage conditions, especially for tropical and subtropical regions. To address these issues, the use of cyclodextrins to solubilize amphotericin B have been tested. Vikmon et al. first described to use of γ-cyclodextrins to solubilize up to 0.65 mg/mL of amphotericin B [21], and since then, several other authors have studied the theoretical and practical aspects of using various cyclodextrins [22–24], including derivatives like 2-hydroxypropyl-γ-cyclodextrin, whose chemical structure is presented Figure 1B. From what has been described, the easiest way to incorporate amphotericin B is to first dissolve the cyclodextrins in an aqueous media, then alkalinise the solution to pH 12 in order to allow the ionic form of amphotericin B to solubilize in the media and incorporate itself into the cyclodextrins. The solution is then brought back to a more tolerable pH. The complexation of amphotericin B using this preparation method has been studied by various authors and is now well documented [23,25,26]. As the first in-vitro tests performed on such formulations seem promising [27,28], it becomes important to know if cyclodextrin complexation with amphotericin B is capable to achieve ready to use formulations with long-term stability.

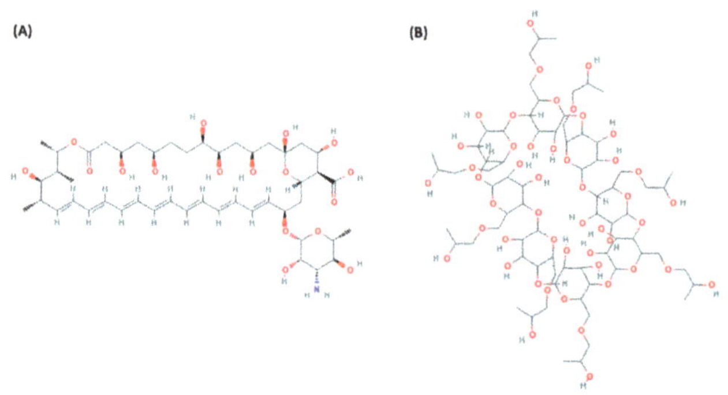

Figure 1. Chemical structure of amphotericin B (**A**) and 2-hydroxypropyl-γ-cyclodextrin (**B**). Publically available from [29].

The objective of this study was therefore to investigate the stability of a formulation of ready-to-use amphotericin B solubilised in 2-hydroxypropyl-γ-cyclodextrins (AB-HP-γ-CD) in low-density polyethylene eyedroppers, for 350 days at 5 °C and 25 °C. A classical ABDC formulation was used as comparator.

2. Materials and Methods

2.1. Preparation of the ABDC Formulation

Amphotericin B deoxycholate powder (obtained from Fungizone® powder for injectable solution vials, Bristol-Myers Squibb, Rueil-Malmaison, France) was reconstituted with sterile 5% glucose (B. Braun Medical, Boulogne Billancourt, France) to obtain a 5 mg/mL solution of AB. After complete dissolution of the powder, the solution was transferred into an empty ethylene-vinyl acetate bag (Baxter, Guyancourt, France) and diluted with a 5% glucose sterile solution to obtain a 2.5 mg/mL amphotericin B solution. All manipulations were performed under the laminar air flow of an ISO 4.8 microbiological safety cabinet.

2.2. Preparation of the AB-HP-γ-CD Formulation

To prepare 500 mL of 2.5 mg/mL solution of amphotericin B, initially 100 g HP-γ-CD (Wacker Chemie AG, Burghausen, Germany) were dissolved in 350 mL water for injection (WFI) (Versylène® Fresenius, Bad Homburg, Germany). After total dissolution, the pH was adjusted to 12 with a 1 N sodium hydroxide solution before adding 1250 mg of amphotericin B base (pharmaceutical grade, Inresa, Bartenheim, France). The mixture was stirred to obtain a clear and orange solution then the pH was readjusted to 7.0 with 1N hydrochloric acid. The solution volume was completed to 500 mL with a NaH_2PO_4/Na_2HPO_4 phosphate buffer solution to obtain a final buffer concentration of 0.02/0.03 mol/L.

As complementary study, a formulation of 2.5 mg/mL HP-γ-CD amphotericin B eye-drops containing 0.5 mg/mL ascorbic acid (0.05%) was also prepared, as following: 100 g of HP-γ-CD was dissolved in 450 mL of WFI adjusted to pH 12 with a NaOH solution, to which 1250 mg of amphotericin B powder were solubilised. After dissolution, 3500 mg of Na2HPO4 and 2500 mg of ascorbic acid were added, and the volume adjusted to 500 mL with WFI.

2.3. Conditioning and Storage

The resulting solutions were sterilely conditioned (4 mL per unit) using a sterile syringe tipped with a 0.22 µm pore size filter (reference SLGP033RS, Milipore SAS, Molsheim CEDEX, France) under the laminar air flow of an ISO 4.8 microbiological safety cabinet into low density polyethylene (LDPE) eyedroppers (CAT, Lorris, France). The eyedroppers were stored at controlled refrigerated temperature (Whirlpool refrigerator) at 5 °C ± 2 °C or in a climate chamber (Binder GmbH, Tuttlingen, Germany) at 25 °C ± 2 °C and 60% residual humidity, until analysis.

2.4. Study Design

The stability of the different amphotericin B eye drops formulations was studied in unopened eyedroppers for up to 350 days at two different temperature 25 °C and 5 °C.

Immediately after conditioning, and then at determined times (3, 7, 14, 28, 56, 168, and 350 days after conditioning), 4 units per tested storage temperature were subjected to the following analyses: visual inspection, osmolality, pH measurements, amphotericin B quantification and breakdown products research. Turbidity measurements were performed at the same analysis times on the pooled volume from the 4 units. Additionally, for the formulation containing ascorbic acid, a chromaticity and luminescence analysis was performed.

Sterility determination assay was realized on 4 extra dedicated units after 0, 28, 168, and 350 days of storage.

2.5. Analyses

2.5.1. Visual Inspection

The multidose eyedroppers were emptied into polycarbonate test tubes and the amphotericin B solutions were visually inspected under white light in front of a matt black panel and a non-glare white panel of an inspection station (LV28, Allen and Co., Liverpool, UK). The aspect and colour of the solutions were noted, and a screening for visible particles, haziness, or gas development was performed.

2.5.2. Osmolality, pH and Turbidity Measurements

For each unit, osmolality was measured using Model 2020 osmometer (Advanced instruments Inc., Radiometer, SAS, Neuilly Plaisance, France). pH measurements were made with a SevenMultiTM pH-meter with an InLabTM Micro Pro glass electrode (Mettler-Toledo, Viroflay, France).

Turbidity was measured using a 2100Q Portable Turbidimeter (Hach Lange, Marne La Vallée, France), by the pooling of four samples per analysed experimental condition and assay time to obtain the necessary volume for the analysis. The results were expressed in Formazin Nephelometric Units (FNU).

2.5.3. Amphotericin B Quantification and Breakdown Products Research

- Chemicals and instrumentation

For each unit, Amphotericin B was quantified and degradation products researched using a liquid chromatography (LC). The LC system that was used was a Prominence-I LC2030C 3D with diode array detection (Shimadzu France SAS, Marne La Vallée, France) and the associated software used to record and interpret chromatograms was LabSolutions™ version 5.82 (Shimadzu France SAS, Marne La Vallée, France). The method that was used was adapted from Chang et al. [30]. The LC separation column used was a C18 a Synergi 4 µm Hydro-RP 80 Å column (Phenomenex, France). The mobile phase in isocratic mode was composed of 29.1/12.8/7.1/51 (*v*/*v*/*v*/*v*) methanol/acetonitril/tetrahydrofuran/EDTA 2.5 mM mixture. All chemicals used for the chromatography analysis were of analytical grade. The flow rate through the column for the analysis was set at 1.5 mL/min, with the column thermo-regulated to a temperature of 30 °C. The eye drops were diluted a 100-fold with deionized water, to a final concentration of 25 µg/mL. The injection volume was of 20 µL and the samples racks were kept at 20 °C. The detection wavelength for quantification was set up at 408 nm and breakdown product detection was performed using DAD detector from 190 to 800 nm.

- Method validation

Linearity was initially verified by preparing one calibration curve daily for three days using five concentrations of amphotericin B (base) solubilised in dimethyl sulfoxide (DMSO) and diluted to 15, 20, 25, 30 and 35 µg/mL. Each calibration curve should have a determination coefficient R^2 equal or higher than 0.999. Homogeneity of the curves was verified using a Cochran test. ANOVA tests were applied to determine applicability of the linear regression model. To verify method precision, six solutions of 25 µg/mL amphotericin B were prepared each day for three days, and analysed and quantified. Repeatability was estimated by calculating the relative standard deviation (RSD) of intraday analysis and intermediate precision was evaluated using RSD of inter-days analysis. Both RSDs should be of less than 5%. Specificity was assessed by comparing UV spectra obtained from the DAD detector. Method accuracy was verified by evaluating the recovery of five theoretical concentrations to experimental values found using mean curve equation, and results should be found within the range of 95–105%. The overall accuracy profile was constructed according to Hubert et al. [31–33]. The matrix effect was evaluated by reproducing the previous methodology with the presence of all the excipients present in the formulations and comparing the calibration curves and intercepts.

Amphotericin B impurities described in the European Pharmacopeia were either used directly from reference product (amphotericin B for peak identification CRS containing impurities A and B, catalogue code Y0001014) or were prepared (impurity B and C) following the procedure described in the Amphotericin B monography [34]. All three impurities were identified using the same method, and their retention times were collected for potential identification and quantification during stability studies.

In order to exclude potential interference of degradation products with amphotericin B quantification, 100 µg/mL amphotericin B (base and deoxycholate) solutions were subjected to the following forced degradation conditions: 0.1, 0.5 and 1N of hydrochloric acid and sodium hydroxide for 60 min at 25 °C; 10 and 30% hydrogen peroxide for 60 and 120 min; and thermal degradation at 60 °C after 1, 2 and 4 h. Susceptibility to light was performed 3 times after solution preparation after 24, 48 and 115 h of radiation exposure using UV-visible (400–800 nm wavelength, colour 640) and UVA (320–400 nm wavelength, colour 09) light. All peaks with a surface ratio higher than 0.1% of reference amphotericin B peak were taken into account for the evaluation, and those for which the surface ratio was higher than 0.2% during at least one forced degradation study were followed.

2.5.4. Chromaticity Analysis

Chromaticity and luminance were measured using a UV-visible spectrophotometer (V670, Jasco France SAS, Lisses, France) using the mode Color Diagnosis of the built-in software (Spectra Manager™, Jasco France SAS, Lisses, France). The xyY CIE colorimetric system was used. Chromaticity was presented as a two dimensional diagram (x and y axes) representing the whole of the colour system independently of luminance. Luminance was defined as the visual sensation of luminosity of a surface measured by the ratio of the colour's luminosity (in $cd.cm^{-2}$) over the luminosity of pure white (reference colour) times 100, its value Y ranging therefore from 0 (no luminosity) to 100 (maximum luminosity).

2.5.5. Sterility Assay

Sterility was assessed using the European Pharmacopeia sterility assay (2.6.1). In brief, the unidose eyedroppers were opened under the laminar airflow of an ISO 4.8 microbiological safety cabinet, and the contents filtered under vacuum using a Nalgene analytical test filter funnel onto a 47 mm diameter cellulose nitrate membrane with a pore size of 0.45 µm (ref 147-0045, Thermo Scientific, Thermo Electron SAS, Courtaboeuf CEDEX, France). The membranes were then rinsed with 500 mL of 0.9% saline solution (Versylene, Fresenius Kabi France, Louvier, France), to remove any antibacterial effect of the solution and divided into two equal parts. Each individual part was transferred to either a fluid thioglycolate medium or a soya bean casein digest medium, and incubated at 30–35 °C or 20–25 °C respectively, for 14 days. The culture medium was then examined for colonies.

2.6. Data Analysi–Acceptability Criteria

The stability of the different amphotericin B formulations was assessed using the following parameters: visual aspect of the solution, presence or absence of visible particles, amphotericin B concentration, presence or absence of breakdown products, pH, osmolality, and turbidity.

The study was conducted following methodological guidelines issued by the International Conference on Harmonisation for stability studies [35], and recommendations issued by the French society of Clinical Pharmacy (SFPC) and Evaluation and Research Group on Protection in Controlled Atmosphere (GERPAC) [36].

A variation of amphotericin B concentration outside the 90–110% interval of initial concentration (including the limits of a 95% confidence interval of the measures) was considered as a being a sign of significant amphotericin B concentration variation. For concentrations fluctuating between a 90–95% or 105–110% range of initial concentration, the risk of instability was assessed in regard to the presence or absence of breakdown products and the variation of the physicochemical parameters. The observed solutions must be limpid, of unchanged colour, and clear of visible signs of haziness or precipitation.

Since there are no standards that define acceptable pH or osmolality variation, pH measures were considered to be acceptable if they did not vary by more than one pH unit from initial value [36]. Osmolality results were interpreted considering clinical tolerance of the preparation and turbidity measurements were considered acceptable if they did not increase by more than 10% from initial values.

3. Results

3.1. Amphotericin B Quantification and Breakdown Products Research

The retention time of Amphotericin B was of 15.49 ± 0.18 min (average ± IC95%) (Figure 2). The chromatographic method used was found linear for concentration ranging from 15 to 35 µg/mL with a mean determination coefficient R^2 equal of 0.999. Average regression equation was y = 73,833x − 73,492 where x is the amphotericin B concentration (µg/mL) and y the surface area of corresponding chromatogram peak. Interception was not significantly different from zero.

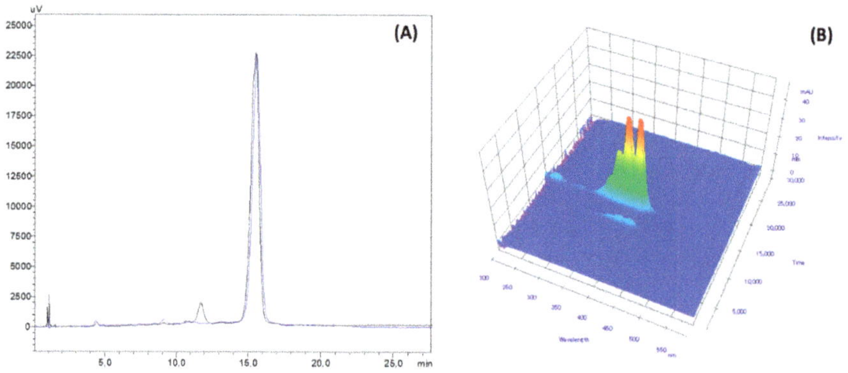

Figure 2. (**A**): Reference chromatogram at 408 nm of a 25 µg/mL amphotericin B base (blue curve) and deoxycholate (black curve) solution and with diode array detector screening (**B**). µV and mAU: units of intensity of signal measured by the UV-visible detector.

The relative mean trueness biases were of less than 1.6%, the mean repeatability RSD coefficient was of 1.33%, and mean intermediate precision RSD coefficient was of 1.31%. The accuracy profile constructed with the data showed that the limits of 95% confidence interval coefficients were all within ±7% of the expected value (see Supplementary Figure S1). The limit of detection was evaluated at 0.5 µg/mL (signal/noise ratio S/N = 21) and the limit of quantification at 5 µg/mL with S/N = 358 and a relative mean trueness of 4.1%.

Forced degradation results are presented Table 1. Amphotericin B showed high sensitivity to both acidic and alkaline conditions (degradations % ranging from 54.8% to 100%), the alkaline condition being the most aggressive, as well as to UV-visible radiations (more than 90% degradation after 24 h) and medium sensitivity to oxidation (20–25% loss after 2 h of contact with H_2O_2 30%). However, amphotericin B proved quite resistant to the heat degradation, showing a loss of about 5% after 4 h at 60 °C. Breakdown products research performed with the diode array detector from wavelengths 190 to 800 nm showed that all breakdown products (18 compounds) that were detected were visible at 408 nm, none of them interfered with the amphotericin peak, and no other compounds were noticed at other wavelengths (see chromatograms provided in supplementary Figures S2–S4). Breakdown products BP8, BP11, and BP12 were identified as being amphotericin B impurities A, B and C (see Supplementary Materials Figures S2–S4 for details). Overall, the method met all criteria for being considered as stability indicating.

Table 1. Amphotericin B forced degradation results for different conditions, in % of reference amphotericin B peak area. BP: Breakdown product. RRT: relative retention time compared to amphotericin B retention time.

Amphotericin B (Base)																			
Compound	RRT Mean	Reference	60 °C			HCl 1 h Contact			NaOH 1 h Contact			H_2O_2 10%		H_2O_2 30%		With UV			
			1 h	2 h	4 h	0.1 N	0.5 N	1 N	0.1 N	0.5 N	1 N	1 h	2 h	1 h	2 h	24 h	48 h	115 h	
BP1	0.07																	0.1%	
BP6	0.17						0.2%				0.1%								
BP7	0.23			0.1%	0.1%														
BP8	0.29	0.5%	0.3%	0.2%	0.2%	0.5%	0.9%			0.1%		0.4%	0.5%	0.3%	0.2%	0.1%			
BP9	0.37	0.1%		0.2%	0.1%								0.1%	0.6%	0.8%				
BP10	0.49	0.1%		0.2%	0.2%		0.1%									0.3%	0.1%		
BP11	0.54		0.2%	0.3%	0.3%					0.1%		0.1%				0.0%			
BP12	0.59	0.9%	0.6%	0.6%	0.6%	0.7%					0.2%	0.1%				0.1%			
BP13	0.70	0.6%				0.8%	0.3%	0.2%	0.5%	0.1%		1.1%	2.3%	11.3%	17.5%	0.1%			
BP14	0.77		0.1%	0.4%	0.8%		2.5%	0.2%		0.1%		2.5%	2.1%	1.1%	0.6%				
BP15	0.85			0.3%	0.3%	0.8%	0.6%	0.2%											
Amphotericin B		100.0%	97.5%	96.4%	94.6%	30.1%	14.8%	1.3%	5.3%	0.9%	0.3%	91.9%	91.6%	81.3%	74.9%	5.2%	0.8%	0.0%	
BP16	1.13											1.1%	1.2%	0.3%	0.8%				
BP17	2.21												0.9%	0.7%	0.9%				
BP18	2.59												1.1%	0.8%	1.4%				

Amphotericin B (Deoxycholate)																			
Compound	RRT Mean	Reference	60 °C			HCl 1 h Contact			NaOH 1 h Contact			H_2O_2 10%		H_2O_2 30%		With UV			
			1h	2h	4h	0.1 N	0.5 N	1 N	0.1 N	0.5 N	1 N	1 h	2 h	1 h	2 h	24 h	48 h	115 h	
BP1	0.07															0.5%	0.5%	0.2%	
BP6	0.17		0.1%	0.1%	0.1%				5.8%	46.6%	43.4%					0.1%			
BP7	0.23		0.1%	0.1%	0.1%					0.3%	0.3%								
BP8	0.29	0.5%	0.2%	0.2%	0.2%	0.2%	1.5%	1.9%	0.1%					0.2%	0.2%	0.4%	0.4%	0.1%	
BP9	0.37									0.1%	0.1%	0.1%		0.4%	0.7%				
BP10	0.49		0.2%	0.2%	0.3%														
BP11	0.54		0.3%	0.4%	0.5%			0.1%											
BP12	0.59	0.2%	0.5%	0.6%	0.6%		0.4%	0.2%								0.3%			
BP13	0.70	0.7%	0.7%	0.7%	0.6%	0.3%	0.6%	0.2%				1.3%	2.1%	9.9%	15.8%	0.6%			
BP14	0.77	6.0%	4.6%	4.1%	3.6%	1.7%	3.9%	7.6%	8.4%	0.2%		1.0%	1.0%	0.6%	0.3%	5.3%	2.6%	0.7%	
BP15	0.85		0.2%	0.2%	0.3%		0.3%	0.3%				0.2%	0.3%	0.3%	0.3%				
Amphotericin B		100.0%	97.7%	97.3%	96.0%	45.2%	36.1%	30.9%	33.8%	0.9%	0.0%	93.6%	93.1%	85.8%	79.3%	6.5%	1.8%	0.0%	
BP16	1.13						0.9%	0.2%				1.0%	1.0%	0.6%	0.8%				
BP17	2.21												0.7%	0.6%	0.5%				
BP18	2.59												1.4%	0.9%	0.9%				

3.2. Physicochemical Stability of ABDC and AB-HP-γ-CD Formulations

At the start of the study (day 0), the AB-HP-γ-CD formulation was a limpid amber coloured solution, whereas the ABDC formulation was a limpid yellow solution (see Supplementary Materials Figure S5 for visual aspect images). Throughout the study, all samples maintained their initial appearance, with no appearance of any visible particulate matter, haziness, or gas development, except for the ABDC formulation stored at 25 °C, for which a haziness was noticed from day 56 onwards. This observation correlated well with the increased turbidity, raising from 11.60 FNU to 162.00 FNU at day 56, then to more than 800 FNU (maximum quantification level) after 168 days of storage. For the ABDC formulation stored at 5 °C turbidity had increased by 5.4% to 12.23 FNU after 168 days and by 124% to 26.00 FNU after 350 days. For the AB-HP-γ-CD formulation, initial turbidity was of 7.31 FNU, and decreased over time to reach 3.40 FNU (53% decrease) after 350 days when stored at 25 °C but increased over time to reach 10.40 FNU (42% increase) when stored at 5 °C.

Concerning pH and osmolality, all results are presented in Table 2. Throughout the study, osmolality did not vary by more than 15 mOsmol/kg (4.6%) and 27 mOsmol/kg (5.8%) from initial value at day 0 (320 and 465 mOsmol/kg) for respectively the ABDC and AB-HP-γ-CD formulations. pH values did not vary by more than 0.39 units except for the ABDC formulation after 336 days of storage at 25 °C, for which a decrease of 0.93 pH units was noticed, however still staying within specifications.

Amphotericin B concentrations decreased over time throughout the study, for both formulations and storage temperatures, but with wide variations between formulations and conservation temperatures (Figure 3).

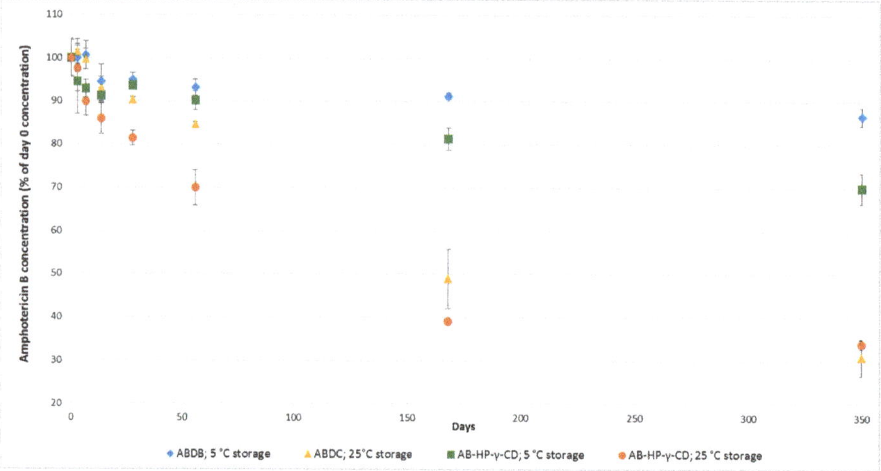

Figure 3. Evolution over time of amphotericin B concentrations for the amphotericin B deoxycholate (ABDC) and amphotericin B 2-hydroxypropyl-γ-cyclodextrin (AB-HP-γ-CD) formulations. $n = 4$, mean ± 95% confidence interval.

Table 2. Evolution over time of pH and osmolality for the amphotericin B deoxycholate and amphotericin B 2-hydroxypropyl-γ-cyclodextrin formulations. $n = 4$, mean ± standard deviation. Osmolality in mOsmol/kg.

Storage Time (Days)	Amphotericin B Deoxycholate				Amphotericin B 2-Hydroxypropyl-γ-Cyclodextrin			
	5 °C Storage		25 °C Storage		5°C Storage		25°C Storage	
	pH	Osmolality	pH	Osmolality	pH	Osmolality	pH	Osmolality
0	7.64 ± 0.02	320 ± 1	7.64 ± 0.02	320 ± 1	7.14 ± 0.02	465 ± 11	7.14 ± 0.02	465 ± 11
3	7.65 ± 0.00	323 ± 1	7.60 ± 0.05	320 ± 1	7.12 ± 0.01	458 ± 4	7.14 ± 0.02	463 ± 9
7	7.63 ± 0.01	320 ± 2	7.59 ± 0.00	321 ± 3	7.00 ± 0.00	457 ± 3	6.99 ± 0.00	458 ± 9
14	7.61 ± 0.01	321 ± 1	7.51 ± 0.01	320 ± 0	7.08 ± 0.01	471 ± 9	7.06 ± 0.02	457 ± 7
28	7.57 ± 0.00	322 ± 3	7.42 ± 0.02	320 ± 1	7.06 ± 0.00	456 ± 12	7.04 ± 0.00	463 ± 6
56	7.55 ± 0.01	325 ± 3	7.35 ± 0.00	326 ± 1	7.06 ± 0.01	466 ± 9	7.02 ± 0.00	465 ± 2
168	7.44 ± 0.01	323 ± 3	7.02 ± 0.01	327 ± 1	7.02 ± 0.00	468 ± 27	6.93 ± 0.01	468 ± 13
350	7.25 ± 0.01	335 ± 1	6.71 ± 0.01	330 ± 4	6.96 ± 0.00	492 ± 31	6.81 ± 0.00	478 ± 60

After 56 days of storage, only the ABDC formulation stored at 5 °C was still within amphotericin B concentration specifications (see acceptability criteria defined in Section 2.6), and remained so up until 168 days of storage included. AB-HP-γ-CD formulation showed higher amphotericin B degradation, having lost 6.45% and 9.78% of amphotericin B after respectively 28 and 56 days when stored at 5 °C, and 18.60% and 30.0% when stored at 25 °C. For both formulations, the temperature had an important impact on degradation, as after 350 days both formulations stored at 25 °C had lost more than 60% of amphotericin B. Concerning breakdown product research, no appearance or increase of compounds already present at day 0 was detected, for neither formulation (see example chromatograms for ABDC and AB-HP-γ-CD formulations at day 168, respectively Figures 4 and 5), except for the AB-HP-γ-CD formulation, for which an increase of breakdown product BP8 (impurity A) was noticed, going from 0.96% at day 0 (in % reference amphotericin B peak area) to 1.44% and 1.37% after six months and 1.69 and 0.70% after 12 months at respectively 5 °C and 25 °C.

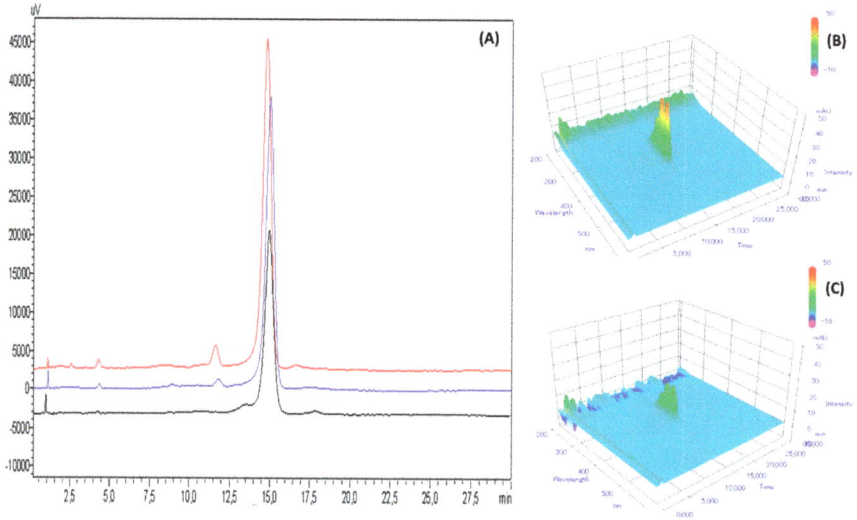

Figure 4. (**A**) Chromatograms at 408 nm of amphotericin B deoxycholate (diluted 1/100th to the theoretical concentration of 25 μg/mL) at day 0 (red curve), after 168 days at 5 °C storage (blue curve) and 25 °C (black curve); with diode array detector screening after 168 days at 5 °C (**B**) and at 25 °C (**C**). μV and mAU: units of intensity of signal measured by the UV-visible detector.

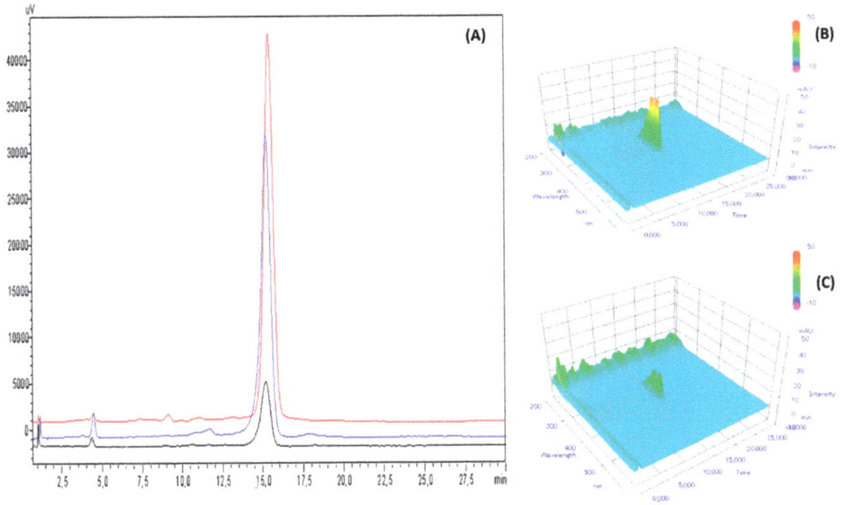

Figure 5. (**A**) Chromatograms at 408 nm amphotericin B solubilised in 2-hydroxypropyl-γ-cyclodextrins (diluted 1/100th to the theoretical concentration of 25 µg/mL) at day 0 (red curve), after 168 days at 5 °C storage (blue curve) and 25 °C (black curve); with diode array detector screening after 168 days at 5 °C (**B**) and at 25 °C (**C**). µV and mAU: units of intensity of signal measured by the UV-visible detector.

3.3. Sterility Assay

None of the four analysed solutions conserved in unopened bottles at day 0, 28, 168, and 350 showed any signs of microbial growth.

3.4. Physicochemical Stability of AB-HP-γ-CD Additionned with 0.5 mg/mL Ascorbic Acid

The addition of ascorbic acid to the formulation did not modify initial visual aspect (limpid amber solution). For both conservation temperatures, turbidity, pH, and osmolality stayed within specifications (Table 3). Concentrations of amphotericin B decreased rapidly, and were out of specifications after 14 and seven days of storage when the formulations were stored respectively at 5 and 25 °C.

Table 3. Evolution of studied parameters for the amphotericin B 2-hydroxypropyl-γ-cyclodextrin formulation added with 0.5 mg/mL of ascorbic acid. $n = 4$; mean ± standard deviation, except for *: $n = 1$. FNU: Formazin Nephelometric Units.

		Turbidity (FNU) *	pH	Osmolality (mOsmol/kg)	Concentration (mg/mL for Day 0 Then % of Day 0 Concentrations)
Before storage	Day 0	3.19	7.08 ± 0.00	423 ± 5	2.47 ± 0.05
Storage at 5 °C	Day 7	3.20	7.09 ± 0.03	452 ± 4	96.54 ± 3.10
	Day 14	3.14	6.95 ± 0.02	449 ± 22	90.09 ± 2.31
	Day 28	3.39	6.79 ± 0.01	450 ± 11	83.93 ± 1.21
Storage at 25 °C	Day 7	3.19	6.84 ± 0.00	453 ± 12	85.08 ± 1.58
	Day 14	3.23	6.64 ± 0.02	479 ± 4	72.41 ± 3.81
	Day 28	3.32	6.38 ± 0.06	468 ± 7	55.32 ± 8.96

Interestingly, in parallel to the decrease in amphotericin B concentrations, an evolution in the colour was visually also noticed (slight darkening and reddening of the solution) with was correlated by an evolution in chromaticity and luminance measurements, which was more pronounced when the formulation was stored at 25 °C (see Figure 6).

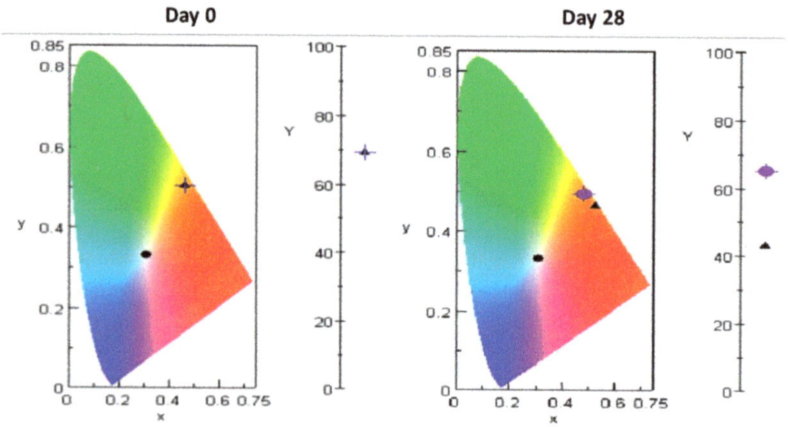

Figure 6. Chromaticity (xy diagram) and luminance (Y) results of the HP-γ-CD amphotericin B formulation containing 0.5 mg/mL ascorbic acid at day 0 and day 28. Blue cross: day 0 results. Purple cross target: storage at 5 °C. Black triangle: storage at 25 °C.

4. Discussion

In this study, we show that amphotericin B solubilised in HP-γ-CD is not as stable as conventional amphotericin B deoxycholate, as amphotericin B loss reached nearly 10 and 20% after respectively 56 and 168 days of storage at 5 °C, whereas for convention ABDC formulation, the loss was of only of 6.89% and 8.70% for the same storage times.

The quantification method used in our study was adapted to our laboratory conditions from a previously published method by Chang et al. that had showed good specificity and resolution between amphotericin B and known impurities [30]. However, as it has not been validated as stability indicating, we performed accelerated degradation tests to verify the absence of interferences with potential breakdown products. The results that were obtained were coherent with those published initially by Chang et al. in terms of retention times and relative retention times, and breakdown studies allowed the detection of multiple compounds, all correctly separated from the main amphotericin B peak. They are also in accordance with the results of a very recent study by Montenegro et al. who also developed a stability indicating liquid chromatography–diode array detector method for amphotericin B quantification [37]. They confirmed that amphotericin B degrades rapidly under acidic, alkaline, oxidative and radiation exposure conditions, detecting 16 breakdown products, and made an interesting tentative shot at identifying some of the compounds using direct injection electrospray ionization mass spectrometry and electrospray ionization tandem mass spectrometry.

During our 350-day stability study, we showed that for both of the tested formulation, amphotericin B concentrations decrease over time; however, different causes could be hypothesised. For the classical deoxycholate formulation, the decrease in amphotericin B active pharmaceutical ingredient (API) happened in parallel to a massive increase in turbidity (especially at 25 °C storage), thus suggesting a physical instability rather than a chemical one, with the precipitation of amphotericin B. This is quite possibly linked to the tendency of amphotericin B to form soluble and insoluble aggregates over time, even at ambient temperature [38–40]. Conversely, for the AB-HP-γ-CD formulation, turbidity did not vary in such a way, yet API concentrations still decreased, with only a slight increase in breakdown product BP8 (impurity A), more visible at 5 °C such suggesting a certain instability of this compound at 25 °C. As the formulation was buffered at was has been described as the optimum pH range (pH 6 to 7) for amphotericin B stability [41], degradation mechanisms other than those mediated by pH are possibly implicated. Indeed, it has been suggested by several authors that amphotericin B decay can happen by autoxidation [42,43], which can also be linked to one of its antifungal activity mechanisms as it is a powerful oxidant [44,45]. Previously, Belhachemi et al. showed that adding ascorbic acid (vitamin C) and α-tocopherol (vitamin E) to amphotericin B improved its therapeutic index [46] and had hypothesised a link with lesser autoxidation, so in a complementary study we investigated if adding ascorbic acid to the AB-HP-γ-CD formulation might help improve its stability. Our results showed that ascorbic acid had no protective effect, and might even hasten the instability process, as after 28 days at 25 °C a 45% loss of API was noticed when in presence of vitamin C, whereas the loss was only 20% without it. The redox potential of ascorbic acid has been reported to be in the range of +0.35 V to +0.50 V [47], so it is possible that if amphotericin B red/ox potential is higher, it will not be protected by ascorbic acid. Another hypothesis could be linked to its high potential to scavenge free radicals [48], meaning that amphotericin B can also be classified as an antioxidant, with an effectiveness superior to that of retinoids but inferior to that of carotenoids [43].

Solubilization of γ cyclodextrin yielded a clear, very light brown solution, without any visible particulate matter. Addition of amphotericin B induced a change of color (light amber for AB-HP-γ-CD and light yellow for ABDC formulations) but remained limpid. Without cyclodextrins, amphotericin B is insoluble in aqueous solutions and a clearly visible precipitate is present. Other authors have confirmed that amphotericin B -γ cyclodextrin solution are limpid and not turbid. Rajagopan et al. observed that a minimum ratio of 1:46 (amphotericin B to γ cyclodextrin) was required for amphotericin B solubilisation, and that at lower ratios the solutions turned cloudy [22]. Kajtar et al. found that while in aqueous solutions amphotericin B forms colloid-like multimolecular aggregates, in the presence of γ-cyclodextrins true solutions can be prepared, which show similar spectral properties as AmB dissolved in organic solvents [25]. During preparation of topical formulations, Ruiz et al. declared that their intermediate preparation of Amphotericin B–CD inclusion complex resulted in a transparent yellow solution [27], which is also consistent with our findings. Interestingly, an evolution in colour was noted in the AB-HP-γ-CD formulation additionned with ascorbic acid, which was better characterized by chromaticity and luminance measurements. Indeed, chromaticity measurements clearly confirmed a slight reddening of the solution, and luminance measurements indicated that the colour was darker. Of course, it cannot be concluded at this stage which compound these modifications are related to (as ascorbic acid is known to undergo a change of colour when oxidized [49]), but these results indicate that colour measurement could be an interesting complement to be performed during stability studies of coloured solutions to track a change of colour, or of uncoloured solutions to detect any beginning coloration. Also, despite the European Pharmacopoeia for the time being only recommending the use of reference colour solutions ranging from brown to greenish-yellow [50] to assess the colouration of liquids, the United States Pharmacopoeia does have a monography describing colour measurement [51], and such a system will be implemented in the European Pharmacopoeia on the 1rst January 2021 as a harmonized text with the United States and Japanese Pharmacopoeias [52].

In 1986, Rajagopan et al. published one of the first studies describing enhanced solubility and inclusion of amphotericin B in γ-cyclodextrin complexes and proposed a mechanism for the formation of the 1:1 inclusion complex [22]. However they did not evaluate amphotericin B stability at physiological pH, only at pH 1.2 and pH 12 and for amphotericin B (base) and complexed with the cyclodextrins and for only up to 350 min. Their results did show that the amphotericin B-γ-cyclodextrin complex was more stable than the base amphotericin B at those extreme pH, but that amphotericin B concentrations (when complexed with γ-cyclodextrins) still did decrease by 10% after 350 min. No comparison with a deoxycholate formulation was made. Other authors have studied the stability of ophthalmic solutions of amphotericin B. Peyron et al. studied the stability of a deoxycholate formulation of 5 mg/mL amphotericin B diluted in dextrose, and found it precipitated after 13 to 16 days at room temperature, but declared it stable after 120 days storage at refrigerated temperature, despite not measuring the turbidity of their solution [19]. More recently, Curti et al. evaluated the physicochemical stability of five anti-infectious eyedrops, including 5 mg/mL amphotericin B, unfortunately without giving any information on the formulation (supposedly in deoxycholate form) in 5% glucose. The data they presented are also in favour of stability for 60 days at 5 °C (end point of the study), but of only 7 days at 25 °C. To the best of our knowledge, there has only been one published study investigating some stability parameters of a 0.5 and 1 mg/mL formulation of amphotericin B in γ cyclodextrins, during a short period of 30 days, at refrigerated and ambient temperatures [24]. The authors declared no API loss at either temperature when diluted in a saline solution, but noticed a 10% decrease of API when diluted in dextrose at the end of the study. At both temperatures, the antifungal activity remained unchanged. However, the study only followed the concentration of amphotericin B and particle size/aggregation effect, and the identity of the container was not mentioned, making it overall difficult to draw complete conclusions about the physicochemical stability of the formulation. The stability of liposomal amphotericin B eye drops at 5 mg/mL has also been studied [53]: the authors found that amphotericin B concentrations remained with a 94–107% range during a six-month study, and mean hydrodynamic diameter of the liposomes also remained stable, at both 5 °C and 25 °C, however one of the limits of the study was that certain parameters like pH, osmolality and turbidy were not indicated as being followed, thus making it difficult to conclude on overall formulation stability.

This study illustrates yet again that preparing adapted formulations of amphotericin B for ophthalmic use is a challenging task. The use of HP-γ-CD effectively allowed the preparation of concentrated amphotericin B solutions, but didn't prevent API loss during long term storage. Recently, Jansook et al. studied the effect of additives like chitosan and phospholipids on γ-CD solubilization of amphotericin B, but have not as yet evaluated the stability of their new formulations [28]. The use of ascorbic acid as an antioxidant to prevent the loss of amphotericin B through possible autoxidation did not increase stability. Tests using different antioxidants like α-carotenoids might be a solution. Eliminating oxygen could also help reduce decay [48], but, although achievable, such a step could complexify the preparation steps, as the apparatus needed is not readily available to all compounding pharmacies. Another solution might be to try alternative excipients, such as polyethoxylated castor oil and polyvinylpyrrolidone, as they have shown to be able to solubilize other lipophilic compounds like cyclosporine A and tacrolimus [54,55]. Otherwise, and for resource-rich countries, the use of high-cost liposomal formulations could provide an acceptable, yet expensive, alternative, albeit without providing a long-term stability solution for ready-to use eye drops of amphotericin B. The search therefore continues.

5. Conclusions

Solutions of amphotericin B solubilised in hydroxypropyl γ cyclodextrins are not physicochemically stable for more than 28 or 56 days at 25 °C or 5 °C, respectively. Adding an antioxidant like ascorbic acid decreases the stability of the formulation. More studies are therefore needed in order to provide an affordable long-term stability solution for ready-to use eye drops of amphotericin B for the treatment of fungal keratitis caused by Fusarium species, Aspergillus species, and Candida species.

Supplementary Materials: The following are available online at http://www.mdpi.com/1999-4923/12/9/786/s1, Figure S1: Accuracy profile of Amphotericin B validation. RTB: relative trueness bias. CI: confidence interval, Figure S2: Chromatograms (at 408 nm wavelength detection) of amphotericin B solutions after forced degradation: (A) acid and alkaline exposure, (B) 24 h (24H) of ultraviolet-visible radiations exposure, (C) oxidative exposure and (D) heat exposure. 4H: after 4 h of heat exposure, Figure S3: Contour maps (diode array detection) of amphotericin B solutions after forced degradation: (A) 0.1N HCl, 1 h contact; (B)) 0.1N NaOH, 1 h contact; (C) 10% H202, 2 h contact; (D) 30% H202, 2 h contact; (E) UV-visible radiations, 24 h contact; (F) heat exposure 60 °C, 4 h contact, Figure S4: Chromatograms of amphotericin B impurities at 408 nm. Blue curve: amphotericin B for peak identification CRS containing impurities A and B; Orange curve: solution prepared following the procedure described in the amphotericin B monography allowing for the preparation of impurities B and C, Figure S5: Visual aspect of the amphotericin B deoxycholate (A) and amphotericin B 2-hydroxypropyl-γ-cyclodextrin (B) formulations, Table S1: all raw data.

Author Contributions: Conceptualization: M.W., M.J., and P.C.; Methodology: F.A.E.K., M.W., Y.B., P.C., and V.S.; Investigation: F.A.E.K. and M.Y.; Verification: F.A.E.K., M.Y., Y.B., and P.C.; Writing—original draft: P.C. and M.Y.; Writing—review & editing: all authors. All authors have read and agreed to the published version of the manuscript.

Funding: This research received no external funding.

Acknowledgments: The authors would like to thank Hélène Confolent, Marie Mula and Françoise Picq for their help in performing the sterility assays, as well as Yoann Le Basle and Agnes Roche for their help in performing some of the physicochemical analyses.

Conflicts of Interest: The authors declare no conflict of interest.

References

1. Green, M.D.; Apel, A.J.G.; Naduvilath, T.; Stapleton, F.J. Clinical outcomes of keratitis. *Clin. Exp. Ophthalmol.* **2007**, *35*, 421–426. [CrossRef] [PubMed]
2. Słowik, M.; Biernat, M.M.; Urbaniak-Kujda, D.; Kapelko-Słowik, K.; Misiuk-Hojło, M. Mycotic infections of the eye. *Adv. Clin. Exp. Med. Off. Organ Wroc. Med. Univ.* **2015**, *24*, 1113–1117. [CrossRef] [PubMed]
3. Bongomin, F.; Gago, S.; Oladele, R.O.; Denning, D.W. Global and Multi-National Prevalence of Fungal Diseases—Estimate Precision. *J. Fungi* **2017**, *3*, 57. [CrossRef] [PubMed]
4. Satpathy, G.; Ahmed, N.H.; Nayak, N.; Tandon, R.; Sharma, N.; Agarwal, T.; Vanathi, M.; Titiyal, J.S. Spectrum of mycotic keratitis in north India: Sixteen years study from a tertiary care ophthalmic centre. *J. Infect. Public Health* **2019**, *12*, 367–371. [CrossRef] [PubMed]
5. Chen, C.-A.; Hsu, S.-L.; Hsiao, C.-H.; Ma, D.H.-K.; Sun, C.-C.; Yu, H.-J.; Fang, P.-C.; Kuo, M.-T. Comparison of fungal and bacterial keratitis between tropical and subtropical Taiwan: A prospective cohort study. *Ann. Clin. Microbiol. Antimicrob.* **2020**, *19*. [CrossRef]
6. Khor, W.-B.; Prajna, V.N.; Garg, P.; Mehta, J.S.; Xie, L.; Liu, Z.; Padilla, M.D.B.; Joo, C.-K.; Inoue, Y.; Goseyarakwong, P.; et al. The Asia Cornea Society Infectious Keratitis Study: A Prospective Multicenter Study of Infectious Keratitis in Asia. *Am. J. Ophthalmol.* **2018**, *195*, 161–170. [CrossRef]
7. Oliveira dos Santos, C.; Kolwijck, E.; van Rooij, J.; Stoutenbeek, R.; Visser, N.; Cheng, Y.Y.; Santana, N.T.Y.; Verweij, P.E.; Eggink, C.A. Epidemiology and Clinical Management of Fusarium keratitis in the Netherlands, 2005–2016. *Front. Cell. Infect. Microbiol.* **2020**, *10*. [CrossRef]
8. Puig, M.; Weiss, M.; Salinas, R.; Johnson, D.A.; Kheirkhah, A. Etiology and Risk Factors for Infectious Keratitis in South Texas. *J. Ophthalmic Vis. Res.* **2020**, *15*, 128–137. [CrossRef]
9. Chew, R.; Woods, M.L. Epidemiology of fungal keratitis in Queensland, Australia. *Clin. Exp. Ophthalmol.* **2019**, *47*, 26–32. [CrossRef]
10. Bograd, A.; Seiler, T.; Droz, S.; Zimmerli, S.; Früh, B.; Tappeiner, C. Bacterial and Fungal Keratitis: A Retrospective Analysis at a University Hospital in Switzerland. *Klin. Mon. Für Augenheilkd.* **2019**, *236*, 358–365. [CrossRef]
11. Thomas, B.; Audonneau, N.C.; Machouart, M.; Debourgogne, A. Fusarium infections: Epidemiological aspects over 10 years in a university hospital in France. *J. Infect. Public Health* **2020**. [CrossRef] [PubMed]
12. Wu, J.; Zhang, W.-S.; Zhao, J.; Zhou, H.-Y. Review of clinical and basic approaches of fungal keratitis. *Int. J. Ophthalmol.* **2016**, *9*, 1676–1683. [CrossRef] [PubMed]
13. Sahay, P.; Singhal, D.; Nagpal, R.; Maharana, P.K.; Farid, M.; Gelman, R.; Sinha, R.; Agarwal, T.; Titiyal, J.S.; Sharma, N. Pharmacologic therapy of mycotic keratitis. *Surv. Ophthalmol.* **2019**, *64*, 380–400. [CrossRef] [PubMed]
14. Manikandan, P.; Abdel-Hadi, A.; Randhir Babu Singh, Y.; Revathi, R.; Anita, R.; Banawas, S.; Bin Dukhyil, A.A.; Alshehri, B.; Shobana, C.S.; Panneer Selvam, K.; et al. Fungal Keratitis: Epidemiology, Rapid Detection, and Antifungal Susceptibilities of Fusarium and Aspergillus Isolates from Corneal Scrapings. *BioMed Res. Int.* **2019**, *2019*, 6395840. [CrossRef] [PubMed]
15. Bourcier, T.; Sauer, A.; Dory, A.; Denis, J.; Sabou, M. Fungal keratitis. *J. Fr. Ophtalmol.* **2017**, *40*, e307–e313. [CrossRef]
16. Mahmoudi, S.; Masoomi, A.; Ahmadikia, K.; Tabatabaei, S.A.; Soleimani, M.; Rezaie, S.; Ghahvechian, H.; Banafsheafshan, A. Fungal keratitis: An overview of clinical and laboratory aspects. *Mycoses* **2018**, *61*, 916–930. [CrossRef]

17. Al-Hatmi, A.M.S.; Bonifaz, A.; Ranque, S.; Sybren de Hoog, G.; Verweij, P.E.; Meis, J.F. Current antifungal treatment of fusariosis. *Int. J. Antimicrob. Agents* **2018**, *51*, 326–332. [CrossRef]
18. Lakhani, P.; Patil, A.; Majumdar, S. Challenges in the Polyene- and Azole-Based Pharmacotherapy of Ocular Fungal Infections. *J. Ocul. Pharmacol. Ther.* **2019**, *35*, 6–22. [CrossRef]
19. Peyron, F.; Elias, R.; Ibrahim, E.; Amarit-Combralier, V.; Bues-Charbit, M.; Balansard, G. Stability of amphotericin B in 5% dextrose ophthalmic solution. *Int. J. Pharm. Compd.* **1999**, *3*, 316–320.
20. Curti, C.; Lamy, E.; Primas, N.; Fersing, C.; Jean, C.; Bertault-Peres, P.; Vanelle, P. Stability studies of five anti-infectious eye drops under exhaustive storage conditions. *Die Pharm.* **2017**, *72*, 741–746. [CrossRef]
21. Vikmon, M.; Stadler-Szöke, Á.; Szejtli, J. Solubilization of amphotericin B with γ-cyclodextrin. *J. Antibiot.* **1985**, *38*, 1822–1824. [CrossRef] [PubMed]
22. Rajagopalan, N.; Chen, S.C.; Chow, W.-S. A study of the inclusion complex of amphotericin-B with γ-cyclodextrin. *Int. J. Pharm.* **1986**, *29*, 161–168. [CrossRef]
23. Jansook, P.; Kurkov, S.V.; Loftsson, T. Cyclodextrins as solubilizers: Formation of complex aggregates. *J. Pharm. Sci.* **2010**, *99*, 719–729. [CrossRef] [PubMed]
24. Serrano, D.R.; Ruiz-Saldaña, H.K.; Molero, G.; Ballesteros, M.P.; Torrado, J.J. A novel formulation of solubilised amphotericin B designed for ophthalmic use. *Int. J. Pharm.* **2012**, *437*, 80–82. [CrossRef]
25. Kajtár, M.; Vikmon, M.; Morlin, E.; Szejtli, J. Aggregation of amphotericin B in the presence of gamma-cyclodextrin. *Biopolymers* **1989**, *28*, 1585–1596. [CrossRef]
26. He, J.; Chipot, C.; Shao, X.; Cai, W. Cyclodextrin-Mediated Recruitment and Delivery of Amphotericin B. *J. Phys. Chem. C* **2013**, *117*, 11750–11756. [CrossRef]
27. Ruiz, H.K.; Serrano, D.R.; Dea-Ayuela, M.A.; Bilbao-Ramos, P.E.; Bolás-Fernández, F.; Torrado, J.J.; Molero, G. New amphotericin B-gamma cyclodextrin formulation for topical use with synergistic activity against diverse fungal species and *Leishmania* spp. *Int. J. Pharm.* **2014**, *473*, 148–157. [CrossRef]
28. Jansook, P.; Maw, P.D.; Soe, H.M.S.H.; Chuangchunsong, R.; Saiborisuth, K.; Payonitikarn, N.; Autthateinchai, R.; Pruksakorn, P. Development of amphotericin B nanosuspensions for fungal keratitis therapy: Effect of self-assembled γ-cyclodextrin. *J. Pharm. Investig.* **2020**, 1–13. [CrossRef]
29. Pubchem. Available online: https://pubchem.ncbi.nlm.nih.gov (accessed on 30 July 2020).
30. Chang, Y.; Wang, Y.-H.; Hu, C.-Q. Simultaneous determination of purity and potency of amphotericin B by HPLC. *J. Antibiot.* **2011**, *64*, 735–739. [CrossRef]
31. Hubert, P.; Nguyen-Huu, J.-J.; Boulanger, B.; Chapuzet, E.; Chiap, P.; Cohen, N.; Compagnon, P.-A.; Dewé, W.; Feinberg, M.; Lallier, M.; et al. Harmonization of strategies for the validation of quantitative analytical procedures: A SFSTP proposal—Part I. *J. Pharm. Biomed. Anal.* **2004**, *36*, 579–586. [CrossRef]
32. Hubert, P.; Nguyen-Huu, J.-J.; Boulanger, B.; Chapuzet, E.; Chiap, P.; Cohen, N.; Compagnon, P.-A.; Dewé, W.; Feinberg, M.; Lallier, M.; et al. Harmonization of strategies for the validation of quantitative analytical procedures: A SFSTP proposal—Part II. *J. Pharm. Biomed. Anal.* **2007**, *45*, 70–81. [CrossRef]
33. Hubert, P.; Nguyen-Huu, J.-J.; Boulanger, B.; Chapuzet, E.; Cohen, N.; Compagnon, P.-A.; Dewé, W.; Feinberg, M.; Laurentie, M.; Mercier, N.; et al. Harmonization of strategies for the validation of quantitative analytical procedures: A SFSTP proposal—Part III. *J. Pharm. Biomed. Anal.* **2007**, *45*, 82–96. [CrossRef]
34. EDQM. Amphotericin B monography. In *European Pharmacopeia*, 10.2 ed.; EDQM, European Pharmacopoeia: Strasbourg, France, 2020.
35. International Conference of Harmonization (ICH) Quality Guidelines: ICH. Guidelines for Stability Q1A to Q1f. Available online: http://www.ich.org/products/guidelines/%20quality/article/quality-guidelines.html (accessed on 18 June 2020).
36. French Society of Clinical Pharmacy (SFPC); Evaluation and Research Group on Protection in Controlled Atmospher (GERPAC). *Methodological Guidelines for Stability Studies of Hospital Pharmaceutical Preparations*; Paris, France. 2013. Available online: https://www.gerpac.eu/IMG/pdf/guide_stabilite_anglais.pdf (accessed on 19 August 2020).
37. Montenegro, M.B.; Souza, S.P.; Leão, R.A.C.; Rocha, H.V.A.; Rezende, C.M.; Souza, R.O.M.A. Methodology Development and Validation of Amphotericin B Stability by HPLC-DAD. *J. Braz. Chem. Soc.* **2020**, *31*, 916–926. [CrossRef]
38. Teresa, L.-F.M.; Ferreira, V.F.N.; Adelaide, F.-A.; Schreier, S. Effect of Aggregation on the Kinetics of Autoxidation of the Polyene Antibiotic Amphotericin B. *J. Pharm. Sci.* **1993**, *82*, 162–166. [CrossRef] [PubMed]

39. Stoodley, R.; Wasan, K.M.; Bizzotto, D. Fluorescence of Amphotericin B-Deoxycholate (Fungizone) Monomers and Aggregates and the Effect of Heat-Treatment. *Langmuir* **2007**, *23*, 8718–8725. [CrossRef]
40. Sawangchan, P. The Effect of Aggregation State on the Degradation Kinetics of Amphotericin B in Aqueous Solution. Ph.D. Thesis, University of Iowa, Iowa City, IA, USA, 2017. [CrossRef]
41. Hamilton-Miller, J.M.T. The effect of pH and of temperature on the stability and bioactivity of nystatin and amphotericin B. *J. Pharm. Pharmacol.* **1973**, *25*, 401–407. [CrossRef] [PubMed]
42. Beggs, W.H. Kinetics of amphotericin B decay in a liquid medium and characterization of the decay process. *Curr. Microbiol.* **1978**, *1*, 301–304. [CrossRef]
43. Osaka, K.; Ritov, V.B.; Bernardo, J.F.; Branch, R.A.; Kagan, V.E. Amphotericin B protects cis-parinaric acid against peroxyl radical-induced oxidation: Amphotericin B as an antioxidant. *Antimicrob. Agents Chemother.* **1997**, *41*, 743–747. [CrossRef]
44. Brajtburg, J.; Powderly, W.G.; Kobayashi, G.S.; Medoff, G. Amphotericin B: Current understanding of mechanisms of action. *Antimicrob. Agents Chemother.* **1990**, *34*, 183–188. [CrossRef]
45. Barwicz, J.; Gruda, I.; Tancrède, P. A kinetic study of the oxidation effects of amphotericin B on human low-density lipoproteins. *FEBS Lett.* **2000**, *465*, 83–86. [CrossRef]
46. Belhachemi, M.H.; Boucherit, K.; Boucherit-Otmani, Z.; Belmir, S.; Benbekhti, Z. Effects of ascorbic acid and α-tocopherol on the therapeutic index of amphotericin B. *J. Mycol. Méd.* **2014**, *24*, e137–e142. [CrossRef] [PubMed]
47. Matsui, T.; Kitagawa, Y.; Okumura, M.; Shigeta, Y. Accurate Standard Hydrogen Electrode Potential and Applications to the Redox Potentials of Vitamin C and NAD/NADH. *J. Phys. Chem. A* **2015**, *119*, 369–376. [CrossRef] [PubMed]
48. Kovacic, P.; Cooksy, A. Novel, unifying mechanism for amphotericin B and other polyene drugs: Electron affinity, radicals, electron transfer, autoxidation, toxicity, and antifungal action. *MedChemComm* **2012**, *3*, 274–280. [CrossRef]
49. Fustier, P.; St-Germain, F.; Lamarche, F.; Mondor, M. Non-enzymatic browning and ascorbic acid degradation of orange juice subjected to electroreduction and electro-oxidation treatments. *Innov. Food Sci. Emerg. Technol.* **2011**, *12*, 491–498. [CrossRef]
50. European Pharmacopoeia. *Degree of Coloration of Liquids*; European Directorate for the Quality of Medecines and Healthcare: Strasbourg, France, 2020. Available online: https://www.drugfuture.com/Pharmacopoeia/EP7/DATA/20202E.PDF (accessed on 6 July 2020).
51. *United States Pharmacopeia USP <1061> Color-Instrumental Measurement, USP 43-NF38 2018*; United States Pharmacopeia: New York, NY, USA, 2018. Available online: https://www.uspnf.com/sites/default/files/usp_pdf/EN/USPNF/usp-nf-commentary/usp-43-nf-38-index.pdf (accessed on 6 July 2020).
52. European Pharmacopoeia Revises General Chapter on Degree of Coloration of Liquids|EDQ-European Directorate for the Quality of Medicines. Available online: https://www.edqm.eu/en/news/european-pharmacopoeia-revises-general-chapter-degree-coloration-liquids (accessed on 6 July 2020).
53. Morand, K.; Bartoletti, A.C.; Bochot, A.; Barratt, G.; Brandely, M.L.; Chast, F. Liposomal amphotericin B eye drops to treat fungal keratitis: Physico-chemical and formulation stability. *Int. J. Pharm.* **2007**, *344*, 150–153. [CrossRef] [PubMed]
54. Chennell, P.; Delaborde, L.; Wasiak, M.; Jouannet, M.; Feschet-Chassot, E.; Chiambaretta, F.; Sautou, V. Stability of an ophthalmic micellar formulation of cyclosporine A in unopened multidose eyedroppers and in simulated use conditions. *Eur. J. Pharm. Sci.* **2017**, *100*, 230–237. [CrossRef]
55. Ghiglioni, D.G.; Martino, P.A.; Bruschi, G.; Vitali, D.; Osnaghi, S.; Corti, M.G.; Beretta, G. Stability and Safety Traits of Novel Cyclosporine A and Tacrolimus Ophthalmic Galenic Formulations Involved in Vernal Keratoconjunctivitis Treatment by a High-Resolution Mass Spectrometry Approach. *Pharmaceutics* **2020**, *12*, 378. [CrossRef]

pharmaceutics

Article

Stability of Ophthalmic Atropine Solutions for Child Myopia Control

Baptiste Berton [1], Philip Chennell [2,*], Mouloud Yessaad [1], Yassine Bouattour [2], Mireille Jouannet [1], Mathieu Wasiak [1] and Valérie Sautou [2]

1 CHU Clermont-Ferrand, Pôle Pharmacie, F-63003 Clermont-Ferrand, France; baptiste-berton@hotmail.fr (B.B.); myessaad@chu-clermontferrand.fr (M.Y.); mjouannet@chu-clermontferrand.fr (M.J.); mwasiak@chu-clermontferrand.fr (M.W.)

2 Université Clermont Auvergne, CHU Clermont-Ferrand, CNRS, SIGMA, ICCF, 63000 Clermont-Ferrand, France; ybouattour@chu-clermontferrand.fr (Y.B.); vsautou@chu-clermontferrand.fr (V.S.)

* Correspondence: pchennell@chu-clermontferrand.fr

Received: 25 June 2020; Accepted: 7 August 2020; Published: 17 August 2020

Abstract: Myopia is an ophthalmic condition affecting more than 1/5th of the world population, especially children. Low-dose atropine eyedrops have been shown to limit myopia evolution during treatment. However, there are currently no commercial industrial forms available and there is little data published concerning the stability of medications prepared by compounding pharmacies. The objective of this study was to evaluate the stability of two 0.1 mg/mL atropine formulations (with and without antimicrobiobial preservatives) for 6 months in two different low-density polyethylene (LDPE) multidose eyedroppers. Analyses used were the following: visual inspection, turbidity, chromaticity measurements, osmolality and pH measurements, atropine quantification by a stability-indicating liquid chromatography method, breakdown product research, and sterility assay. In an in-use study, atropine quantification was also performed on the drops emitted from the multidose eyedroppers. All tested parameters remained stable during the 6 months period, with atropine concentrations above 94.7% of initial concentration. A breakdown product (tropic acid) did increase slowly over time but remained well below usually admitted concentrations. Atropine concentrations remained stable during the in-use study. Both formulations of 0.1 mg/mL of atropine (with and without antimicrobial preservative) were proved to be physicochemically stable for 6 months at 25 °C when stored in LDPE bottles, with an identical microbial shelf-life.

Keywords: atropine; ophthalmic solution; stability; myopia

1. Introduction

Myopia (or short-sightedness) is an ophthalmic condition that leads to blurred long-distance vision, generally characterized by a refractive error of −0.5 or −1 diopters. Overall, it has been estimated that currently 1.4 billion people in the world are myopic (22.9% of the population), and crude estimations suggest that, by 2050, there will be 4.7 billion people affected (nearly 50% of world population) [1]. The prevalence of myopia is variable between countries, affecting for example about 30% of young adults in Europe [2], 59% in North America [3], to more than 95% in some student populations of Asian countries [4,5], with onset of the disease occurring during childhood and adolescence. Many risk factors have been suggested or clearly identified, such as time spent performing close-vision activities, such as reading or looking at smart-device screens [6], lack of physical exercise, or exposure to sunlight [3,7], often all linked to higher education rates [8]. If left uncorrected, myopia has been shown to have major consequences on children's level of education, quality of life, and personal and psychological well-being [9], and its economic impact on society has been estimated at US$244 billion from global potential productivity loss [10]. Several recommendations have been proposed to limit the onset of myopia, like encouraging children spending time outside, limiting close-vision activities, and adapting light conditions [11], but whilst fundamental, they might not be sufficient or easily implemented. Current therapeutic options all have limitations; for example, orthokeratology (reshaping of the cornea by a hard, hydrophilic, gas-permeable contact lens worn during sleep and removed during the day) does not stop disease progression to returning to its previous rate after treatment discontinuation and requires high levels of patient compliance [12]. The use of correction glasses or lenses does not address the root-cause, refractive surgery is only curative, and its cost-effectiveness is still uncertain [13]. Pharmacological treatments have however shown some very promising potential. Of these, mydriatic agents such as atropine or tropicamide gained interest early on [14], with atropine being the most studied. Its biological action has been surmised as involving a complex interplay with receptors on different ocular tissues at multiple levels, leading to a decrease in change in the cycloplegic refraction and axial length elongation [15]. Initially tested at 1% concentration during the ATOM1 trial, atropine eyedrops were proved to be effective in controlling myopic progression but caused important visual side effects resulting from cycloplegia and mydriasis [16]. Since then, several clinical trials have evaluated the safety and efficiency of atropine eye drops at lower concentrations. The ATOM2 trial studied myopia progression in 400 children 2 years after treatment with 0.01%, 0.1%, and 0.5% and found the 0.01% concentration to be the concentration causing the least side effects for comparable efficacy in controlling myopia progression [17,18]. Very recently, the LAMP phase 2 trial report confirmed that concentrations ranging from 0.01% to 0.05% were well tolerated in 383 children after two years of treatment, with patients experiencing rare and mild side effects [19], even if the need for photochomratic glasses was higher than 30% for treated patients. The ATOM1, ATOM2, and LAMP trials were all conducted on Asian patients, and some have highlighted the need for high-quality evidence from European populations on atropine effectiveness in controlling myopia progression [20]. However, a smaller study on European paediatric patients also concluded that 0.01% atropine eye drops slowed the rate of myopia progression whilst retaining a favourable safety profile [21].

Despite all this recent and very favourable clinical data, there is still currently no commercially available low dose formulation of atropine eyedrops. In order to treat patients, hospital and compounding pharmacies could produce the desired ophthalmic solution, but the lack of long-term validated stability data severely limits their conservation period by imposing short expiration dates after preparation [22,23]. Indeed, few studies have been published concerning atropine eyedrops stability, but the analyses were either lacking several tests or suffered from shortcomings concerning breakdown product research [24–26]. As single-dose container technology is not readily available to compounding pharmacies, multidose eyedroppers (often in low dose polypropylene) are the most used container and therefore the most studied [27–30]. However, not all of those devices possess a system allowing their content to be preservative-free, and their contents must therefore be preserved. Because 0.1 mg/mL is the concentration with currently the most data concerning safety and efficacy, the aim of this study was therefore to assess the physicochemical stability and to control the sterility of two 0.1 mg/mL atropine ophthalmic solutions (with and without an antimicrobial conservative) in two different low-density polyethylene (LDPE) multidose eyedroppers (one with a sterility-preserving technology allowing the absence of an antimicrobial preservative in the formulation and the other without such a system in order to allow choice of container depending on stability data) at 25 °C for six months in unopened eyedroppers.

2. Materials and Methods

2.1. Preparation and Storage of Atropine Solution Formulations

Two different formulations of 0.1 mg/mL (0.01%) atropine ophthalmic solutions were prepared:

- atropine solution with an antimicrobial preservative (cetrimide) for use with ethylene oxide sterilized white opaque LDPE squeezable multidose eyedroppers (reference VPLA25B10; Laboratoire CAT®, Lorris, France)
- atropine solution without the preservative for use within gamma-sterilized white opaque LDPE squeezable multidose eyedropper (reference 10002134) equipped with sterility preserving Novelia® caps (reference 20050772; Nemera, La Verpillère, Cedex France).

The details of each formulation are presented in Table 1. All compounds that were used were of pharmaceutical grade.

Table 1. Composition of the tested atropine ophthalmic formulations. q.s: quantity sufficient.

Chemical Components	Formulation (mg)	
	Without Preservative	With Preservative
Atropine sulphate (batch 18276508, exp. 31/01/2021, Inresa, France)	100	100
Natrium dihydrogenophosphate dihydrate (NaH_2PO_4) (batch 190298040, exp. 30/11/2021, Inresa, France)	7800	7800
Dinatrium monohydrogenophosphate dodecahydrate (Na_2HPO_4) (batch 18129611, exp. 30/04/2023, Inresa, France)	4480	4480
Cetrimide (batch 16F08-B01-334049, exp. 05/2020, Fagron, Netherlands)		100
Sodium chloride (NaCl) 0.9% (Versylene®; Fresenius Kabi France, Louviers, France)	q.s 1000 mL	q.s 1000 mL

The formulations were prepared by dissolving atropine into the 0.9% sodium chloride solution at room temperature under gentle agitation before adding the hydrogenophosphate buffer and, finally, if needed, the preservative (cetrimide). For the purpose of the study, batch size was 1 L for both formulations. Cetrimide at a concentration of 0.01% was chosen because it is a preservative commonly used for the antimicrobial preservation of ophthalmic solutions, with an efficacy similar to benzalkonium chloride [31,32].

The obtained atropine solutions were filtered through a 0.22-µm filter (Stericup® Sterile Vacuum Filtration Systems, Merck Millipore, MC2, Clermont-Ferrand, France) and then sterilely distributed (6 mL per unit, for a maximum filling capacity of 8 mL for both multidose eyedroppers) into the eyedroppers under the laminar airflow of an ISO 4.8 microbiological safety cabinet using a conditioning pump (Repeater pump, Baxter, Guyancourt, France). The solution was distributed into the two different low-density polyethylene (LDPE) eyedroppers.

2.2. *Study Design*

The stability of the 0.1 mg/mL atropine solutions was studied for 180 days at 25 °C in unopened eyedroppers and in simulated use conditions for 6 days.

2.2.1. Stability of 0.1 mg/mL Atropine in Unopened Multidose Eyedroppers

The eyedroppers containing atropine were stored upwards in an ICH Q1B compliant climate chamber (BINDER GmbH, Tuttlingen, Germany) at 25 °C ± 2 °C and 60 ± 5% residual humidity until analysis.

Immediately after preparation (day 0) and at days 8, 15, 30, 90, and 180, five units per kind of eyedropper were submitted to the following analyses: visual inspection, chromaticity analysis, atropine quantification, breakdown products (BPs) research (i.e., looking specifically for products resulting from the degradation of atropine), osmolality, pH, and turbidity. Sterility was also assessed using five units for each kind of eyedropper and storage temperature immediately after preparation and after 60 and 180 days of storage. Initial day 0 analyses were performed immediately after conditioning within 4 h after the end of the preparation of the solutions to have results as representative as possible of initial conditions (least degradation or modification of parameters).

2.2.2. Evaluation of Atropine Concentrations in Eye Drops during Simulated Use

Thirty eyedroppers were subjected to simulated patient use: every day for 6 days, one drop from each eyedroppers was manually emitted (i.e., the drop was squeezed out of the bottle as if to be administered to the eye, but instead of being administered, it was collected for analysis) at room temperature. Atropine quantification was then realized in triplicate from 10 collected and pooled drops. In between use, the bottles were stored vertically at 25 °C.

2.3. Analyses Performed on the Atropine Solutions

2.3.1. Visual Inspection

The multidose eyedroppers were emptied into glass test tubes, and the atropine solutions were visually inspected under day light and under polarized white light from an inspection station (LV28, Allen and Co., Liverpool, UK). Aspect and colour of the solutions were noted, and a screening for visible macroparticles, haziness, or gas development was performed.

2.3.2. Chromaticity Analysis

Chromaticity and luminance were measured with a UV-visible spectrophotometer (V670, Jasco®, Lisses, France) using the mode Color Diagnosis of the built-in software (Spectra Manager®, version 2.12.00). The xyY CIE colorimetric system was used. Chromaticity was presented as a two-dimensionl diagram (x and y axes) representing the whole the colour system independently of luminance. uminance is defined as the visual sensation of luminosity of a surface measured by the ratio of the colour's luminosity (in $cd{\cdot}cm^{-2}$) over the luminosity of pure white (reference colour) times 100; its value Y ranges therefore between 0 (no luminosity) and 100 (maximum luminosity).

2.3.3. Atropine Quantification and BPs Research

Chemicals and Instrumentation

For each unit, atropine was quantified and BPs were detected using the liquid chromatography (LC) method described by the European Pharmacopeia, Atropine monography [33]. The LC system that was used was a Prominence-I LC2030C 3D with diode array detection (Shimadzu France SAS, Marne La Vallée, France), and the associated software used to record and interpret chromatograms was LabSolutions® version 5.82. The LC separation column used was a C18 Synergi® Fusion-RP 80 (150 × 4.6 mm, 4 μm) with an associated guard column (Phenomenex, Le Pecq, France).

The mobile phase was a gradient mixture of phases A and B. Phase A consisted of an aqueous solution of 3.5 g of sodium dodecyl sulphate (SDS) (CAS 1561-21-3, purity > 99%, Sigma-Aldrich, St. Louis, MO, USA) in 606 mL of a 7 g/L solution of potassium dihydrogen phosphate (CAS 10049-21-5, purity > 99%, Sigma-Aldrich, St. Louis, MO, USA) previously adjusted to pH 3.3 with orthophosphoric acid (20,624.295, purity > 85%, Normapur, Prolabo, Paris, France) and mixed with 320 mL of acetonitrile (34851-2, purity > 99.9%, Honeywell, Charlotte, NC, USA). The final pH of phase A was of 3.9. Phase B consisted of 100% acetonitrile. The gradient used is presented in Table 2. All solvents were of analytical grade.

The flow rate through the column for the analysis was set at 1 mL/min, with column thermo-regulation set to a temperature of 30 °C. The injection volume was of 20 μL. The quantification wavelength was set up at 210 nm. BP detection was realized by screening with a diode array detector (DAD) detector from 190 nm to 800 nm.

Table 2. Gradient used for the liquid chromatography (LC) mobile phase.

Time (min)	Mobile Phase (%)	
	A	B
0	95	5
2	95	5
20	70	30
21	95	5
25	95	5

Method Validation

Linearity was initially verified by preparing one calibration curve daily for three days using five concentrations of atropine (European Pharmacopoeia reference standard Y0000878 (Sigma-Aldrich, MC2, Clermont-Ferrand, France) at 10, 20, 60, 100, and 140 µg/mL, diluted in deionized water. Each calibration curve should have a determination coefficient R^2 equal or higher than 0.999. Homogeneity of the curves was verified using a Cochran test. ANOVA tests were applied to determine applicability. Each day for three days, six solutions of atropine 0.1 mg/mL were prepared, analysed, and quantified using a calibration curve prepared the same day. To verify the method precision, repeatability was estimated by calculating relative standard deviation (RSD) of intraday analysis and intermediate precision was evaluated using an RSD of inter-days analysis. Both RSDs should be less than 5%. Specificity was assessed by comparing the UV spectra DAD detector. Method accuracy was verified by evaluating the recovery of five theoretical concentrations to experimental values found using mean curve equation, and results should be found within the range of 95–105%. The overall accuracy profile was constructed according to Hubert et al. [34–36].

The matrix effect was evaluated by reproducing the previous methodology with the presence of all excipients present in the formulation (including the preservative) and by comparing the calibration curves and intercepts.

Atropine impurities described in European Pharmacopeia (atropine impurity B CRS, atropine for peak identification CRS (containing impurities A, D, E, F, G, and H) and tropic acid R (impurity C)) were identified with the same method. Their retention times were collected for potential identification and quantification during stability studies.

In order to exclude potential interference of degradation products with atropine quantification, atropine 0.1 mg/mL solutions was subjected to the following forced degradation conditions: 0.1, 0.5, and 1 N hydrochloric acid for 150 min at 25 °C; 0.1, 0.5, and 1 N chloride acid for 150 min at 90 °C; 0.1, 0.5, and 1 N sodium hydroxide for 30 min at 25 °C; 15% hydrogen peroxide for 60 min at 60 °C and 90 °C; and 30% hydrogen peroxide for 60 and 180 min at 90 °C. Susceptibility to light was performed 3 times after solution preparation for 180 min and 4 and 8 days using an UVA light in climatic chamber (25 °C).

Tropic acid was quantified at 210 nm using the same method as for atropine quantification in the presence of a phosphate buffer, using a calibration curve ranging from 0.1 to 5.0 µg/mL validated using the same methodology as previously described for the validation of the atropine quantification method.

2.3.4. Osmolality, pH, and Turbidity Measurements

For each unit, pH measurements were made using a SevenMultiTM pH-meter with an InLabTM Micro Pro glass electrode (Mettler-Toledo, Viroflay, France). Measures were preceded and followed by instrument validation using standard buffer solution of pH 4 and pH 7 (HANNAH® Instrument, Tannerries, France). Osmolality was measured for each solution using an osmometer Model 2020 Osmometer® (Advanced instruments Inc., Radiometer, SAS, Neuilly Plaisance, France). Turbidity was measured using a 2100Q Portable Turbidimeter (Hach Lange, Marne La Vallée, France), by pooling the five samples per analysed experimental condition and assay time to obtain the necessary volume for the analysis. The results were expressed in Formazin Nephelometric Units (FNU).

2.3.5. Sterility Assay

Sterility was assessed using the European Pharmacopoeia sterility assay (2.6.1). Multidose eyedroppers were opened under the laminar air flow of an ISO 4.8 microbiological safety cabinet, and the contents were filtered under vacuum using a Nalgene® analytical test filter funnel onto a 47-mm diameter cellulose nitrate membrane with a pore size of 0.45 mm (ref 147-0045, Thermo Scientific, purchased from MC2, Clermont-Ferrand CEDEX, France). The membranes were then rinsed with 500 mL deionized water (Versylene®; Fresenius Kabi, France, Louviers, France) and divided into two equal parts. Each individual part was transferred to each of a fluid thioglycolate and soya tripcase medium and incubated at 30–35 °C or 20–25 °C, respectively, for 14 days. The culture medium was then examined for colonies.

2.4. Data Analysis—Acceptability Criteria

The stability of diluted atropine solutions was assessed using the following parameters: visual aspect of the solution, turbidity, pH, osmolality, atropine concentration, and presence or absence of BPs.

The study was conducted following methodological guidelines issued by the International Conference on Harmonisation for stability studies [37] and recommendations issued by the French Society of Clinical Pharmacy (SFPC) and by the Evaluation and Research Group on Protection in Controlled Atmosphere [38]. A variation of concentration outside the 90–110% range of initial concentration (including the limits of a 95% confidence interval of the measures) was considered as being a sign of instability. Presence of BPs and the variation of the physicochemical parameters were also considered a sign of atropine instability but were interpreted with regards to quantities found in commercial ophthalmic atropine solution (see Supplementary data file S1). The observed solutions must be limpid, of unchanged colour, and clear of visible signs of haziness or precipitation. Since there are no standards that define acceptable pH or osmolality variation, pH measures were considered acceptable if they did not vary by more than one pH unit from the initial value [38], and osmolality results were interpreted considering clinical tolerance of the preparation.

3. Results

3.1. Atropine Quantification and Breakdown Products (BP) Research

Atropine retention time was of 9.7 ± 0.3 min (Figure 1). The chromatographic method used was found linear for concentrations ranging from 0.5 to 140 μg/mL. Average regression equation was $y = 22429.5x - 13.6$, where x is the atropine concentration (in μg/mL) and y is the surface area of the corresponding chromatogram peak. Interception was not significantly different from zero, and average determination coefficient R^2 of three calibration curves was 0.99999. No matrix effect was detected.

The relative mean trueness bias coefficients were less than 2.75%, except for the 0.5 μg/mL calibration point, for which it was of 3.75%. Mean repeatability RSD coefficient and mean intermediate precision RSD coefficient were less than 2%. The accuracy profile constructed with the data showed that the limits of 95% confidence interval coefficients were all within 3% of the expected value, except for the 10 μg/mL calibration point, for which the lower range limit was −8.8%. The limit of detection was evaluated at 0.05 μg/mL (signal-to-noise ratio of 3.03 and experimentally confirmed by visual analysis of the chromatograms), and the limit of quantification was fixed at 0.5 μg/mL, even if the signal-to-noise ratio was 46, thus potentially indicating that a lower quantification limit could be reached.

No impurities were visible in the initial atropine solution on the reference chromatogram at 210 nm in Figure 1. All the impurities specified by the European Pharmacopeia were detected and identified in Figure 2. The chromatograms presented show separately different impurities as they come from different European Pharmacopoeia reference solutions and were thus analysed sequentially in order to be able to correctly identify each peak using the relative retention times provided in the atropine monography. They were all visible at 210 nm, which allowed maximum sensitivity. No other impurities were detected at other wavelengths.

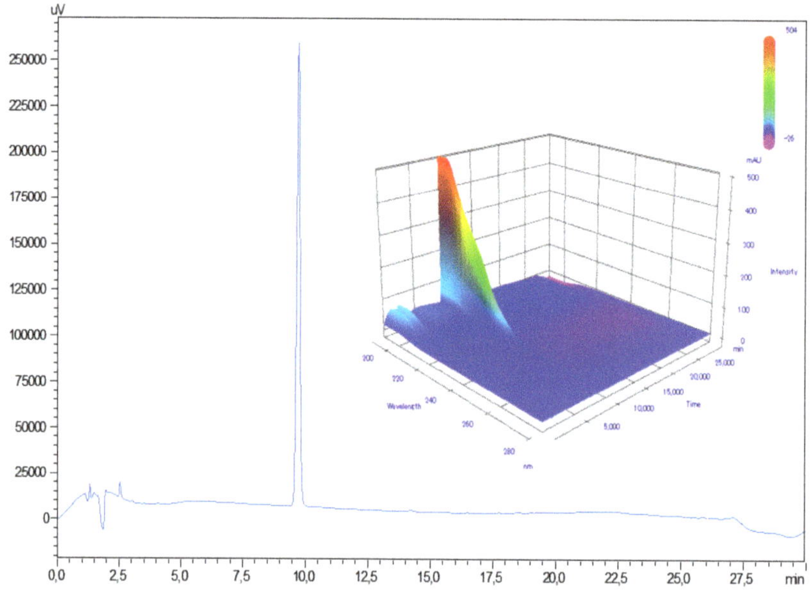

Figure 1. Reference chromatogram of a 0.1 mg/mL atropine solution at 210 nm and with diode array detector screening.

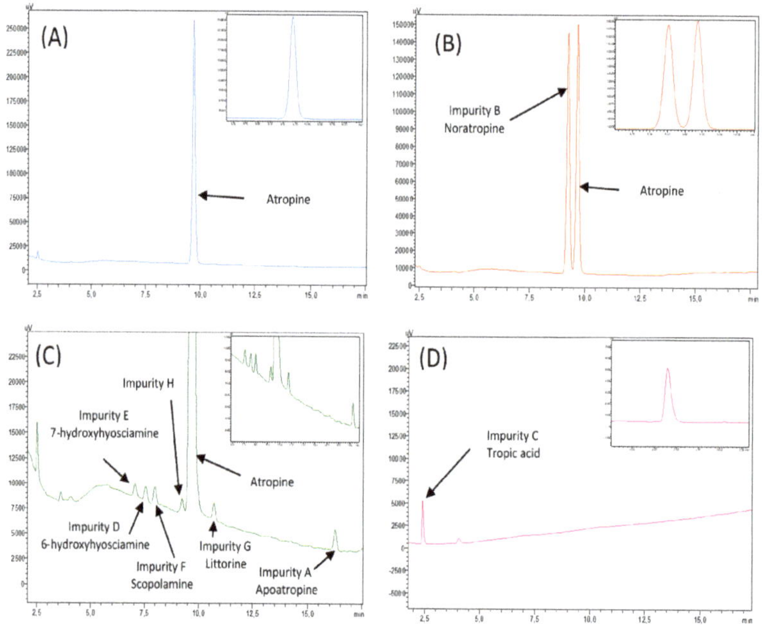

Figure 2. Chromatograms of atropine impurities at 210 nm: (**A**) reference atropine chromatogram, (**B**) chromatogram of the atropine impurity B CRS solution, (**C**) chromatogram of atropine for the peak identification CRS (containing impurities A, D, E, F, G, and H) solution, and (**D**) chromatogram of the tropic acid R (impurity C) solution. The insets represent a close up of the chromatograms.

A summary of the impurity retention times and relative retention times (relative to atropine) is presented in Table 3.

Table 3. Atropine impurities retention times and relative retention times.

	Impurity Retention Times	
	Experimental Absolute Retention Time (min)	**Relative Retention Time**
Atropine	9.7	1
Impurity A	16.2	1.7
Impurity B	9.3	0.9
Impurity C	2.5	0.3
Impurity D	7.6	0.8
Impurity E	7.1	0.7
Impurity F	8.0	0.8
Impurity G	10.8	1.1
Impurity H	9.3	0.9

After forced degradation, BPs were detected with a resolution higher than 1.5 of the atropine peak to all its BPs and particularly in alkaline forced conditions. No BPs were detected when atropine solutions were exposed to UVA light, and atropine concentration did not vary after 8 days of UV-Vis exposure. After 1 h at 15% H_2O_2 exposure at 60 °C, no loss of atropine concentration was detected. After 1 h at 90°, a loss of 7.9% of atropine was noticed, without any breakdown products being detected. Chromatogram results are showed in Figure 3.

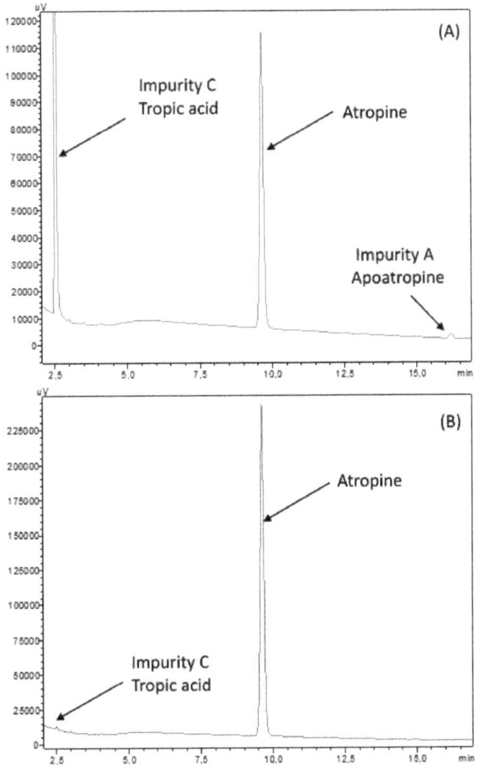

Figure 3. Chromatograms at 210 nm of breakdown products (BPs) obtained after forced degradation: (**A**) alkaline conditions of NaOH 0.5 N for 0.5 h and (**B**) acid conditions of HCl 0.1 N for 1 h at 90 °C.

Detailed results of tropic acid quantification are presented in Supplementary data.

3.2. Stability of Atropine in Unopened Multidose Eyedroppers

3.2.1. Physical Stability

All samples stayed limpid and uncoloured; chromaticity and luminance were unchanged during the study for both tested kind of eyedroppers; and there was no appearance of any visible particulate matter, haziness, or gas development. Initial turbidity was 0.33 and 0.32 FNU respectively for the atropine formulation with and without preservatives and did not vary by more than 0.6 FNU for the formulation with antimicrobial preservative or 0.32 FNU for the formulation without preservative (Table 4).

Table 4. Evolution of turbidity over time. $n = 1$ (pooled volume from 5 units). FNU: Formazin Nephelometric Units.

	Turbidity (FNU)						
	Day 0	**Day 8**	**Day 15**	**Day 30**	**Day 60**	**Day 90**	**Day 180**
Atropine solution with preservative conditioned in LDPE CAT® eyedroppers	0.33	0.31	0.27	0.78	0.78	0.43	0.93
Atropine solution without preservative conditioned LDPE NOVELIA® eyedroppers	0.32	0.31	0.26	0.54	0.44	0.34	0.64

3.2.2. Chemical Stability

Evolution of pH and osmolality throughout the study is presented Table 5. Throughout the study, osmolality did not vary by more than 3.7% (15 mOsm/kg) of the initial osmolality (412 and 398 mOsm/kg respectively for the atropine solution with and without preservatives) after 6 months of storage at 25 °C. Moreover, pH did not vary by more than 1.8% (0.1 pH unity) of the initial pH (6.1 for both solutions).

Table 5. Evolution of pH and osmolality over time ($n = 5$, mean ± 95% confidence interval).

		Day 0	Day 8	Day 15	Day 30	Day 60	Day 90	Day 180
Atropine solution with preservative conditioned in LDPE CAT® eyedroppers	pH	6.10 ± 0.01	6.11 ± 0.01	6.13 ± 0.02	6.13 ± 0.01	6.13 ± 0.02	6.21 ± 0.04	6.12 ± 0.01
	Osmolality (mOsm/kg)	412 ± 16	400 ± 6	403 ± 14	393 ± 14	400 ± 5	413 ± 11	418 ± 23
Atropine solution without preservative conditioned LDPE NOVELIA® eyedroppers	pH	6.10 ± 0.01	6.11 ± 0.01	6.13 ± 0.01	6.14 ± 0.02	6.13 ± 0.01	6.21 ± 0.01	6.09 ± 0.01
	Osmolality (mOsm/kg)	399 ± 2	401 ± 6	409 ± 6	405 ± 2	415 ± 15	408 ± 10	405 ± 7

For all studied conditions, mean atropine concentrations did not vary by more than 5.7% of mean initial concentrations (as presented in Figure 4). By extrapolation of the degradation rate using a linear regression, it could be estimated that atropine concentrations would remain higher than 90% of the original concentration for about 300 days.

Chromatographs showed no sign of BPs until day 8 for both types of LDPE eyedroppers at 25 °C. After 15 days of storage, one BP appeared, presenting a retention time of 2.10 min (relative retention time of 0.2; Figure 5A) seemingly not detected during forced degradation assays but close to that of tropic acid (Figure 5B). However, when diluting the know impurity tropic acid in a phosphate buffer of the same nature and concentration of the one used for the atropine formulation, its retention time changed to be identical to that of the breakdown product (Figure 5C), thus indicating that it is highly likely that the misidentified breakdown product is in fact tropic acid.

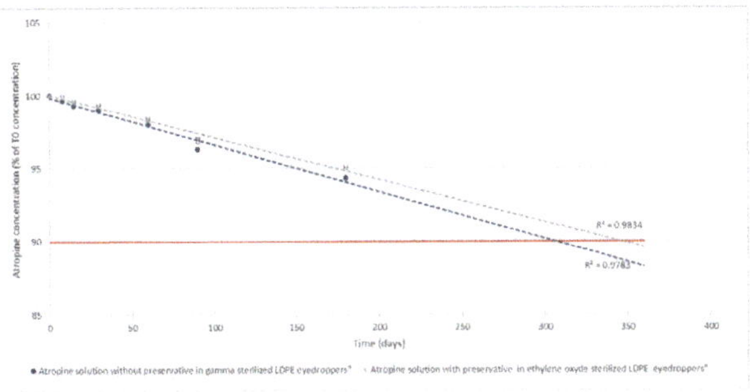

Figure 4. Evolution of atropine concentration over time (n = 5, mean ± 95% confidence interval): the grey curve is the atropine solution with preservatives conditioned in low-density polyethylene (LDPE) CAT® eyedroppers. The blue curve is the atropine solution without preservatives conditioned in LDPE NOVELIA® eyedroppers. The red line is 90% of the initial concentration. The dotted lines are the calculated linear regression of the evolution of atropine concentrations.

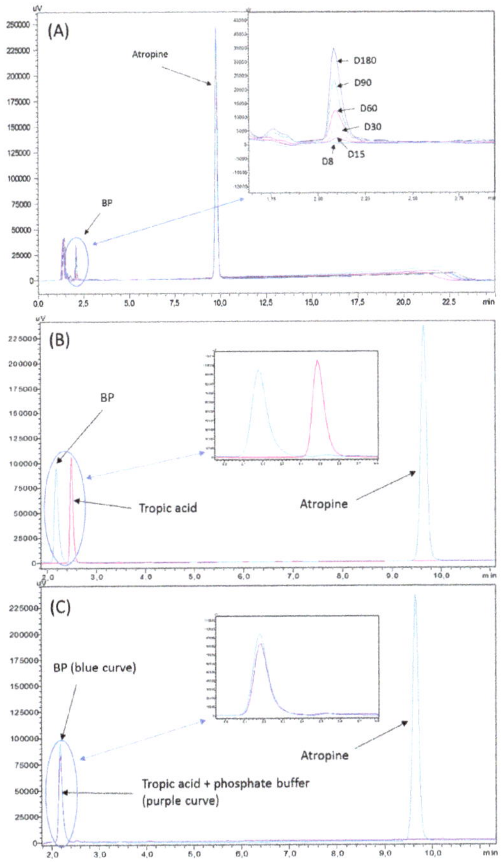

Figure 5. Chromatograms of (**A**) the increased area under curve of the breakdown product, (**B**) superposition of chromatograms of tropic acid diluted in water and an atropine solution containing the breakdown product, and (**C**) superposition of chromatograms of tropic acid diluted in phosphate buffer and an atropine solution containing the breakdown product.

Figure 6 shows the increase of tropic acid concentrations during the 6 months of the study. After 6 months, tropic acid concentrations were 3.5 and 3.4 µg/mL, respectively, for both the formulation with and without the preservative.

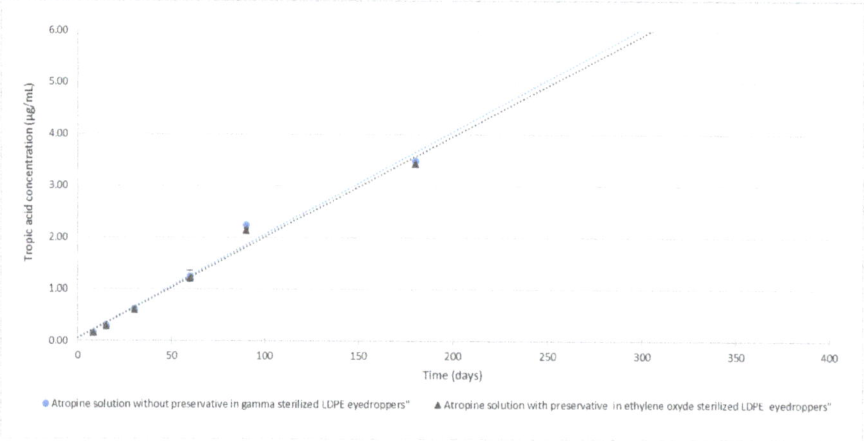

Figure 6. Evolution of breakdown product (tropic acid) concentration during time ($n = 5$, mean ± 95% confidence interval): The grey curve is the atropine solution with preservative conditioned in LDPE CAT® eyedroppers. The blue curve is the atropine solution without preservative conditioned LDPE NOVELIA® eyedroppers. The dotted lines are the linear regression of the evolution of breakdown product concentrations.

3.2.3. Sterility Assay

None of the five analysed solutions conserved in unopened bottles at day 0, day 60, and day 180 showed any signs of microbial growth.

3.3. Atropine Concentrations in Eye Drops During Simulated Use

During 6 days of drop sampling, no variation exceeding ±5% of initial concentration was found for any of the studied conditioned as presented in Figure 7.

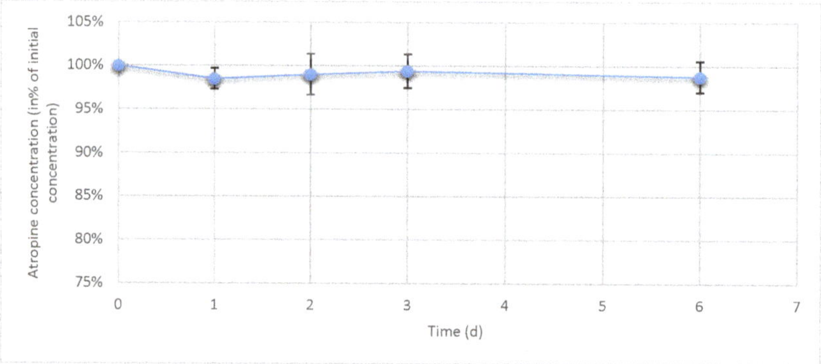

Figure 7. Evolution of atropine concentration in the emitted drops during simulated use ($n = 3$ times 10 pooled drops, mean ± 95% confidence interval).

4. Discussion

Our study presents new data on the physicochemical stability of 2 formulations (with and without antimicrobial preservatives) of a 0.1 mg/mL atropine solution conditioned in two differently sterilized LDPE eyedroppers (gamma radiations and ethylene oxide) which can be used to prevent myopia progression in children.

The method used for the quantification of atropine was the one described in the European Pharmacopeia, atropine monography, and the use of atropine impurities allowed the identification of 2 breakdown products that appeared during forced degradation to validate the method as being stability-indicating: tropic acid (impurity C) and apoatropine (impurity A). These two compounds have already been widely described as being the main instability by-products occurring during either hydrolysis (tropic acid and tropine) or dehydration (apoatropine) [39]. Our forced degradation results are coherent with previously described data suggesting higher stability in acidic conditions and lower half-life in neutral (pH 7–8) or alkaline (pH > 8) conditions [40]. Using the same chromatographic method, we were also able to quantify tropic acid, which presented a retention time of 2.5 min in the absence of a phosphate buffer. However, in the presence of the phosphate buffer used in the formulations, its retention time was reduced to about 2 min. This could be explained by a local modification of pH induced by the buffer (pH of the formulation = 6.1) leading to tropic acid being deprotonated (the pKa of tropic acid being of 4.3 [41]) and thus being less retained by the stationary C18 column than when injected without the buffer, as the pH will therefore be imposed by the mobile phase (pH 3.9) and tropic acid will be in unionized protonated form. The choice of the quantification wavelength at 210 assured maximum sensitivity with minor influence of the mobile phase, and the absence of dilution of the formulations before chromatographic analysis also meant that we were able to detect minute quantities of breakdown products in the ophthalmic solutions.

For both of the tested formulations, all parameters were in favour of a physicochemical stability of 6 months. No modifications of visual aspect, chromaticity, or luminance were detected. Chromaticity analyses would have helped to detect minute modifications of colour [42], invisible to the naked eye, but as such, the solutions remained colourless throughout the study. Turbidity analyses did not reveal the formation of any additional particles, and the pH and osmolality values also remained within specifications and were compatible with an ophthalmic administration route. Atropine concentrations also remained within specifications after 6 months of storage (maximum loss of 5.3% of initial mean concentration), thus conserving good therapeutic efficiency during the conservation period. However, they did decrease for both formulations following a linear degradation rate, leading to increasing concentrations of tropic acid which reached a maximum of 3.5 µg/mL after 6 months of storage. Comparatively, the concentrations of tropic acid found in commercialised atropine ophthalmic specialities were 6 to 11 times higher (21.4 and 40.2 µg/mL versus 3.5 µg/mL) (see Supplementary data file S1). This information is therefore in favour of a limited clinical impact of the appearance of tropic acid in the formulations during storage, even if studies evaluating the possible toxicity of tropic acid during chronic use could be performed to verify this point. By extrapolation of the evolution of measured atropine concentration over time, assuming it will follow in the worst case a zero-order reaction [43], it could be hypothesised that a 10% decrease would be reached within 300 to 350 days. As the degradation of atropine is linked to the hydrolysis of the ester function in an aqueous media, the equilibrium state will likely not be reached immediately, therefore making this hypothesis plausible, but it would however need to verify if precise data past 6 months is needed. Also, if longer stabilities are one day required, refrigerated conservation conditions could be tested (as lower temperatures will lead a slower breakdown rate by slowing down atropine hydrolysis), or alternatively, the pH of the formulation could be reduced to reach the maximum stability range of atropine (pH comprised between 3 and 4) [44,45]. However, this could decrease ophthalmic tolerance, especially for paediatric patients, which is the target population for which these formulations are designed. In the formulations we tested, the pH was buffered to a more physiological value (around pH 6), thus hopefully limiting potential unpleasantness for the children during administration and therefore increasing therefore adherence to treatment as well as suppressing any potential modifications of pH that have already been reported during the use of gamma-sterilized LDPE eyedroppers [28].

The sterility assay that we performed in our work followed the European Pharmacopeia sterility monography [46] and, in our case (for our preparation conditions), did not reveal any microbial contamination in units stored for up to 6 months. Microbiological testing of the final product is an essential test to be able to assign a microbiological shelf-life (along with prerequisites such as controlled cleanroom environment, validated preparation conditions, and integrity testing of the container and closure [47]). Concerning the container and closure system, the gamma-sterilized eyedroppers were provided with a closure system (Novelia® caps) which does not allow unfiltered air to penetrate the eyedropper, is commercially guaranteed to preserve sterility of the content more than a month [48], as well as has been tested for various hospital-prepared ophthalmic solutions either after one month of simulated use or after freezing and thawing [27,29].

During the simulated use study, atropine was quantified in the emitted drops to evaluate any potential loss of API by sorption (adsorption or absorption), as it has been shown that such a phenomena can occur during the first few days of treatment initiation with certain APIs and ophthalmic delivery devices [49]. During the 6-day study, atropine concentrations in the emitted drops remained stable (no variation exceeding of ±5% of initial concentration), therefore excluding any clinically significant loss of atropine. Such information is of high clinical value, as it correlates directly with the drop volume to determine the quantity received by the patient and needs to be known by prescribers. It also indicates that the preservative-free formulation can be used safely with the sterility preserving device that was tested (using Novelia® caps). As antimicrobial preservatives are known to cause potential side effects, especially during long-term treatments [50–52], this information is also of high clinical value.

The stability of atropine in aqueous solutions has been studied over the years, mainly for injectable usage and at concentrations higher than 1 mg/mL, but there is little pertinent data regarding the stability of more diluted forms. Driver et al. followed atropine concentrations of 0.4 mg/mL atropine sulphate solution stored at room temperature for up to 8 days and did not notice any change in concentrations [24], but no other physicochemical parameters were evaluated and the exhaustive composition of the formulation was not detailed. More recently, the physicochemical stability of a 0.1 mg/mL atropine sulphate solution prepared by diluting 10 mg/mL commercial atropine single doses in 0.9% sodium chloride was evaluated for 6 months at room temperature [25]. The authors reported less than 5% loss of atropine and did not mention any breakdown product detection, but the wavelength of their chromatographic method was set up at 250 nm, which is not the wavelength recommended by the European Pharmacopoeia for the analysis of atropine (210 nm) and is less advantageous for the detection of breakdown products in minute quantities. Saito et al. also reported a physicochemical stability of 6 months of 1% commercial atropine solutions diluted in 0.9% saline solution to concentrations of 0.1 mg/mL as well as higher concentrations ranging up to 5 mg/mL [26]. Despite using a tandem mass spectrometry liquid chromatography method initially developed for the quantification of atropine in plasma for clinical and forensic purposes [53], the authors did not mention the presence specifically of tropic acid or of any other breakdown products, possibly because the method they used was not validated as stability-indicating or because breakdown products were not even researched, as the research or quantification of such products was not included in their acceptability criteria.

Stability studies are of vital importance to be able to assign a shelf-life to medications; however, they must be conducted properly to avoid any misinterpretation or incomplete conclusions [54]. Several guidelines exist, such as those prepared by the International Conference on Harmonisation for stability studies [37], by the US Pharmacopoeia [55], or by international consensus by learned societies [38,56,57]. In our case, we validated a European Pharmacopoeia monography initially designed for the quality control of API atropine as being stability-indicating and capable of detecting and identifying potential breakdown products. Our results are concordant with previously published data concerning the stability of low concentration atropine solutions with regards to the concentration of atropine; however, we showed that atropine degradation is present and does lead to increased concentrations of tropic acid, a known breakdown product. Very little information is available about the toxicity of tropic acid and even less is available about any potential ocular toxicity. In the human body, atropine metabolism produces small (3%) amounts of tropic acid [58] and atropine is mostly excreted unchanged in the urines. During ophthalmic administrations in rabbits, it has been shown that atropine has good ocular bioavailability via both transcorneal and transconjunctival-scleral routes [59]. Unfortunately and to the best of our knowledge, atropine metabolism in the eye has not been studied despite there being a clear incentive to do so, like for other drugs [60]. There is therefore very little information available about the possibility of the natural formation of tropic acid in the eye after atropine topical application or, as stated previously, about tropic acid's ophthalmic toxicity. In this work, we found that concentrations of tropic acid reached 3.5 μg/mL in the atropine formulations we tested, those concentrations being 6 to 11 times lower than the quantities we also detected in commercial atropine ophthalmic formulations available on the marked. As such, it could be considered safe to administer the tested formulations after 6 months of conservation.

5. Conclusions

This study brings new information about the behaviour and stability of low-dose atropine ophthalmic solutions, showing that 0.1 mg/mL atropine solutions buffered at a physiological pH, with or without antimicrobial preservative, are physiochemically stable for 6 months at 25 °C when stored in LDPE bottles, with an identical microbial shelf-life.

Supplementary Materials: The following are available online at http://www.mdpi.com/1999-4923/12/8/781/s1, Supplementary data file S1 (containing the additional data described in the manuscript and all raw data).

Author Contributions: Conceptualization: M.W., M.J. and P.C.; methodology: B.B., M.W., Y.B., P.C. and V.S.; investigation: B.B. and M.Y.; verification: B.B., M.Y., Y.B. and P.C.; writing—original draft: B.B. and P.C.; writing—review and editing: all authors. All authors have read and agreed to the published version of the manuscript.

Funding: This research received no external funding.

Acknowledgments: The authors would like to thank Hélène Confolent, Marie Mula, and Françoise Picq for their help in performing the sterility assays.

Conflicts of Interest: The authors declare no conflict of interest.

References

1. Holden, B.A.; Fricke, T.R.; Wilson, D.A.; Jong, M.; Naidoo, K.S.; Sankaridurg, P.; Wong, T.Y.; Naduvilath, T.J.; Resnikoff, S. Global Prevalence of Myopia and High Myopia and Temporal Trends from 2000 through 2050. *Ophthalmology* **2016**, *123*, 1036–1042. [CrossRef] [PubMed]
2. Williams, K.M.; Verhoeven, V.J.M.; Cumberland, P.; Bertelsen, G.; Wolfram, C.; Buitendijk, G.H.S.; Hofman, A.; van Duijn, C.M.; Vingerling, J.R.; Kuijpers, R.W.A.M.; et al. Prevalence of refractive error in Europe: The European Eye Epidemiology (E3) Consortium. *Eur. J. Epidemiol.* **2015**, *30*, 305–315. [CrossRef] [PubMed]
3. Theophanous, C.; Modjtahedi, B.S.; Batech, M.; Marlin, D.S.; Luong, T.Q.; Fong, D.S. Myopia prevalence and risk factors in children. *Clin. Ophthalmol.* **2018**, *12*, 1581–1587. [CrossRef] [PubMed]
4. Ding, B.-Y.; Shih, Y.-F.; Lin, L.L.K.; Hsiao, C.K.; Wang, I.-J. Myopia among schoolchildren in East Asia and Singapore. *Surv. Ophthalmol.* **2017**, *62*, 677–697. [CrossRef] [PubMed]
5. Xie, Z.; Long, Y.; Wang, J.; Li, Q.; Zhang, Q. Prevalence of myopia and associated risk factors among primary students in Chongqing: Multilevel modeling. *BMC Ophthalmol.* **2020**, *20*, 146. [CrossRef]
6. Dirani, M.; Crowston, J.G.; Wong, T.Y. From reading books to increased smart device screen time. *Br. J. Ophthalmol.* **2019**, *103*, 1–2. [CrossRef]
7. Wen, L.; Cao, Y.; Cheng, Q.; Li, X.; Pan, L.; Li, L.; Zhu, H.; Lan, W.; Yang, Z. Objectively measured near work, outdoor exposure and myopia in children. *Br. J. Ophthalmol.* **2020**. [CrossRef]

8. Nickels, S.; Hopf, S.; Pfeiffer, N.; Schuster, A.K. Myopia is associated with education: Results from NHANES 1999–2008. *PLoS ONE* **2019**, *14*, e0211196. [CrossRef]
9. Congdon, N.; Burnett, A.; Frick, K. The impact of uncorrected myopia on individuals and society. *Commun. Eye Health* **2019**, *32*, 7–8.
10. Naidoo, K.S.; Fricke, T.R.; Frick, K.D.; Jong, M.; Naduvilath, T.J.; Resnikoff, S.; Sankaridurg, P. Potential lost productivity resulting from the global burden of myopia: Systematic review, meta-analysis, and modeling. *Ophthalmology* **2019**, *126*, 338–346. [CrossRef]
11. Spillmann, L. Stopping the rise of myopia in Asia. *Graefes Arch. Clin. Exp. Ophthalmol.* **2020**, *258*, 943–959. [CrossRef] [PubMed]
12. Modjtahedi, B.S.; Ferris, F.L.; Hunter, D.G.; Fong, D.S. Public health burden and potential interventions for myopia. *Ophthalmology* **2018**, *125*, 628–630. [CrossRef] [PubMed]
13. Tran, K.; Ryce, A. *Laser Refractive Surgery for Vision Correction: A Review of Clinical Effectiveness and Cost-Effectiveness*; CADTH Rapid Response Reports; Canadian Agency for Drugs and Technologies in Health: Ottawa, ON, Canada, 2018.
14. Sankaridurg, P.; Conrad, F.; Tran, H.; Zhu, J. Controlling Progression of Myopia: Optical and pharmaceutical strategies. *Asia Pac. J. Ophthalmol.* **2018**, *7*, 405–414. [CrossRef]
15. Upadhyay, A.; Beuerman, R.W. Biological Mechanisms of Atropine Control of Myopia. *Eye Contact Lens* **2020**, *46*, 129–135. [CrossRef] [PubMed]
16. Chua, W.-H.; Balakrishnan, V.; Chan, Y.-H.; Tong, L.; Ling, Y.; Quah, B.-L.; Tan, D. Atropine for the treatment of childhood myopia. *Ophthalmology* **2006**, *113*, 2285–2291. [CrossRef]
17. Chia, A.; Chua, W.-H.; Cheung, Y.-B.; Wong, W.-L.; Lingham, A.; Fong, A.; Tan, D. Atropine for the treatment of childhood myopia: Safety and efficacy of 0.5%, 0.1%, and 0.01% doses (atropine for the treatment of myopia 2). *Ophthalmology* **2012**, *119*, 347–354. [CrossRef]
18. Chia, A.; Lu, Q.-S.; Tan, D. Five-Year Clinical Trial on Atropine for the treatment of myopia 2: Myopia control with atropine 0.01% eyedrops. *Ophthalmology* **2016**, *123*, 391–399. [CrossRef]
19. Yam, J.C.; Jiang, Y.; Tang, S.M.; Law, A.K.P.; Chan, J.J.; Wong, E.; Ko, S.T.; Young, A.L.; Tham, C.C.; Chen, L.J.; et al. Low-concentration atropine for myopia progression (LAMP) study: A randomized, double-blinded, placebo-controlled trial of 0.05%, 0.025%, and 0.01% atropine eye drops in myopia control. *Ophthalmology* **2019**, *126*, 113–124. [CrossRef]
20. Azuara-Blanco, A.; Logan, N.; Strang, N.; Saunders, K.; Allen, P.M.; Weir, R.; Doherty, P.; Adams, C.; Gardner, E.; Hogg, R.; et al. Low-dose (0.01%) atropine eye-drops to reduce progression of myopia in children: A multicentre placebo-controlled randomised trial in the UK (CHAMP-UK)-study protocol. *Br. J. Ophthalmol.* **2019**. [CrossRef]
21. Sacchi, M.; Serafino, M.; Villani, E.; Tagliabue, E.; Luccarelli, S.; Bonsignore, F.; Nucci, P. Efficacy of atropine 0.01% for the treatment of childhood myopia in European patients. *Acta Ophthalmol.* **2019**, *97*, e1136–e1140. [CrossRef]
22. Akers, M.J. Formulation and Stability of Solutions. *Int. J. Pharm. Compd.* **2016**, *20*, 137–141. [PubMed]
23. Vigneron, J.; D'Huart, E.; Demoré, B. Stability studies in oncology: A marketing tool for pharmaceutical companies, a scientific mission for hospital pharmacists. *Eur. J. Oncol. Pharm.* **2019**, *2*, e12. [CrossRef]
24. Driver, R.P.; Brula, J.M.; Bezouska, C.A. The stability of atropine sulfate solutions stored in plastic syringes in the operating room. *Anesth. Analg.* **1999**, *89*, 1056. [CrossRef] [PubMed]
25. Farenq, P.O.; Jobard, M.; Cros, C.; Bezia, C.; Brandely-Piat, M.-L.; Batista, R. Physical, Chemical and Microbiological Stability Study of 0.1 mg mL^{-1} Atropine Eye Drops. In Proceedings of the 22th European GERPAC Conference, Hyères, France, 2–4 October 2019.
26. Saito, J.; Imaizumi, H.; Yamatani, A. Physical, chemical, and microbiological stability study of diluted atropine eye drops. *J. Pharm. Health Care Sci.* **2019**, *5*, 25. [CrossRef] [PubMed]
27. Chennell, P.; Delaborde, L.; Wasiak, M.; Jouannet, M.; Feschet-Chassot, E.; Chiambaretta, F.; Sautou, V. Stability of an ophthalmic micellar formulation of cyclosporine A in unopened multidose eyedroppers and in simulated use conditions. *Eur. J. Pharm. Sci.* **2017**, *100*, 230–237. [CrossRef] [PubMed]
28. Bouattour, Y.; Chennell, P.; Wasiak, M.; Jouannet, M.; Sautou, V. Stability of an ophthalmic formulation of polyhexamethylene biguanide in gamma-sterilized and ethylene oxide sterilized low density polyethylene multidose eyedroppers. *PeerJ* **2018**, *6*. [CrossRef]

29. Roche, M.; Lannoy, D.; Bourdon, F.; Danel, C.; Labalette, P.; Berneron, C.; Simon, N.; Odou, P. Stability of frozen 1% voriconazole eye-drops in both glass and innovative containers. *Eur. J. Pharm. Sci.* **2020**, *141*, 105102. [CrossRef]
30. Ghiglioni, D.G.; Martino, P.A.; Bruschi, G.; Vitali, D.; Osnaghi, S.; Corti, M.G.; Beretta, G. Stability and safety traits of novel cyclosporine a and tacrolimus ophthalmic galenic formulations involved in vernal keratoconjunctivitis treatment by a high-resolution mass spectrometry approach. *Pharmaceutics* **2020**, *12*, 378. [CrossRef]
31. Velpandian, T. Preservatives for topical ocular drug formulations. In *Pharmacology of Ocular Therapeutics*; Velpandian, T., Ed.; Springer International Publishing: Cham, Germany, 2016; pp. 419–430, ISBN 978-3-319-25498-2.
32. Dao, H.; Lakhani, P.; Police, A.; Kallakunta, V.; Ajjarapu, S.S.; Wu, K.-W.; Ponkshe, P.; Repka, M.A.; Narasimha Murthy, S. Microbial stability of pharmaceutical and cosmetic products. *AAPS Pharm. Sci. Tech.* **2018**, *19*, 60–78. [CrossRef]
33. European Pharmacopeia. *Edition 10.2 Atropine Sulfate Monography*; United States Pharmacopeia: New York, NY, USA, 2020.
34. Hubert, P.; Nguyen-Huu, J.-J.; Boulanger, B.; Chapuzet, E.; Chiap, P.; Cohen, N.; Compagnon, P.-A.; Dewé, W.; Feinberg, M.; Lallier, M.; et al. Harmonization of strategies for the validation of quantitative analytical procedures: A SFSTP proposal—Part I. *J. Pharm. Biomed. Anal.* **2004**, *36*, 579–586. [CrossRef]
35. Hubert, P.H.; Nguyen-Huu, J.-J.; Boulanger, B.; Chapuzet, E.; Chiap, P.; Cohen, N.; Compagnon, P.-A.; Dewé, W.; Feinberg, M.; Lallier, M.; et al. Harmonization of strategies for the validation of quantitative analytical procedures: A SFSTP proposal—Part II. *J. Pharm. Biomed. Anal.* **2007**, *45*, 70–81. [CrossRef] [PubMed]
36. Hubert, P.H.; Nguyen-Huu, J.-J.; Boulanger, B.; Chapuzet, E.; Cohen, N.; Compagnon, P.-A.; Dewé, W.; Feinberg, M.; Laurentie, M.; Mercier, N.; et al. Harmonization of strategies for the validation of quantitative analytical procedures: A SFSTP proposal—Part III. *J. Pharm. Biomed. Anal.* **2007**, *45*, 82–96. [CrossRef]
37. International Conference of Harmonization (ICH) Quality Guidelines. Guidelines for Stability Q1A to Q1f. Available online: http://www.ich.org/products/guidelines/%20quality/article/quality-guidelines.html (accessed on 18 July 2016).
38. French Society of Clinical Pharmacy (SFPC); Evaluation and Research Group on Protection in Controlled Atmospher (GERPAC). *Methodological Guidelines for Stability Studies of Hospital Pharmaceutical Preparations*; SFPC: Paris, France, 2013.
39. Kirchhoff, C.; Bitar, Y.; Ebel, S.; Holzgrabe, U. Analysis of atropine, its degradation products and related substances of natural origin by means of reversed-phase high-performance liquid chromatography. *J. Chromatogr. A* **2004**, *1046*, 115–120. [CrossRef] [PubMed]
40. Schier, J.G.; Ravikumar, P.R.; Nelson, L.S.; Heller, M.B.; Howland, M.A.; Hoffman, R.S. Preparing for Chemical Terrorism: Stability of Injectable Atropine Sulfate. *Acad. Emerg. Med.* **2004**, *11*, 329–334. [CrossRef] [PubMed]
41. Chemicalize-Instant Cheminformatics Solutions. Available online: https://chemicalize.com/app/calculation/tropic%20acid (accessed on 7 June 2020).
42. Choudhury, A.K.R. *Principles of Colour and Appearance Measurement: Object Appearance, Colour Perception and Instrumental Measurement*; Elsevier: Amsterdam, The Netherlands, 2014; ISBN 978-0-85709-924-2.
43. Waterman, K.C.; Adami, R.C. Accelerated aging: Prediction of chemical stability of pharmaceuticals. *Int. J. Pharm.* **2005**, *293*, 101–125. [CrossRef]
44. Connors, K.A.; Amidon, G.L.; Stella, V.J. *Chemical Stability of Pharmaceuticals: A Handbook for Pharmacists*, 2nd ed.; John Wiley & Sons: Hoboken, NJ, USA, 1986; ISBN 978-0-471-87955-8.
45. American Society of Health-System Pharmacists. *Handbook on Injectable Drugs*, 20th ed.; ASHP: Bethesda, MA, USA, 2018; ISBN 978-1-58528-615-7.
46. European Pharmacopeia. *Monography 2.6.1 Sterility*; United States Pharmacopeia: New York, NY, USA, 2020.
47. Crauste-Manciet, S.; Krämer, I.; Lagarce, F.; Sautou, V.; Beaney, A.; Smith, J.; Fenton-May, V.; Hecq, J.-D.; Sadeghipour, F.; Brun, P.L. GERPAC Consensus Conference—Guidance on the Assignment of Microbiological Shelf-life for Hospital Pharmacy Aseptic Preparations. *Pharm. Technol. Hosp. Pharm.* **2020**, *5*. [CrossRef]
48. Nemera. Ophthalmic-Preservative-free multidose eyedropper. *Drug Deliv. Mag.* **2018**, *82*, 16–20.
49. Le Basle, Y.; Chennell, P.; Sautou, V. A Sorption Study between Ophthalmic Drugs and Multi Dose Eyedroppers in Simulated Use Conditions. *Pharm. Technol. Hosp. Pharm.* **2017**, *2*, 181–191. [CrossRef]

50. Coroi, M.C.; Bungau, S.; Tit, M. Preservatives from The Eye Drops and the Ocular Surface. *Rom. J. Ophthalmol.* **2015**, *59*, 2–5.
51. Ramli, N.; Supramaniam, G.; Samsudin, A.; Juana, A.; Zahari, M.; Choo, M.M. Ocular surface disease in glaucoma: Effect of polypharmacy and preservatives. *Optom. Vis. Sci.* **2015**, *92*, e222–e226. [CrossRef]
52. Steven, D.W.; Alaghband, P.; Lim, K.S. Preservatives in glaucoma medication. *Br. J. Ophthalmol.* **2018**, *102*, 1497–1503. [CrossRef] [PubMed]
53. Koželj, G.; Perharič, L.; Stanovnik, L.; Prosen, H. Simple validated LC–MS/MS method for the determination of atropine and scopolamine in plasma for clinical and forensic toxicological purposes. *J. Pharm. Biomed. Anal.* **2014**, *96*, 197–206. [CrossRef] [PubMed]
54. Trissel, L.A. Avoiding common flaws in stability and compatibility studies of injectable drugs. *Am. J. Hosp. Pharm.* **1983**, *40*, 1159–1160. [CrossRef] [PubMed]
55. United States Pharmacopeia. *USP <1150> Pharmaceutical Stability*; USP 43-NF38; United States Pharmacopeia: New York, NY, USA, 2018.
56. Association of Southeast Asian Nations. Asean Guidelines on Stability Study of Drug Product. Update Review. In Proceedings of the 9th ACCSQ-PPWg Meeting, Manila, Phillìphines, 21–24 February 2005.
57. Bardin, C.; Astier, A.; Vulto, A.; Sewell, G.; Vigneron, J.; Trittler, R.; Daouphars, M.; Paul, M.; Trojniak, M.; Pinguet, F. Guidelines for the practical stability studies of anticancer drugs: A European consensus conference. *Eur. J. Hosp. Pharm.* **2012**, *19*, 278–285. [CrossRef]
58. Van der Meer, M.J.; Hundt, H.K.; Müller, F.O. The metabolism of atropine in man. *J. Pharm. Pharmacol.* **1986**, *38*, 781–784. [CrossRef]
59. Wang, L.Z.; Syn, N.; Li, S.; Barathi, V.A.; Tong, L.; Neo, J.; Beuerman, R.W.; Zhou, L. The penetration and distribution of topical atropine in animal ocular tissues. *Acta Ophthalmol.* **2019**, *97*, e238–e247. [CrossRef]
60. Argikar, U.A.; Dumouchel, J.L.; Kramlinger, V.M.; Cirello, A.L.; Gunduz, M.; Dunne, C.E.; Sohal, B. Do We Need to Study Metabolism and Distribution in the Eye: Why, When, and Are We There Yet? *J. Pharm. Sci.* **2017**, *106*, 2276–2281. [CrossRef]

pharmaceutics

MDPI

Article

Uptake Study in Lysosome-Enriched Fraction: Critical Involvement of Lysosomal Trapping in Quinacrine Uptake But Not Fluorescence-Labeled Verapamil Transport at Blood-Retinal Barrier

Yoshiyuki Kubo *,†, Miki Yamada †, Saki Konakawa †, Shin-ichi Akanuma and Ken-ichi Hosoya *

Department of Pharmaceutics, Graduate School of Medicine and Pharmaceutical Sciences, University of Toyama, 2630 Sugitani, Toyama 930-0194, Japan; s1560205@ems.u-toyama.ac.jp (M.Y.); s1560221@ems.u-toyama.ac.jp (S.K.); akanumas@pha.u-toyama.ac.jp (S.-i.A.)

* Correspondence: kuboyosh@pha.u-toyama.ac.jp (Y.K.); hosoyak@pha.u-toyama.ac.jp (K.-i.H.); Tel.: +81-76-434-7505 (Y.K. & K.-i.H.)

† These authors contribute equally to this work.

Received: 8 July 2020; Accepted: 6 August 2020; Published: 8 August 2020

Abstract: Lysosomal trapping at the blood–retinal barrier (BRB) was investigated through quinacrine and fluorescence-labeled verapamil (EFV) uptake. Quinacrine uptake by conditionally immortalized rat retinal capillary endothelial (TR-iBRB2) cells suggested saturable and non-saturable transport processes in the inner BRB. The reduction of quinacrine uptake by bafilomycin A1 suggested quinacrine distribution to the acidic intracellular compartments of the inner BRB, and this notion was also supported in confocal microscopy. In the study using the lysosome-enriched fraction of TR-iBRB2 cells, quinacrine uptake was inhibited by bafilomycin A1, suggesting the lysosomal trapping of quinacrine in the inner BRB. Pyrilamine, clonidine, and nicotine had no effect on quinacrine uptake, suggesting the minor role of lysosomal trapping in their transport across the inner BRB. Bafilomycin A1 had no effect on EFV uptake, and lysosomal trapping driven by the acidic interior pH was suggested as a minor mechanism for EFV transport in the inner BRB. The minor contribution of lysosomal trapping was supported by the difference in inhibitory profiles between EFV and quinacrine uptakes. Similar findings were observed in the outer BRB study with the fraction of conditionally immortalized rat retinal pigment epithelial (RPE-J) cells. These results suggest the usefulness of lysosome-enriched fractions in studying lysosomal trapping at the BRB.

Keywords: blood-retinal barrier; cationic drug; transport; lysosomal trapping

1. Introduction

The blood–retinal barrier (BRB) has two barrier structures, the inner and outer BRB, separating the neural retina and circulating blood [1–3]. The study of transport mechanisms at the BRB is assumed to be essential for improving drug therapy of retinal diseases because the efficient and safe delivery of drugs to the retina is a major challenge [1–3]. The retinal capillary endothelial and pigment epithelial cells are main constituents of the inner and outer BRB, respectively [3]. These cells are largely responsible for the transcellular blood-to-retina transport of nutrients and drugs, and the paracellular transport is limited by tight junctions [3]. Previous progress in the study of the BRB achieved using in vivo and in vitro methods has demonstrated the critical roles of blood-to-retina transport across the BRB in the retinal homeostasis [2,3]. Furthermore, these studies have clearly shown that nutrient transport at the BRB involves various membrane transporters, such as glucose transporter (GLUT1/SLC2A1), taurine transporter (TAUT/SLC6A6), creatine transporter (CRT/SLC6A8), cationic amino acid transporter (CAT1/SLC7A1), equilibrative nucleoside transporter (ENT2/SLC29A2), and riboflavin transporter (RFVTs/SLC52A) [3–11].

In addition, recent advances in the study of the BRB have revealed the involvement of novel transport systems in the blood-to-retina transport of cationic drugs, such as pyrilamine, nicotine, propranolol, clonidine and verapamil at the inner and outer BRB [12–17]. These transport systems are considered to be promising in the efficient and safe delivery of drugs to the retina, because they recognize cationic drugs, such as desipramine, imipramine, memantine, and clonidine, whose neuroprotective effects on cerebral ischemia and optic nerve injury have been reported [18–20]. Therefore, the combination of neuroprotective cations and transport systems at the BRB is expected to be beneficial in the effective therapy of neurological dysfunction of the retina, such as macular degeneration and diabetic retinopathy with severe symptoms, including blindness [3,12].

Furthermore, functional studies have revealed the temperature-dependent and saturable characteristics of the carrier-mediated cationic drug transport systems at the inner BRB, suggesting that they involve unknown membrane transporters expressed at the BRB [12–17]. In addition, cumulative evidence demonstrates that the substrate candidates of the systems include several cationic amphiphilic drugs that possibly undergo lysosomal trapping and are sequestrated in lysosomes, which are acidic organelles [21–23]. Uptake studies using a typical lysosomotropic agent, LysoTracker® Red DND-99 (LysoTracker Red; LTR, p*Ka* = 7.5, Log *P* = 2.1) [23–25], suggested that lysosomal trapping takes place in the retinal capillary endothelial cells (inner BRB) and that the uptake of LTR involves saturable and non-saturable transport processes in the inner BRB [26]. Inhibition studies suggested that lysosomal trapping has a minor effect on the transport of clonidine, nicotine, pyrilamine and verapamil at the inner BRB [26]. Furthermore, this suggestion was also supported by in vivo and in vitro studies with a fluorescence-labeled verapamil, EverFluor FL verapamil (EFV), which clearly demonstrated the permeation of verapamil from circulating blood to the retina [27].

However, further studies are still essential to determine the influence of lysosomal trapping in the BRB because it has been reported to significantly affect cationic drug distribution in the lung and liver [28–30]. In the present study, lysosomal trapping at the BRB was investigated using quinacrine as a test compound because it is suggested to be a lysosomotropic agent of antimalaria with intrinsic fluorescence by its physicochemical properties (p*Ka* = 10.3, Log *P* = 5.2). The accumulation of quinacrine in acidic intracellular compartments was reported to be inhibited by bafilomycin A1, a specific inhibitor of vacuolar (V)-ATPase [31–33], supporting the notion that quinacrine is a useful test compound for the study of lysosomal trapping. In the uptake study, we used the lysosome-enriched fraction prepared from the in vitro model cell line of the inner and outer BRB, which was also tried for EFV to investigate the influence of lysosomal trapping on the blood-to-retina transport of cationic drugs at the BRB.

2. Materials and Methods

2.1. Materials

LTR, EFV and quinacrine were purchased from Thermo Fisher Scientific (Waltham, MA, USA), Setareh Biotech (Eugene, OR, USA) and Merk (St. Louis, MO, USA), respectively. Optiprep™, an iodixanol solution for the purification of biological particles, was obtained from Abbott Diagnostics Technologies AS (Oslo, Norway), and protease inhibitor cocktail was purchased from Merk. Conditionally immortalized rat retinal capillary endothelial (TR-iBRB2) cells and rat retinal pigment epithelial (RPE-J) cells were established by Hosoya et al and Nabi et al, respectively [34,35], and these were used as in vitro model cell lines of inner and outer BRB, respectively. The fetal bovine serum (FBS) used for these cultures was purchased from SAFC Bioscience (Lenexa, KS, USA). Chemicals of reagent-grade used in this study were commercially obtained, and the supplemental information (Supplementary Materials) shows the buffer composition. The bafilomycin A1 used to study the effect of acidic interior pH was obtained from LC Laboratories (Woburn, MA, USA), while ammonium chloride (NH_4Cl) and carbonyl cyanide-p-trifluoromethoxyphenylhydrazone (FCCP) were obtained from Merk.

2.2. Methods

2.2.1. Cellular Uptake Analysis

Cellular uptake analysis was designed as described in our previous reports [13–16]. BioCoat™ Collagen I Cellware 24-well culture dishes (Corning, Corning, NY, USA) were used for TR-iBRB2 cells. Before the assay, the cells were rinsed with extracellular fluid (ECF)-buffer warmed to 37 °C. The uptake assay was initiated by adding ECF-buffer containing 5 μM test compound, and was terminated by washing with ice-cold ECF-buffer three times. The fluorescent intensity of test compounds taken up by the cell was determined using SpectraMax i3 microplate detection system (Molecular Devices, San Jose, CA, USA) after cell disruption using an ultrasonic homogenizer. The cellular uptake was expressed as the cell-to-medium ratio (cell/medium) calculated using the following equation:

$$\text{Cell/medium ratio} = (\text{fluorescence intensity in the cells})/(\text{fluorescence intensity in the medium}) \quad (1)$$

The nonlinear least-squares regression analysis program (MULTI) was used for data analysis [36], and kinetic parameters, such as the Michaelis constant (K_m), maximal uptake rate (V_{max}), and non-saturable uptake rate (K_d), for cell uptake were estimated by fitting data obtained in the cellular uptake analysis to the following equation, where the test compound concentration and uptake rate are S and V, respectively.

$$V = (V_{max} \times S)/(K_m + S) + K_d \times S \quad (2)$$

2.2.2. Confocal Microscopy of Fluorescent Compounds

The fluorescence distribution in TR-iBRB2 cells was analyzed as described in our previous report, and BioCoat™ Collagen I eight-well culture slides were used for culturing TR-iBRB2 cells (4500 cells/slide) for 48 hr at 33 °C [27,37]. Prior to confocal microscopy, the cells were incubated in ECF-buffer containing the test compound for 30 min. The incubation was terminated by washing the cells with ice-cold ECF-buffer, and cells were treated with phosphate-buffered saline (PBS) containing 4% paraformaldehyde (PFA) for 20 min in the dark. The slides were treated with VECTASHIELD mounting medium (Vector Laboratories, Burlingame, CA, USA), followed by confocal microscopy using a TCS-SP5 confocal microscope (Leica Microsystems, Wetzlar, Germany).

2.2.3. Preparation of Lysosome-Enriched Fraction

BioCoat™ Collagen I Cellware 10 mm dishes (Corning) were used for culturing TR-iBRB2 and RPE-J cells, and the lysosome-enriched fractions were prepared as described in our previous reports [7,8,38]. Cells were rinsed with PBS and collected in suspension buffer (25 mM sucrose, 10 mM HEPES, 1 mM ethylenediaminetetraacetic acid (EDTA), 0.1% protease inhibitor cocktail, pH 7.4) using a cell lifter (Corning), followed by centrifugation for 5 min at 200× g and 4 °C. The cells were suspended in suspension buffer, homogenized using a Teflon glass homogenizer (2500 rpm, 10 strokes), and then centrifuged for 10 min at 800× g at 4 °C. The resultant post nuclear supernatant was collected and layered on top of a discontinuous gradient composed of 12%, 15%, and 18% iodixanol (Optiprep™) in suspension buffer, followed by centrifugation for 3 h at 178,000× g at 4 °C in a near-vertical rotor, NVT65, and Optima L70 (Beckman Coulter, Brea, CA). The gradient solutions were collected into eleven fractions using 18G syringe needles, and their densities were determined using a digital refractometer (Atago, Tokyo, Japan). The fractions were also assayed for acid phosphatase activity for the isolation of the lysosome-enriched fraction and *p*-nitrophenylphosphate was used as a substrate to measure *p*-nitrophenol, a reaction product, using a GeneQuant 1300 spectrophotometer (GE Healthcare, Chicago, IL, USA).

2.2.4. Uptake Assay of Cationic Drugs in Lysosome-Enriched Fraction

The lysosome-enriched fraction was rinsed in intracellular fluid (ICF)-buffer (140 mM K-gluconate, 4 mM NaCl, 2 mM K_2HPO_4, 2 mM $MgCl_2$, 0.39 mM $CaCl_2$, 1 mM ethylene glycol tetraacetic acid (EGTA), and 10 mM HEPES, pH 7.2) by centrifuging twice for 30 min at 20,000× *g* at 4 °C to remove the suspension buffer [38,39]. The assay was initiated by suspending the lysosome-enriched fraction in 100 μM ICF-buffer containing the test compounds at 37 °C and was terminated by adding 1000 μL ice-cold ICF-buffer. The assay mixture was centrifuged for 30 min at 20,000× *g* and 4 °C, and the resultant pellet was solubilized by adding 100 μL 1% Triton X-100 for 8 h, followed by fluorescence determination at excitation and emission wavelengths (λ_{ex} and λ_{em}, respectively) of 420 nm and 500 nm for quinacrine and 480 nm and 510 nm for EFV, respectively using SpectraMax i3 microplate detection system. The uptake in the lysosome-enriched fraction was expressed as fraction-to-medium ratio (fraction/medium) calculated using the following equation:

$$\text{Fraction/medium ratio} = (\text{fluorescence intensity in the lysosome-enriched fraction}) / (\text{fluorescence intensity in the medium}) \quad (3)$$

In addition, the inhibition in uptake by the lysosome-enriched fraction was expressed as relative uptake (percentage of control, %) calculated with the following equation.

$$\text{Relative uptake (\%)} = (\text{fraction/medium ratio in the presence of inhibitor}) / (\text{fraction/medium ratio in the absence of inhibitor}) \quad (4)$$

2.2.5. Statistical Analysis

In the determination of significant difference for two groups and for several groups was carried out using an unpaired two-tailed Student's t-test was taken for two groups and a one-way analysis of variance (ANOVA) followed by Dunnett's test, respectively. In the least-square regression analysis, the kinetic parameter was expressed as mean values ± standard deviation (S.D.). Unless otherwise indicated, data represent mean values ± standard error of the mean (S.E.M.).

3. Results

3.1. Uptake of Quinacrine by TR-iBRB2 Cells

The uptake of quinacrine was examined using TR-iBRB2 cells as the in vitro model cell line of the inner BRB. The time-course study showed a time-dependent linear increase of quinacrine at 37 °C after at least 30 min (Figure 1A), and the initial uptake rate was calculated to be 445 ± 51 μL/(min·mg protein). The uptake of quinacrine at 30 min was calculated to be 1640 ± 170 μL/(min·mg protein), which was 540 times greater than the cellular volume (≈3 μL/{mg protein}). In TR-iBRB2 cells, quinacrine uptake was significantly reduced by 45% at 4 °C (Figure 1A), and significantly increased by 31% at pH 8.4, while the uptake exhibited no significant change in K^+- or Li^+-replacement buffer (Figure 1B).

In the study of concentration-dependence, quinacrine uptake by TR-iBRB2 cells exhibited a saturable process with K_m and V_{max} values of 1.87 ± 0.61 μM and 189 ± 50 μmol/(min·mg protein), respectively, and a non-saturable process with a K_d value of 29.7 ± 3.0 μL/(min·mg protein) (Figure 1C). The contribution of saturable and non-saturable processes was estimated to be 52% and 48%, respectively at a concentration of 5 μM. In addition, pretreatment of TR-iBRB2 cells with bafilomycin A1 significantly reduced quinacrine uptake by 76% (Figure 1D).

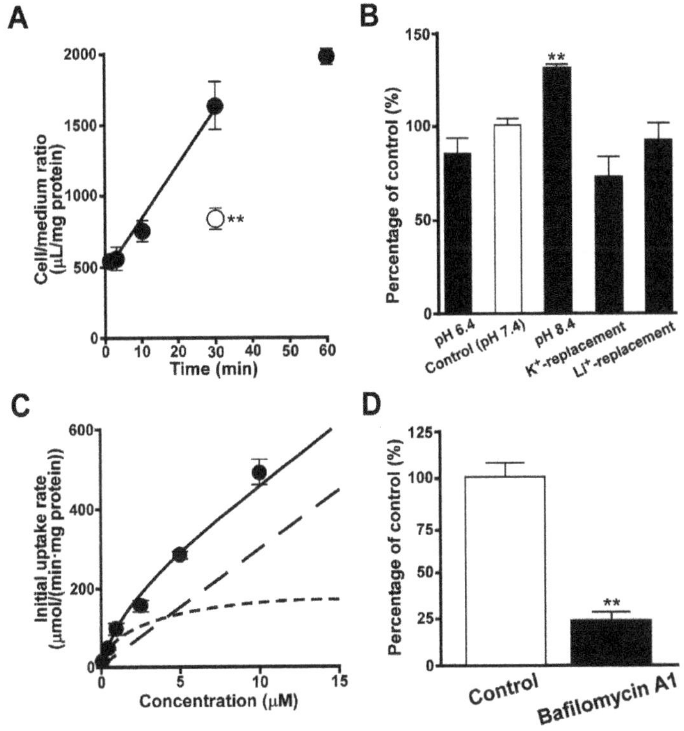

Figure 1. Quinacrine uptake by TR-iBRB2 cells. (**A**) Time-dependent uptake of quinacrine (5 μM) by TR-iBRB2 cells was investigated at 37 °C (closed circles) and 4 °C (open circles). (**B**) The effects of Na^+, extracellular pH and membrane potential were examined at 37 °C for 30 min. (**C**) Concentration-dependent uptake was examined at 37 °C for 30 min, over the concentration range 1–10 μM. Dotted and dashed lines represent a saturable and non-saturable transport process, respectively. (**D**) The effects of bafilomycin A1 was examined. Before quinacrine uptake at 37 °C for 30 min, cells were treated with 100 nM bafilomycin A1 at 37 °C for 30 min. Each column and point represent the mean ± S.E.M. (n = 3–4). Significant difference for two groups and for several groups was taken using an unpaired two-tailed Student's t-test was taken for two groups and a one-way analysis of variance (ANOVA) followed by Dunnett's test, respectively. ** $p < 0.01$, significantly different from the control (37 °C, pH 7.4).

3.2. Effect of Intracellular pH on Quinacrine Uptake by TR-iBRB2 Cells

The uptake of quinacrine at various intracellular pH conditions was examined in TR-iBRB2 cells, and acute treatment with NH_4Cl reduced it by 47% while pretreatment with NH_4Cl had no significant effect on the uptake (Figure 2A). In addition, quinacrine uptake by TR-iBRB2 cells was reduced by 48% in the presence of FCCP, a H^+ ionophore (Figure 2A). Confocal microscopy showed the punctate fluorescence signal of quinacrine (green) taken up by TR-iBRB2 cells, and its intracellular distribution was similar to that of LTR (red), a typical compound that undergoes lysosomal trapping (Figure 2B). In addition, the punctate fluorescence signal of quinacrine was attenuated by treatment with bafilomycin A1 or NH_4Cl (Figure 2C).

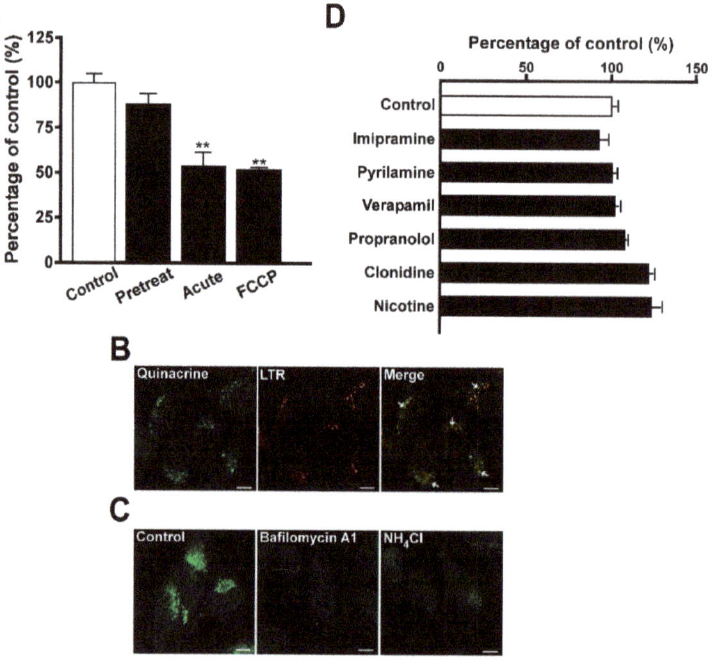

Figure 2. Effect of intracellular pH modulators on quinacrine uptake by TR-iBRB2 cells. (**A**) The quinacrine uptake was examined in the presence or absence of 30 mM NH_4Cl at 37 °C for 30 min. In a pretreat condition, cells were treated with 30 mM NH_4Cl, and the uptake of quinacrine (5 μM) was performed in the absence of NH_4Cl. In an acute condition, cells were treated with ECF-buffer, and quinacrine uptake was performed in the presence of 30 mM NH_4Cl. The uptake was also examined in the presence of 50 μM FCCP at 37 °C for 30 min. (**B**) Confocal microscopy was carried out to investigate the intracellular distribution of quinacrine and LTR. The uptake of quinacrine (5 μM, green) and LTR (300 nM, red) was carried out at 37 °C for 30 min. (**C**) Confocal microscopy was carried out to investigate the intracellular distribution of quinacrine in the presence of intracellular pH modulator, such as 100 nM bafilomycin A1 and 30 mM NH_4Cl. The uptake of quinacrine (5 μM, green) was carried out at 37 °C for 30 min. (**D**) Inhibitory effect of cationic drugs on quinacrine uptake was examined in the presence of bafilomycin A1. After the treatment of TR-iBRB2 cells with 100 nM bafilomycin A1 at 37 °C for 30 min, quinacrine uptake was examined in the presence of 100 μM cationic drug at 37 °C for 30 min. Each column represents the mean ± S.E.M. (n = 3–4). ** $p < 0.01$, significantly different from the control. FCCP, Carbonyl cyanide-*p*-trifluoromethoxyphenylhydrazone. Scale bar, 10 μm.

3.3. Inhibition of Quinacrine Uptake by TR-iBRB2 Cells

The inhibitory effect of compounds on the uptake of quinacrine by TR-iBRB2 cells was examined. The uptake was significantly decreased by various cationic drugs such as desipramine, imipramine, propranolol, verapamil, pyrilamine and nicotine, but was not changed by *p*-aminohippuric acid (PAH), choline, L-carnitine and cimetidine (Table 1). When TR-iBRB2 cells were treated with 100 nM bafilomycin A1, no significant effect was observed in the uptake of quinacrine in the presence of imipramine, amiodarone, pyrilamine, verapamil, propranolol, clonidine, and nicotine (Figure 2D).

Table 1. Inhibitory Effect of Quinacrine Uptake.

Compounds	Relative Uptake (% of Control)		
	TR-iBRB2 Cells	Lysosome-Enriched Fraction of TR-iBRB2 Cells	Lysosome-Enriched Fraction of RPE-J Cells
Control	100 ± 3	100 ± 3	100 ± 11
Desipramine	47.9 ± 2.2 **	47.2 ± 1.9 **	64.4 ± 0.9 **
Imipramine	55.2 ± 2.7 **	49.6 ± 5.0 **	61.8 ± 2.9 **
Propranolol	55.4 ± 2.5 **	65.8 ± 1.8 **	76.8 ± 3.8 *
Verapamil	64.7 ± 1.2 **	42.4 ± 1.3 **	57.3 ± 2.1 **
Pyrilamine	72.6 ± 2.3 **	87.1 ± 5.0	66.0 ± 2.4 **
Clonidine	90.3 ± 6.6	106 ± 11	89.4 ± 6.8
Nicotine	79.5 ± 6.0 **	106 ± 2	97.1 ± 7.1
Choline	98.7 ± 3.3	N.D.	N.D.
Cimetidine	88.3 ± 1.9	N.D.	N.D.
L-Carnitine	98.5 ± 8.9	N.D.	N.D.
PAH	97.6 ± 8.2	N.D.	N.D.

By using TR-iBRB2 cells and lysosome-enriched fractions, the uptake of quinacrine (300 nM) was examined in the presence of compounds (100 μM) for 30 min at 37 °C. Each value represents the means ± S.E.M. (n = 3–8). * $p < 0.05$, ** $p < 0.01$, significantly different from the control (absence of inhibitor). N.D., not determined. PAH, p-aminohippuric acid; N.D., not determined.

3.4. Uptake of Quinacrine in Lysosome-Enriched Fraction

The uptake of quinacrine in the lysosome-enriched fraction of TR-iBRB2 cells was significantly reduced by 53%, 50%, 34%, and 58% in the presence of desipramine, imipramine, propranolol and verapamil, respectively whereas pyrilamine, clonidine and nicotine had no effect (Table 1). The uptake of quinacrine in the lysosome-enriched fractions of TR-iBRB2 cells was examined following pretreatment with 100 nM bafilomycin A1, which significantly reduced the uptake (Figure 3A). The uptake of quinacrine in lysosome-enriched fractions of RPE-J cells was also examined, and it was significantly reduced by 36%, 38%, 23%, 43%, and 34% in the presence of desipramine, imipramine, propranolol, verapamil, and pyrilamine, respectively, whereas clonidine and nicotine had no effect (Table 1).

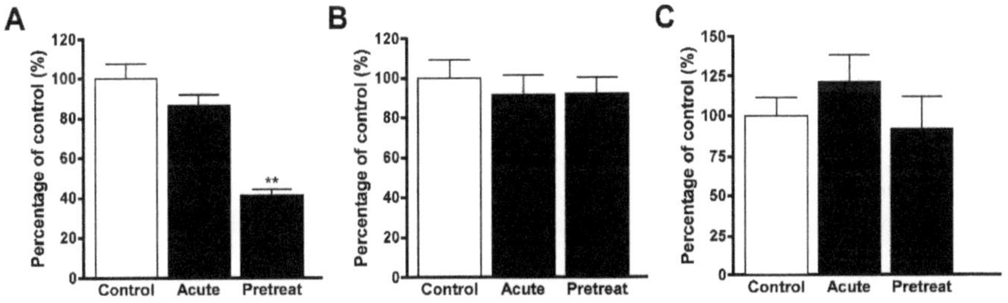

Figure 3. Effect of lysosomal pH on quinacrine and EFV uptake in lysosome-enriched fractions. (**A**) The uptake of quinacrine (5 μM) in the fraction of TR-iBRB2 cells was examined in the presence or absence of 100 nM bafilomycin A1 at 37 °C for 30 min. (**B**) The uptake of EFV (1 μM) in the fraction of TR-iBRB2 cells was examined in the presence or absence of 100 nM bafilomycin A1 at 37 °C for 30 min. (**C**) The uptake of EFV (1 μM) in the fraction of RPE-J cells was examined in the presence or absence of 100 nM bafilomycin A1 at 37 °C for 30 min. Bafilomycin A1 is an inhibitor of V-ATPase that attenuate the lysosomal acidic interior pH, and the uptake was examined in the presence or absence of 100 nM bafilomycin A1 at 37 °C for 30 min. In a pretreat condition, fractions were treated with 100 nM bafilomycin A1, and the uptake was performed in the absence of bafilomycin A1. In an acute condition, fractions were treated with ICF-buffer, and the uptake was performed in the presence of 100 nM bafilomycin A1. Each column represents the mean ± S.E.M (n = 4). ** $p < 0.01$, significantly different from the control.

3.5. Uptake of EFV in Lysosomal-Enriched Fraction

The uptake of EFV was examined in the lysosome-enriched fractions of TR-iBRB2 cells, and desipramine significantly reduced it by 38%. Imipramine and verapamil also reduced the uptake by 32% and 28%, respectively, indicating their tendency to inhibit the uptake, whereas no effect was shown by propranolol, pyrilamine, clonidine and nicotine (Table 2). The uptake of EFV by lysosome-enriched fractions of RPE-J cells was significantly reduced by 35% and 49% in the presence of desipramine and verapamil, respectively, whereas no effect was shown by imipramine, propranolol, pyrilamine, clonidine and nicotine (Table 2). EFV uptake was also examined in the presence of bafilomycin A1, and no significant alteration was observed in the lysosome-enriched fraction of TR-iBRB2 and RPE-J cells in the presence of 100 nM bafilomycin A1 (Figure 3B,C).

Table 2. Inhibitory effect of EFV uptake.

Compounds	Relative Uptake (% of Control)		
	TR-iBRB2 Cells [27]	Lysosome-Enriched Fraction of TR-iBRB2 Cells	Lysosome-Enriched Fraction of RPE-J Cells
Control	100 ± 3	100 ± 3	100 ± 7
Desipramine	47.9 ± 2.2 **	61.8 ± 1.9 *	65.5 ± 5.8 *
Imipramine	55.2 ± 2.7 **	68.5 ± 2.8	82.5 ± 11.0
Propranolol	55.4 ± 2.5 **	108 ± 13	114 ± 7
Verapamil	64.7 ± 1.2 **	71.5 ± 3.0	51.0 ± 3.8 **
Pyrilamine	72.6 ± 2.3 **	143 ± 1	122 ± 12
Clonidine	90.3 ± 6.6	132 ± 7	98.6 ± 4.1
Nicotine	79.5 ± 6.0 **	147 ± 23	110 ± 10

By using TR-iBRB2 cells and lysosome-enriched fractions, the uptake of EFV (1 μM) by was examined in the presence of compounds (100 μM) at 37 °C for 3 min. Each value represents the means ± S.E.M. ($n = 4$). * $p < 0.05$, ** $p < 0.01$, significantly different from the control (absence of inhibitor). EFV, EverFluor FL Verapamil. Data for EFV uptake by TR-iBRB2 cells was presented by reference to previous report [27].

4. Discussion

P-glycoprotein (P-gp/Mdr1/Abcb1) is known to be a representative efflux transporter at the blood-brain barrier, and involved in restricting the distribution of lipophilic and cationic drugs to the brain [40]. P-gp was also reported to be localized at the luminal membrane of the retinal capillary endothelial cells [41], suggesting its possible contribution to the restriction of drug distribution to the retina. However, the study of relationship between the BRB permeability and the lipophilicity of compounds showed a greater in vivo retinal uptake of verapamil, a substrate of P-glycoprotein [42], revealing the influx transport of verapamil at the BRB and the different barrier function between the BRB and the blood-brain barrier (BBB). Furthermore, the carrier-mediated blood-to-retina transport of cationic drugs at the BRB has been reported [13–17], and is suggested to be promising for the establishment of the safe and efficient delivery of cationic drugs to the retina where neurological dysfunctions are caused by severe retinal diseases such as macular degeneration and diabetic retinopathy [3,12]. In addition, lysosomal trapping has been implied to exert the undesirable influence on the blood-to-retina transport of cationic neuroprotectants across the BRB since its unignorable influence had been suggested in the accumulating reports [28–30]. The study using a representative lysosomotropic agent, LTR, suggested that lysosomal trapping only partially influenced transport of cationic amphiphilic drugs in the BRB [26], and this was also supported by the study using EFV [27]. In the present study, lysosome-enriched fraction was used to investigate the influence of lysosomal trapping on quinacrine and EFV uptake in the inner and outer BRB in detail.

The study of quinacrine uptake by TR-iBRB2 cells showed an initial uptake rate of 445 μL/(min·mg protein), and suggested that quinacrine uptake was concentrated in the retinal capillary endothelial cells. This was because the quinacrine uptake at 30 min (1640 μL/[min·mg protein]) indicated that the cellular concentration of quinacrine was approximately 273 μM, which was clearly higher than that of the uptake buffer (5 μM) (Figure 1A). The uptake study at 4 °C showed that the quinacrine uptake was significantly reduced by 45% (Figure 1A), and this result implied the unignorable contribution of lysosomal trapping to quinacrine uptake in the inner BRB because the 45% reduction in cellular uptake of quinacrine seems to be insufficient to support the unilateral contribution of carrier-mediated transport. In addition, the experiment in TR-iBRB2 cells suggested that quinacrine uptake in the inner BRB occurs in an Na^+- and membrane potential-insensitive manner (Figure 1B), and showed a sensitivity to extracellular pH. In addition, there was a 1.31-fold higher quinacrine uptake at pH 8.4 than at pH 7.4, whereas no significant change was observed in the uptake at pH 6.4 (Figure 1B). Based on the Henderson–Hasselbalch equation, the uptake of nonionized quinacrine at pH 8.4 was estimated to be 9.84-fold higher than that at pH 7.4, indicating that quinacrine uptake by TR-iBRB2 cells could not be explained by the pH-partition hypothesis. Furthermore, this observation suggests that passive diffusion in accordance with the physicochemical characteristics is not enough to explain the uptake of quinacrine in the inner BRB. This idea is closely supported by the estimation of K_m, V_{max}, and K_d values 1.87 μM, 189 μmol/(min·mg protein), and 29.7 μL/(min·mg protein), respectively, revealing the involvement of saturable and non-saturable processes in quinacrine uptake in the inner BRB (Figure 1C). Similarly, the transport was also reported to include saturable and non-saturable processes in the acidic intracellular compartments or at the plasma membrane of the inner BRB for the uptake of LTR, a typical lysosomotropic agent [26]. The results obtained for quinacrine and LTR demonstrate the difficulty involved in the study of lysosomal trapping using cellular uptake analysis, suggesting the possible advantage of using lysosomal fractions.

Bafilomycin A1 is a known specific inhibitor of V-ATPase, which is expressed in acidic intracellular compartments, including the lysosome, and contributes to maintaining their acidic interior pH [24]. Pretreatment with bafilomycin A1 significantly reduced quinacrine uptake by TR-iBRB2 cells (Figure 1D), suggesting that quinacrine uptake is largely influenced by the interior acidic pH in the inner BRB. In addition, the acute treatment of cells with NH_4Cl or FCCP is known to cancel the H^+-gradient between the lysosomes and cytosol [23–25], and TR-iBRB2 cells showed a significant decrease in quinacrine uptake following acute treatment with NH_4Cl or FCCP, whereas pretreatment with NH_4Cl had no effect (Figure 2A), supporting that the acidic interior pH is important in quinacrine uptake in the inner BRB. In addition to the saturable and non-saturable transport processes, the present results suggest that the characteristics of quinacrine transport were similar to those of LTR reported previously [26], and this was also supported by the results of the confocal microscopy because the fluorescence signals of quinacrine and LTR were shown to merge, suggesting quinacrine was distributed to the lysosome (Figure 2B). Confocal microscopy with bafilomycin A1 or NH_4Cl also supported the sequestration of quinacrine in acidic intracellular compartments at the inner BRB because the punctate quinacrine distribution was shown to be attenuated in TR-iBRB2 cells treated with these agents (Figure 2C).

The inhibition study suggested that quinacrine possibly interacted with cationic amphiphilic drugs, except for clonidine, in the retinal capillary endothelial cells because the uptake of quinacrine by TR-iBRB2 cells was significantly reduced by desipramine, imipramine, propranolol, verapamil pyrilamine, and nicotine (Table 1). The study using bafilomycin A1 suggested that the interaction predominantly takes place in acidic intracellular compartments, including the lysosomes, and not at the plasma membrane, since TR-iBRB2 cells treated with bafilomycin A1 showed no significant change in quinacrine uptake in the presence of cationic drugs (Figure 2D). This observation clearly suggests the importance of studies with lysosomes in understanding the influence of lysosomal trapping on the transport of cationic drug at the BRB.

The uptake of quinacrine in the lysosome-enriched fractions of TR-iBRB2 cells was significantly inhibited by treatment with bafilomycin A1 (Figure 3A), and this was consistent with the results obtained in the cellular uptake with TR-iBRB2 cells (Figure 1D), supporting the distribution of quinacrine to lysosomes. The results of the inhibition study using several cationic drugs suggested that quinacrine interacted with desipramine, imipramine, propranolol and verapamil at the lysosome of the inner BRB, because quinacrine uptake in the lysosome-enriched fraction of TR-iBRB2 cells was significantly inhibited by these cationic drugs (Table 1). In addition, pyrilamine, clonidine, and nicotine had no effect on the uptake of quinacrine in the fractions of TR-iBRB2 cells (Table 1), and these results suggests that the interaction of these drugs in the lysosome is minor. These results also provide evidence that clearly supports previous reports of the carrier-mediated blood-to-retina transports of these agents across the inner BRB [13–15]. Similar results were also obtained with the lysosome-enriched fractions of RPE-J cells, used as an in vitro model cell line of the outer BRB (Table 1), and these results suggest the interaction of quinacrine with desipramine, imipramine, verapamil, and pyrilamine, and the blood-to-retina transport of clonidine and nicotine across the outer BRB.

Furthermore, the lysosome-enriched fraction of TR-iBRB2 cells was used to study the uptake of EFV, which was not changed by treatment with bafilomycin A1 (Figure 3B). This result was very similar to the outcome of our recent study of EFV uptake by TR-iBRB2 cells treated with bafilomycin A1 [27], and the similarity suggests that the interior acidic pH is not essential for EFV transport in the inner BRB (Figure 3B), showing that its transport characteristics differ from those of quinacrine. In the inhibition study, EFV uptake in TR-iBRB2 cell fractions was not altered in the presence of the cationic drugs (Table 2), suggesting a minor interaction between EFV and cationic drugs in lysosomes. The inhibition profile obtained was not consistent with that of quinacrine (Tables 1 and 2), and these results suggests that the transport characteristics for EFV definitely differ from those of quinacrine in the inner BRB. These results also suggest the minor contribution of lysosomal trapping driven by acidic interior pH in EFV transport at the inner BRB, supporting the carrier-mediated blood-to-retina transport of EFV across the inner BRB [27]. In the lysosome-enriched fraction of RPE-J cells, EFV uptake was significantly inhibited by verapamil, whereas it was almost similar to those obtained in the fraction of TR-iBRB2 cells (Table 2 and Figure 3C). These results still suggest the clear difference between EFV transport characteristics and those of quinacrine in the outer BRB, supporting the fact that lysosomal trapping only partially influences EFV transport across the outer BRB as reported previously [27].

5. Conclusions

The cellular uptake study suggests that quinacrine was distributed to the acidic intracellular compartments of the inner BRB, and this was also supported by the confocal microscopy results. The inhibition of cellular uptake suggested the possible interaction of quinacrine with cationic drugs in lysosomes of the inner BRB, implying the importance of uptake studies in lysosomes. The adoption of the lysosome-enriched fraction in the uptake study suggested the lysosomal trapping of quinacrine in the BRB, and supported that lysosomal trapping exerts a minor influence on the transport of several cationic drugs at the BRB while its influence at varying degrees is also implied on the transport of other drugs. The study of EFV transport in lysosome-enriched fractions also suggested the minor influence of lysosomal trapping driven by interior acidic pH on the transport of EFV across the BRB. This observation also provides evidence supporting the blood-to-retina transport of verapamil across the BRB [15,17,27]. The present findings are expected to improve our understanding of the blood-to-retina transport of cationic amphiphilic drugs across the BRB, thereby contributing to the establishment of a new strategy for safe and efficient drug delivery to the retina.

Supplementary Materials: The Supplemental information are available online at http://www.mdpi.com/1999-4923/12/8/747/s1.

Author Contributions: Y.K., S.-i.A., and K.-i.H.: conception and design; M.Y. and S.K.: collection and assembly of data; Y.K., M.Y., and S.K.: data analysis and interpretation; Y.K. and K.-i.H.: writing manuscript. All authors have read and agreed to the published version of the manuscript.

Funding: This study was supported in part by Grant-in-Aids for Scientific Research (B) [KAKENHI: 20H03403], Scientific Research (C) [KAKENHI: 19K07160] and Scientific Research (C) [KAKENHI: 20K07173] from the Japan Society for Promotion of Science, and Research Grants from the Tamura Science and Technology Foundation.

Conflicts of Interest: The authors declare no conflict of interest.

References

1. Cunha-Vaz, J.G.; Shakib, M.; Ashton, N. Studies on the permeability of the blood-retinal barrier. I. On the existence, development, and site of a blood-retinal barrier. *Br. J. Ophthalmol.* **1966**, *50*, 441453. [CrossRef] [PubMed]
2. Hosoya, K.; Tomi, M.; Tachikawa, M. Strategies for therapy of retinal diseases using systemic drug delivery: Relevance of transporters at the blood-retinal barrier. *Expert. Opin. Drug. Deliv.* **2011**, *8*, 1571–1587. [CrossRef] [PubMed]
3. Kubo, Y.; Akanuma, S.; Hosoya, K. Recent advances in drug and nutrient transport across the blood-retinal barrier. *Expert. Opin. Drug. Metab. Toxicol.* **2018**, *14*, 513–531. [CrossRef] [PubMed]
4. Takata, K.; Kasahara, T.; Kasahara, M.; Ezaki, O.; Hirano, H. Ultracytochemical localization of the erythrocyte/ HepG2-type glucose transporter (GLUT1) in cells of the blood-retinal barrier in the rat. *Investig. Ophthalmol. Vis. Sci.* **1992**, *33*, 377–383.
5. Kubo, Y.; Akanuma, S.; Hosoya, K. Impact of SLC6A transporters in physiological taurine transport at the bloodretinal barrier and in the liver. *Biol. Pharm. Bull.* **2016**, *39*, 1903–1911. [CrossRef]
6. Kubo, Y.; Obata, A.; Akanuma, S.; Hosoya, K. Impact of cationic amino acid transporter 1 on blood-retinal barrier transport of L-ornithine. *Investig. Ophthalmol. Vis. Sci.* **2015**, *56*, 5925–5932. [CrossRef]
7. Kubo, Y.; Yahata, S.; Miki, S.; Akanuma, S.; Hosoya, K. Blood-to-retina transport of riboflavin via RFVTs at the inner blood-retinal barrier. *Drug. Metab. Pharmacokinet.* **2017**, *32*, 92–99. [CrossRef]
8. Kubo, Y.; Miki, S.; Akanuma, S.; Hosoya, K. Riboflavin transport mediated by riboflavin transporters (RFVTs/SLC52A) at the rat outer blood-retinal barrier. *Drug. Metab. Pharmacokinet.* **2019**, *34*, 380–386. [CrossRef]
9. Nagase, K.; Tomi, M.; Tachikawa, M.; Hosoya, K. Functional and molecular characterization of adenosine transport at the rat inner blood-retinal barrier. *Biochim. Biophys. Acta.* **2006**, *1758*, 13–19. [CrossRef]
10. Nakashima, T.; Tomi, M.; Katayama, K.; Tachikawa, M.; Watanabe, M.; Terasaki, T.; Hosoya, K.I. Blood-to-retina transport of creatine via creatine transporter (CRT) at the rat inner blood-retinal barrier. *J. Neurochem.* **2004**, *89*, 1454–1461. [CrossRef]
11. Liu, L.; Liu, X. Roles of Drug Transporters in Blood-Retinal Barrier. In *Drug Transporters in Drug Disposition, Effects and Toxicity. Advances in Experimental Medicine and Biology*; Liu, X., Pan, G., Eds.; Springer: Singapore, 2019; p. 1140.
12. Kubo, Y.; Akanuma, S.; Hosoya, K. Influx transport of cationic drug at the blood-retinal barrier: Impact on the retinal delivery of neuroprotectants. *Biol. Pharm. Bull.* **2017**, *40*, 1139–1145. [CrossRef] [PubMed]
13. Tega, Y.; Kubo, Y.; Yuzurihara, C.; Akanuma, S.; Hosoya, K. Carrier-mediated transport of nicotine across the inner blood-retinal barrier: Involvement of a novel organic cation transporter driven by an outward H(+) gradient. *J. Pharm. Sci.* **2015**, *104*, 3069–3075. [CrossRef] [PubMed]
14. Kubo, Y.; Tsuchiyama, A.; Shimizu, Y.; Akanuma, S.; Hosoya, K. Involvement of carrier-mediated transport in the retinal uptake of clonidine at the inner blood-retinal barrier. *Mol. Pharm.* **2014**, *11*, 3747–3753. [CrossRef] [PubMed]
15. Kubo, Y.; Kusagawa, Y.; Tachikawa, M.; Akanuma, S.; Hosoya, K. Involvement of a novel organic cation transporter in verapamil transport across the inner blood-retinal barrier. *Pharm. Res.* **2013**, *30*, 847–856. [CrossRef] [PubMed]
16. Kubo, Y.; Shimizu, Y.; Kusagawa, Y.; Akanuma, S.; Hosoya, K. Propranolol transport across the inner blood-retinal barrier: Potential involvement of a novel organic cation transporter. *J. Pharm. Sci.* **2013**, *102*, 3332–3342. [CrossRef] [PubMed]
17. Han, Y.H.; Sweet, D.H.; Hu, D.N.; Pritchard, J.B. Characterization of a novel cationic drug transporter in human retinal pigment epithelial cells. *J. Pharmacol. Exp. Ther.* **2001**, *296*, 450–457.
18. Molinuevo, J.L.; Lladó, A.; Rami, L. Memantine: Targeting glutamate excitotoxicity in Alzheimer's disease and other dementias. *Am. J. Alzheimers Dis. Other Demen.* **2005**, *20*, 77–85. [CrossRef]
19. Martini, D.; Monte, M.D.; Ristori, C.; Cupisti, E.; Mei, S.; Fiorini, P.; Filippi, L.; Bagnoli, P. Antiangiogenic effects of β2 -adrenergic receptor blockade in a mouse model of oxygen-induced retinopathy. *J. Neurochem.* **2011**, *119*, 1317–1329. [CrossRef]
20. Yoles, E.; Wheeler, L.A.; Schwartz, M. Alpha2-adrenoreceptor agonists are neuroprotective in a rat model of optic nerve degeneration. *Investig. Ophthalmol. Vis. Sci.* **1999**, *40*, 65–73.

21. Nadanaciva, S.; Lu, S.; Gebhard, D.F.; Jessen, B.A.; Pennie, W.D.; Will, Y. A high content screening assay for identifying lysosomotropic compounds. *Toxicol, In Vitro.* **2011**, *25*, 715–723. [CrossRef]
22. Kazmi, F.; Hensley, T.; Pope, C.; Funk, R.S.; Loewen, G.J.; Buckley, D.B.; Parkinson, A. Lysosomal sequestration (trapping) of lipophilic amine (cationic amphiphilic) drugs in immortalized human hepatocytes (Fa2N-4 cells). *Drug. Metab. Dispos.* **2013**, *41*, 897–905. [CrossRef] [PubMed]
23. Lemieux, B.; Percival, M.D.; Falgueyret, J.P. Quantitation of the lysosomotropic character of cationic amphiphilic drugs using the fluorescent basic amine Red DND-99. *Anal. Biochem.* **2004**, *327*, 247–251. [CrossRef] [PubMed]
24. Yoshimori, T.; Yamamoto, A.; Moriyama, Y.; Futai, M.; Tashiro, Y. Bafilomycin A1, a specific inhibitor of vacuolar-type H^+-ATPase, inhibits acidification and protein degradation in lysosomes of cultured cells. *J. Biol. Chem.* **1991**, *266*, 17707–17712. [PubMed]
25. Ohkuma, S.; Moriyama, Y.; Takano, T. Identification and characterization of a proton pump on lysosomes by fluorescein-isothiocyanate-dextran fluorescence. *Proc. Natl. Acad. Sci. USA.* **1982**, *79*, 2758–2762. [CrossRef]
26. Kubo, Y.; Seko, N.; Usui, T.; Akanuma, S.; Hosoya, K. Lysosomal trapping is present in retinal capillary endothelial cells: Insight into its influence on cationic drug transport at the inner blood-retinal barrier. *Biol. Pharm. Bull.* **2016**, *39*, 1319–1324. [CrossRef]
27. Kubo, Y.; Nakazawa, A.; Akanuma, S.; Hosoya, K. Blood-to-retina transport of fluorescence-labeled verapamil at the blood-retinal Barrier. *Pharm. Res.* **2018**, *35*, 93. [CrossRef]
28. Daniel, W.A.; Wójcikowski, J. Contribution of lysosomal trapping to the total tissue uptake of psychotropic drugs. *Pharmacol. Toxicol.* **1997**, *80*, 62–68. [CrossRef]
29. Ishizaki, J.; Yokogawa, K.; Ichimura, F.; Ohkuma, S. Uptake of imipramine in rat liver lysosomes in vitro and its inhibition by basic drugs. *J. Pharmacol. Exp. Ther.* **2000**, *294*, 1088–1098.
30. Logan, R.; Kong, A.C.; Krise, J.P. Time-dependent effects of hydrophobic amine-containing drugs on lysosome structure and biogenesis in cultured human fibroblasts. *J. Pharm. Sci.* **2014**, *103*, 3287–3296. [CrossRef]
31. Marceau, F.; Bawolak, M.T.; Bouthillier, J.; Morissette, G. Vacuolar ATPase-mediated cellular concentration and retention of quinacrine: A model for the distribution of lipophilic cationic drugs to autophagic vacuoles. *Drug. Metab. Dispos.* **2009**, *37*, 2271–2274. [CrossRef]
32. Roy, C.; Gagné, V.; Fernandes, M.J.; Marceau, F. High affinity capture and concentration of quinacrine in polymorphonuclear neutrophils via vacuolar ATPase-mediated ion trapping: Comparison with other peripheral blood leukocytes and implications for the distribution of cationic drugs. *Toxicol. Appl. Pharmacol.* **2013**, *270*, 77–86. [CrossRef] [PubMed]
33. Parks, A.; Charest-Morin, X.; Boivin-Welch, M.; Bouthillier, J.; Marceau, F. Autophagic flux inhibition and lysosomogenesis ensuing cellular capture and retention of the cationic drug quinacrine in murine models. *PeerJ.* **2015**, *3*, e1314. [CrossRef] [PubMed]
34. Hosoya, K.; Tomi, M.; Ohtsuki, S.; Takanaga, H.; Ueda, M.; Yanai, N.; Obinata, M.; Terasaki, T. Conditionally immortalized retinal capillary endothelial cell lines (TR-iBRB) expressing differentiated endothelial cell functions derived from a transgenic rat. *Exp. Eye Res.* **2001**, *72*, 163–172. [CrossRef] [PubMed]
35. Nabi, I.R.; Mathews, A.P.; Cohen-Gould, L.; Gundersen, D.; Rodriguez-Boulan, E. Immortalization of polarized rat retinal pigment epithelium. *J. Cell Sci.* **1993**, *104*, 37–49. [PubMed]
36. Yamaoka, K.; Tanigawara, Y.; Nakagawa, T.; Uno, T. A pharmacokinetic analysis program (multi) for microcomputer. *J. Pharmacobiodyn.* **1981**, *4*, 879–885. [CrossRef]
37. Kinoshita, Y.; Nogami, K.; Jomura, R.; Akanuma, S.-I.; Abe, H.; Inouye, M.; Kubo, Y.; Hosoya, K.-I. Investigation of receptor-mediated cyanocobalamin (vitamin B12) transport across the inner blood-retinal barrier using fluorescence-labeled cyanocobalamin. *Mol. Pharm.* **2018**, *15*, 3583–3594. [CrossRef]
38. Kawaguchi, K.; Okamoto, T.; Morita, M.; Imanaka, T. Translocation of the ABC transporter ABCD4 from the endoplasmic reticulum to lysosomes requires the escort protein LMBD1. *Sci. Rep.* **2016**, *6*, 30183. [CrossRef]
39. Cang, C.; Zhou, Y.; Navarro, B.; Seo, Y.-J.; Aranda, K.; Shi, L.; Battaglia-Hsu, S.; Nissim, I.; Clapham, D.E.; Ren, D. mTOR regulates lysosomal ATP-sensitive two-pore Na(+) channels to adapt to metabolic state. *Cell* **2013**, *152*, 778–790. [CrossRef]
40. Erdő, F.; Denes, L.; de Lange, E. Age-associated physiological and pathological changes at the blood-brain barrier: A review. *J. Cereb. Blood Flow Metab.* **2017**, *37*, 4–24. [CrossRef]

41. Hosoya, K.; Tomi, M. Advances in the cell biology of transport via the inner blood-retinal barrier: Establishment of cell lines and transport functions. *Biol. Pharm. Bull.* **2005**, *28*, 1–8. [CrossRef]
42. Hosoya, K.; Yamamoto, A.; Akanuma, S.; Tachikawa, M. Lipophilicity and transporter influence on blood-retinal barrier permeability: A comparison with blood-brain barrier permeability. *Pharm. Res.* **2010**, *27*, 2715–2724. [CrossRef] [PubMed]

pharmaceutics

MDPI

Article

Biopharmaceutical Assessment of Dexamethasone Acetate-Based Hydrogels Combining Hydroxypropyl Cyclodextrins and Polysaccharides for Ocular Delivery

Roseline Mazet [1,2], Xurxo García-Otero [3,4], Luc Choisnard [1], Denis Wouessidjewe [1], Vincent Verdoot [5], Frédéric Bossard [5], Victoria Díaz-Tomé [3,6], Véronique Blanc-Marquis [1], Francisco-Javier Otero-Espinar [3], Anxo Fernandez-Ferreiro [6,7,*] and Annabelle Gèze [1,*]

1 University Grenoble Alpes, CNRS, DPM, 38000 Grenoble, France; rmazet@chu-grenoble.fr (R.M.); luc.choisnard@univ-grenoble-alpes.fr (L.C.); denis.wouessi@univ-grenoble-alpes.fr (D.W.); veronique.blanc-marquis@univ-grenoble-alpes.fr (V.B.-M.)

2 Pharmacy Unit, Grenoble University Hospital, 38000 Grenoble, France

3 Department of Pharmacology, Pharmacy, Pharmaceutical Technology and Industrial Pharmacy Institute, Faculty of Pharmacy, University of Santiago de Compostela (USC), 15782 Santiago de Compostela, Spain; xurxo.garcia.otero@gmail.com (X.G.-O.); victoriadiaztome@gmail.com (V.D.-T.); francisco.otero@usc.es (F.-J.O.-E.)

4 Molecular Imaging Group, Health Research Institute of Santiago de Compostela (IDIS), 15706 Santiago de Compostela, Spain

5 University Grenoble Alpes, CNRS, Grenoble INP, LRP, 38000 Grenoble, France; vincent.verdoot@univ-grenoble-alpes.fr (V.V.); frederic.bossard@univ-grenoble-alpes.fr (F.B.)

6 Clinical Pharmacology Group, Health Research Institute of Santiago de Compostela (IDIS), 15706 Santiago de Compostela, Spain

7 Pharmacy Department, Clinical University Hospital Santiago de Compostela (SERGAS), 15706 Santiago de Compostela, Spain

* Correspondence: anxordes@gmail.com (A.F.-F.); annabelle.geze@univ-grenoble-alpes.fr (A.G.); Tel.: +33-476-63-53-01 (A.G.)

Received: 20 May 2020; Accepted: 24 July 2020; Published: 30 July 2020

Abstract: We previously developed two optimized formulations of dexamethasone acetate (DXMa) hydrogels by means of special cubic mixture designs for topical ocular administration. These gels were elaborated with hydroxypropyl-β-CD (HPβCD) and hydroxypropyl-γ-CD (HPγCD) and commercial hydrogels in order to enhance DXMa water solubility and finally DXMa's ocular bioavailability and transcorneal penetration. The main objective of this study was to characterize them and to evaluate in vitro, ex vivo, and in vivo their safety, biopermanence, and transcorneal permeation. Gels A and B are Newtonian fluids and display a viscosity of 13.2 mPa.s and 18.6 mPa.s, respectively, which increases their ocular retention, according to the in vivo biopermanence study by PET/CT. These hydrogels could act as corneal absorption promoters as they allow a higher transcorneal permeation of DXMa through porcine excised cornea, compared to DEXAFREE® and MAXIDEX®. Cytotoxicity assays showed no cytotoxic effects on human primary corneal epithelial cells (HCE). Furthermore, Gel B is clearly safe for the eye, but the effect of Gel A on the human eye cannot be predicted. Both gels were also stable 12 months at 25 °C after sterilization by filtration. These results demonstrate that the developed formulations present a high potential for the topical ocular administration of dexamethasone acetate.

Keywords: dexamethasone acetate; cyclodextrins; eye drops; hydrogels; rheology; cytotoxicity studies; transcorneal permeation; radiolabeled ocular biopermanence

1. Introduction

Dexamethasone (DXM) is one of the most prescribed anti-inflammatory drug in the treatment of acute and chronic eye inflammation due to its high potency and effectiveness [1]. DXM acts by binding with the corticosteroid receptors present in the human trabecular meshwork cells and inhibits phospholipase-A2 and thus prostaglandins synthesis. DXM eye drops, as MAXIDEX® 1 mg/mL DXM (Novartis Pharma, Rueil-Malmaison, France) and DEXAFREE® 1 mg/mL DXM phosphate (Laboratoires Théa, Clermont-Ferrand, France) are effective in treating postoperative inflammation, keratitis, uveitis [2], and prevention of corneal graft rejection [3]. Despite the many advantages offered by this route of administration, these marketed formulations present a major disadvantage by requiring frequent administrations (up to six times/day) [2]. This is due to the presence of various anatomical and physiological barriers, which leads to a poor bioavailability of the ophthalmic drugs; only 1–5% of drug instilled reaches in aqueous humor [4].

In order to enhance DXM bioavailability, the lipophilic derivative DXM acetate (DXMa), currently unavailable for ophthalmic topical use, could be very interesting. Indeed, DXMa has shown to readily permeate the cornea and be hydrolyzed into DXM during absorption [5]. Furthermore, Leibowitz et al. demonstrated that the acetate form was more effective compared to the phosphate derivative in suppressing inflammation in the cornea. This therapeutic effect was not associated with a greater propensity to increase intraocular pressure, one of the most frequent side effects of glucocorticoids [6].

Furthermore, for the topical administration of DXMa into the eyes, we previously developed, by means of experimental designs, two optimized formulations based on HPβCD or HPγCD/DXMa solutions and marketed gels, with the aim of increasing DXMa bioavailability and reducing instillation frequency. HPβCD or HPγCD have considerably enhanced DXMa solubility in water, 500, and 1550-fold [7]. CELLUVISC® (sodium carboxymethylcellulose) and VISMED® (sodium hyaluronate) have both been used as an artificial tear in order to stabilize the tear film on the ocular surface [8]. Carboxymethylcellulose (CMC) and sodium hyaluronic (NaHA) present great advantages to be mucoadhesive, biodegradable, and biocompatible [9]. These properties exhibit an enhancement of the precorneal residence time and a reduction in the nasolacrymal drainage due to increased viscosity [10]. In addition, NaHA has been shown to modulate the inflammation response of the ocular surface in dry eye syndrome [11].

In the present study, the optimized formulations were characterized. The ocular in vitro cytotoxicity and mucoadhesion properties were evaluated as well as ex vivo transcorneal permeation of DXMa. Furthermore, in vivo precorneal drug kinetics were investigated by radiolabeling with ^{18}F-FDG in order to show the benefits of the newly designed formulations.

2. Materials and Methods

2.1. Materials

DXMa was purchased from LA COOPER (Melun, France). Hydroxypropyl-γ-cyclodextrin (HPγCD, W8HP, DS = 0.6, and Mw = 1576 Da) was a kind gift from ASHLAND (Schaffhausen, Switzerland) and hydroxypropyl-β-cyclodextrin (HPβCD, KLEPTOSE DS = 0.63 and Mw = 1391 Da) was obtained from ROQUETTE (Lestrem, France). CELLUVISC® (sodium carboxymethylcellulose) and VISMED® (sodium hyaluronate) are marketed gels used for the treatment of dry eye syndrome. DEXAFREE® (DXM sodium phosphate 1% solution eye drops), MAXIDEX® (DXM 0.1% suspension eye drops) and BSS® (Alcon Laboratories, Rueil-Malmaison, France) are human authorized ocular medicines. Normal human primary corneal epithelial cells (ATCC PCS 700-010), medium (ATCC PCS-700-030), growth kit (ATCC PCS-700-040), PBS (ATCC 30-2200), trypsin EDTA (ATCC PCS-999-003 and 005), and antibiotics (gentamicin, streptomycin, and amphotericin BATC PCS-999-002) were obtained from LGC standard - ATCC® (Molsheim, France). Thioglycollate with resazurine medium and Tryptic soy broth were obtained from BIOMERIEUX (Craponne, France). ALAMARBLUE® was purchased from BIO-RAD (Marnes-la-Coquette, France) and DMSO from SIGMA-ALDRICH (Lyon,

France). Purified water was prepared by DIRECT-Q®3UV water purifier (MILLIPORE, Molsheim, France). All other solvents and chemicals were of HPLC and analytical grade, respectively.

2.2. Methods

2.2.1. Gel Composition

The composition of optimized mixed Gels A and B were obtained by means of experimental design, as previously described [7] (Table 1).

In a first step, the cyclodextrin derivative was introduced in sterile water (600 mg/mL) and agitated at room temperature. Then, the DXMa powder was added to the cyclodextrin solution. After complete drug dissolution, the DXMa (10 mg/mL)/HPβCD (600 mg/mL) and DXMa (30 mg/mL)/HPγCD (600 mg/mL) were obtained. In a second step, CELLUVISC® (sodium carboxymethylcellulose) and/or VISMED® (sodium hyaluronate) were added to the DXMa/CD aqueous solutions in order to obtain the final Gels A and B, according to the ratio described in Table 1.

Table 1. Composition of optimized mixed Gels A and B.

Mixed Gels	Components	Quantity (g)
Optimized mixed Gel A	VISMED®	0.300
	HPβCD 600 mg/mL with DXMa	0.700
	Optimized mixed Gel A contains 7 mg/g of DXMa and an osmolality of 449 mOsm/kg	
Optimized mixed Gel B	CELLUVISC®	0.151
	VISMED®	0.085
	HPγCD 600 mg/mL with DXMa	0.764
	Optimized mixed Gel B contains 20 mg/g of DXMa and an osmolality of 425 mOsm/kg	

2.2.2. Sterilization Step

Two different methods were investigated with Gels A and B (i.e., autoclaving, SANO CLAV from ADOLF WOLF, Überkingen, Germany) at 121 °C during 20 min or double sterilizing filtration (CME or PVDF 0.22 µm filter, ROTH, Karlsruhe, Germany) and conditioned in sterile vials under laminar air flow of an ISO 4.8 microbiological safety cabinet.

2.2.3. Physicochemical Characterizations

Drug Quantification

The drug quantification methodology was adapted from that previously reported [7,12] and validated in DXMa concentrations according to ICH Q2 (R1) guidelines in order to evaluate specificity, linearity, repeatability, intermediate fidelity, and limit of detection (LOD) and limit of quantification (LOQ) [13]. Quantitative determination were performed on a reversed-phase, high-performance liquid chromatographic (HPLC) component system LC 2010 AHT (SHIMADZU, Kyoto, Japan) consisting of a pump with degasser, an autosampler, a UV–VIS detector, and a column XTERRA®MS C8, 5 µm particles, and 150 × 4.6 mm with a C8 cartridge. The mobile phase made of methanol:water (70:30 v/v) was set at the rate of 1.2 mL/min. The column was thermo-regulated at 25 °C. The detection wavelength was set up at 240 nm.

Method Validation

The method was validated according to the International Conference on Harmonization (ICH) guideline Q2 (R1) "Validation of Analytical Procedures" [13].

Linearity and Accuracy Studies

Five standard samples at different concentration values were prepared using 0.1 mg/mL DXMa as a solution stock. Table 2 contains the different sample concentration levels for Gels A and B.

Table 2. Sample concentration levels of DXMa for Gels A and B.

Gels	Level 80%	Level 90%	Level 100%	Level 110%	Level 120%
Gel A (µg/mL)	56	63	70	77	84
Gel B (µg/mL)	160	180	200	220	240

These calibration levels were analyzed twice a day during three days [14]. The peak area was plotted against the concentration at each level and a calibration curve was generated by a linear least square regression analysis by checking the pre-required assumptions.

Specificity

The specificity of the developed method was first established by verifying that all the components of gels were separated from the DXMa chromatographic peak. In complement, to exclude potential interference of degradation products with DXMa quantification, DXMa 1 mg/mL solutions, Gel A, and Gel B were subjected to forced degradation conditions, according to SFSTP guidelines [15]: 0.5 N hydrochloric acid or sodium hydroxide, at 80 °C for 60 min, in 3% hydrogen peroxide at 80 °C for 4 h and under visible and ultraviolet light for 6 h.

Precision

Intra-day (repeatability) and inter-day (intermediate) precision assays were determined by preparing a model solution at a 100% concentration level (70 µg/mL for Gel A and 200 µg/mL for Gel B). Each solution was analyzed six times a day for three days.

Limit of detection (LOD) and limit of quantification (LOQ) were estimated from the standard deviation of the response as well as the slope, according to ICH guidelines. The estimated results were not empirically verified.

Rheological Measurements

Rheological characteristics of both gels were examined at various shear rates using an ARES-G2 rheometer from TA Instruments (New Castle, PA, USA) equipped with a Couette system (cup diameter 33.985 mm, upper cylinder diameter 32 mm, and APS kit) from TA Instruments (New Castle, USA). The measuring corresponded to 1.0620 according to ISO 3219. The gap length was 2 mm and the sample volume of >5.2 mL. The temperature was controlled at 35 °C by a Peltier jaquette.

The steady-state flow experiments were performed in the range of 0.11 to 100 s^{-1}. The frequency sweep method was performed between 0.1 Hz and 10 Hz, with a shear strain of 10% for both formulations, while the table of shear rate method was performed by increasing the shear rate from 0.1 to 100 s^{-1}, at 35 °C. The shear stress was measured by this method and the apparent viscosity was calculated by dividing the shear stress by the shear rate. An oscillatory amplitude sweep and frequency testing were performed using this equipment.

The amplitude sweep conditions used were shear strain between 0.1% and 100% with the frequency of 0.1 Hz. Amplitude tests showed that 10% deformation corresponded to a value in the linear range. In the frequency testing, the frequency range used was between 0.1–10 Hz with a shear strain of 10%.

2.2.4. Mucoadhesion

In this study, mucin was rehydrated with water by gentle stirring until complete dissolution to yield a dispersion of 10% (w/w) at 20–25 °C. The mucoadhesion was evaluated by the effect of mucin on zeta potential (ZP) values of Gel A ± mucin (1:1), Gel B ± mucin (1:1). A volume of 40 µL of Gel A, Gel B, and mucin were diluted in either 2 mL of sterile purified water [16–18]. The ZP values of the different mixtures were measured using a Zetasizer Nanoseries Nano ZS (Malvern Instruments, Malvern, UK) at 35 °C. All the experiments were done in triplicate.

2.2.5. Cytotoxicity Studies

Two different cellular toxicity assays were used based on cell viability in relation to mitochondrial enzymes [19] (i.e., the methylthiazolyldiphenyl-tetrazolium bromide conversion (MTT) and ALAMAR BLUE® assays). The experiments were performed using normal human primary corneal epithelial cells (HCEC) obtained from ATCC® and maintained in an incubator (37 °C and 5% CO_2 saturation). HCEC were kept in corneal epithelial cell growth culture medium with gentamicin and amphotericin B, without fetal bovine serum. All experiments were performed in between steps 4 and 8. Three thousand cells per well (96 wells per plates) were incubated for 24 h at 37 °C and 5% CO_2 in order to have between 80 and 90% of cell confluence, according to ATCC® protocol. Subsequently, during the MTT assay, the original culture medium was aspirated and different concentrations (25 µL/200 µL, and 0.25 µL/200 µL) of different formulations: Gels A and B with or without DXMa, HPβCD (600 mg/mL) and HPγCD (600 mg/mL) aqueous solutions, DEXAFREE® eye drop solution, and MAXIDEX® eye drop suspension were added to different wells and incubated for 30 min and 2 h. Each concentration was tested in three individual wells. After 30 min, 2 h, and 24 h, the supernatant was removed and 200 µL of MTT solution (5 mg/mL in PBS and then diluted to 1/10 in complete medium) was added to each well and then incubated for 3 h at 37 °C to allow the formation of formazan crystals. The medium was then removed, and blue formazan was eluted from cells by 200 µL of DMSO. The plates were shaken in order to solubilize the crystals of formazan. The liquid was aspirated to another new 96-wells plate and measured directly at 590 nm with Clariostar (BMG Labtech, Champigny sur Marne, France). Each plate was duplicated. The cell viability values were compared using a well-known t-test procedure with $\alpha = 5\%$. Additionally, the ALAMAR BLUE® was performed after 2 h of incubation at 37 °C, 5% CO_2, with the IC50 concentrations as determined by the MTT assay. A total of 20 µL of ALAMAR BLUE® reagent were added in each well before 2 h of incubation at 37 °C, 5% CO_2. Fluorescence was measured with an excitation wavelength at 530–560 nm and emission wavelength at 590 nm with Clariostar (BMG Labtech, Champigny sur Marne, France). Each plate was duplicated.

The % of reduction of ALAMAR BLUE® can be calculated by Equation (1):

$$\begin{aligned}&\%\ \text{Reduction}\\&= \frac{(\text{Experimental RFU value})-(\text{Negative control RFU value})}{(100\%\ \text{reduced positive control RFU value})-(\text{Negative control RFU value})} \times 100,\end{aligned} \quad (1)$$

2.2.6. Ex Vivo Evaluation of the Corneal Permeation

The transcorneal permeation experiment was performed for Gels A and B, DEXAFREE®, and MAXIDEX® using Franz diffusion cells with an available diffusion area of 1.131 cm^2. The porcine corneas were recovered from the slaughterhouse in accordance with ethical regulations. The corneas were removed and then mounted onto diffusion cells, with the epithelial layer exposed to the donor chamber. The latter was filled with 0.4 g of each ophthalmic formulation; whereas the receptor chamber was filled with 13 mL artificial tear fluid Balanced Salt Solution (BSS) According to Wen et al. [20], the experiment was performed at 35 ± 1 °C in a thermostatic water bath with a moderate speed of rotation maintained for 24 h. Three corneas per formulation (n = 3) were used. A 1 mL sample was removed at predetermined time intervals (15 min, 30 min, 1 h, 2 h, and 4 h) and replaced with an equal volume of fresh medium to maintain the sink conditions. The withdrawn samples from the receptor chamber were analyzed by HPLC. The cumulative amount of drug appearing in the receptor compartment (Qn) was plotted as a function of time (t_n) and calculated using Equation (2):

$$Qn = V_0\left(C_n + \frac{V}{V_0}\sum_{i=1}^{n-1} C_i\right) = V_0C_n + V\sum_{i=1}^{n-1} C_i, \quad (2)$$

C_n: Drug concentration at t time points (µg.mL^{-1}), C_i: Drug concentration at sampling points, V_0: Volume of the medium in the receiving chamber, and V: sampling volume.

The corneal hydration level (% HL) was measured with a relative humidity analyzer MB45 OHAUS® (Parsippany, NJ, USA).

2.2.7. In Vivo Evaluation of the Residence Time on the Ocular Surface

In vivo studies were carried out on male Sprague-Dawley rats with an average weight of 250 g supplied by the animal facility at University of Santiago de Compostela (Spain). The animals were treated according to the laboratory guidelines [21]. The experiments were approved by the Galician Network Committee for Ethics Research following the Spanish and European Union (EU) rules (86/609/CEE, 2003/65/CE, 2010/63/EU, RD 1201/2005 and RD53/2013)The project identification code was IDIS12072017, 12/07/2017 was approved by the Health Research Institute of Santiago de Compostela institutional review board. The animals were kept in individual cages at controlled conditions of temperature and humidity (22 °C and 60%) with free access to water and food, with day–night cycles regulated by artificial light. Each component of the optimized formulations, in other words, CELLUVISC®, VISMED®, DXMa (10 mg/g)/HPβCD (600 mg/mL), and DXMa (30 mg/g)/HPγCD (600 mg/mL) aqueous solutions; Gel A and Gel B were radiolabeled by incorporating 100 µL ^{18}F-fluorodeoxyglucose (^{18}F-FDG) in a volume of 1 mL of either hydrogel or cyclodextrin based aqueous solution until homogenization, according to the methodology followed in previous studies [22]. Randomly taken samples from each labeled component were measured using a high-precision dose calibrator (Atomlab 500, Biodex Medical System, Inc., New-York, NY, USA) in order to control radiotracer uniformity. Positron emission tomography and computerized tomography (PET/CT) images were acquired using the Albira PET/CT Preclinical Imaging System (Bruker Biospin, Woodbridge, CT, USA). The anesthetized animals were positioned into the imaging bed and 7.5 µL of each formulation labeled with^{18}F-FDG was instilled into the conjunctival sac of eye using a micropipette. The administered radioactivity was 0.35 ± 0.08 MBq. Therefore, the ^{18}F-FDG labeled component (CELLUVISC®, VISMED®), DXMa (10 mg/g)/HPβCD (600 mg/mL), and DXMa (20 mg/g)/HPγCD (600 mg/mL) aqueous solutions as well as the ^{18}F-FDG labeled optimized gels (A or B) were tested. Immediately after administration, static PET frames of 10 min were acquired and the animal was awakened. Then, single frames of 10 min at 0.5, 1, 2, 3, and 5 h after instillation were acquired, anesthetizing the animal 5 min before obtaining the images and then waking it up. Three eyes of three animals were tested for each formulation. The results were corrected to radioactive decay. Graphical representations of radioactivity versus time were obtained. The % remaining formulations on ocular surface was calculated as the ratio of radioactivity at time t in ocular surface/initial radioactivity. The fitting of the remaining formulation versus time to a monoexponential decay equation using a single compartmental model was performed using pKSolver [23]. A non-compartmental analysis was also performed calculating the mean residence time (MRT) and the total area under the curve (AUC) of the remaining formulations (%) versus time. All data were expressed as mean value ± standard deviation (SD). Statistical analyses were performed using one-way ANOVA test, and the level of significance was set at 5%.

2.2.8. Stability Studies

Both formulations were prepared using sterile water, HPβCD, HPγCD, DXMa, VISMED®, and CELLUVISC® under laminar air flow of an ISO 4.8 microbiological safety cabinet. A total of 2 mL of each gel was conditioned into a 5 mL glass vial previously autoclaved, closed with a polypropylene cap, and sealed with an aluminum ring. Two batches of each gel were prepared and submitted to a double filtration with PVDF 0.22 µm filters.

The stability of each gel was studied in unopened multidose eyedroppers for 12 months at 25 °C in a climate chamber (BINDER GmbH, Tuttlingen, Germany). Four units per formulation were subjected to visual inspection, DXMa quantification, sterility, osmolality, and pH measurements at times 0, 14, and 30 days, 2, 6, 9, and 12 months. More precisely, for each unit, color and aspect were checked. DXMa was quantified by HPLC and the degradation product sought using a stability indicating method [13]. Gels A and B were previously diluted by 1/100 with the mobile phase. Osmolality was measured using a 2020 freezing point osmometer (Advanced Instruments, Norwood, United States). pH measurements were made with a SevenMulti® pH-meter with an InLab electrode (Mettler-Toledo, Viroflay, France). The sterility test was carried out according to the European Pharmacopeia sterility assay (2.6.1) [24]. Briefly, the multidose eyedroppers were opened under the laminar air flow of an ISO 4.8 microbiological safety cabinet and the content was divided into two equal parts, each transferred in a fluid thioglycollate with resazurine medium and Tryptic soy broth and incubated at 30–35 °C and 20–25 °C, respectively for 14 days. The culture medium was examined every day.

3. Results and Discussion

3.1. *Drug Quantification Before and After Sterilization*

Pure DXMa and DXMa formulated in Gels A and B presented a retention time of 3.2 ± 0.2 min and their chromatograms are presented in Supplementary Materials (Figure S1).

Method Validation Studies

The RP-HPLC method used to analyze the DXMa in Gels A and B was validated according to current ICH Q2(R1) [13]. The performed validation tests proved the suitability of the method for its intended purposes. Validation tests including specificity, linearity and range parameter, accuracy, precision, LOQ, and LOD. Original validation data are reported in the Supplementary Materials.

3.2. *Sterilization Step*

Two different methods were investigated with Gels A and B (i.e., autoclaving, SANO CLAV from ADOLF WOLF, Überkingen, Germany) at 121 °C during 20 min or double sterilizing filtration (CME or PVDF 0.22 µm filter, ROTH, Karlsruhe, Germany). The sterile filtered product was packaged in sterile vials under laminar air flow of an ISO 4.8 microbiological safety cabinet. The choice of the sterilization steps is primordial and was evaluated in terms of change in chromatographic profile and in % of drug loss. As seen in Supplementary Materials Figures S5 and S6, a peak of degradation product appeared and the DXMa peak was reduced. Therefore it excludes autoclaving as a sterilization method of DMXa. DXMa seems to be heat labile, and a similar result is reported in the literature for dexamethasone sodium phosphate [25].

The CME filters were discarded because they led after filtration to a loss of 12.9 ± 0.5% DXMa with Gel A and 5.3 ± 0.3% with Gel B, while the filter PVDF resulted in only a loss of 0.6 ± 0.02% DXMa with Gel A and 0.4 ± 0.02% with Gel B. The PVDF filters were therefore retained and were confirmed by demonstrating the repeatability of the sterilization step without a great loss of DXMa. Indeed, six samples of each gel were prepared and DXMa was quantified by HPLC before and after the double filtration steps with PVDF 0.22 µm filters. The relative percentage of standard deviation (RSD) of drug quantification was calculated from these quantifications. For both formulations, the drug loss was <0.3% and the repeatability RSD values were 0.96% (Gel A) and 0.95% (Gel B). The RSD (%) values were found to be <1%, which were considered acceptable.

3.3. *Rheological Measurements*

The administration of an ophthalmic formulation should not influence the pseudoplastic nature of precorneal film, or the influence should be negligible. Figure 1a,b present the dynamic viscosity of each formulation as a function of shear rate (0.11–100 s^{-1}) at 35 °C, measuring five points per decade and with 20 s equilibration time. The both formulations exhibited Newtonian behavior. At shear gradients greater than 70–80 s^{-1}, centrifugal forces and turbulences come into play, which results in a fall in axial force. The apparent rheofluidifying behavior past 100 s^{-1} is therefore an artifact caused by these centrifugal forces. For shear rates of less than 1 s^{-1}, the crust formed by the eye drops when drying opposes a resistance to the rotational movement of the geometry, which is no longer negligible compared to the measured torque, which explains the slight rise in the curve between 0.1 and 1 s^{-1}.

Below 0.3 s^{-1}, this crust makes measurements imprecise and so between 0.3 and 100 s^{-1}, Gels A and B present a Newtonian behavior, Gel A displays a viscosity of 13.2 mPa s ± 10%, and Gel B a viscosity of 18.6 mPa s ± 10% (Figure 1). As demonstrated by Zaki et al., the retention on eye surface began to increase only after a viscosity exceeding a critical value of about 10 mPa s [26].

Although increasing fluid viscosity improves the residence time, it may also cause discomfort and damage to ocular epithelia due to an increase in the shear stresses during blinking. Carboxymethylcellulose and sodium hyaluronate are well known for their viscosifying properties. Furthermore, sodium hyaluronate, present in Gel A, Gel B, and VISMED®, is a shear thinning fluid. Sodium hyaluronate should contribute to enhance viscosity while avoiding excessive stresses during blinking [27]. Additionally, these viscosities, lower than 30 mPa.s, are well tolerated by patients because it does not lead to blurred vision and foreign body sensation, resulting in a faster elimination due to reflex tears and blinks [28].

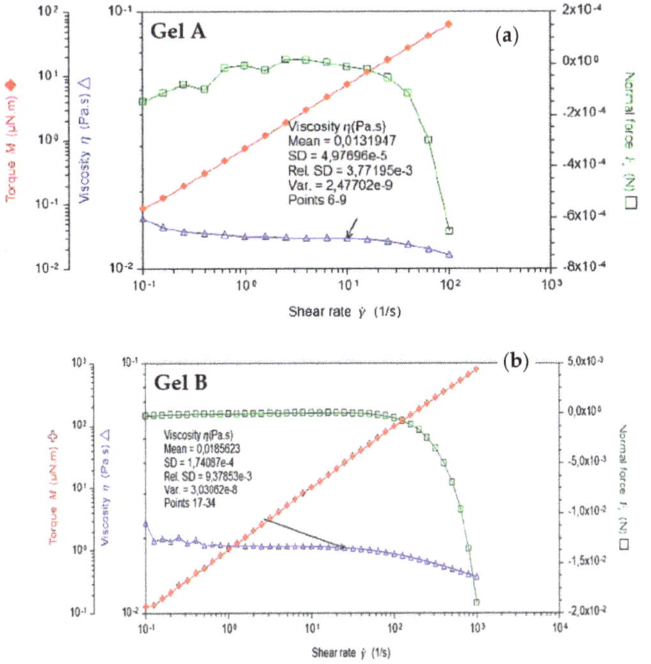

Figure 1. Dynamic viscosity of (**a**) Gel A and (**b**) Gel B performed in the range of 0.11 to 100 s^{-1} at 35 °C.

Before oscillation frequency sweep, an amplitude sweep test was performed to define the fluid's linear-viscoelastic region (LVER), and 10% at least for both formulations. Indeed, for Gel A, the amplitude sweep test performed at 1 Hz between 0.1 and 100% did not indicate any output of the linear domain. For Gel B, the oscillation measured between 0.1 and 100% of deformation did not show any upper limit and so, caution should be used to avoid not being below 1.5% deformation with this rheometer (Supplementary Materials Figure S7). At 0.1 Hz, the storage module was negligible, which explains why some points are missing on the graphs (negative values cannot be displayed on a logarithmic scale). For both at low amplitudes, the signal becomes lower than the sensitivity of the material (0.05 μNm).

With these results, Gels A and B can be further characterized using a frequency sweep, proving more information about the effect of colloidal forces [29]. Figure 2 presents oscillation frequency performed between 0.1–10 Hz with a shear strain of 10% at 35 °C. Both formulations exhibited fluid-like mechanism spectra with G″ modulus even greater than G′, being both frequency dependent.

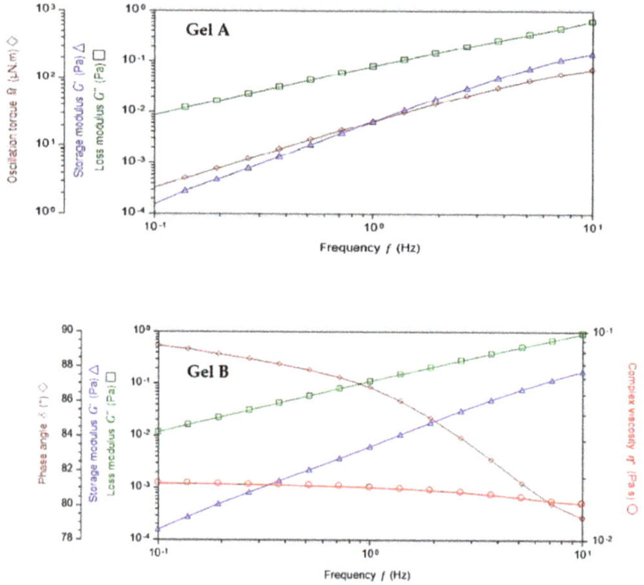

Figure 2. Oscillation frequency performed with Gels A and B between 0.1–10 Hz with a shear strain of 10% at 35 °C.

Mucoadhesion

Zeta potential (ZP) value is related to the measurement of the surface charge that a specific material possesses or acquires when suspended in a fluid. This study demonstrated that the ZP values of Gel A and Gel B are quite different. Indeed, Gel B ZP value (−41.1 ± 2.3 mV) is much more negative than Gel A (−23.9 ± 0.7 mV) (Figure 3). These negative values are in accordance with the anionic nature of the hyaluronic acid due to the presence of carboxylic groups. HA is present in VISMED®, Gel A, and Gel B. The mucins also presented a negative ZP value due to their carboxyl and sulfate groups. The obtained value was quite different from the one described in the literature, which was approximately −10 mV [16]. This difference could be explained by a different degree of hydration [30]. When the mucin 5% (w/v) suspension was added to Gel B, an increase of the negative charge was observed, showing the reduction in electrostatic repulsion, and indirectly an interaction of the vehicle with the mucins [31].

3.4. Cytotoxicity Studies

3.4.1. MTT

To evaluate in vitro cell toxicity of Gels A and B with or without DXMa, HPβCD (600 mg/mL) and HPγCD (600 mg/mL) aqueous solutions, DEXAFREE® and MAXIDEX®, HCE cells grown in the presence of each formulation were evaluated by quantitative determination of living cells, after 30 min, 2 h, and 24 h at 5 and 0.05% concentration (Figure 4). The results were analyzed according to the Organization for Economic Co-operation and Development (OECD) guidelines for short time exposure in vitro test method [32] (Table 3).

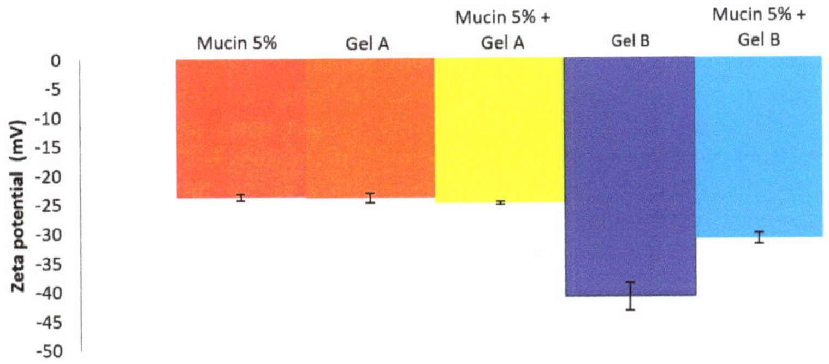

Figure 3. Zeta potential values (mean ± SD, n = 3) of mucin 5%, Gel A, Gel B, and mucin 5% + Gel A or Gel B.

Table 3. Prediction model inspired by the short time exposure according to the Organization for Economic Co-operation and Development (OECD) guidelines [32].

Cell Viability		UN GHS Classification	Applicability	DXMa Formulation Vehicles
At 5%	At 0.05%			
>70%	>70%	No category	No serious damage nor eye irritation effect	Gel B
				HPγCD aqueous solution (600 mg/mL)
≤70%	>70%	No prediction can be made	No prediction can be made, eventual eye irritation	Gel A
				HPβCD aqueous solution (600 mg/mL)
≤70%	≤70%	Category 1	Serious eye damage	None

As shown in Figure 4, Gel B showed an acceptable level of cytotoxicity to HCE cells and is considered rather well tolerated by HCEC with a cell viability higher than 70% at 5% and 0.05% at 30 min (p value < 0.001) and 24 h. In addition, DEXAFREE® presented a similar cytotoxicity profile after 30 min and 24 h (p value = 0.035). In contrast, Gel A was classified in the non-predictable category since the cell viability was lower than 70% at 5% (p-value < 0.001) and higher than 70% at 0.05% (p-value = 0.022) at 30 min and 24 h. A similar cytotoxicity profile was observed in the case of the reference suspension MAXIDEX®. A cell viability lower than 70% at 5% (p-value = 0.01) and higher than 70% at 0.05% (p-value = 0.04) at 30 min and 24 h. The cytotoxic effect of Gel A was time and concentration dependent and seems to be caused mainly by the HPβCD (600 mg/mL) aqueous solution. Indeed, the cell viability of Gel A with or without DXMa and HPβCD (600 mg/mL) aqueous solution were relatively similar at each time and each concentration with values decreasing from around 30%, 15%, and 10% at 30 min, 2 h, and 24 h, respectively. Furthermore, each CD derivative at the concentration of 600 mg/mL presents a cytotoxic effect more or less pronounced. These observations could be attributed to the known capacity of CDs to extract and solubilize cholesterol from membranes, potentially causing destruction of phospholipid bilayers [33]. One can note that in the present study, HPγCD had a much less pronounced effect than HPβCD, showing a cell viability higher than 65%, against lower than 30% for HPβCD (p-value < 0.001 at 30 min). Moreover, the cytotoxicity of HPβCD is enhanced with increasing exposure time [34]. These differences may be attributed to the higher propensity of the βCD derivative to solubilize cholesterol from membranes compared to γCD [33]. Moreover, the clear decreased cytotoxicity observed in the case of Gel B may be related to the lower extent of free cavities available for complexation in the case of HPγCD for which a higher complexation efficiency value was previously described [7], allowing Gel B to be relatively safe for HCEC. Therefore, in the future, it will be possible to consider a lower concentration of HPβCD in Gel A in order to improve ocular tolerance [34], even if this means reducing the solubilized DXMa fraction.

3.4.2. ALAMAR BLUE® Assay

To complete the in vitro cell biocompatibility study, the ALAMAR BLUE® assay was performed by using fluorescence, which is proportional to the number of cells with metabolic activity (Figure 5). Gel B, Gel B without DXMa, and HPγCD showed acceptable levels of metabolic activity as DEXAFREE®, with a cell viability even >70% after 2 h of exposure. Unfortunately Gel A, Gel A without DXMa, and HPβCD (600 mg/mL) showed a low metabolic activity of <30%, which could cause serious eye damage. According to these results, we can demonstrate different biocompatibility profiles between Gel A and Gel B, probably related to the difference in biocompatibility profile between HPβCD and HPγCD. Hence, Gel B is considered as biocompatible and the formulation of Gel A might be optimized regarding the effect of HPβCD on HCEC.

3.5. Ex Vivo Evaluation of the Corneal Permeation

Ex vivo permeation of Gel A, Gel B, DEXAFREE®, and MAXIDEX® were evaluated using the excised porcine cornea. The amount of DXMa permeated through the excised cornea from Gel B was higher than that of the other formulations (Figure 6). With Gel B, a maximum of 71.71 μg of DXMa permeates (i.e., 0.89% amount of the drug applied) and was nearly 3.2-fold higher than DEXAFREE® and 4-fold higher than MAXIDEX®. Gel A also presented a good corneal permeation with a maximum of 40.48 μg (i.e., 1.44% amount of the drug applied), which is 1.8-fold higher than DEXAFREE® and 2.5-fold higher than MAXIDEX®. This suggests that both Gels A and B might be more effective than reference marketed formulations to treat corneal inflammations. Moreover, these results are associated with a good corneal hydration level between 76 and 80%.

Dexamethasone is a highly potent long acting drug requiring a far lower dosage compared to other intermediate and short acting glucocorticoids (i.e., nearly five times lower than prednisolone, methylprednisolone, and 25 times lower than hydrocortisone) to elicit a biological response [35,36]. As demonstrated by Djalilian et al., dexamethasone inhibits inflammatory cytokines in human corneal epithelial cells and fibroblast cell lines with a concentration range of 0.1 to 10 μM [37]. The marketed formulation DEXAFREE® contains 1 mg/mL drug (i.e., 1.9 mM). As previously described, Gel B released DXMa allowing a maximum drug amount of 63.4 μg/cm^2 to be permeated across the excised cornea. In addition, Gel A allowed a permeated drug amount of 36.07 μg/cm^2.

Therefore, considering the normal tear volume to be about 6 to 10 μL, assuming no tear drainage and similar release behavior as observed in 13 mL of PBS, 71.71 μg and 40.48 μg of DXMa (Mw = 434.5 g/mol) in 10 μL of tears would theoretically be almost 16.6 mM and 9.3 mM, which is about 8- and 5-fold higher than the concentration provided by DEXAFREE®. These latter results warranted to be clinically relevant and within the therapeutic index [37].

3.6. In Vivo Evaluation of the Residence Time on the Ocular Surface

The biopermanence of Gels A and B, DXMa (10 mg/mL)/HPβCD (600 mg/mL), DXMa (30 mg/mL)/ HPγCD (600 mg/mL), VISMED®, and CELLUVISC® was characterized on the ocular surface of rats by ^{18}F-FDG radiolabeling followed by radioactivity in PET over 5 h (300 min) (Figure 7). It is a non-invasive tool for pharmacokinetic studies of clearance of topical ocular drug delivery systems [22,38]. In the present study, all the formulations tested presented a higher residence than the control solution of Balanced Salt Solution (BSS), whose composition is close to tears. Indeed, in Figure 8, it can be observed that after 30 min of contact, 23% of the BSS remained in the ocular surface against 60 to 100% remaining doses for the other formulations.

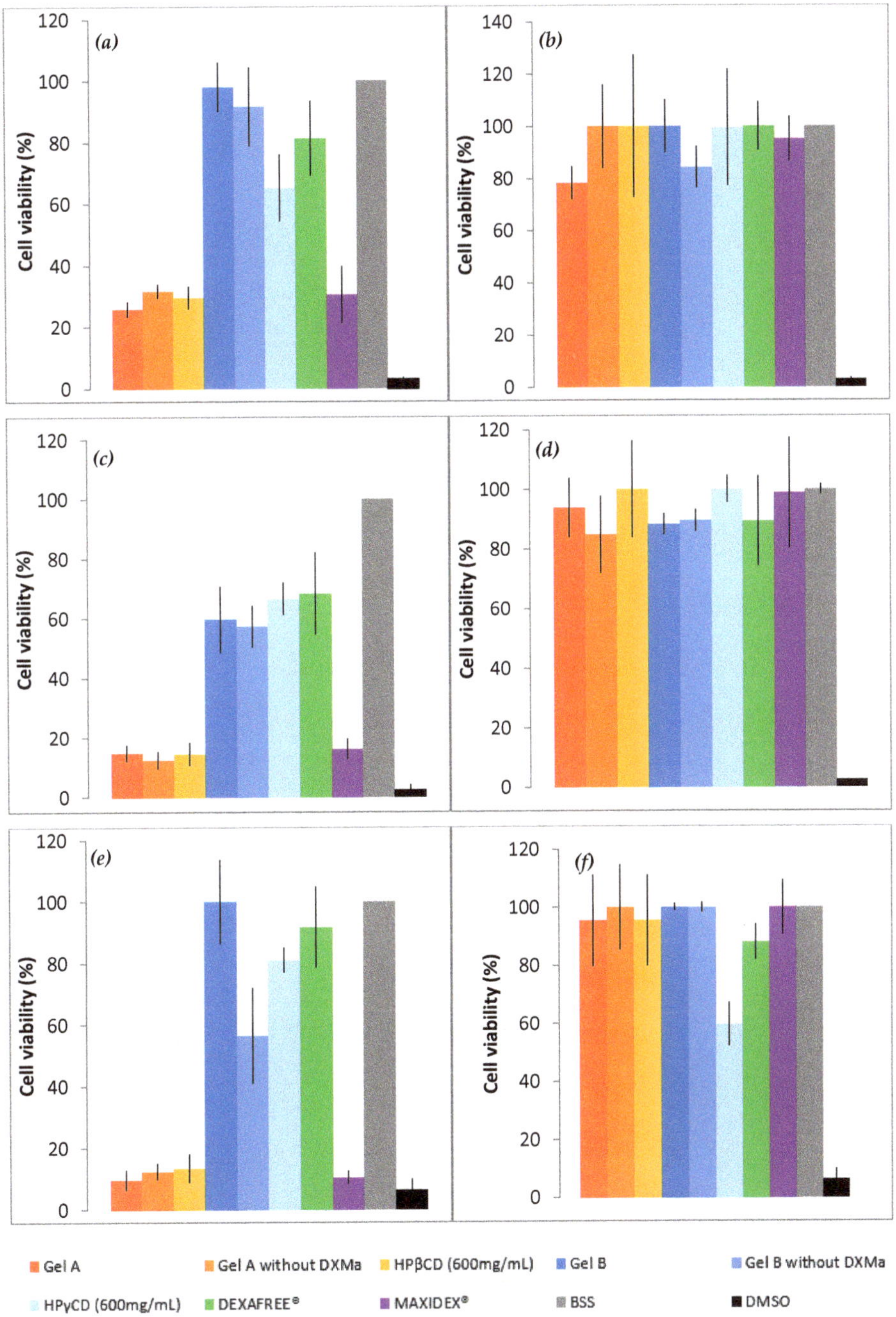

Figure 4. Cell viability of Gels A and B with or without DXMa, HPβCD (600 mg/mL) and HPγCD (600 mg/mL) aqueous solutions, DEXAFREE®, and MAXIDEX®. (**a**) 5% concentration during 30 min, (**b**) 0.05% during 30 min, (**c**) 5% during 2 h, (**d**) 0.05% during 2 h, (**e**) 5% during 24 h, (**f**) 0.05% during 24 h.

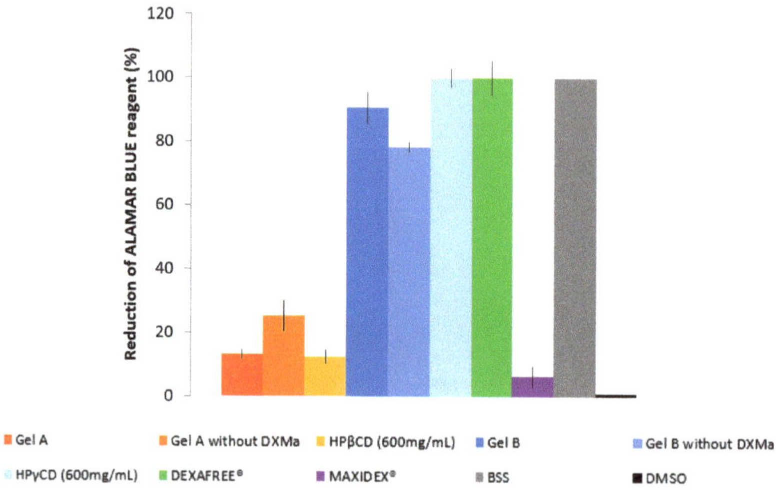

Figure 5. Reduction of ALAMAR BLUE® reagent (%) of Gels A and B with or without DXMa, HPβCD (600 mg/mL) and HPγCD (600 mg/mL) aqueous solutions, DEXAFREE®, and MAXIDEX®.

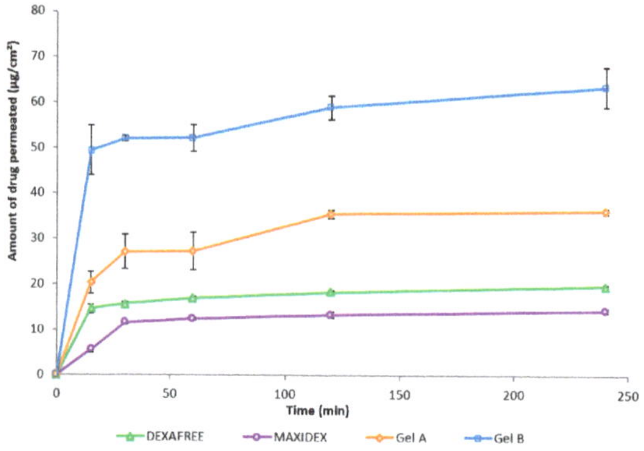

Figure 6. Amount of drug permeated (mean ± SD, n = 3) through the excised cornea of Gels A and B, DEXAFREE®, and MAXIDEX® as a function of time.

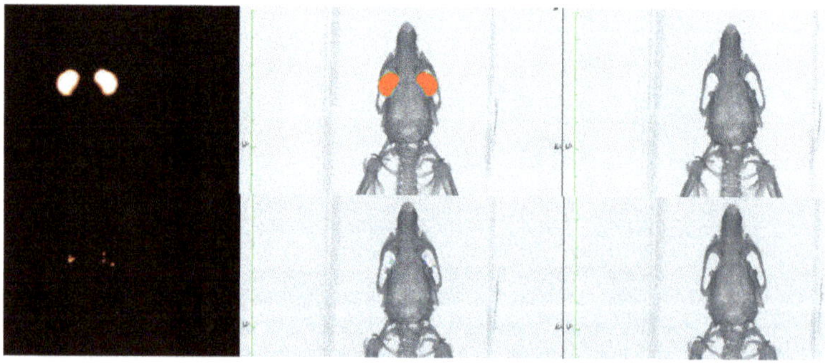

Figure 7. PET (**left**), CT (**right**), and fused image PET/CT (**center**) of the rat eyes immediately after administration (**top**) and 300 min post-administration (**bottom**).

These observations are in accordance with the PET data described by Luaces-Rodriguez et al. in the case of tacrolimus eye drops [39]. According to the literature, increasing fluid viscosity increases the residence time to some extent by delaying the tear action [26]. This is in agreement with our observations since the reference marketed gels, sodium carboxymethylcellulose and sodium hyaluronate, are more viscous than the other components, and presented a higher ocular residence time with a MRT of 197 and 134 min, respectively. Furthermore, the CD solutions presented a slight viscosity of around 6 mPa.s, which resulted in a significant increase in $T_{1/2}$ and MRT values when compared to BSS. The MRT value for Gel B (112 min) was between the values obtained for CELLUVISC® (197 min), VISMED® (134 min), and DXMa/HPγCD solution (101 min). In addition, the presence of both CMC and HA, associated with higher gel B viscosity, seems to promote ocular remanence. The low MRT value of 67 min obtained in the case of Gel A is rather surprising with respect to the observed HPβCD solution MRT value (118 min). This would merit further investigation since a high variability in the results was observed. Furthermore, sodium hyaluronate, present in Gel A, Gel B, and VISMED®, is a shear thinning fluid. Sodium hyaluronate contributes to enhance viscosity while avoiding excessive stress during blinking [27].

The data summarized in Table 4 show that pharmacokinetic parameters such as $T_{1/2}$, MRT, and k are significantly different between each gel and BSS at $p < 0.05$.The data collected from 3 to 240 min were significantly different between Gels A and B, DXMa (10 mg/mL)/HPβCD (600 mg/mL), DXMa (30 mg/mL)/HPγCD (600 mg/mL), VISMED®, and CELLUVISC® at $p < 0.05$.

Table 4. Ocular biopermanence parameters measured in vivo for Gels A and B, DXMa (10 mg/mL)/HPβCD (600 mg/mL), DXMa (30 mg/mL)/HPγCD (600 mg/mL), VISMED®, and CELLUVISC® versus Balanced Salt Solution (BSS).

Components	Viscosity at 35 °C (mPa.s)	k (min^{-1})	$T_{1/2}$ (min)	MRT (min)	R^2
CELLUVISC®	167–260	0.007 ± 0.003	136.5 ± 95.5	196.9 ± 137.8	0.9738
VISMED®	16.8	0.008 ± 0.003	92.7 ± 26.7	133.7 ± 38.5	0.9404
Gel B	18.6	0.0096 ± 0.036	77.4 ± 28.8	111.6 ± 41.5	0.9837
Gel A	13.2	0.015 ± 0.002	46.6 ± 4.8	67.2 ± 6.9	0.9365
DXMa/HPβCD (10 mg/mL/600 mg/mL)	6.4	0.015 ± 0.014	81.7± 59.0	117.9± 85.2	0.9866
DXMa/HPγCD (30 mg/mL/600 mg/mL)	6.5	0.11 ± 0.003	70.2 ± 21.9	101.3 ± 31.6	0.9697
BSS	1.5	0.046 ± 0.015	16.0 ± 5.2	23.1 ± 7.6	0.9965

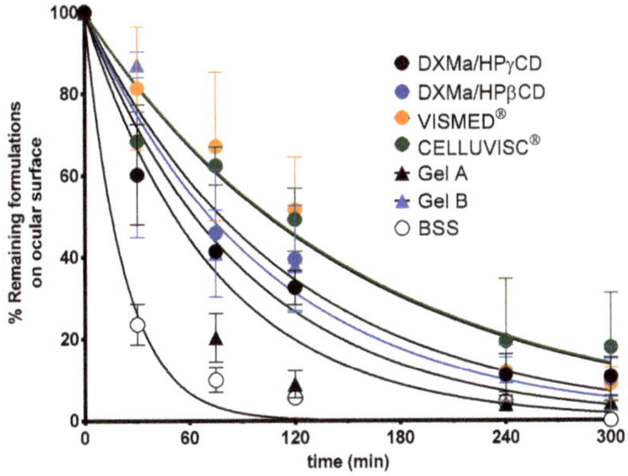

Figure 8. Ocular biopermanence of Gels A and B, DXMa (10 mg/mL)/HPβCD (600 mg/mL), DXMa (30 mg/mL)/HPγCD (600 mg/mL), VISMED®, and CELLUVISC® versus BSS.

3.7. Stability

The stability of Gels A and B was assessed using the following parameters: visual inspection, presence or absence of visible particles, DXMa concentration, presence or absence of breakdown products, pH, and osmolality. The study was conducted according to ICH Q1A (R2) methodological guidelines for stability studies [15,40]. A variation of DXMa concentration outside 90–110% intervals of the initial concentration was considered as a sign of a significant DXMa concentration variation. The observed gels must be limpid, of unchanged color, and clear with no visible signs of haziness or precipitation. pH values were considered to be acceptable if they did not vary by more than one pH unit from the initial value.

Gels A and B stayed limpid and there was no appearance of any visible particulate matter, haziness, or gas development. Every Gel A presented a slightly yellowish tinge throughout the study.

The DXMa concentrations during 12 months are presented in Figure 9. Throughout the dosage times, Gel A and B stored at 25 °C did not vary by more than 10% of the initial concentrations, with low variability as 95% confidence intervals.

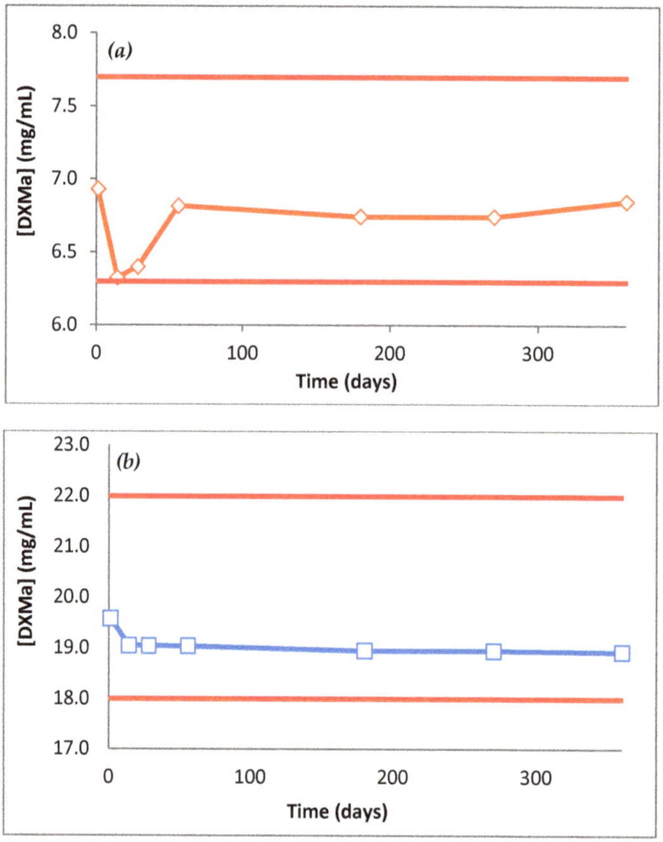

Figure 9. DXMa concentrations (mg/mL) of (**a**) Gel A and (**b**) Gel B as a function of time.

For each gel, pH did not vary by more than 0.3 pH units from D0 to M12. pH Gel A was 7.5 and pH Gel B was 7.0. At 12 months, osmolality of Gel A and B had not varied by more than 2.5% of initial osmolality. Both pH and osmolality did not vary during 12 months and stayed within an acceptable physiological range.

Since autoclaving led to DXMa degradation, Gels A and B were sterilized by a validated filtration methodology. The samples of gels conserved at 25 °C in unopened bottles at day 0, 14 days, 30 days and 2, 6, 9, and 12 months did not show any signs of microbiological growth (< 1UFC), meeting the requirements of the 2.6.1 European Pharmacopeia.

4. Conclusions and Future Prospects

In conclusion, the data provided in this study demonstrate that the use of hydrogels combined with hydrosoluble cyclodextrins is relatively safe, increases ocular retention, and could act as penetration promoters for DXMa. Indeed, both gels present a good corneal permeation, which was 3.22-fold higher than DEXAFREE® and 4.04-fold higher than MAXIDEX® for Gel B and 1.8-fold higher than DEXAFREE® and 2.5-fold higher than MAXIDEX® for Gel A. Furthermore, they were stable at 25 °C during 12 months after filtration sterilization. These good results have to be confirmed in vivo with pharmacokinetic, efficacy, and tolerance studies.

Supplementary Materials: The following are available online at http://www.mdpi.com/1999-4923/12/8/717/s1, Figure S1. A, B, C and D show the chromatogram of DXMa for Gel A diluted to 70 µg/mL, DXMa in Gel A diluted to 70 µg/mL and DXMa for Gel B diluted to 200 µg/mL and DXMa in Gel B diluted to 200 µg/mL obtained with the chromatographic methods used. Figure S2. Calibration curves for DXMa in Gel A and Gel B (3 days/5 levels a day). Figure S3. Chromatograms obtained for DXMa in Gel A after applying different stress conditions. (a) No stress, (b) HCl 0.5 N at 80 °C during 1 h, (c) NaOH 0.5 N at 80 °C during 1 h, (d) H_2O_2 3% at 80 °C during 4 h and (e) UV light for 6 h. Figure S4. Chromatograms obtained for DXMa in Gel B after applying different stress conditions. (a) No stress, (b) HCl 0.5 N at 80 °C during 1 h, (c) NaOH 0.5 N at 80 °C during 1 h, (d) H_2O_2 3% at 80 °C during 4 h and (e) UV light for 6 h. Figure S5. Chromatograms before and after autoclaving Gel A. Figure S6. Chromatograms before and after autoclaving Gel B. Figure S7. Amplitude sweep test performed with Gel B at 0.1, 1 and 10 Hz at 35 °C. Table S1. Calibration curves of DXMa in Gel A and Gel B. Table S2. Limit of detection and quantification for Gels A and B.

Author Contributions: R.M., X.G.-O., L.C., V.V., F.B., V.B.-M., V.D.-T., F.-J.O.-E., and A.F.-F. contributed to a part of the experimental work. X.G.-O. also participated as the first signatory in the development of the ocular remanence work. R.M., L.C., D.W., and A.G., designed all the studies, oversaw all the experiments and contributed to drafting the manuscript and intellectually to the development of the project. All authors have read and agreed to the published version of the manuscript.

Funding: This research received no external private funding.

Acknowledgments: This work was supported by Labex ARCANE (ANR-11-LABX-0003-01) and Institut de Chimie Moléculaire de Grenoble (FR 2607) and the Glyco@Alps program (ANR-15-IDEX-02). A.F.-F. acknowledges the support obtained from the Instituto de Salud Carlos III (ISCIII) through its research grants (JR18/00014). X.G.-O. acknowledges the financial support of the IDIS (Health Research Institute of Santiago de Compostela) (predoctoral research fellowships).

Conflicts of Interest: The authors declare no conflicts of interest.

References

1. Ohira, A.; Hara, K.; Jóhannesson, G.; Tanito, M.; Ásgrímsdóttir, G.M.; Lund, S.H.; Loftsson, T.; Stefánsson, E. Topical dexamethasone γ-cyclodextrin nanoparticle eye drops increase visual acuity and decrease macular thickness in diabetic macular oedema. *Act. Ophthalmol.* **2015**, *93*, 610–615. [CrossRef]
2. Rodríguez Villanueva, J.; Rodríguez Villanueva, L.; Guzmán Navarro, M. Pharmaceutical technology can turn a traditional drug, dexamethasone into a first-line ocular medicine. A global perspective and future trends. *Int J. Pharm.* **2017**, *516*, 342–351. [CrossRef]
3. Pan, Q.; Xu, Q.; Boylan, N.J.; Lamb, N.W.; Emmert, D.G.; Yang, J.-C.; Tang, L.; Heflin, T.; Alwadani, S.; Eberhart, C.G.; et al. Corticosteroid-loaded biodegradable nanoparticles for prevention of corneal allograft rejection in rats. *J. Control. Release* **2015**, *201*, 32–40. [CrossRef] [PubMed]
4. Hughes, P.M.; Olejnik, O.; Chang-Lin, J.-E.; Wilson, C.G. Topical and systemic drug delivery to the posterior segments. *Adv. Drug Deliv. Rev.* **2005**, *57*, 2010–2032. [CrossRef] [PubMed]
5. Usayapant, A.; Karara, A.H.; Narurkar, M.M. Effect of 2-hydroxypropyl-beta-cyclodextrin on the ocular absorption of dexamethasone and dexamethasone acetate. *Pharm. Res.* **1991**, *8*, 1495–1499. [CrossRef] [PubMed]

6. Leibowitz, H.M.; Kupferman, A.; Stewart, R.H.; Kimbrough, R.L. Evaluation of dexamethasone acetate as a topical ophthalmic formulation. *Am. J. Ophthalmol.* **1978**, *86*, 418–423. [CrossRef]
7. Mazet, R.; Choisnard, L.; Levilly, D.; Wouessidjewe, D.; Gèze, A. Investigation of combined cyclodextrin and hydrogel formulation for ocular delivery of dexamethasone acetate by means of experimental designs. *Pharmaceutics* **2018**, *10*, 249. [CrossRef] [PubMed]
8. Guillon, M.; Maissa, C.; Ho, S. Evaluation of the effects on conjunctival tissues of optive eyedrops over one month usage. *Cont. Lens Anterior Eye* **2010**, *33*, 93–99. [CrossRef]
9. Chatterjee, B.; Amalina, N.; Sengupta, P.; Kumar Mandal, U. Mucoadhesive polymers and their mode of action: A recent update. *J. Appl. Pharm. Sci.* **2017**, *7*, 195–203. [CrossRef]
10. Achouri, D.; Alhanout, K.; Piccerelle, P.; Andrieu, V. Recent advances in ocular drug delivery. *Drug Dev. Ind. Pharm.* **2013**, *39*, 1599–1617. [CrossRef]
11. Oh, H.J.; Li, Z.; Park, S.-H.; Yoon, K.C. Effect of hypotonic 0.18% sodium hyaluronate eyedrops on inflammation of the ocular surface in experimental dry eye. *J. Ocul. Pharm. Ther.* **2014**, *30*, 533–542. [CrossRef] [PubMed]
12. Urban, M.C.C.; Mainardes, R.M.; Gremião, M.P.D. Development and validation of HPLC method for analysis of dexamethasone acetate in microemulsions. *Braz. J. Pharm. Sci.* **2009**, *45*, 87–92. [CrossRef]
13. Borman, P.; Elder, D. Q2(R1) Validation of Analytical Procedures. In *ICH Quality Guidelines*; Teasdale, A., Elder, D., Nims, R.W., Eds.; ICH: Geneva, Switzerland, 2017. [CrossRef]
14. Space, J.S.; Opio, A.M.; Nickerson, B.; Jiang, H.; Dumont, M.; Berry, M. Validation of a dissolution method with HPLC analysis for lasofoxifene tartrate low dose tablets. *J. Pharm. Biomed. Anal.* **2007**, *44*, 1064–1071. [CrossRef] [PubMed]
15. Sautou, V.; Bossard, D.; Chedru-Legros, V.; Crauste-Manciet, S.; Fleury-Souverain, S.; Lagarce, F.; Odou, P.; Roy, S.; Sadeghipour, F.; Sautou, V. *Methodological Guidelines for Stability Studies of Hospital Pharmaceutical Preparations*, 1st ed.; GERPAC, SFPC, Eds.; 2013; p. 75. Available online: https://www.gerpac.eu/IMG/pdf/guide_stabilite_anglais.pdf (accessed on 20 February 2018).
16. Graça, A.; Gonçalves, L.M.; Raposo, S.; Ribeiro, H.M.; Marto, J. Useful In vitro techniques to evaluate the mucoadhesive properties of hyaluronic acid-based ocular delivery systems. *Pharmaceutics* **2018**, *10*, 110. [CrossRef] [PubMed]
17. Silva, M.M.; Calado, R.; Marto, J.; Bettencourt, A.; Almeida, A.J.; Gonçalves, L.M.D. Chitosan nanoparticles as a mucoadhesive drug delivery system for ocular administration. *Mar. Drugs* **2017**, *15*, 370. [CrossRef]
18. da Silva, S.B.; Ferreira, D.; Pintado, M.; Sarmento, B. Chitosan-based nanoparticles for rosmarinic acid ocular delivery—In vitro tests. *Int. J. Biol. Macromol.* **2016**, *84*, 112–120. [CrossRef]
19. Rönkkö, S.; Vellonen, K.-S.; Järvinen, K.; Toropainen, E.; Urtti, A. Human corneal cell culture models for drug toxicity studies. *Drug Deliv. Transl. Res.* **2016**, *6*, 660–675. [CrossRef]
20. Wen, Y.; Ban, J.; Mo, Z.; Zhang, Y.; An, P.; Liu, L.; Xie, Q.; Du, Y.; Xie, B.; Zhan, X.; et al. A potential nanoparticle-loaded in situ gel for enhanced and sustained ophthalmic delivery of dexamethasone. *Nanotechnology* **2018**, *29*, 425101. [CrossRef]
21. National Research Council (US) Committee for the Update of the Guide for the Care and Use of Laboratory Animals. *Guide for the Care and Use of Laboratory Animals*, 8th ed.; The national academies collection: Reports funded by national institutes of health; National Academies Press: Washington, DC, USA, 2011; ISBN 978-0-309-15400-0.
22. Fernández-Ferreiro, A.; Silva-Rodríguez, J.; Otero-Espinar, F.J.; González-Barcia, M.; Lamas, M.J.; Ruibal, A.; Luaces-Rodriguez, A.; Vieites-Prado, A.; Sobrino, T.; Herranz, M.; et al. Positron emission tomography for the development and characterization of corneal permanence of ophthalmic pharmaceutical formulations. *Invest. Ophthalmol. Vis. Sci.* **2017**, *58*, 772–780. [CrossRef]
23. Zhang, Y.; Huo, M.; Zhou, J.; Xie, S. PKSolver: An add-in program for pharmacokinetic and pharmacodynamic data analysis in Microsoft Excel. *Comput. Methods Programs Biomed.* **2010**, *99*, 306–314. [CrossRef]
24. *European Phramacopoeia*, 9.8th ed.; EDQM: Strasbourg, France, 2019.
25. McEvoy, G.K. *American Society of Health-System Pharmacists. AHFS Drug information 2007*; American Society of Health-System Pharmacists: Bethesda, MD, USA, 2007; ISBN 978-1-58528-161-9.
26. Zaki, I.; Fitzgerald, P.; Hardy, J.G.; Wilson, C.G. A comparison of the effect of viscosity on the precorneal residence of solutions in rabbit and man. *J. Pharm. Pharmcol.* **1986**, *38*, 463–466. [CrossRef]

27. Snibson, G.R.; Greaves, J.L.; Soper, N.D.; Prydal, J.I.; Wilson, C.G.; Bron, A.J. Precorneal residence times of sodium hyaluronate solutions studied by quantitative gamma scintigraphy. *Eye* **1990**, *4*, 594–602. [CrossRef] [PubMed]
28. Salzillo, R.; Schiraldi, C.; Corsuto, L.; D'Agostino, A.; Filosa, R.; De Rosa, M.; La Gatta, A. Optimization of hyaluronan-based eye drop formulations. *Carbohydr. Polym.* **2016**, *153*, 275–283. [CrossRef] [PubMed]
29. Franck, A. *Understanding Rheology of Structured Fluids*; TA Instruments: New Castle, DE, USA, 2004; pp. 1–11. Available online: http://scholar.google.com/scholar?hl=en&btnG=Search&q=intitle: Understanding+Rheology+of+Structured+Fluids#2%5Cnhttp://scholar.google.com/scholar?hl=en&btnG= Search&q=intitle (accessed on 27 March 2018).
30. Madsen, F.; Eberth, K.; Smart, J.D. A rheological examination of the mucoadhesive/mucus interaction: The effect of mucoadhesive type and concentration. *J. Control. Release* **1998**, *50*, 167–178. [CrossRef]
31. Ludwig, A. The use of mucoadhesive polymers in ocular drug delivery. *Adv. Drug Deliv. Rev.* **2005**, *57*, 1595–1639. [CrossRef]
32. OECD. *Guideline for the Testing of Chemicals—Short Time Exposure in Vitro Test Method*; Organisation for Economic Co-operation and Development: Paris, France, 2018; p. 19. Available online: https://www.oecd-ilibrary.org/environment/test-no-491-short-time-exposure-in-vitro-test-method-for-identifying-i-chemicals-inducing-serious-eye-damage-and-ii-chemicals-not-requiring-classification-for-eye-irritation-or-serious-eye-damage_9789264242432-en (accessed on 27 March 2018).
33. Piel, G.; Piette, M.; Barillaro, V.; Castagne, D.; Evrard, B.; Delattre, L. Study of the relationship between lipid binding properties of cyclodextrins and their effect on the integrity of liposomes. *Int. J. Pharm.* **2007**, *338*, 35–42. [CrossRef]
34. Fernández-Ferreiro, A.; Fernández Bargiela, N.; Varela, M.S.; Martínez, M.G.; Pardo, M.; Piñeiro Ces, A.; Méndez, J.B.; Barcia, M.G.; Lamas, M.J.; Otero-Espinar, F. Cyclodextrin–polysaccharide-based, in situ-gelled system for ocular antifungal delivery. *Beilstein J. Org. Chem.* **2014**, *10*, 2903–2911. [CrossRef]
35. Zoorob, R.J.; Cender, D. A different look at corticosteroids. *Am. Fam. Physician* **1998**, *58*, 443–450.
36. Behl, G.; Iqbal, J.; O'Reilly, N.J.; McLoughlin, P.; Fitzhenry, L. Synthesis and characterization of poly(2-hydroxyethylmethacrylate) contact lenses containing chitosan nanoparticles as an ocular delivery system for dexamethasone sodium phosphate. *Pharm. Res.* **2016**, *33*, 1638–1648. [CrossRef]
37. Djalilian, A.R.; Nagineni, C.N.; Mahesh, S.P.; Smith, J.A.; Nussenblatt, R.B.; Hooks, J.J. Inhibition of inflammatory cytokine production in human corneal cells by dexamethasone, but not cyclosporin. *Cornea* **2006**, *25*, 709–714. [CrossRef]
38. Castro-Balado, A.; Mondelo-García, C.; González-Barcia, M.; Zarra-Ferro, I.; Otero-Espinar, F.J.; Ruibal-Morell, Á.; Aguiar, P.; Fernández-Ferreiro, A. Ocular biodistribution studies using molecular imaging. *Pharmaceutics* **2019**, *11*, 237. [CrossRef] [PubMed]
39. Luaces-Rodríguez, A.; Touriño-Peralba, R.; Alonso-Rodríguez, I.; García-Otero, X.; González-Barcia, M.; Rodríguez-Ares, M.T.; Martínez-Pérez, L.; Aguiar, P.; Gómez-Lado, N.; Silva-Rodríguez, J.; et al. Preclinical characterization and clinical evaluation of tacrolimus eye drops. *Eur. J. Pharm. Sci.* **2018**, *120*, 152–161. [CrossRef] [PubMed]
40. ICH. Stability testing of new drug substances and products Q1A (R2). In *Proceedings of the International Conference on Harmonisation*; ICH: Geneva, Switzerland, 2003; pp. 1–20. Available online: https://www.ema.europa.eu/en/documents/scientific-guideline/ich-q-1-r2-stability-testing-new-drug-substances-products-step-5_en.pdf (accessed on 27 March 2018).

pharmaceutics

Article

Fasudil Loaded PLGA Microspheres as Potential Intravitreal Depot Formulation for Glaucoma Therapy

Raphael Mietzner [1], Christian Kade [2], Franziska Froemel [3], Diana Pauly [4], W. Daniel Stamer [5], Andreas Ohlmann [6], Joachim Wegener [2,7], Rudolf Fuchshofer [3] and Miriam Breunig [1,*]

1 Department of Pharmaceutical Technology, University of Regensburg, Universitaetsstrasse 31, 93040 Regensburg, Germany; raphael.mietzner@chemie.uni-regensburg.de
2 Institute of Analytical Chemistry, Chemo- and Biosensors, University of Regensburg, Universitaetsstrasse 31, 93040 Regensburg, Germany; christian.kade@ur.de (C.K.); joachim.wegener@ur.de (J.W.)
3 Department of Human Anatomy and Embryology, University of Regensburg, Universitaetsstrasse 31, 93040 Regensburg, Germany; franziska.froemel@vkl.uni-regensburg.de (F.F.); rudolf.fuchshofer@vkl.uni-regensburg.de (R.F.)
4 Experimental Ophthalmology, University Hospital Regensburg, Franz Josef Strauss Allee 11, 93053 Regensburg, Germany; diana.pauly@ukr.de
5 Department of Ophthalmology, Duke University, Durham, NC 27710, USA; william.stamer@dm.duke.edu
6 Department of Ophthalmology, Ludwig-Maximilians-University Munich, Mathildenstrasse 8, 80336 Munich, Germany; andreas.ohlmann@med.uni-muenchen.de
7 Fraunhofer Research Institution for Microsystems and Solid State Technologies EMFT, Universitaetsstrasse 31, 93040 Regensburg, Germany
* Correspondence: miriam.breunig@chemie.uni-regensburg.de; Tel.: +49-(0)-941-943-4828

Received: 26 June 2020; Accepted: 23 July 2020; Published: 27 July 2020

Abstract: Rho-associated protein kinase (ROCK) inhibitors allow for causative glaucoma therapy. Unfortunately, topically applied ROCK inhibitors suffer from high incidence of hyperemia and low intraocular bioavailability. Therefore, we propose the use of poly (lactide-co-glycolide) (PLGA) microspheres as a depot formulation for intravitreal injection to supply outflow tissues with the ROCK inhibitor fasudil over a prolonged time. Fasudil-loaded microspheres were prepared by double emulsion solvent evaporation technique. The chemical integrity of released fasudil was confirmed by mass spectrometry. The biological activity was measured in cell-based assays using trabecular meshwork cells (TM cells), Schlemm's canal cells (SC cells), fibroblasts and adult retinal pigment epithelium cells (ARPE-19). Cellular response to fasudil after its diffusion through vitreous humor was investigated by electric cell-substrate impedance sensing. Microspheres ranged in size from 3 to 67 µm. The release of fasudil from microspheres was controllable and sustained for up to 45 days. Released fasudil reduced actin stress fibers in TM cells, SC cells and fibroblasts. Decreased collagen gel contraction provoked by fasudil was detected in TM cells (~2.4-fold), SC cells (~1.4-fold) and fibroblasts (~1.3-fold). In addition, fasudil readily diffused through vitreous humor reaching its target compartment and eliciting effects on TM cells. No negative effects on ARPE-19 cells were observed. Since fasudil readily diffuses through the vitreous humor, we suggest that an intravitreal drug depot of ROCK inhibitors could significantly improve current glaucoma therapy particularly for patients with comorbid retinal diseases.

Keywords: drug delivery; glaucoma; ROCK inhibitor; fasudil; PLGA microspheres; intravitreal injection; trabecular meshwork; Schlemm's canal; retinal pigment epithelium; Electric Cell-Substrate Impedance Sensing

1. Introduction

With the advent of rho-associated protein kinase (ROCK) inhibitors netarsudil (Rhopressa^{TM}) and ripasudil (Glanatec^{TM}), a promising new class of drugs has been introduced for glaucoma management [1,2]. In contrast to standard treatment with prostaglandin analogs or β-blockers that reduce the intraocular pressure (IOP) but fail to tackle the root cause of IOP elevation, ROCK inhibitors target cells in the conventional outflow pathway [3]. They increase the outflow facility by acting on cells of the trabecular meshwork (TM) and Schlemm's canal (SC). Mechanistically, they reduce stress fiber and focal adhesion formation, actomyosin contractility and the expression of various extracellular matrix (ECM) proteins. ROCK inhibitors are applied as eye drops and are therefore associated with high incidence of conjunctival hyperemia and possibly subconjunctival hemorrhage [3]. Moreover, short corneal residence time and poor corneal penetration strongly limit the bioavailability of topically applied drugs in the aqueous humor to a typical range of about 0.1% to 5% [4–6]. In addition, an application frequency of up to two times a day is associated with poor compliance; thus about 20% of patients discontinue therapy with eye drops after three years [4,7,8].

A delivery system that provides ROCK inhibitors to the cells of the TM and SC in a controlled and continuous fashion would significantly increase therapeutic success. To date, only a small number of sustained delivery devices have been developed, and these have been limited to traditional glaucoma drugs [9]. For example, a silicone ring placed on the cornea into the conjunctival fornix releases bimatoprost over a period of six months [9]. Reliable placement and stable localization of the ring over six months may be an issue, and the corneal barrier still poses a major hurdle for drug absorption. Recently, a bimatoprost-containing biodegradable implant for intracameral application received first approval in the USA [10]. This device tremendously increases bioavailability at the target site [11]. However, besides the risk of decellularization of corneal endothelia [10], such a freely movable device may bear the risk migrating into the posterior segment. Other preclinical approaches aim to place a drug depot subconjunctivally or supra-choroidally, but several tissue barriers severely reduce the amount of drug that reaches its place of action, and rapid drug elimination into the circulation increases off-target effects [12].

We propose to create an intravitreal depot of ROCK inhibitors because the vitreous offers space for a huge drug reservoir of about 100 μL and intravitreal injections have become routine in the clinic [6,13,14]. Intravitreal depot formulations have gained significant attention for the delivery of antibodies or small molecules to the posterior eye [15–17], however, they have not been exploited to deliver drug to the cells in the anterior chamber. This transport route is feasible since small molecules are eliminated from the vitreous via both the anterior chamber and the retina [13,18]. We hypothesize that the ROCK inhibitor will be transported to the anterior chamber after release from such an intravitreal depot (Scheme 1). The great advantages of this strategy are that there is no ocular surface exposure and the portion of the drug that reaches the retina may be beneficial. In fact, ROCK inhibitors have been demonstrated to have neuroprotective effects on cells of the retina [19].

In this study, poly (lactic-co-glycolic acid) (PLGA) microspheres containing the ROCK inhibitor fasudil were developed. We selected PLGA as the material for the depot formulation because it is a biodegradable polymer and because PLGA microspheres are well tolerated in the rat vitreous up to a concentration of two milligrams per milliliter [20]. Depending on microsphere size, polymer composition and concentration, PLGA microspheres allow for releasing small molecules up to 90 days [20,21] which would be a convenient dosing interval for glaucoma treatment. We demonstrated the principal feasibility of our approach by diffusion experiments of fasudil through porcine vitreous ex vivo as well as measurements of the functionality of TM and SC cells that received fasudil released from microspheres. Fibroblasts were included as well because during glaucoma development, cells of the TM experience a change from a mesenchymal- to myofibroblast-like phenotype [22]. In addition, a potential adverse effect of fasudil on adult retinal pigment epithelium cells (ARPE 19 cells) was investigated.

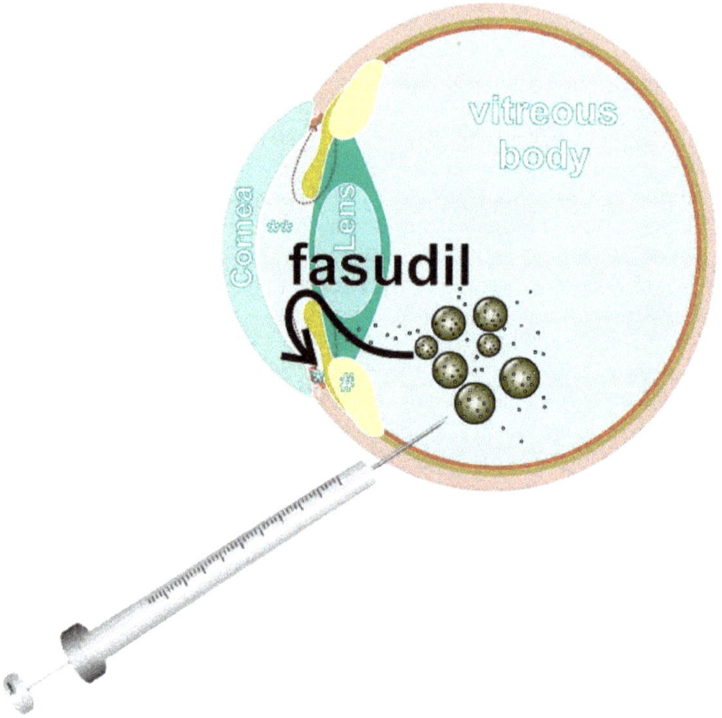

Scheme 1. Fasudil-loaded microspheres injected into the vitreous body. After intravitreal injection, microspheres agglomerate and subsequently sediment at the site of injection leaving a free visual axis [23]. As the depot formulation degrades, fasudil (small dots) is released and transported to its target site in the anterior chamber (**) of the eye, taking advantage of natural water movement patterns in the eye. Red dashed arrow indicates the flow of the aqueous humor. The dimensions do not correspond to reality. #: ciliary body; *: Trabecular meshwork and Schlemm's canal. With permission adapted from Mietzner et al. [4].

2. Materials and Methods

2.1. Materials

Ester-terminated PLGA (ratio 50:50; Resomer® RG 503) was acquired from Evonik (Darmstadt, Germany). Fasudil HCl was supplied by Selleck chemicals (Houston, TX, USA). Dichloromethane (DCM) was purchased from Sigma-Aldrich (Taufkirchen, Germany). Ultrapure water was obtained from a Millipore system (Millipore, Schwalbach, Germany). Polyvinyl alcohol (PVA; Mowiol 8–88) was obtained from Kuraray Specialities Europe GmbH (Hattersheim am Main, Germany). Tween-20 was purchased from SERVA Electrophoresis GmbH (Heidelberg, Germany). Dulbecco's modified Eagle's medium (DMEM) for cell culture was purchased from Pan Biotech GmbH (Aidenbach, Germany).

2.2. Preparation of Fasudil-Loaded PLGA Microspheres

PLGA microspheres were prepared by double emulsion solvent evaporation technique. Two modifications of the water-in-oil-in-water (W/O/W) and one solid-in-oil-in-water (S/O/W) emulsification manufacturing method were applied. The main characteristics of the methods are summarized in Table 1: S/O/W microspheres (S) were prepared according to Xu et al. with slight modifications [24]. First, fasudil was crushed with a mortar and micronized by two cycles of jet milling (MC One®, Jetpharma SA, Balerna, Switzerland) at 6 bar and room temperature (microsphere size ≈ 1 μm). Micronized fasudil HCl (20 mg) was added to 1 mL DCM containing 200 mg PLGA and dispersed for one minute by probe ultrasonication (Digital Sonifier Model 250-D Branson, MO, USA) in an ice–water bath. Then, 10 mL of 1% (*w*/*v*) PVA solution were added to the primary dispersion and homogenized (7000 rotations per minute (rpm); 30 s) at room temperature using a T18 digital Ultra-Turrax equipped with an S 18N–10G dispersing tool (IKA Labortechnik, Staufen, Germany). The resulting S/O/W multi-emulsion was rapidly poured into 90 mL of 1% (*w*/*v*) PVA solution and stirred for three hours using a magnetic stirrer (700 rpm). The resulting microspheres were collected by centrifugation (3000 rpm) and washed three times with ultrapure water. The PLGA microspheres were finally lyophilized with an LMC-2 freeze-dryer (Christ, Osterode am Harz, Germany) and stored at −20 °C until use.

Table 1. Parameters for the Preparation of the Microsphere Formulations.

Sample	Method	Volume of Inner Aqueous Phase (mL)	Fasudil (mg)	Volume of DCM (mL)	PLGA (mg)	Stirring Speed (rpm)
W1	W/O/W	1	20	8	200	20,000
W2	W/O/W	0.5	5	3	200	10,000
S	S/O/W	–	20	1	200	7000

DCM: dichloromethane; PLGA: poly (lactic-co-glycolic acid).

The first variant of the W/O/W microspheres (W1) was prepared according to Ramazani et al. with some modifications [25]. First 1 mL of inner water phase (ultrapure water) containing 20 mg fasudil HCl was added to 8 mL DCM containing 200 mg PLGA (25 mg/mL) and homogenized in an icewater bath at 20,000 rpm for 1 min using the same Ultra-Turrax as previously described. Next, 15 mL of 250-mM Tris HCl buffer (pH 9.0) containing 1% (*w*/*v*) PVA was added to the initial W/O emulsion and homogenized again for 1 min using the same homogenizer and conditions as before. The resulting W/O/W emulsion was poured into 85 mL of the same buffer (pH 9.0) containing 1% (*w*/*v*) PVA and stirred for 3 h using a magnetic stirrer at 700 rpm to allow the solvent to evaporate. Afterwards, the procedure was the same as for S microspheres.

The second variant of the W/O/W microspheres (W2) was prepared by dissolving fasudil HCl (5 mg) in 500 μL of ultrapure water. Then, 3 mL of DCM containing 200 mg PLGA (67 mg/mL) was added to the initial fasudil solution and homogenized at 10,000 rpm for 1 min using the Ultra-Turrax. This primary W/O emulsion was subsequently added to 10 mL of 1% (*w*/*v*) PVA solution and homogenized again at 10,000 rpm for 1 min. The resulting W/O/W emulsion was poured into 90 mL of 1% (*w*/*v*) PVA solution and stirred again for 3 h using a magnetic stirrer at 700 rpm, allowing the solvent to evaporate. Afterwards, the procedure was the same as for the other two samples (W1 and S). Three independent batches of each microsphere type were produced.

2.3. *Characterization of Fasudil-Loaded PLGA Microspheres*

2.3.1. Size Determination

The volume weighted mean diameter (reported as microsphere size in the following) and microsphere size distribution of the microspheres were determined by laser diffraction spectroscopy after the washing step in the manufacturing procedure. Analyses were performed with a Mastersizer 2000 (Malvern Panalytical Ltd., Malvern, UK) equipped with a Hoydro 2000 μ dispersion unit. For the measurement, microspheres were dispersed in ultrapure water (≈8 mg/mL) and were added into the dispersion unit, which was floated with ultrapure water, until the obscuration was higher than 5%. The stirring speed was set to 500 rpm. To determine the uniformity of the microsphere sizes, span values were calculated according to the following equation:

$$Span = \left(\frac{d90 - d10}{d50}\right) \quad (1)$$

d90, d10 and d50 are the microsphere diameters at 90%, 10% and 50% of the cumulative size, respectively. Data were obtained by three independent samples, presented as mean ± standard deviation.

2.3.2. Morphologic Characterization

The surface morphology of fasudil-loaded microspheres was observed with a Zeiss LEO 1530 Gemini scanning electron microscope (Carl Zeiss Microscopy GmbH, Oberkochen, Germany). Lyophilized microspheres were placed to conductive pads (Plano GmbH, Wetzlar, Germany) stuck to aluminum specimen stubs. The samples were sputtered with gold two times for two minutes using a Polaron E5100 coating unit (Polaron Equipment, Ltd., Hertfordshire, UK).

2.3.3. Fasudil Quantification

Fasudil was quantified by high performance liquid chromatography (HPLC) using a 1260 Infinity II LC system (Agilent Technologies, Inc., Santa Clara, CA, USA) equipped with a binary pump and a diode array detector. Analyses were performed using a reverse phase C_{18} column (150 mm × 5 mm; 5-µm microsphere size; Eclipse XDB-C18, Agilent Technologies, Inc., Santa Clara, CA, USA) preceded by a C_{18} security guard cartridge (Phenomenex, Inc., Torrance, CA, USA) at 40 °C. The mobile phase was composed of ultrapure water (eluent A) and methanol (eluent B; HPLC grade, Merck, Darmstadt, Germany), both containing 0.03% (*v*/*v*) trifluoroacetic acid (HPLC grade, Sigma-Aldrich GmbH, Taufkirchen, Germany). Fasudil was eluted by a gradient at a flow rate of 0.8 mL/min. The gradient used was as follows: 0.0–0.5 min constant at 85% (*v*/*v*) eluent A; 0.5–6.5 min 85–40% (*v*/*v*) eluent A (linear gradient); 6.5–7.0 min changed to 5% (*v*/*v*) eluent A; 7.0–17.0 min constant at 5% (*v*/*v*) eluent A; 17.0–17.10 min changed to 85% (*v*/*v*) eluent A; 17.10–27.10 min constant at 85% (*v*/*v*) eluent A. The injection volume was 5 µL for encapsulation efficiency (% EE) measurements and 10 to 12 µL for in vitro release studies. Each sample was injected three times. The absorbance of fasudil was measured at $\lambda = 320$ nm.

2.3.4. Encapsulation Efficiency

Fasudil content of microspheres was quantified by dissolving lyophilized fasudil-loaded microspheres (20–40 mg) in DCM (1 mL), followed by precipitation of PLGA by the addition of methanol (3 mL). The obtained dispersion was mixed, centrifuged (9000 G; 10 min), and the supernatant was filtered for fasudil quantification by HPLC-UV-Vis. To calculate the percentage encapsulation efficiency (% EE) and drug loading (% DL), the following equations were used:

$$\%\,EE = \left(\frac{actual\ drug\ content}{theoretical\ drug\ content}\right) \times 100 \quad (2)$$

$$\%\,DL = \left[\frac{drug\ (mg)}{drug + polymer}\right] \times 100 \quad (3)$$

Three independent samples were analyzed and are presented as mean ± standard deviation.

2.3.5. In Vitro Drug Release

Fasudil-loaded microspheres (20–50 mg) of three independent batches were dispersed in 1 mL of Dulbecco's phosphate-buffered saline (DPBS) containing 0.02% Tween-20 in 2-mL centrifuge tubes and placed in a shaking water bath incubator (37 °C). Tween-20 was added to improve the wettability and to avoid floating of microspheres. At several points over a time period of 50 days, samples were centrifuged and 500 to 850 μL of the supernatants were replaced by the same volume of fresh buffer. The pellet was redispersed, placed back in the incubator and collected supernatants were stored at −80 °C until fasudil quantification. Data were obtained from three independent samples and are expressed as mean ± standard deviation. Because the amount of released fasudil was rather low, the drug was pooled from the release medium of all three microsphere types for subsequent experiments.

2.3.6. Mass Spectrometric (MS) Analysis of Fasudil

Analyses were performed with an Agilent 1290 Infinity HPLC system (Agilent Technologies, Inc., Santa Clara, CA, USA), interfaced to an Agilent 6540 Quadrupole time-of-flight (Q-TOF) mass spectrometer with a dual electrospray ionization (ESI) source (Agilent Technologies, Inc., Santa Clara, CA, USA). A Phenomenex (Torrance, CA, USA) Luna Omega 1.6 μm C18 column (pore size 100 Å; 100 × 2.1 mm) was used for separation at 40 °C. The mobile phase was composed of ultrapure water (eluent A) and acetonitrile (eluent B), both containing 0.1% (*v*/*v*) formic acid. The elution was performed under gradient conditions at a flow rate of 0.6 mL/min. The flow gradient used was as follows: 0–4 min 95–2% (*v*/*v*) eluent A (linear gradient); 4–5 min constant at 2% (*v*/*v*) eluent A; 5–5.10 min changed to 95% (*v*/*v*) eluent A. Mass spectrometric analyses were carried out in positive ion mode.

2.3.7. Preparation of Released Fasudil for Cell Experiments

To investigate the biologic activity of fasudil released from microspheres (released fasudil), parallel to in vitro release studies, fasudil-loaded microspheres were incubated in ultrapure water containing 0.02% Tween-20 for several days. The supernatant was collected and lyophilized. The lyophilized product was reconstituted in ultrapure water, and after adjusting the pH to 7.3, the solution was sterile filtered, and the amount of fasudil was determined by the previously described method. Finally, the solution was diluted to the desired concentration with DPBS. The same procedure was followed for control microspheres (unloaded microspheres) except for fasudil quantification.

2.4. *Cellular Effect of Fasudil*

2.4.1. Cell Culture

Primary human trabecular meshwork cells (TM cells) and Schlemm's canal cells (SC cells) were used until passage numbers 7 and 12, respectively. Primary cultures of human foreskin fibroblasts were used until passage 13. TM and SC cells were characterized according to established methods [26,27]. Procedures for securing human tissue were humane, included proper consent and approval accordingly to the Declaration of Helsinki. Primary cells were cultivated in DMEM (supplemented with 4.5 g/L glucose for fibroblasts and 1 g/L glucose for TM and SC cells) containing 10% (*v*/*v*) fetal bovine serum (FBS; Thermo Fisher Scientific, Waltham, MA, USA), 100 units/mL penicillin and 100 μg/mL streptomycin. Immortalized human TM cells (HTM-N) were used for electric cell–substrate impedance sensing (ECIS) and were made available by Iok-Hou Pang and Louis DeSantis (Alcon Research Laboratories, Fort Worth, TX, USA). They were cultured according to published protocols [28]. Human male adult retinal pigment epithelium cells (ARPE-19 cells, American Type Culture Collection, #CRL-2302 passage 25) were cultivated in Transwell® inserts for 4–6 weeks in DMEM containing 4.5 g/L glucose supplemented with 1% FCS (Pan Biotech GmbH, Aidenbach, Germany), 100 units/mL penicillin, 100 μg/mL streptomycin and 1 mM sodium pyruvate. If not otherwise stated, cells were incubated for 24 h in medium containing 0.35% FBS supplemented with unencapsulated fasudil (free fasudil; 25 μM) or released fasudil (25 μM), respectively. Both, DPBS and medium collected from blank microspheres served as negative controls for free and released fasudil, respectively. Since there was no significant difference between both controls, only one representative control is shown. A serum concentration of 0.35% was chosen because it is equivalent to the amount of protein in the aqueous humor [29]. Fasudil at a concentration of 25 μM was used because it is a widely applied concentration and was well tolerated by the cells (c.f. supplementary materials: Figure S1) [30,31]. Cells were not directly incubated with the microspheres, but rather with the release media containing fasudil. Since the loading with fasudil was too low, an immensely high number of microspheres would be necessary to elicit cellular effects. In this case, a strong acidification of the culture medium would have occurred due to PLGA's degradation products glycolic and lactic acid.

2.4.2. Fluorescence Labeling of Actin Cytoskeleton

Cells were placed into 8-well μ-slides (ibidi GmbH, Gräfelfing, Germany) at a density of 2×10^4 cells/well. After fasudil exposure, as described above, cells were washed once with 0.1×-PBS, fixed in 4% paraformaldehyde for 5 min at room temperature and washed twice with 0.1×-PBS for 5 min. To stain actin stress fibers, fixed cells were incubated in the dark with phalloidin–fluorescein isothiocyanate (FITC–phalloidin; Invitrogen, Molecular Probes, Eugene, OR, USA) for 1 h at room temperature. Afterwards, cells were rinsed three times with 0.1×-PBS and embedded in Dako Fluorescence Mounting Medium (Agilent Technologies, Santa Clara, CA, USA). Nuclei of ARPE19 cells were labeled additionally by 4′,6-diamidino-2-phenylindole (DAPI). The fluorescence of fibroblast, TM and SC cells was visualized using an LSM 510 Meta confocal microscope (Carl Zeiss AG, Göttingen, Germany)). To visualize ARPE19 cells, an Axio Imager Z1 fluorescence microscope (Carl Zeiss AG, Göttingen, Germany) was used.

2.4.3. Collagen Gel Contraction Assay

The collagen gel contraction assay was carried out with slight modifications according to Su et al. [32]: Fibroblasts, TM cells, and SC cells were trypsinized (Pan Biotech GmbH, Aidenbach, Germany) and resuspended at a density of 1.5×10^5 cells/mL in DMEM containing 0.35% FBS and 1.17 mg/mL of rat tail collagen type I (4.00 mg/mL in 0.02-N acetic acid; BD Bioscience, San Jose, CA, USA; (adjusted with 0.02-N acetic acid for the desired concentration). To allow the gel to solidify at optimal conditions, 1-M sodium hydroxide solution was added to adjust the solution to neutral pH. Then, 500 μL of the collagen-cell mixture were transferred to each well of a 24-well plate. The mixture was incubated at 37 °C under 5% CO_2 for one hour. After the gel solidified, 500 μL of DMEM containing 0.35% FBS supplemented with controls, free or released fasudil for a final concentration of 25 μM was pipetted onto the collagen gels. Gels were carefully dissociated from the wall of the culture wells using a hypodermic needle. After 0, 24, 48 and 72 h, culture wells were tangentially illuminated and photographed (EOS 750D, Canon, Tokyo, Japan) from above with a fixed distance in front of a dark background. The areas of the matrices were measured using ImageJ software (version 1.52d, U.S. National Institutes of Health, Bethesda, MD, USA) [33]. For normalization, the mean areas measured in controls was set at 1 ($n = 4$).

2.4.4. Electric Cell–Substrate Impedance Sensing (ECIS)

The impact of fasudil on HTM-N cells was monitored by noninvasive impedance readings. A schematic illustration of the experimental setup is shown in Section 3.5. HTM-N cells were seeded in 8-well plates milled into a poly(methyl methacrylate) block with a well diameter of 16 mm each. In order to allow for ECIS measurements, the bottom of the well was made from a polycarbonate (Lexan®) base substrate coated with a gold electrode layout generated by sputter deposition of gold and subsequent photolithographic patterning. The bottom plate with the electrode layout was glued to the 8-well block using a biocompatible silicon adhesive. Cells were either treated directly by replacing half of culture medium with fresh culture medium containing controls, free or released fasudil for a final concentration of 25 μM; or samples were premixed with 200 μL vitreous body of fresh enucleated porcine eyes (purchased from a local slaughterhouse) by vortexing them and putting them into 6.5 mm Transwells® with a polycarbonate membrane holding 108 pores per cm^2 of 0.4 μm pore diameter each (Corning, Inc., Corning, NY, USA). The height of the vitreous body in the insert was 6 mm. Experiments were performed at 37 °C under 5% CO_2. Relay bank, lock-in amplifier and software for the ECIS data acquisition and analysis were obtained from Applied BioPhysics (Troy, NY, USA).

The impedance values of each well were recorded at an alternating current frequency of 8 kHz every 4 min over the entire time of analysis. Impedance values are presented as the values captured along the experimental time course normalized to the impedance values recorded immediately before addition of test substances. Two independent experiments were performed. Due to the 8-well-format of the experimental setup, all fasudil containing samples (free- and released fasudil) were performed in triplicate and control samples were performed in duplicate.

2.5. Statistical Analysis

All data are presented as means ± standard deviation. Standard deviations of normalized mean values were calculated according to the rules of error propagation. Multiple *t*-tests with the Holm–Sidak method (in Section 3) were performed using GraphPad Prism 6.0c (GraphPad Software, San Diego, CA, USA) to assess statistical significance (statistical significance assigned at $p < 0.05$).

3. Results

3.1. Manufacture and Characterization of Fasudil-Loaded Microspheres

Because fasudil is a water-soluble drug, the double emulsion solvent evaporation technique was chosen for its encapsulation into PLGA microspheres. Two modifications of the water-in-oil-in-water (W/O/W) and one solid-in-oil-in-water (S/O/W) emulsification methods were applied to obtain three different microsphere species with individual sizes. These will be denoted as W1, W2 and S in the following. The W1 and W2 method differed in polymer concentration (W1: 25 mg/mL; W2; 67 mg/mL), emulsifying stirring speed (W1: 20,000 rpm; W2: 10,000 rpm) and pH of the external aqueous phase (W1: adjusted to pH 9.0; W2: not controlled). In the S preparation, the polymer concentration was 200 mg/mL and solid fasudil was incorporated into the PLGA matrix instead of dissolved fasudil, since fasudil was not soluble in DCM due to its hydrophilic nature. The W1 batch had the smallest size of about 3.4 µm, followed by W2—with a size of about 18.2 µm and S with a size of about 66.9 µm (Figure 1 and Table 2). All three microsphere types were spherical in shape as evaluated by scanning electron microscopy (SEM) (Figure 1). W1 and W2 microspheres had overall smooth and nonporous surfaces. Single W2 and S microspheres showed tiny holes on their surfaces. The surfaces of S microspheres were covered in circular dents. The encapsulation efficacy of all three batches was below 5% (Table 1). SEM images demonstrated that no free, unencapsulated fasudil was resting on the surface of microspheres.

Table 2. Size, span, encapsulation efficiency (EE), drug loading (DL) and drug content of fasudil-loaded microspheres. Values expressed as mean (± standard deviation) of three independent batches.

Sample	Microsphere Size (µm) †	Size (µm)			Span *	EE (%)	DL (%)	Content (µg/mg Microsphere)
		d (10)	d (50)	d (90)				
W1	3.4 (± 0.6)	1.1 (±0.1)	2.7 (±0.1)	4.5 (±0.6)	1.7 (±0.1)	2.5 (±0.2)	0.2 (±0.0)	2.3 (±0.2)
W2	18.2 (± 2.7)	6.0 (±1.0)	14.7 (±0.7)	32.2 (±4.7)	1.8 (±0.4)	2.3 (±1.0)	0.1 (±0.0)	0.6 (±0.3)
S	66.9 (± 16.0)	30.7 (±1.0)	51.4 (±4.3)	118.6 (±56.4)	1.7 (±1.1)	3.9 (±1.6)	0.4 (±0.2)	3.7 (±1.3)

† mean microsphere size expressed as volume weighted mean diameter D [4.3] * Span = width of the microsphere size distribution: Span = (d90 − d10/d50. d90, d10 and d50 are the microsphere diameters at 90%, 10% and 50% of the cumulative size, respectively.

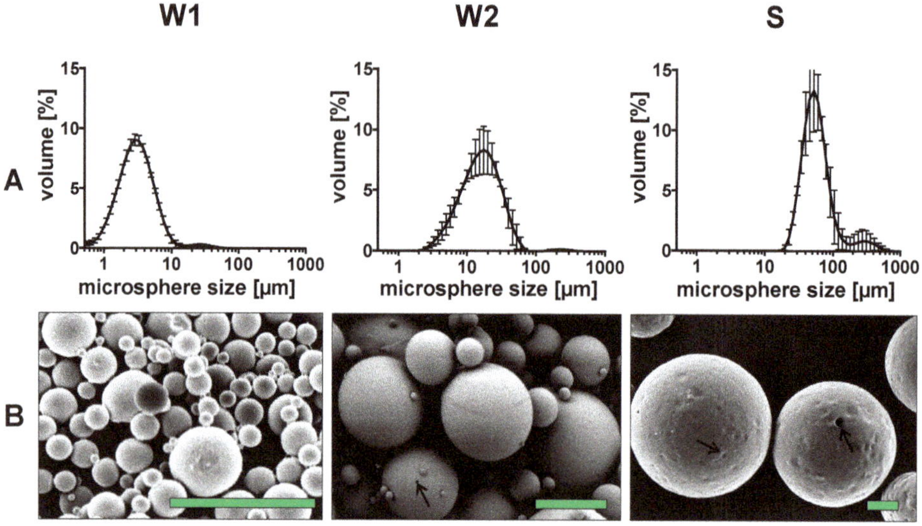

Figure 1. Microsphere size distribution and shape of microspheres. (**A**) Volume microsphere size distribution of W1, W2 and S microspheres was measured by laser light diffraction. The W1 batch had the smallest microsphere size of about 3.4 µm, followed by W2 (18.2 µm) and S with a microsphere size of about 66.9 µm. Error bars represent the standard deviation (SD) of the volume microsphere size of three independent batches; (**B**) Shape of the microspheres was visualized by scanning electron microscopy (SEM). All microsphere types had a round shape. W1 microspheres were quite smooth and nonporous. In contrast, some W2 and S microspheres exhibited holes (white arrows) on their surface, and S microspheres additionally showed circular dents as indicated by the blue arrow. Bars indicate 10 µm.

3.2. Fasudil Release from Microspheres Can Be Tailored under Maintenance of its Structure

The release of fasudil depended strongly on the microsphere size of the microspheres (Figure 2). The smallest microspheres (W1) had a high burst release of about 65% during the first 3 days, and the monophasic release was completed after only 20 days. Medium-sized W2 microspheres also showed a high burst release of about 40%, which was followed by a sustained release period over 35 days. In contrast, the S microspheres showed a typical triphasic sustained release, over about 45 days starting with a burst release of only about 20% followed by a plateau from day 1 to day 10 where no fasudil was released up to day 10 and followed by an almost linear release from day 17 to day 38.

To determine whether the fasudil was chemically unmodified after release from microspheres, HPLC-mass spectrometry (HPLC-MS) analysis was performed. Figure 3a shows the HPLC-MS total ion chromatogram of fasudil that was not encapsulated into microspheres as reference (indicated as free fasudil), and Figure 3b shows fasudil after it was released from microspheres (indicated as released fasudil). Both, free and released fasudil had the same retention time of 0.89 min. The MS-spectra of free and released fasudil matched very well (Figure 3c,d). Both showed a molecular peak at 291.1 *m*/*z* and a fragment ion peak at 146.6 *m*/*z* indicating that fasudil remained structurally intact during the encapsulation process and release.

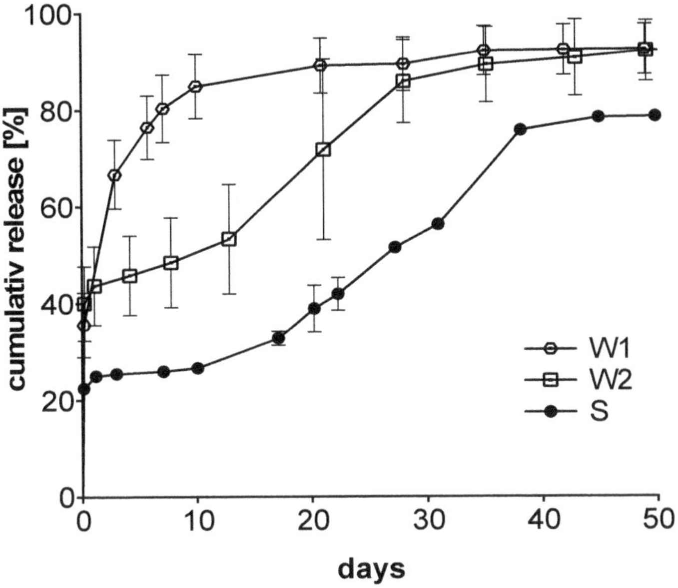

Figure 2. Cumulative release of fasudil from poly (lactide-*co*-glycolide) (PLGA) microspheres. Release experiments were performed in Dulbecco's phosphate-buffered saline (DPBS) containing 0.02% Tween-20 at 37 °C. Increasing microsphere size is indicated by the gray triangle with the inscription "size." The burst release of fasudil was reduced with increasing microsphere size. In the same order, the release period was extended. Data are expressed as mean ± standard deviation of cumulative released fasudil of three independent batches.

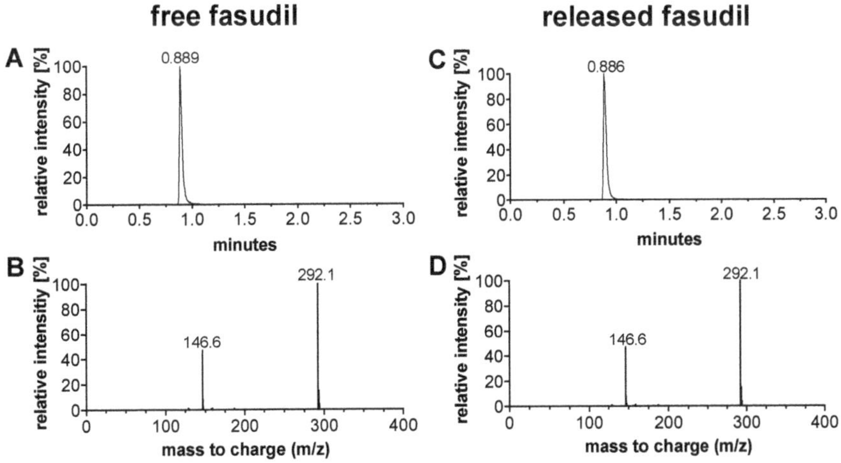

Figure 3. Integrity of fasudil before encapsulation and after release from PLGA microspheres. (**A**,**B**) HPLC-MS total ion chromatogram and electrospray mass spectrum of free fasudil. (**C**,**D**) HPLC-MS total ion chromatogram and electrospray mass spectrum of released fasudil. Both, free and released fasudil had a retention time of 0.89 min and the molecular peak was at 292.1 *m*/*z*.

3.3. *Released Fasudil Reduces Actin Stress Fiber Formation*

ROCK inhibitors decrease the outflow resistance in the anterior chamber of the eye due to their effects on the cytoskeleton of TM and SC cells [4,34]. TM and SC cells as well as fibroblasts were treated with free fasudil and fasudil released from microspheres. After staining the actin cytoskeleton with FITC–phalloidin, cells were studied by fluorescence microscopy (Figure 4). Untreated TM and SC cells and fibroblasts displayed numerous thick and longitudinally arranged actin stress fibers. The stress fibers of TM cells and fibroblasts were thicker than those of SC cells, which had a more cortical actin at baseline. In contrast, fasudil treatment (free or released) caused a dramatic reduction of actin stress fibers, and rather a cortical actin cytoskeleton remained. In all cell types, the effect of fasudil released from microspheres was comparable to free fasudil, corroborating that fasudil was not affected by the encapsulation procedure and still biologically active after release.

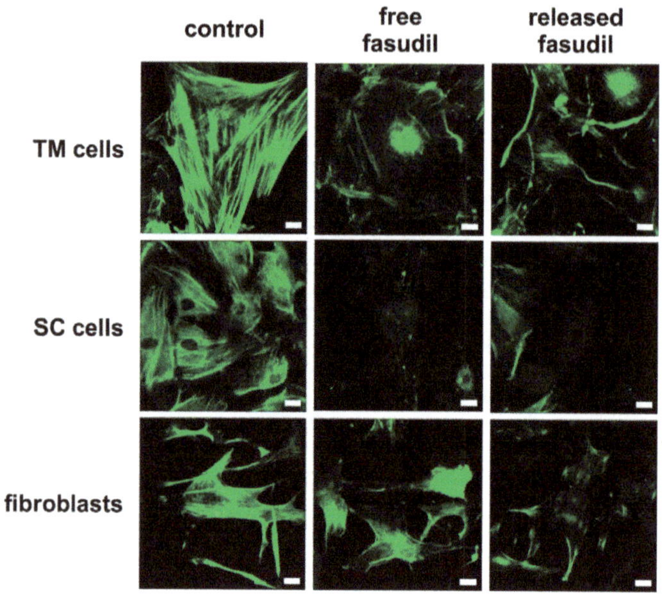

Figure 4. Free and released fasudil disrupt actin stress fibers. Representative fluorescence microscopic images of the actin cytoskeleton. Human using trabecular meshwork (TM) and Schlemm's canal (SC) cells and fibroblasts were incubated for 24 h with free or released fasudil at a concentration of 25 µM. This concentration was chosen because it is widely used in literature and well tolerated by all three cell types at a serum concentration of 0.35% (c.f. supplementary materials Figure S1) [30,31]. Actin cytoskeleton was labeled with FITC–phalloidin and visualized by fluorescence microscopy. Free and released fasudil caused a reduction of actin stress fibers and induced an actin reorientation compared to controls. Scale bar indicates 20 µm.

3.4. *Released Fasudil Reduces Cell Contractility*

To functionally measure the effect on actomyosin contractility, TM and SC cells as well as fibroblasts were embedded in a three-dimensional collagen type I gel and treated with free or released fasudil. Because cells have an inherent contractility, the gel matrix moves together over time. As a consequence, the gel surface area decreases. The more pronounced the cell contractility is, the smaller is the gel surface area and vice versa. The gel surface area was analyzed over time and served as a measure for cell contractility [35,36]. Gel area and cell contractility behave inversely, which means the smaller the gel area, the higher is the cell contractility. The gels initially filled the entire well, but over time and without fasudil treatment, the surface area of control gels decreased due to the contractility of embedded cells (Figure 5a, left column). Control gels with embedded TM cells had the smallest surface area after an assay time of 72 h, followed by those with SC cells and fibroblasts. In contrast, with fasudil treatment (free or released), the gel surface area remained nearly constant or only slightly decreased over 72 h (Figure 5a, middle and right columns). Due to the stronger gel contraction observed for TM cells under control conditions, the impact of fasudil was more pronounced for TM cells than for fibroblast and SC cells. This became even more apparent in the semi-quantitative analysis in Figure 5b. After 48 h, for example, the projected gel area relative to the control was the highest when TM cells (~2.4-fold) were embedded, followed by SC cells (~1.4-fold) and finally fibroblasts (~1.3-fold). For each cell type, no significant difference ($p > 0.05$) between free or released fasudil-treated cells was observed.

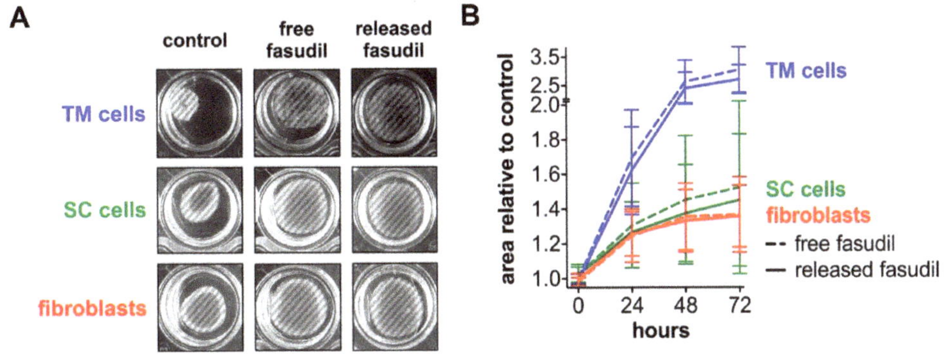

Figure 5. Free and released fasudil reduce contractility of fibroblasts, TM and SC cells embedded in collagen gels. (**A**) Representative images of control gels and gels that were incubated with free or released fasudil at a concentration of 25 μM after 48 h. The projected gel surface is highlighted by the hatched area. Control gels with embedded TM cells had the smallest surface area. The surface areas of gels with SC cells or fibroblast were similar. After incubation with fasudil, the surface area was much larger irrespective of the cell type. (**B**) Semiquantitative analysis of mean areas of collagen gels incubated with free or released fasudil normalized to controls at 0, 24, 48 and 72 h. For each cell type, no significant difference ($p < 0.05$) between free or released fasudil treated gels was observed. Y-axis is discontinued between 2.0 and 2.5. Data are expressed as normalized mean ± standard deviation of the mean ($n = 4$).

3.5. *Fasudil Diffuses through Vitreous Humor and Alters Cell Junctions*

Fasudil-loaded microspheres are intended to be injected into the vitreous body. To test whether released fasudil diffuses through the vitreous body to affect target cells in the anterior chamber, an experimental setup was developed that measures the cellular response only after successful fasudil diffusion through vitreous humor (Figure 6a). In this setup, the cellular response over time is measured by electric cell–substrate impedance sensing (ECIS) and serves as a measure for changes in cell–cell and cell–matrix junctions induced by cytoskeletal rearrangements (e.g., loss of stress fibers) [37,38]. A direct incubation of immortalized TM (HTM-N) cells with either free or released fasudil resulted in an immediate drop of impedance values from basal values by about 18% within 50 min (Figure 6b). The impedance signal showed a modest recovery over the next four hours. There was no statistically significant difference ($p < 0.05$) between free and released fasudil at any timepoint. In contrast, when fasudil was mixed with vitreous body and its contact to the cell monolayer was only possible after diffusion through the gel-like vitreous, the cellular impedance decreased over a much longer time period of about three hours to final values that were comparable to those after a direct treatment with fasudil. Again, no significant differences ($p < 0.05$) were observed between free and released fasudil.

The observed impedance changes indicate that TM cells experience a significant weakening of their cell–cell and/or cell–matrix adhesion in good agreement with the fasudil-induced loss of stress fibers.

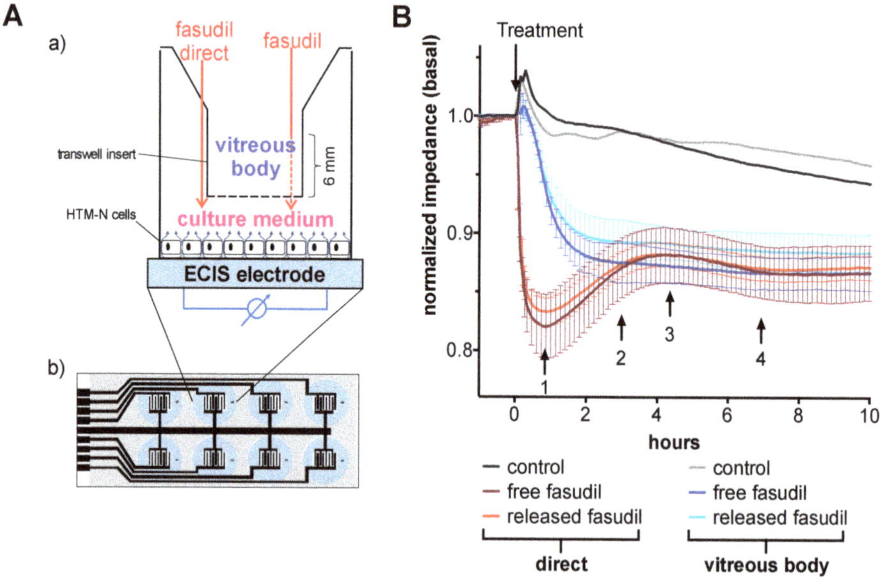

Figure 6. Free and released fasudil diffuse through the vitreous body and induce changes in cell–cell and cell–matrix junctions of immortalized TM cells. (**A**) Schematic illustration of the experimental setup of the vitreous diffusion assay in combination with electric cell–substrate impedance sensing (ECIS). (**a**) Cells were seeded in a culture well with integrated gold-film electrodes to allow for impedance measurements. Impedance was recorded at an alternating current frequency of 8 kHz. Cells were treated with free or released fasudil at a final concentration of 25 µM. Fasudil was either directly added to the cells (solid red arrow) or first mixed with vitreous humor, which was then placed in a Transwell® insert (dashed red arrow). Small blue arrows represent the current flow. (**b**) The bottom of the well was fabricated from a polycarbonate-based substrate (gray) with an interdigitated gold electrode layout (black). Each blue cycle represents one culture well. The dimensions are not drawn to scale; (**B**) Time-dependent changes of the impedance of immortalized TM cells (HTM-N cells) are shown. Values were normalized to impedance values immediately before addition of fasudil. Incubation with fasudil started at timepoint 0 h (indicated by arrow and "Treatment"). Cells that were directly incubated with fasudil (red curves) showed an immediate reduction of the impedance from basal values. In contrast, impedance slowly decreased over an extended time period, when a diffusion of fasudil through the vitreous was necessary (blue curves). All samples treated with fasudil (free or released) were performed in triplicate and control sample was performed in duplicate. Error bars show the standard deviation of normalized ECIS data. One representative experiment of two independent ones is shown. At indicated timepoints (black arrows with numbers), no statistical differences ($p < 0.05$) between free and released fasudil were observed.

3.6. Released Fasudil Does Not Influence Retinal Pigment Epithelial Cells

Fasudil that is released in the vitreous body may also come in contact with cells of the posterior chamber of the eye. Therefore, the effect of fasudil—either free or released—on the actin cytoskeleton of ARPE-19 cells was investigated. After staining the actin cytoskeleton with FITC–phalloidin, cells were visualized by fluorescence microscopy (Figure 7). Both untreated cells and cells that were treated with fasudil showed characteristics of a healthy retinal pigment epithelium (RPE), including defined cell borders, a cobblestone-like monolayer and a well-organized actin cytoskeleton, suggesting that fasudil at a concentration of 25 μM did not negatively affect ARPE-19 cells.

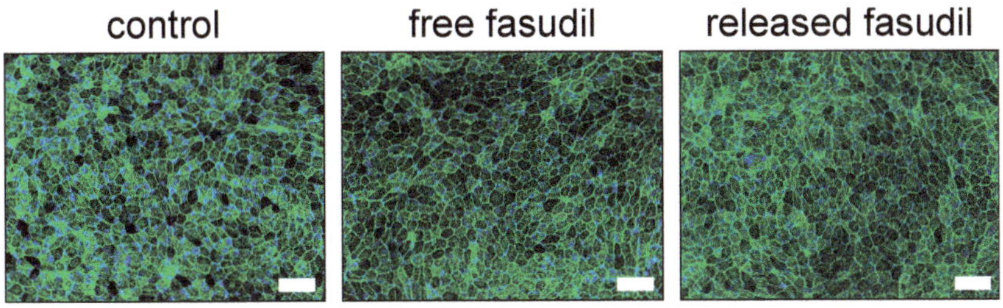

Figure 7. Free and released fasudil do not negatively affect retinal pigment epithelium cells (ARPE-19). ARPE-19 cells were incubated for 24 h with free or released fasudil at a concentration of 25 μM. The actin cytoskeleton was labeled with FITC–phalloidin (green) and the cell nuclei were stained with DAPI (blue). All samples had features characteristic of retinal pigment epithelium (RPE) including defined cell borders, an overall cobblestone appearance and a well-organized actin cytoskeleton. Representative fluorescence microscopic images of ARPE-19 cells are shown. Scale bar indicates 50 μm.

4. Discussion

ROCK inhibitors are considered as promising drug class for glaucoma therapy because they allow for causative treatment. To date, only eye drop formulations of ROCK inhibitors are available on the market. To deal with the issues associated with these formulations, including conjunctival hyperemia, subconjunctival hemorrhage and low intraocular bioavailability, we propose a depot formulation for intravitreal application. We incorporated the ROCK inhibitor fasudil into PLGA microspheres. PLGA is an advantageous material choice because it is approved by the Food and Drug Administration and the European Medicines Agency for intravitreal application [39] and it is commonly used to fabricate devices for controlled and sustained delivery of small and large drug molecules [40]. In contrast to non-biodegradable delivery devices for glaucoma therapy like the implant iDose made from titanium, which must be removed after the travoprost-loaded reservoir is empty, its biodegradability and high biocompatibility makes PLGA favorable for intraocular application.

Three modifications of the double emulsion solvent evaporation technique were applied to produce microspheres of different sizes of about 3, 18 and 70 μm (W1, W2 and S microspheres, respectively). One important parameter to control the microsphere size was the stirring speed during the first step of microsphere formation. Stirring is necessary because it provides the energy to disperse the immiscible oily PLGA phase and the aqueous drug-containing phase into each other [41]. As expected, the mean microsphere size was inversely proportional to the stirring speed. The second parameter to control microsphere size was the polymer concentration; microsphere size increased with increasing PLGA concentration. S microspheres were produced with the highest polymer concentration of 200-mg/mL and thus yielded the largest microsphere size, while W1 microspheres were the smallest and had the lowest polymer concentration (25 mg/mL) [42,43]. Size of the microspheres may have an influence on their intravitreal tolerability. Due to a higher specific surface area, smaller microspheres may show slightly more adverse effects [44]. We suggest fabrication under aseptic conditions to obtain a sterile ocular drug formulation. The encapsulation efficacy of fasudil into PLGA microspheres was only about 4%. It is known that hydrophilic molecules like fasudil with a log$P$-value around zero (log$P$ = 0.16 [45]) are difficult to encapsulate into PLGA polymer matrices, which are relatively lipophilic [46]. The main reason for the poor encapsulation efficacy is that fasudil shows a free solubility in water (up to ~200 mg/mL [47]), which favors its distribution from the lipophilic polymer matrix to the external aqueous phase. As a consequence, fasudil was already "released" from the PLGA matrix before microsphere creation was complete. Unfortunately, varying process parameters such as increasing the pH to reduce the solubility of the weakly basic fasudil (pK_a = 9.7 [48]) in the external water phase (as was performed for the W1 microspheres) did not improve the encapsulation efficacy [25]. In addition, the encapsulation of fasudil in its solid form, as done for the S microspheres, did not avoid its partitioning into the water phase during the manufacturing process.

Nevertheless, varying process parameters produced microspheres with different release characteristics in terms of initial release and time profile. A characteristic feature of microspheres manufactured by emulsion solvent evaporation technique is their initial burst release [49], which was particularly prominent for the smallest W1 microspheres with about 65% of the drug being released in the burst phase. This can be attributed to the high specific surface area of smaller microspheres and the shorter diffusion length that the drug must overcome to be transported from the microsphere matrix to the surrounding medium [49]. Because W2 and S microspheres were larger, the diffusion barrier to fasudil increased, resulting in initial burst releases of only about 40% and 20%, respectively. Additionally, the release duration of fasudil was prolonged to about 35 and 45 days, respectively. The PLGA concentration was the lowest for W1 (25 mg/mL) followed by W2 (66.7 mg/mL) and S (200 mg/mL) during microsphere formation. To decrease mobility and sedimentation of fasudil crystals and thus preventing drug loss towards the surrounding aqueous phase during microspheres hardening, a high polymer concentration was chosen for S microspheres to increase the viscosity. Furthermore, the polymer concentration has a huge impact on initial burst release [50]. With decreasing polymer concentration, the internal porosity is increased and vice versa [50]. A high internal porosity allows water to penetrate much easier and deeper into the polymer matrix within a shorter time frame and thus shortens the diffusion distance of the drug [50]. Additionally, hydrophilic drugs such as fasudil favor water penetration into microspheres upon drug leaching leading to higher burst release and shorter release duration [40,50]. Further possibilities to reduce the extend of burst release would be the use of a polymer with a higher molecular weight or to add additives such as alginate or chitosan to the internal aqueous phase [51,52]. S microspheres showed the typical triphasic profile, which is controlled by drug diffusion within the polymer matrix and polymer erosion [53,54]. PLGA degrades by hydrolysis into its acidic monomers, lactic and glycolic acid, and thus, the surrounding medium in which fasudil is released acidifies [55,56]; however, the integrity of fasudil was not negatively affected. Therefore, PLGA is a suitable carrier for fasudil as it does not affect its chemical structure.

Through several downstream mediators, ROCK promotes the phosphorylation of the myosin light chain and thereby facilitates the assembly and formation of actin stress fibers and focal adhesions [3,57,58]. In addition, cells of the TM undergo a switch from a mesenchymal- to a myofibroblast-like phenotype during the progression of glaucoma disease [58]. Therefore, fibroblasts were included in this study, in addition to cultures of TM and SC cells, to analyze the biologic activity of fasudil released from microspheres. Cytochemical staining clearly showed that treatment with free or released fasudil resulted in a reduction of actin stress fibers in all three cell types. Due to individual phenotypes of the three cell types and the use of primary cells from different human donors with unknown previous diseases, the number and extent of the stress fibers varied between TM and SC cells and fibroblasts. However, all three cell types showed the same trend upon fasudil treatment. Our observations were similar to effects observed in ROCK inhibitor-treated cells found in literature [31,57,59,60]. It must be kept in mind that our experimental setup measuring cellular effects of released fasudil has some limitations, since cells were only treated with a fixed dose of previously released fasudil and were not incubated directly with fasudil loaded microspheres which would reflect more the in vivo conditions.

ROCK also regulates the cellular contractility by modulating the actomyosin contraction in the outflow tissues [3,57,58]. Increased contractility of TM and particularly of SC cells alters the outflow resistance in glaucoma [61]. The impact of free and released fasudil on the cellular contractility was investigated using a collagen gel contraction assay. Treatment with fasudil caused a decrease in contraction of the collagen gel of the embedded cell type. These observations suggest reduced cellular contractility or at least altered interactions between the embedded cells and the collagen when fasudil was applied. Effects similar to those observed in our study have been reported for TM cells and fibroblasts [38,62,63]. Similar to TM cells, SC cells have a smooth muscle-like morphology and are therefore also highly contractile [61,64]. The reduced contractility of SC cells in presence of fasudil should therefore be based on a similar mechanism as for TM cells.

The present microsphere formulation is intended to be injected into the vitreous body. During PLGA degradation, fasudil most likely distributes throughout the vitreous body. Small, hydrophilic molecules like fasudil are eliminated from the vitreous humor either by the anterior or posterior route [22]. It is known that hydrophilic drugs are drained predominantly via the anterior route to the trabecular meshwork. We developed an experimental setup to emulate the situation in the vitreous body and evaluate whether released fasudil disseminates freely within the vitreous humor without significant retention. In this vitreous body diffusion model, fasudil only affects the cells after successful diffusion through the vitreous humor. ECIS measurements were used to monitor the cell response with a time resolution of minutes. The general principle of ECIS is to cultivate adherent cells on gold-film electrodes which allows to measure the changes of the cellular impedance as a function of time. The impedance is determined by the cell type-specific architecture and by the tightness of cell–cell and cell–matrix contacts [65]. It can be measured in a very sensitive and non-invasive manner with high resolution [65]. Our ECIS data clearly demonstrate that fasudil successfully diffuses through the vitreous humor and is thus able to induce changes in cell junctions of TM cells located in a second compartment that is separated from vitreous by a permeable membrane. Despite the diffusion-related time delay through the vitreous humor, the final changes in cell junctions were comparable to those of cells directly treated with fasudil. Our results suggest that the decrease in impedance after treatment with a ROCK inhibitor is attributed to loss of actin stress fibers and focal adhesions. Bischoff et al. treated endothelial cells with the more potent ROCK inhibitor Y-27632 and found a similar impedance time course to those we observed for TM cells directly treated with fasudil [66]. The novelty of our setup is that it includes the diffusion of fasudil through vitreous humor before its cellular effect is monitored by ECIS. Another advantage is that by altering the composition of the gel matrix, the ability of molecules to diffuse through other tissues is assessable in a similar way. Finally, in this study, up to 16 samples were measured simultaneously, and further scaleup to high-throughput formats is easy to realize.

As already mentioned, the remaining fraction of released fasudil will most likely be eliminated via the retina. Besides their neuroprotective effects on retinal ganglion cells [19], ROCK inhibitors are under investigation for the treatment of several vitreoretinal diseases [67]. This could be very beneficial for some glaucoma patients because the prevalence of comorbid retinal disease is higher in patients with primary open-angle glaucoma (15.7%) [68]. For example, intravitreally injected fasudil reduced retinal hypoxia and RPE barrier breakdown in Goto Kakizaki type 2 diabetic rats [69]. Ni et al. investigating the effect of a ROCK inhibitor (Y-27632) on ARPE19 cells, observed increased proliferation and reduced apoptosis of RPE cells [70]. In our study, ARPE19 cells appeared unaffected by treatment with free and released fasudil. Therefore, we assume that intravitreal delivery of a ROCK inhibitor could have a doubly beneficial effect: both on TM and SC cells in the anterior chamber and on retinal cells in the posterior eye.

Regarding the in vivo applicability, a critical question must be raised—are PLGA microspheres a suitable depot for ROCK inhibitors? Subrizi et al. developed a simple equation to calculate the drug dose (D) of an ocular depot formulation necessary for a desired dosing interval (τ) [6]. The equation also takes the drug clearance (CL), bioavailability (F) and the desired steady-state concentration ($C_{ss,av}$) into account:

$$D = CC_{ss,av} \times CL \times (\tau/F), \tag{4}$$

This equation allows to predict whether a formulation is suitable as an intraocular delivery device. With regard to our formulation, we used the following parameters and inserted them into the equation: For steady-state concentration $C_{ss,av}$ of fasudil at the target site we assumed 25 µM since it is a widely used concentration in literature and well-tolerated by TM and SC cells [30,31]. The CL of hydrophilic and small molecules from the vitreous is 0.28 mL/h according to literature [6]. For the dosing interval τ, we assumed 30 days based on the mean release duration of fasudil from our microspheres. However, it should be mentioned that longer dosing intervals would be attractive to improve patient compliance. Finally, the bioavailability was considered to be 100% because after intravitreal injection, no tissue barriers must be overcome (F = 1.0). According to this calculation, a total amount of about 1.7 mg fasudil would be required for a 30 day dosing interval. Taking the encapsulation efficacy and the drug loading of the microspheres into account, about 460 mg of microspheres would have to be applied per dosing interval. This polymer amount would correspond to a final intraocular PLGA concentration of 115 mg/mL in humans (volume of human vitreous body: four milliliters [13]). The maximum tolerated concentration of PLGA in the rat vitreous was determined to be about 10 mg/mL [20], thus a total microsphere dose of 460 mg would most likely be too high for intraocular use. According to these considerations, a higher drug content of at least 42.5 µg/mg would be necessary for this application interval. Particularly, when longer dosing intervals are desired, a higher encapsulation efficiency is needed to keep the amount of polymer as low as possible. Because the technical options to increase the encapsulation efficacy of fasudil into PLGA microspheres in an aqueous environment are exhausted, other encapsulation strategies or the encapsulation of other ROCK inhibitors must be considered. The prodrug netarsudil, for example would bring two advantages: first, it is more lipophilic (log$P$ = 3.77 [45]) compared to fasudil, which would improve its encapsulation into the lipophilic PLGA matrix. Second, netarsudil is more potent compared to fasudil (netarsudil: K_i value $_{(ROCK2)}$ = 1 nM [60]; versus fasudil: K_i value $_{(ROCK2)}$ = 330 nM [71]). At least a significant portion of intravitreally released netarsudil will be metabolized to netarsudil–M1 by esterases present in the vitreous humor [72–74]. While the lipophilic netarsudil will most likely be eliminated from the vitreous via the posterior route across the retina, the active metabolite netarsudil–M1 (log$P$ = 1.19 [45]) will be eliminated via both pathways—the posterior and anterior route [13]. The extent of elimination across the retina depends largely on the localization of the formulation in the vitreous and poses therefore an adjusting screw to control the elimination pathway. In addition, netarsudil–M1 is a more potent ROCK inhibitor compared to netarsudil with a K_i value $_{(ROCK2)}$ of 0.2 nM [60], and therefore an even lower concentration will be necessary at the target site to achieve similar effects. We started with fasudil because it is available in sufficient quantities for this type of proof-of-concept study.

5. Conclusions

We successfully developed fasudil-loaded PLGA microspheres of different sizes. For one preparation we achieved a controllable sustained release behavior. The biologic activity of released fasudil was successfully demonstrated in several cell-based assays using TM and SC cells as well as fibroblasts. A finding of utmost importance was that the proposed intravitreal application route is feasible, since fasudil is able to overcome the barrier of the vitreous humor and subsequently elicit the desired cellular effect. Because ROCK inhibitors have positive concomitant effects on retinal cells, an intravitreal delivery system could have additional advantages, particularly for glaucoma patients with comorbid retinal diseases. Unfortunately, the encapsulation efficiency of fasudil into the microspheres was quite low, thereby limiting their in vivo applicability. Possibilities to address this issue are to prepare microspheres by altering the lactic to glycolic acid ratio, e.g., with the Resomer® RG 501 H (ratio 45:55). Moreover, spray-drying the microspheres in a nonaqueous system or the manufacture of microspheres using microfluidics could significantly improve the encapsulation efficiency [46]. A completely different approach could be the covalent attachment of fasudil to polyacid poly(L-glutamic acid) based layer-by-layer thin films [75]; or the use of lipid based implants manufactured by compression or extrusion [76,77]. Alternatively, a more lipophilic and potent ROCK inhibitor such as netarsudil could be used, which would be more easily encapsulated into lipophilic polymers such as PLGA and achieve similar efficacy with a lower dose. Our results suggest that intravitreal delivery of a ROCK inhibitor as a dual-purpose drug depot could significantly supplement and improve current glaucoma therapy.

Supplementary Materials: The following are available online at http://www.mdpi.com/1999-4923/12/8/706/s1, Figure S1: Fasudil at a concentration of 25 μM is well tolerated by HTM-N cells, TM cells, SC cells and fibroblasts.

Author Contributions: R.M., C.K. and F.F. are PhD candidates from the University of Regensburg. M.B., R.F. and J.W. are professors at the University of Regensburg and D.P. is a group leader at the University Hospital Regensburg. A.O. is a group leader at the Ludwig-Maximilians-University Munich and W.D.S. is professor at the Duke University. Conceptualization, M.B.; methodology, R.M., M.B., R.F., J.W.; validation, R.M. and C.K.; formal analysis, R.M. and C.K.; investigation, R.M., C.K. and D.P.; resources, M.B., R.F., D.P. and W.D.S.; data curation, R.M.; writing—original draft preparation, R.M.; writing—review and editing, M.B., R.M., R.F., J.W., D.P., W.D.S., A.O., C.K. and F.F.; visualization, R.M.; supervision, M.B. and R.F.; project administration, M.B. and R.M.; funding acquisition, M.B., R.F. and W.D.S. All authors have read and agreed to the published version of the manuscript.

Funding: This research was supported by Deutsche Forschungsgemeinschaft (DFG; Grant BR3566/3–1 and FU734/4–1) and by U.S. National Institutes of Health (Grant EY022359 and EY019696).

Acknowledgments: The authors thank Renate Liebl, Silvia Babl and Margit Schimmel for excellent technical support. The authors thank Katherine Fein for careful proofreading of the manuscript and Evelyn König for artwork.

Conflicts of Interest: The authors declare no conflicts of interest.

References

1. Garnock-Jones, K.P. Ripasudil: First global approval. *Drugs* **2014**, *74*, 2211–2215. [CrossRef] [PubMed]
2. Hoy, S.M. Netarsudil Ophthalmic Solution 0.02%: First Global Approval. *Drugs* **2018**, *78*, 389–396. [CrossRef] [PubMed]
3. Tanna, A.P.; Johnson, M. Rho Kinase Inhibitors as a Novel Treatment for Glaucoma and Ocular Hypertension. *Ophthalmology* **2018**, *125*, 1741–1756. [CrossRef] [PubMed]
4. Mietzner, R.; Breunig, M. Causative glaucoma treatment: Promising targets and delivery systems. *Drug Discov. Today* **2019**, *24*, 1606–1613. [CrossRef] [PubMed]
5. Janagam, D.R.; Wu, L.; Lowe, T.L. Nanoparticles for drug delivery to the anterior segment of the eye. *Adv. Drug Deliv. Rev.* **2017**, *122*, 31–64. [CrossRef] [PubMed]
6. Subrizi, A.; Del Amo, E.M.; Korzhikov-Vlakh, V.; Tennikova, T.; Ruponen, M.; Urtti, A. Design principles of ocular drug delivery systems: Importance of drug payload, release rate, and material properties. *Drug Discov. Today* **2019**, *24*, 1446–1457. [CrossRef]
7. Pita-Thomas, D.W.; Goldberg, J.L. Nanotechnology and glaucoma: Little particles for a big disease. *Curr. Opin. Ophthalmol.* **2013**, *24*, 130–135. [CrossRef]
8. Konstas, A.G.; Maskaleris, G.; Gratsonidis, S.; Sardelli, C. Compliance and viewpoint of glaucoma patients in Greece. *Eye (Lond.)* **2000**, *14*, 752–756. [CrossRef]
9. Szigiato, A.-A.; Podbielski, D.W.; Ahmed, I.I.K. Sustained drug delivery for the management of glaucoma. *Expert Rev. Ophthalmol.* **2017**, *12*, 173–186. [CrossRef]
10. Shirley, M. Bimatoprost Implant: First Approval. *Drugs Aging* **2020**, *37*, 457–462. [CrossRef]
11. Seal, J.R.; Robinson, M.R.; Burke, J.; Bejanian, M.; Coote, M.; Attar, M. Intracameral Sustained-Release Bimatoprost Implant Delivers Bimatoprost to Target Tissues with Reduced Drug Exposure to Off-Target Tissues. *J. Ocul. Pharmacol. Ther.* **2019**, *35*, 50–57. [CrossRef] [PubMed]
12. Li, S.K.; Hao, J.; Liu, H.; Lee, J.H. MRI study of subconjunctival and intravitreal injections. *J. Pharm. Sci.* **2012**, *101*, 2353–2363. [CrossRef] [PubMed]
13. Del Amo, E.M.; Rimpela, A.K.; Heikkinen, E.; Kari, O.K.; Ramsay, E.; Lajunen, T.; Schmitt, M.; Pelkonen, L.; Bhattacharya, M.; Richardson, D.; et al. Pharmacokinetic aspects of retinal drug delivery. *Prog. Retin. Eye Res.* **2017**, *57*, 134–185. [CrossRef] [PubMed]
14. Rimpela, A.K.; Kiiski, I.; Deng, F.; Kidron, H.; Urtti, A. Pharmacokinetic Simulations of Intravitreal Biologicals: Aspects of Drug Delivery to the Posterior and Anterior Segments. *Pharmaceutics* **2018**, *11*, 9. [CrossRef]
15. Lau, C.M.L.; Yu, Y.; Jahanmir, G.; Chau, Y. Controlled release technology for anti-angiogenesis treatment of posterior eye diseases: Current status and challenges. *Adv. Drug Deliv. Rev.* **2018**, *126*, 145–161. [CrossRef]
16. Kaji, H.; Nagai, N.; Nishizawa, M.; Abe, T. Drug delivery devices for retinal diseases. *Adv. Drug Deliv. Rev.* **2018**, *128*, 148–157. [CrossRef]

17. Glendenning, A.; Crews, K.; Sturdivant, J.; deLong, M.A.; Kopczynski, C.; Lin, C.W. Sustained Release, Biodegradable PEA Implants for Intravitreal Delivery of the ROCK/PKC Inhibitor AR-13503. *Investig. Ophthalmol. Vis. Sci.* **2018**, *59*, 5672.
18. Del Amo, E.M.; Urtti, A. Rabbit as an animal model for intravitreal pharmacokinetics: Clinical predictability and quality of the published data. *Exp. Eye Res.* **2015**, *137*, 111–124. [CrossRef]
19. Akaiwa, K.; Namekata, K.; Azuchi, Y.; Sano, H.; Guo, X.; Kimura, A.; Harada, C.; Mitamura, Y.; Harada, T. Topical Ripasudil Suppresses Retinal Ganglion Cell Death in a Mouse Model of Normal Tension Glaucoma. *Investig. Ophthalmol. Vis. Sci.* **2018**, *59*, 2080–2089. [CrossRef]
20. Zhao, M.; Rodriguez-Villagra, E.; Kowalczuk, L.; Le Normand, M.; Berdugo, M.; Levy-Boukris, R.; El Zaoui, I.; Kaufmann, B.; Gurny, R.; Bravo-Osuna, I.; et al. Tolerance of high and low amounts of PLGA microspheres loaded with mineralocorticoid receptor antagonist in retinal target site. *J. Control. Release* **2017**, *266*, 187–197. [CrossRef]
21. Chen, W.; Palazzo, A.; Hennink, W.E.; Kok, R.J. Effect of Particle Size on Drug Loading and Release Kinetics of Gefitinib-Loaded PLGA Microspheres. *Mol. Pharm.* **2017**, *14*, 459–467. [CrossRef] [PubMed]
22. Braunger, B.M.; Fuchshofer, R.; Tamm, E.R. The aqueous humor outflow pathways in glaucoma: A unifying concept of disease mechanisms and causative treatment. *Eur. J. Pharm. Biopharm.* **2015**, *95*, 173–181. [CrossRef] [PubMed]
23. Cardillo, J.A.; Souza-Filho, A.A.; Oliveira, A.G. Intravitreal Bioerudivel sustained-release triamcinolone microspheres system (RETAAC). Preliminary report of its potential usefulnes for the treatment of diabetic macular edema. *Arch. Soc. Esp. Oftalmol.* **2006**, *81*, 675–677, 679–681. [PubMed]
24. Xu, Q.; Crossley, A.; Czernuszka, J. Preparation and characterization of negatively charged poly(lactic-co-glycolic acid) microspheres. *J. Pharm. Sci.* **2009**, *98*, 2377–2389. [CrossRef]
25. Ramazani, F.; Chen, W.; Van Nostrum, C.F.; Storm, G.; Kiessling, F.; Lammers, T.; Hennink, W.E.; Kok, R.J. Formulation and characterization of microspheres loaded with imatinib for sustained delivery. *Int. J. Pharm.* **2015**, *482*, 123–130. [CrossRef] [PubMed]
26. Keller, K.E.; Bhattacharya, S.K.; Borras, T.; Brunner, T.M.; Chansangpetch, S.; Clark, A.F.; Dismuke, W.M.; Du, Y.; Elliott, M.H.; Ethier, C.R.; et al. Consensus recommendations for trabecular meshwork cell isolation, characterization and culture. *Exp. Eye Res.* **2018**, *171*, 164–173. [CrossRef]
27. Stamer, W.D.; Roberts, B.C.; Howell, D.N.; Epstein, D.L. Isolation, culture, and characterization of endothelial cells from Schlemm's canal. *Investig. Ophthalmol. Vis. Sci.* **1998**, *39*, 1804–1812.
28. Pang, I.H.; Shade, D.L.; Clark, A.F.; Steely, H.T.; DeSantis, L. Preliminary characterization of a transformed cell strain derived from human trabecular meshwork. *Curr. Eye Res.* **1994**, *13*, 51–63. [CrossRef]
29. Tripathi, R.C.; Millard, C.B.; Tripathi, B.J. Protein composition of human aqueous humor: SDS-PAGE analysis of surgical and post-mortem samples. *Exp. Eye Res.* **1989**, *48*, 117–130. [CrossRef]
30. Pitha, I.; Oglesby, E.; Chow, A.; Kimball, E.; Pease, M.E.; Schaub, J.; Quigley, H. Rho-Kinase Inhibition Reduces Myofibroblast Differentiation and Proliferation of Scleral Fibroblasts Induced by Transforming Growth Factor beta and Experimental Glaucoma. *Transl. Vis. Sci. Technol.* **2018**, *7*, 6. [CrossRef]
31. Kaneko, Y.; Ohta, M.; Inoue, T.; Mizuno, K.; Isobe, T.; Tanabe, S.; Tanihara, H. Effects of K-115 (Ripasudil), a novel ROCK inhibitor, on trabecular meshwork and Schlemm's canal endothelial cells. *Sci. Rep.* **2016**, *6*, 19640. [CrossRef] [PubMed]
32. Su, S.; Chen, J. Collagen Gel Contraction Assay, 2015. Protocol Exchange Website. Available online: https://protocolexchange.researchsquare.com/article/nprot-4169/v1 (accessed on 24 July 2000).
33. Schneider, C.A.; Rasband, W.S.; Eliceiri, K.W. NIH Image to ImageJ: 25 years of image analysis. *Nat. Methods* **2012**, *9*, 671–675. [CrossRef]
34. Wang, S.K.; Chang, R.T. An emerging treatment option for glaucoma: Rho kinase inhibitors. *Clin. Ophthalmol.* **2014**, *8*, 883–890. [CrossRef] [PubMed]
35. Tsuno, A.; Nasu, K.; Kawano, Y.; Yuge, A.; Li, H.; Abe, W.; Narahara, H. Fasudil inhibits the proliferation and contractility and induces cell cycle arrest and apoptosis of human endometriotic stromal cells: A promising agent for the treatment of endometriosis. *J. Clin. Endocrinol. Metab.* **2011**, *96*, E1944–E1952. [CrossRef] [PubMed]
36. Junglas, B.; Kuespert, S.; Seleem, A.A.; Struller, T.; Ullmann, S.; Bosl, M.; Bosserhoff, A.; Kostler, J.; Wagner, R.; Tamm, E.R.; et al. Connective tissue growth factor causes glaucoma by modifying the actin cytoskeleton of the trabecular meshwork. *Am. J. Pathol.* **2012**, *180*, 2386–2403. [CrossRef] [PubMed]

37. Sperber, M.; Hupf, C.; Lemberger, M.-M.; Goricnik, B.; Hinterreiter, N.; Lukic, S.; Oberleitner, M.; Stolwijk, J.A.; Wegener, J. Monitoring the Impact of Nanomaterials on Animal Cells by Impedance Analysis: A Noninvasive, Label-Free, and Multimodal Approach. In *Measuring Biological Impacts of Nanomaterials*; Wegener, J., Ed.; Springer International Publishing: Cham, Switzerland, 2015; pp. 45–108.
38. Ramachandran, C.; Patil, R.V.; Combrink, K.; Sharif, N.A.; Srinivas, S.P. Rho-Rho kinase pathway in the actomyosin contraction and cell-matrix adhesion in immortalized human trabecular meshwork cells. *Mol. Vis.* **2011**, *17*, 1877–1890.
39. Stein, S.; Auel, T.; Kempin, W.; Bogdahn, M.; Weitschies, W.; Seidlitz, A. Influence of the test method on in vitro drug release from intravitreal model implants containing dexamethasone or fluorescein sodium in poly (d,l-lactide-*co*-glycolide) or polycaprolactone. *Eur. J. Pharm. Biopharm.* **2018**, *127*, 270–278. [CrossRef]
40. Han, F.Y.; Thurecht, K.J.; Whittaker, A.K.; Smith, M.T. Bioerodable PLGA-Based Microparticles for Producing Sustained-Release Drug Formulations and Strategies for Improving Drug Loading. *Front. Pharmacol.* **2016**, *7*, 185. [CrossRef]
41. Ravi, S.; Peh, K.K.; Darwis, Y.; Murthy, B.K.; Singh, T.R.; Mallikarjun, C. Development and characterization of polymeric microspheres for controlled release protein loaded drug delivery system. *Indian J. Pharm. Sci.* **2008**, *70*, 303–309. [CrossRef] [PubMed]
42. Nafea, E.H.; El-Massik, M.A.; El-Khordagui, L.K.; Marei, M.K.; Khalafallah, N.M. Alendronate PLGA microspheres with high loading efficiency for dental applications. *J. Microencapsul.* **2007**, *24*, 525–538. [CrossRef]
43. Emami, J.; Hamishehkar, H.; Najafabadi, A.R.; Gilani, K.; Minaiyan, M.; Mahdavi, H.; Mirzadeh, H.; Fakhari, A.; Nokhodchi, A. Particle size design of PLGA microspheres for potential pulmonary drug delivery using response surface methodology. *J. Microencapsul.* **2009**, *26*, 1–8. [CrossRef] [PubMed]
44. Thackaberry, E.A.; Farman, C.; Zhong, F.; Lorget, F.; Staflin, K.; Cercillieux, A.; Miller, P.E.; Schuetz, C.; Chang, D.; Famili, A.; et al. Evaluation of the Toxicity of Intravitreally Injected PLGA Microspheres and Rods in Monkeys and Rabbits: Effects of Depot Size on Inflammatory Response. *Investig. Ophthalmol. Vis. Sci.* **2017**, *58*, 4274–4285. [CrossRef] [PubMed]
45. Tetko, I.V.; Gasteiger, J.; Todeschini, R.; Mauri, A.; Livingstone, D.; Ertl, P.; Palyulin, V.A.; Radchenko, E.V.; Zefirov, N.S.; Makarenko, A.S.; et al. Virtual computational chemistry laboratory–design and description. *J. Comput. Aided Mol. Des.* **2005**, *19*, 453–463. [CrossRef] [PubMed]
46. Ramazani, F.; Chen, W.; van Nostrum, C.F.; Storm, G.; Kiessling, F.; Lammers, T.; Hennink, W.E.; Kok, R.J. Strategies for encapsulation of small hydrophilic and amphiphilic drugs in PLGA microspheres: State-of-the-art and challenges. *Int. J. Pharm* **2016**, *499*, 358–367. [CrossRef] [PubMed]
47. Gupta, N.; Ibrahim, H.M.; Ahsan, F. Peptide-micelle hybrids containing fasudil for targeted delivery to the pulmonary arteries and arterioles to treat pulmonary arterial hypertension. *J. Pharm. Sci.* **2014**, *103*, 3743–3753. [CrossRef] [PubMed]
48. Gupta, V.; Gupta, N.; Shaik, I.H.; Mehvar, R.; McMurtry, I.F.; Oka, M.; Nozik-Grayck, E.; Komatsu, M.; Ahsan, F. Liposomal fasudil, a rho-kinase inhibitor, for prolonged pulmonary preferential vasodilation in pulmonary arterial hypertension. *J. Control. Release* **2013**, *167*, 189–199. [CrossRef]
49. Rosca, I.D.; Watari, F.; Uo, M. Microparticle formation and its mechanism in single and double emulsion solvent evaporation. *J. Control. Release* **2004**, *99*, 271–280. [CrossRef]
50. Mao, S.; Xu, J.; Cai, C.; Germershaus, O.; Schaper, A.; Kissel, T. Effect of WOW process parameters on morphology and burst release of FITC-dextran loaded PLGA microspheres. *Int. J. Pharm* **2007**, *334*, 137–148. [CrossRef]
51. Jaraswekin, S.; Prakongpan, S.; Bodmeier, R. Effect of poly(lactide-co-glycolide) molecular weight on the release of dexamethasone sodium phosphate from microparticles. *J. Microencapsul.* **2007**, *24*, 117–128. [CrossRef]
52. Zheng, C.; Liang, W. A one-step modified method to reduce the burst initial release from PLGA microspheres. *Drug Deliv.* **2010**, *17*, 77–82. [CrossRef]
53. Kimura, H.; Ogura, Y.; Moritera, T.; Honda, Y.; Tabata, Y.; Ikada, Y. In vitro phagocytosis of polylactide microspheres by retinal pigment epithelial cells and intracellular drug release. *Curr. Eye Res.* **1994**, *13*, 353–360. [CrossRef] [PubMed]

54. Fredenberg, S.; Wahlgren, M.; Reslow, M.; Axelsson, A. The mechanisms of drug release in poly(lactic-co-glycolic acid)-based drug delivery systems—A review. *Int. J. Pharm.* **2011**, *415*, 34–52. [CrossRef] [PubMed]
55. Shameem, M.; Lee, H.; DeLuca, P.P. A short term (accelerated release) approach to evaluate peptide release from PLGA depot-formulations. *AAPS PharmSciTech* **1999**, *1*, E7. [CrossRef] [PubMed]
56. Fu, K.; Pack, D.W.; Klibanov, A.M.; Langer, R. Visual evidence of acidic environment within degrading poly(lactic-co-glycolic acid) (PLGA) microspheres. *Pharm. Res.* **2000**, *17*, 100–106. [CrossRef] [PubMed]
57. Liu, W.T.; Zhang, Y.Y.; Ye, W.; Lu, Z.Z. Effects of fasudil on the cytoskeleton of trabecular meshwork cells and outflow facility in bovine eyes. *Int. J. Clin. Exp. Med.* **2017**, *10*, 2326–2335.
58. Rao, P.V.; Pattabiraman, P.P.; Kopczynski, C. Role of the Rho GTPase/Rho kinase signaling pathway in pathogenesis and treatment of glaucoma: Bench to bedside research. *Exp. Eye Res.* **2017**, *158*, 23–32. [CrossRef]
59. Honjo, M.; Tanihara, H.; Inatani, M.; Kido, N.; Sawamura, T.; Yue, B.Y.; Narumiya, S.; Honda, Y. Effects of rho-associated protein kinase inhibitor Y-27632 on intraocular pressure and outflow facility. *Investig. Ophthalmol. Vis. Sci.* **2001**, *42*, 137–144.
60. Lin, C.W.; Sherman, B.; Moore, L.A.; Laethem, C.L.; Lu, D.W.; Pattabiraman, P.P.; Rao, P.V.; deLong, M.A.; Kopczynski, C.C. Discovery and Preclinical Development of Netarsudil, a Novel Ocular Hypotensive Agent for the Treatment of Glaucoma. *J. Ocul. Pharmacol. Ther.* **2018**, *34*, 40–51. [CrossRef]
61. Stamer, W.D.; Braakman, S.T.; Zhou, E.H.; Ethier, C.R.; Fredberg, J.J.; Overby, D.R.; Johnson, M. Biomechanics of Schlemm's canal endothelium and intraocular pressure reduction. *Prog. Retin. Eye Res.* **2015**, *44*, 86–98. [CrossRef]
62. Koga, T.; Koga, T.; Awai, M.; Tsutsui, J.; Yue, B.Y.; Tanihara, H. Rho-associated protein kinase inhibitor, Y-27632, induces alterations in adhesion, contraction and motility in cultured human trabecular meshwork cells. *Exp. Eye Res.* **2006**, *82*, 362–370. [CrossRef]
63. Honjo, M.; Tanihara, H.; Kameda, T.; Kawaji, T.; Yoshimura, N.; Araie, M. Potential role of Rho-associated protein kinase inhibitor Y-27632 in glaucoma filtration surgery. *Investig. Ophthalmol. Vis. Sci.* **2007**, *48*, 5549–5557. [CrossRef]
64. Stamer, W.D.; Clark, A.F. The many faces of the trabecular meshwork cell. *Exp. Eye Res.* **2017**, *158*, 112–123. [CrossRef] [PubMed]
65. Lukic, S.; Wegener, J. Impedimetric Monitoring of Cell-Based Assays. 2015. Available online: https://onlinelibrary.wiley.com/doi/abs/10.1002/9780470015902.a0025710 (accessed on 24 July 2000).
66. Bischoff, I.; Hornburger, M.C.; Mayer, B.A.; Beyerle, A.; Wegener, J.; Furst, R. Pitfalls in assessing microvascular endothelial barrier function: Impedance-based devices versus the classic macromolecular tracer assay. *Sci. Rep.* **2016**, *6*, 23671. [CrossRef] [PubMed]
67. Yamaguchi, M.; Nakao, S.; Arima, M.; Wada, I.; Kaizu, Y.; Hao, F.; Yoshida, S.; Sonoda, K.H. Rho-Kinase/ROCK as a Potential Drug Target for Vitreoretinal Diseases. *J. Ophthalmol.* **2017**, *2017*, 8543592. [CrossRef] [PubMed]
68. Griffith, J.F.; Goldberg, J.L. Prevalence of comorbid retinal disease in patients with glaucoma at an academic medical center. *Clin. Ophthalmol.* **2015**, *9*, 1275–1284. [CrossRef]
69. Rothschild, P.R.; Salah, S.; Berdugo, M.; Gelize, E.; Delaunay, K.; Naud, M.C.; Klein, C.; Moulin, A.; Savoldelli, M.; Bergin, C.; et al. ROCK-1 mediates diabetes-induced retinal pigment epithelial and endothelial cell blebbing: Contribution to diabetic retinopathy. *Sci. Rep.* **2017**, *7*, 8834. [CrossRef]
70. Ni, Y.; Qin, Y.; Fang, Z.; Zhang, Z. ROCK Inhibitor Y-27632 Promotes Human Retinal Pigment Epithelium Survival by Altering Cellular Biomechanical Properties. *Curr. Mol. Med.* **2017**, *17*, 637–646. [CrossRef]
71. Ono-Saito, N.; Niki, I.; Hidaka, H. H-series protein kinase inhibitors and potential clinical applications. *Pharmacol. Ther.* **1999**, *82*, 123–131. [CrossRef]
72. Luaces-Rodriguez, A.; Gonzalez-Barcia, M.; Blanco-Teijeiro, M.J.; Gil-Martinez, M.; Gonzalez, F.; Gomez-Ulla, F.; Lamas, M.J.; Otero-Espinar, F.J.; Fernandez-Ferreiro, A. Review of Intraocular Pharmacokinetics of Anti-Infectives Commonly Used in the Treatment of Infectious Endophthalmitis. *Pharmaceutics* **2018**, *10*, 66. [CrossRef]
73. Attar, M.; Shen, J.; Kim, M.; Radojicic, Q.-C. Cross-Species and Cross-Age Comparison of Esterase Mediated Metabolism in Vitreous Humor: Human versus Rabbit, Dog and Monkey. *Investig. Ophthalmol. Vis. Sci.* **2013**, *54*, 5404.

74. Heikkinen, E.M.; Del Amo, E.M.; Ranta, V.P.; Urtti, A.; Vellonen, K.S.; Ruponen, M. Esterase activity in porcine and albino rabbit ocular tissues. *Eur. J. Pharm. Sci.* **2018**, *123*, 106–110. [CrossRef]
75. Hsu, B.B.; Park, M.H.; Hagerman, S.R.; Hammond, P.T. Multimonth controlled small molecule release from biodegradable thin films. *Proc. Natl. Acad. Sci. USA* **2014**, *111*, 12175–12180. [CrossRef] [PubMed]
76. Kreye, F.; Siepmann, F.; Siepmann, J. Drug release mechanisms of compressed lipid implants. *Int. J. Pharm* **2011**, *404*, 27–35. [CrossRef] [PubMed]
77. Sax, G.; Kessler, B.; Wolf, E.; Winter, G. In-vivo biodegradation of extruded lipid implants in rabbits. *J. Control. Release* **2012**, *163*, 195–202. [CrossRef] [PubMed]

Pharmaceutics 2020, 12, 703
pharmaceutics
MDPI

Review

Intravitreal Dexamethasone Implant as a Sustained Release Drug Delivery Device for the Treatment of Ocular Diseases: A Comprehensive Review of the Literature

Claudio Iovino [1,*,†], Rodolfo Mastropasqua [2,†], Marco Lupidi [3,4,5,†], Daniela Bacherini [6,†], Marco Pellegrini [7,†], Federico Bernabei [7,†], Enrico Borrelli [8,†], Riccardo Sacconi [8,†], Adriano Carnevali [9,†], Rossella D'Aloisio [10,†], Alessio Cerquaglia [3,†], Lucia Finocchio [6,11,†], Andrea Govetto [12,13,†], Stefano Erba [12,†], Giacinto Triolo [12,†], Antonio Di Zazzo [14,†], Matteo Forlini [15,†], Aldo Vagge [16,†] and Giuseppe Giannaccare [9,†]

1 Department of Surgical Sciences, Eye Clinic, University of Cagliari, 09124 Cagliari, Italy
2 Institute of Ophthalmology, University of Modena and Reggio Emilia, 41121 Modena, Italy; rodolfo.mastropasqua@unimore.it
3 Department of Surgical and Biomedical Sciences, Section of Ophthalmology, University of Perugia, S. Maria della Misericordia Hospital, 06129 Perugia, Italy; marco.lupidi@ospedale.perugia.it (M.L.); alessio.cerquaglia@studenti.unipg.it (A.C.)
4 Fondazione per la Macula Onlus, DINOMGI., University Eye Clinic, 16132 Genova, Italy
5 Centre de l'Odéon, 113 Boulevard St Germain, 75006 Paris, France
6 Department of Neurosciences, Psychology, Drug Research and Child Health, Eye Clinic, University of Florence, AOU Careggi, 50139 Florence, Italy; d.bacherini@unifi.it (D.B.); luciafinocchio@gmail.com (L.F.)
7 Ophthalmology Unit, S. Orsola-Malpighi University Hospital, University of Bologna, 40138 Bologna, Italy; marco.pellegrini9@studio.unibo.it (M.P.); federico.bernabei2@studio.unibo.it (F.B.)
8 Department of Ophthalmology, Hospital San Raffaele, University Vita Salute San Raffaele, 20132 Milan, Italy; enrico.borrelli@hsr.it (E.B.); sacconi.riccardo@hsr.it (R.S.)
9 Department of Ophthalmology, University "Magna Graecia", 88100 Catanzaro, Italy; adrianocarnevali@unicz.it (A.C.); giuseppe.giannaccare@unicz.it (G.G.)
10 Department of Medicine and Science of Ageing, Ophthalmology Clinic, University "G. d'Annunzio" Chieti-Pescara, 66100 Chieti, Italy; rossella.daloisio@unich.it
11 Moorfields Eye Hospital NHS Foundation Trust, London EC1V2PD, UK
12 Fatebenefratelli-Oftalmico Hospital, ASST-Fatebenefratelli-Sacco, 63631 Milan, Italy; andrea.govetto@UHBristol.nhs.uk (A.G.); stefano.erba@asst-fbf-sacco.it (S.E.); giacinto.triolo@asst-fbf-sacco.it (G.T.)
13 Bristol Eye Hospital, University Hospitals Bristol NHS Foundation Trust, Bristol BS12LX, UK
14 Ophthalmology Complex Operative Unit, Campus Bio Medico University Hospital, 00128, Rome, Italy; a.dizazzo@unicampus.it
15 Domus Nova Hospital, 48121 Ravenna, Italy; matteo.forlini@iss.sm
16 University Eye Clinic, DINOGMI, Polyclinic Hospital San Martino IRCCS, 16132 Genoa, Italy; aldo.vagge@unige.it
* Correspondence: claudioiovino88@gmail.com; Tel.: +39-070-609-2319
† Member of the Young Ophthalmologists Reviews Study Group (YORSG).

Received: 15 June 2020; Accepted: 22 July 2020; Published: 26 July 2020

Abstract: Drug delivery into the vitreous chamber remains a great challenge in the pharmaceutical industry due to the complex anatomy and physiology of the eye. Intravitreal injection is the mainstream route of drug administration to the posterior segment of the eye. The purpose of this review is to assess the current literature about the widening use of the intravitreal 0.7 mg dexamethasone (Dex) implant, and to provide a comprehensive collection of all the ocular disorders that benefit from Dex administration. Although anti-vascular endothelial growth-factors (VEGFs) have been largely indicated as a first-choice level, the Dex implant represents an important treatment option, especially in selected cases, such as vitrectomized eyes or patients in whom anti-VEGF failed or are contraindicated. In this article, the safety profile as well as the list of the possible complications related to intravitreal Dex injection are also discussed.

Keywords: corticosteroids; drug delivery systems; intravitreal dexamethasone implant; intravitreal injections; Ozurdex

1. Introduction

Intravitreal injection is nowadays considered the best accepted means of delivering drugs directly to the retina and choroid [1]. However, it is difficult to achieve and maintain significant levels of drugs into the vitreous cavity, and frequent injections are often needed.

The sustained-release of intravitreal 0.7 mg dexamethasone (Dex) implant (Ozurdex®, Allergan Pharmaceuticals, Irvine, CA, USA) with a biodegradable capsule of lactic acid and glycolytic acid polymers has been shown to overcome this drawback, being effective for 3–6 months [2,3].

As a corticosteroid, intravitreal Dex has been shown to suppress inflammation by inhibiting multiple inflammatory cytokines, resulting in decreased capillary leakage and the migration of inflammatory cells, edema, and fibrin deposition [4]. The United States (US) Food and Drug Administration (FDA) approved Ozurdex for the treatment of macular edema (ME), related to the following diseases: central or branch retinal vein occlusion (CRVO or BRVO, 2009), non-infectious posterior uveitis (NIU, 2010) and diabetic retinopathy (DR, 2014) [4].

To date, published reviews, articles and collected literature data about the approved use of Dex implant confirm its efficacy [4–6]. Nevertheless, in recent years several additional studies further confirmed the potential benefits of intravitreal Dex for various ocular pathologies with inflammatory etiopathogenesis and ME (Figure 1).

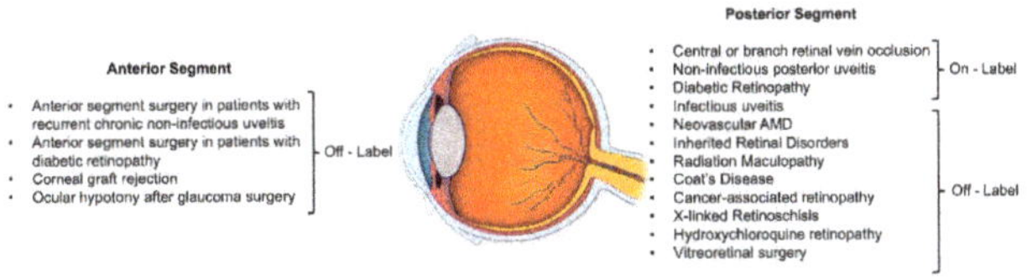

Figure 1. Ocular disorders that can benefit from Intravitreal Dexamethasone Injection.

The purpose of this review is to assess the current literature about the widening use of Dex implant, and to further provide a comprehensive collection of all the ocular disorders that benefit from Dex administration. The safety profile and the list of the possible complications related to intravitreal Ozurdex injection are also discussed.

2. Methods

PubMed databases from January 2009 to March 2020 were searched by using the terms "dexamethasone intravitreal implant" and "Ozurdex". Studies were limited to the English language. Registered randomized controlled studies (RCTs), prospective and retrospective, randomized and nonrandomized, single center and multicenter studies, case series and case reports were included. Anatomical and functional outcomes, as well as complications, were analyzed and discussed.

3. Dex Implant Mechanism of Action and Pharmacokinetic

Drug distribution in the posterior segment of the eye is a crucial step in the treatment of ocular pathologies. Dex implant contains micronized, preservative-free Dex 0.7 mg in a biodegradable copolymer of polylactic-co-glycolic acid that releases active ingredients within the vitreous chamber for up to 6 months [7]. Corticosteroids have multiple levels of action, modifying tight junction integrity, inhibiting different molecules involved in inflammation and vascular permeability process, such as Intercellular adhesion molecule-1 (ICAM-1), interleukin-6, stroma-derived factor-1, as well as vascular endothelial growth-factor (VEGF). Intravitreal Dex also targets prostaglandins and leukotrienes production blocking phospholipase A2 and paracellular permeability of Muller cells by downregulating aquaporin 4 levels [7]. A decrease of 30% in some vasoactive proteins (persephin, pentraxin 3, hepatocyte growth factor, insulin-like growth factor binding proteins, endocrine gland-VEGF) has been reported after Dex implant [7].

Dex concentrations in the retina and vitreous humor reach a plateau within days of administration and are maintained at high levels for 2 months before declining over subsequent months. A dual-phase pharmacokinetic has been described, related to the fragmentation of the implant [8]. From days 7 to 60, high concentrations of Dex in the vitreous were detected in monkeys' eyes, whereas at days 90 to 180, Dex release was sustained at low concentrations. From days 210 to 270, Dex was below the limit of quantification [8]. Although the study was conducted in monkey eyes, the steady state concentrations of Dex achieved in monkeys are expected to be similar to those in humans [8]. Indeed, the biphasic pharmacokinetic profile resembles that obtained with the systemic pulse administration of corticosteroids and is consistent with the sustained duration of action of DEX implant seen in clinical studies. Of note, the time-point of the evaluation of Dex efficacy can account for differences in terms of functional and anatomical outcomes influencing the interpretation of the findings from different studies. Considering the Ozurdex efficacy profile, a scheduled visit at the end of the first phase is recommended to eventually consider the need for a second implant. The pharmacokinetics of 0.7 mg Ozurdex is similar in non-vitrectomized and vitrectomized eyes [9].

4. Dex Implant in Retinal Vein Occlusion

4.1. Pathogenesis of Retinal Vein Occlusion and Inflammation

Retinal vein occlusion (RVO) has been identified as the second main cause of vision loss in the working age population, following DR [10]. The known risk factors include systemic hypertension, diabetes mellitus (DM), smoking, hyperlipidemia, systemic vascular diseases, hypercoagulable states and ocular hypertension [10]. Two different types of RVO are described based on the site of occlusion: CRVO with a prevalence of 0.1–0.4% and BRVO with a prevalence of 0.6–1.1% [10].

Two main mechanisms are involved in RVO pathophysiology: (i) inner blood-retina barrier breakdown due to venous pressure rise, which is a consequence of mechanical/ischemic damage; (ii) pro-inflammatory cytokine dysregulation with consequent increase in vascular permeability and capillary network impairment [11].

Several inflammatory molecules have been identified to play an important role in the RVO pathogenesis. ICAM-1, P-selectin and E-selectin are involved in leukocyte recruitment and their adhesion to retinal blood vessel surface [10]. Moreover, high levels of VEGF and ICAM-1 in the vitreous cavity have been associated with ischemic CRVO, suggesting their role in the pathogenesis of the disease [10].

Intraretinal exudation of fluid, lipids and blood contribute to vision-threatening ME, which is a common complication of both BRVO and CRVO [12,13].

Over the years, several treatments have been proposed for ME secondary to RVO, including grid laser photocoagulation, pars plana vitrectomy (PPV), intravitreal anti-VEGF and systemic and intravitreal corticosteroids [12]. The rationale of using anti-inflammatory therapies, such as intravitreal Dex, is supported by the pathophysiology of the disease, as described above [14]. Being a water-soluble biodegradable corticosteroid with anti-inflammatory properties, Ozurdex is able to inhibit VEGF, prostaglandin and inflammatory molecule synthesis [15].

4.2. Evidence of the Efficacy of Dex Implant in RVO

Despite the proven efficacy of anti-VEGF in RVO resolution [16], some patients do not improve at all (20%) or even worsen (6.9%), probably due to the high variability of VEGF levels strictly related to retinal ischemia grade [17,18].

Ozurdex was approved in June 2009 by the US FDA for ME secondary to RVO, based on a phase III sham-controlled study with 6-month follow-up [19]. The GENEVA trial highlighted its beneficial effects in the treatment of 1267 patients suffering from BRVO or CVRO. In detail, 30% of patients enrolled achieved a gain of at least 15 letters visual acuity (VA) during the first 6 months of the trial compared to sham. The mean decrease in central macular thickness (CMT) was significantly higher after Dex implant as well, compared to the sham group. The GENEVA trial was extended in an open-label manner at 6 further months and, although a second implant was performed, the safety and tolerability profiles were preserved [14]. Comparable results were shown in Chinese population, where Ozurdex determined a significant improvement of functional and anatomical parameters in both BRVO and CRVO in comparison to sham [20].

Based on data collected from GENEVA trial, Danis et al. found a significant negative linear correlation between changes in CMT and in VA, with the greatest VA improvement in eyes that achieved and maintained CMT decrease at 90 and 180 days after Dex implant [21].

The SOLO study was the first multicenter trial evaluating functional and anatomical findings in patients with RVO after a unique Dex implantation with a 6-month follow-up in a real life clinical setting [22].

Early re-treatment (before 6 months) was suggested since the peak of functional and anatomical efficacy were seen at 8 weeks, with a progressive reduction in efficacy in the subsequent period. Specifically, the mean time-point of reinjection was 17.50 ± 4.20 weeks and 17.68 ± 4.20 weeks in BRVO and CRVO, respectively. Of note, in the first two months, BRVO and CRVO showed a different response to treatment with better outcomes in the BRVO group, probably related to the natural progression of the disease, which is more favorable than CRVO [22].

The onset and duration of VA improvement after Ozurdex implant in eyes with RVO have been further investigated in another study [23]. The authors reported a peak of clinical activity at 60 days (starting at 7 days), that began to decrease at 3 months [23].

A prompt treatment with intravitreal Dex in patients with RVO is associated with better clinical outcomes [24,25]. Longer ME duration at the time of first treatment was associated with significantly lower likelihood of achieving a VA gain (15 letters or more) and CMT reduction (200 micron or more) at 6-month follow-up, particularly in BRVO [25].

Ferrini et al. reported an immediate effect of the Dex implant at 24 h after the injection, while the mean time of edema relapse was identified as approximately 4.6 months [24].

In a real world setting multicenter open-label phase IV clinical study in the US (SHASTA STUDY, 26 sites, n = 289) patients were treated with two or more Ozurdex injections for ME secondary to RVO [26]. The mean time between two consecutive Dex implants was 5.6 months and multiple treatments demonstrated high durability and safety. A similar significant reduction in CMT was obtained between re-treatments and, as expected, intraocular pressure (IOP) increased more frequently in patients with a known history of IOP response to steroid treatment [26].

These results suggest that an accurate patient anamnesis is mandatory before starting the corticosteroid treatment. Similarly, Querques et al. reported a mean interval time of re-treatment of 4.7 ± 1.1 months and 5.1 ± 1.5 months after the first and the second implant, respectively [27].

Interestingly, the correlation between clinical improvements and angiographic findings in patients receiving intravitreal Dex for RVO, was also investigated [28]. Changes in macular leakage correlated significantly with CMT decrease in both BRVO and CRVO patients. Moreover, the proportion of eyes with active neovascularization increased from baseline to day 180 in the sham group, but remained unchanged in subjects receiving Dex injections [28].

As known, anti-VEGF agents are considered as first line treatment in eyes with RVO, although the number of injections is definitely higher and sometimes patients may not show a good clinical response [18,29].

Two multicenter RCTs investigated the efficacy and safety at 6 months of intravitreal Dex versus Ranibizumab (Rzb) 0.5 mg for the treatment of CRVO (COMRADE C study) [30] and BRVO (COMRADE B) [31].

Patients treated with Rzb showed a higher VA gain and a lower degree of retinal ischemia at 6 months [30,31]. Moreover, the results from the 1 year COMBRADE extension study provided an additional 6 months of data, revealing that BRVO and CRVO had a better response to continuous Rzb treatment in comparison to Dex in terms of VA, and this was true especially for BRVO form [32]. However, all the aforementioned studies had an important limitation because patients in the Ozurdex group were not re-treated during the 6-month follow-up [30–32]. As previously mentioned, Ozurdex effect peaks at 3 months and re-injection should be considered earlier than 6 months. Therefore, adopting a Dex Pro Re Nata (PRN) regimen may have provided a more robust comparison between the two treatments groups.

In a real-life study, the authors reported a significant improvement in VA with a significant reduction in CMT from baseline to week six after Dex treatment in both BRVO and CRVO [33]. Enrolled subjects were divided into three subgroups, based on ME duration. At week 12, the mean change was +9.5 Early Treatment Diabetic Retinoapthy Study (ETDRS) letters in patients with ME duration <90 days, +7.3 letters in those with ME duration between 90 and 180 days and +5.4 letters in those with ME duration >180 days. Furthermore, a very good tolerability of Dex treatment was detected in 84% of patients, while a moderate tolerability in 6% [33].

These data further support the evidence that a prompt treatment with Ozurdex in patients with RVO is associated with better clinical outcomes [24,25,33,34]. This is valid also for patients unsuccessfully treated with Rzb and aflibercept and switched to DEX [35].

A 12-month multicenter RCT (COMO study) compared anti-VEGF with multiple Dex injections in BRVO [36]. In brief, a mean of 2.5 Ozurdex injections and 8.0 Rzb injections were performed during the 12-month follow-up. The authors demonstrated that intravitreal Dex effect could be maintained only if a retreatment was performed at 4–5 months after the first implant. The use of Ozurdex was associated with an increased risk of IOP elevation and cataract progression, but a lower injection burden, compared to Rzb [36].

Of note, Kumar et al. compared the efficacy and safety of four different injection therapeutic schemes: three monthly Rzb injections (Group 1); combination of one intravitreal Rzb + laser photocoagulation (Group 2); Dex implant (Group 3); combination of one Dex implant + laser photocoagulation (Group 4) [37].

Improvements in the BCVA and CMT were comparable initially in all groups, but Rzb alone (Group 1) showed significantly higher BCVA gains at 6 months. No additional advantage of the combination with laser photocoagulation was found in both Rzb and Dex treatments [37].

In the RANIDEX study, Rzb and Dex implant were found to be both safe and effective at the 12-month follow-up in patients with ME, secondary to CRVO, with no statistically significant differences in VA and CMT changes [38].

Similar results were reported by Gado et al., who showed no significant differences at 6 months in terms of VA and CMT in patients with CRVO receiving either Ozurdex implant or bevacizumab [39].

5. Dex Implant in Posterior Non-Infectious Uveitis

5.1. *Pathogenesis of Posterior Non-Infectious Uveitis*

Posterior NIUs include a wide range of inflammatory conditions, affecting the uveal tissue. ME is a common complication and represents one of the leading causes of vision loss among patients affected by NIUs and its prevalence varies depending on the diagnostic technique and the underlying cause, ranging from 20% to 70% [40]. The treatment of NIUs and associated ME is still very challenging. Since inflammation is the main pathogenic event in these disorders, corticosteroids, either systemic or regional, represent the mainstay of treatment [5]. Although effective, the use of systemic corticosteroids is limited due to numerous adverse effects [41]. Intravitreal drug delivery allows us to obtain rapid and high concentrations of the drug into the eye, with a lower incidence of drug related systemic adverse events [42].

5.2. Evidence of the Efficacy of Dex in Posterior Non-Infectious Uveitis

Several studies showed the efficacy of Ozurdex in controlling inflammation in NIUs. The HURON trial initially investigated the safety and efficacy of a single Dex injection for the treatment of NIUs, showing a significant improvement of vitreous inflammation and VA, persisting for up to 6 months [2]. Throughout the 26-week study, the percentage of eyes in the 0.7-mg Dex implant group requiring IOP-lowering medications was 23% or less, but none needed surgical intervention for glaucoma [2].

Lightman and coauthors further confirmed the benefits of a single Dex implant in patients with NIUs for up to 6 months, reporting a significant BCVA improvement [43].

Dex implant has been proven effective and well tolerated in patients with persistent ME, resulting from uveitis or Irvine–Gass syndrome, producing significant improvements in VA and fluorescein leakage at 3 months [44].

A shorter duration of Dex implant of approximately 3 to 4 months was reported by Myung et al., albeit only four consecutive patients were included in their retrospective study [45].

A significant increase in VA and decrease in CMT and vitreous haze (VH) were observed in patients with NIUs treated with Ozurdex and followed up for at least 1 year [46]. In this study multiple injections yielded comparable visual and anatomical outcomes to single injections, and mean IOP did not change significantly during follow-up [46]. The efficacy and safety of repeated DEX implants in patients with NIUs were further confirmed by several studies, with a median duration of therapeutic effect of 6 months and a transient rise in mean IOP always well managed by topical medication [46–49].

Recent evidence suggests that Intravitreal Dex has a better safety profile and a slightly longer-lasting effect than intravitreal triamcinolone acetonide (TA) [50,51].

Of note, in a multicenter RCT it has been shown that both intravitreal TA and intravitreal Dex implants were superior to periocular TA for treating uveitic ME [52]. The risk of IOP elevation was mild and did not differ significantly between the two intravitreal treatments [52].

Significant improvements in mean CMT and VA were reported in eyes with well-controlled NIUs and persistent ME [53–55]. Of note, due to good clinical response, some patients reduced the daily systemic corticosteroid dosage [55]. A significant systemic corticosteroid sparing effect of the Ozurdex implant was further highlighted by Fabiani and coauthors, who reported a prompt resolution of the ME and vasculitis without any safety issue [56].

Ratra et al., investigated the role of Dex in nonresponsive ME secondary to chronic NIUs in adults and children, reporting a significant VA improvement and a good safety profile [57]. Moreover, a single injection of Ozurdex was safe and effective, as an additional treatment to systemic immunomodulatory drugs, in the treatment of refractory Behcet posterior uveitis for a 6-month period [58,59]. In a recent retrospective study, 20 patients with ocular sarcoidosis were successfully treated with intravitreal Dex injection, and only 35% of them required a second injection during the follow-up period (median 16.5 months) [60].

Ozurdex constitutes an efficacious treatment option against uveitic ME in eyes that received pars plana vitrectomy (PPV) as well, and it appears to have similar dissolution rates in vitrectomized and non-vitrectomized eyes [61]. The latter showed higher IOP increase following Dex implant than vitrectomized eyes, showing the need for close IOP monitoring [61]. Nevertheless, Dex efficacy has also been proven in challenging cases, as in a patient with NIU tamponated with silicon oil after PPV [62], and in eight patients with chronic NIU and uveitic glaucoma successfully treated with a combined surgery of Ozurdex + Ahmed drainage device [63].

Worthy of note, the Dex implant has been additionally noted to be safe and efficacious in the management of pediatric NIUs, where repeated implantations resulted in continuous control of the inflammation, allowing for the reduction in systemic immunosuppression with few systemic complications [64,65].

In 16 eyes of patients with recalcitrant Juvenile idiopathic arthritis-associated active uveitis (mean age of 17 ± 6.7), the injection of sustained-release Dex achieved the control of anterior inflammation and the resolution of ME [66].

However, further data are required to establish the safety profile of the implant in the pediatric age group [67].

DEX implant showed promising results in controlling disease activity and progression in a group of inflammatory disorders named as white dot syndromes responsible for NUI [68–72]. The main outcomes of these studies are summarized in Table 1.

Table 1. Characteristics of studies evaluating efficacy and safety of DEX implant in White Dot Syndrome.

Author (Year)	Design	Condition	Eyes (*n*)	DEX Injections (Time Interval Range)	Follow up (Months)	Main Outcomes	Complications
Miserocchi et al. (2017) [68]	Retrospective case series	Serpiginous Choroiditis	8	Single (5 eyes), Repeated (3 eyes; 5–8 months)	18	Stabilization of serpiginous lesions, Decrease in systemic corticosteroids	Transient IOP increase (3 eyes), Cataract progression (2 eyes)
Mora-Cantallops et al. (2019) [72]	Case report	Acute Posterior Multifocal Placoid Pigment Epitheliopathy	1	Single	6	Stabilization of inflammatory lesions, Increased BCVA	Transient IOP increase
Barnes et al. (2018) [71]	Retrospective case series	Acute Zonal Occult Outer Retinopathy	6	Single	14–63	Stabilization of inflammatory lesions, Increased BCVA	Transient IOP increase, Cataract progression
Walsh et al. (2017) [69]	Retrospective case series	Birdshot Chorioretinopathy	6	Single (2 eyes), Repeated (4 eyes; 4–6 months)	12–36	Stabilization of inflammatory lesions, Reduced macular edema, Increased BCVA	IOP increase (2 eyes)
Bajwa et al. (2018) [70]	Retrospective case series	Birdshot Chorioretinopathy	6	Single (2 eyes), Repeated (4 eyes; 4–6 months)	12–36	Stabilization of the disease (2 eyes), Increased BCVA	IOP increase (2 eyes), Cataract progression (3 eyes)

DEX: Dexamethasone intravitreal implant, IOP: Intraocular pressure, BCVA: Best corrected visual acuity.

Moreover, in two cases of bilateral idiopathic retinal vasculitis–aneurysms–neuroretinitis syndrome, the Dex implant was successfully employed to control ME in addition to panretinal photocoagulation (PRP), systemic corticosteroids, and PPV [73]; or in addition to PRP and systemic aziathioprine [74].

6. Dex Implant in Diabetic Retinopathy

6.1. Pathogenesis of Diabetic Macular Edema and Inflammation

DR represents the leading cause of visual loss and blindness in adults of working age in developed countries [75]. Central visual loss in patients affected by DR can be related to both ME and macular ischemia, with an estimated prevalence of around 20% [76].

Hyperglycemia is certainly a major cause of early microvascular changes in diabetes, causing endothelial dysfunction and the breakdown of the blood–retinal barrier.

Albeit VEGF-mediated pathways play a crucial role in DR and diabetic macular edema (DME) pathogenesis, DME shows typical features of local, low-grade chronic inflammation. Elevated levels of inflammatory markers have been detected in vitreous samples drawn from DME patients [4]. The setting of a localized, chronic and self-perpetuating inflammation is the key point of the pathogenesis of DME.

Anti-VEGF agents represent the first-line therapy for DME patients, on account of their safety and clear efficacy [77]. Nevertheless, there are patients in whom anti-VEGF drugs are contraindicated (e.g., pregnancy, high cardiovascular risk) or have demonstrated poor efficacy in improving visual function and reducing DME [78]. Therefore, intravitreal steroids, especially a sustained-release device, such as the Ozurdex implant, play a central role in the treatment of DME.

6.2. Evidence of the Efficacy of Dex in Diabetic Macular Edema

The Diabetic Retinopathy Clinical Research Network (DRCR.net) Protocol I study, evaluating intravitreal TA or Rzb in combination with laser treatment, demonstrated similar efficacy of both drugs in pseudophakic eyes [76]. Nevertheless, Dex has higher anti-inflammatory potency than TA and less side effects because of its higher aqueous solubility and lower lipophilicity, ensuring, therefore, a poor impact on trabecular meshwork and lens tissues [78]. The safety and efficacy of the Dex implant have been evaluated in two large, multicenter Phase III RCTs and the 3-year results of both trials were reported in the MEAD study [76,79,80]. VA improvement and macular volume reduction over the 3-year evaluation were significant with both 0.7 mg and 0.35 mg Dex (vs. sham procedure). Moreover, treatment with Ozurdex slowed the progression of DR, delaying by approximately 12 months the onset of two-step progression in Diabetic Retinopathy Disease Severity Score [79].

The safety profile of Dex implant resulted in a better safety profile compared to other intraocular steroids. In the Dex implant groups the IOP increase was usually transient, and no significant IOP changes were present after 3 years, without any cumulative effect due to repeated implants [80]. Additionally, there were no differences between the Dex arms and sham in systemic serious adverse events [80].

A subgroup analysis of the MEAD study revealed that Dex implant 0.7 mg was effective in improving VA and anatomical outcomes in the eyes of previously treated patients (with laser, anti-VEGF, TA or a combination) with a similar safety profile as compared to the overall study population [81].

Mastropasqua et al., evaluated morphological and functional changes, by means of optical coherence tomography (OCT), microperimetry and electrophysiology, in patients with DME treated with the Ozurdex implant over a follow-up of 12 months [82]. VA, macular sensitivity and central retinal thickness (CRT) substantially improved 1 month after Dex implant administration and persisted for up to 5 months. Nevertheless, there were no improvements in electro-functional parameters, which remained stable after DEX implant for up to 4 months [82].

A similar finding was reported in a short-scale prospective, multicenter, randomized study comparing the efficacy of a single Dex implant versus Dex implant, followed by retreatment on the PRN regimen over a 6-month follow-up period [83].

Lo Giudice et al., investigated the very early effect of Ozurdex implant in patients with DME [84]. More than 30% of the maximal reduction in CRT was already achieved within 3 h after injection and more than 60% within 3 days. BCVA followed at a slower rate the CRT reduction, improving significantly 7 days after treatment [84].

Interestingly, Dex implant was demonstrated to be effective even in improving other functional aspects, such as color vision. The analysis of both red-green (RG) and yellow-blue (YB) color thresholds variation after Dex implant was performed in 14 patients with DME [85]. Twenty-four weeks after injection, the RG threshold improved significantly, while YB ones remained substantially unchanged after treatment. The authors hypothesized that the DEX implant may have a direct neurotrophic effect on the retina, promoting the assessment of chromatic sensitivity as an important biomarker for monitoring DR evolution and treatment response.

Several trials were conducted in order to directly compare Ozurdex with anti-VEGFs in terms of efficacy and safety in the setting of DME [6]. In the BEVORDEX study, 42 eyes were randomized to receive bevacizumab every 4 weeks and 46 eyes were randomized to receive a Dex implant every 16 weeks in a PRN treatment regimen [86]. Patients treated with Ozurdex showed better anatomical outcomes with fewer injections (2.7 vs. 8.6). Nevertheless, these data did not translate to better VA outcomes (1% of Dex implant eyes lost 10 letters or more—mostly because of cataracts—whereas none of the 42 bevacizumab eyes did). Both drugs were able to induce a considerable regression of macular hard exudates without a statistically significant difference at 12 and 24 months between groups, albeit exudates regression seemed to be faster in Dex-treated eyes [87].

The patient-centered effectiveness of treatment, evaluated in 48 patients with the Impact of Vision Impairment Questionnaire at baseline and 24 months after, was similar in both groups ($p > 0.1$) [88]. Moreover, a post-hoc analysis of the trial highlighted how the mean retreatment interval was more than double in Dex arm compared with bevacizumab-treated eyes [89].

Ozurdex has been demonstrated to be non-inferior even to Rzb in the treatment of DME [6]. In a randomized, multicenter 12-month study, Dex implant administered every 5 months induced similar changes in VA, CRT and leakage reduction on FA when compared to Rzb [90].

Favorable results have also been reported with Dex implant in patients non-responsive to anti-VEFG or in vitrectomized eyes with DME [91–94].

In a real-world setting, eyes with DME considered refractory to anti-VEGF therapy after three monthly injections, which were switched to Dex implant, had better visual and anatomical outcomes at 12 months than those that continued treatment with anti-VEGF therapy [92,94]. In a study including 55 vitrectomized eyes, Ozurdex was found to be significantly effective in reducing CRT and vascular leakage and in improving BCVA [94].

Several trials have been conducted in order to determine if Dex implant used in combination with anti-VEGF or laser treatment could increase the anatomical and functional outcomes in persistent DME [95,96]. When compared to laser treatment alone, a significantly higher percentage of patients treated with Dex implant 1 month before laser treatment achieved at least a 10-letter improvement in VA from baseline at week 1 and at months 1 and 9 ($p < 0.007$) [95]. The CRT reduction was significantly higher in the combination group than in the laser group, and the combination treatment was well tolerated. Nevertheless, this difference was no more significant at 12 months.

Dex implant did not allow for the achievement of better visual outcomes at 12 months when compared to bevacizumab in monotherapy, whereas CRT significantly decreased in the combination group compared to the bevacizumab group [96].

Similar results have been reported for the combination therapy of Dex implant with Rzb [97]. General limitations of these trials were the confounding effect due to the lens status, which influenced the evaluation of final functional outcomes [96,97].

The rationale for combination therapy with Dex implant and anti-VEGFs has been recently strengthened by a small-size study determining the effect of both drug classes on aqueous humour cytokine expression [98]. Even though there were high inter-individual differences in cytokine concentrations in both treatment groups, monthly Rzb seemed to have a long-acting impact on VEGF and placental growth-factor levels, whereas Ozurdex showed a fast-acting action on other soluble inflammatory mediators [98].

7. Dex Implant in Neovascular Age-Related Macular Degeneration

Evidence of the Efficacy of Dex in Age-Related Macular Degeneration

Age-related macular degeneration (AMD) may be complicated by the proliferation of different types of macular neovascularization. The presence of an exudative neovascular lesion characterizes the exudative or neovascular form of AMD [99,100]. Although antiangiogenic therapy is considered the gold standard of treatment for exudative neovascular AMD, previous reports have also employed corticosteroids in the treatment of these patients [101–107]. The use of corticosteroids is based on the assumption that inflammation is known to play a major role in the AMD pathogenesis [103,108].

A combined therapy (Dex + Rzb) may lead to an overall reduction in required Rzb injections [101,104]. Rezar-Dreindl and colleagues investigated 40 eyes with recurrent or persistent neovascular AMD [104]. Included subjects were divided into two subgroups: the first group received intravitreal Rzb with a PRN treatment regimen, while the second group received a combination of intravitreal Dex implant and Rzb. Patients receiving the combo therapy required less Rzb retreatments with consistent functional outcomes.

Conversely, Chaundhary and coauthors reported no significant advantages from the combination therapy of Dex + Rzb vs. Rzb alone [103].

The role of the Ozurdex implant was further investigated in patients with neovascular AMD resistant to anti-VEFG [105]. The authors showed significant improvements in patients receiving a single Dex injection combined with Rzb or aflibercept if compared to anti-VEGF alone [105]. These findings suggest a potential role of corticosteroids in the treatment of selected cases of neovascular AMD.

8. Dex Implant in Inherited Retinal Disorders

Evidence of the Efficacy of Dex in Inherited Retinal Disorders

The use of Dex implant in patients affected by an inherited retinal disorder is usually limited to patients affected by CME secondary to retinitis pigmentosa (RP). Cystoid macular edema (CME) is a relatively common complication of RP, developing in about 20% of patients [109,110]. Table 2 summarizes characteristics and main outcomes of case reports or small series evaluating the efficacy and safety of DEX implant in RP [111–115].

Table 2. Characteristics of retrospective studies evaluating efficacy and safety of DEX implant in Retinitis Pigmentosa.

Author (Year)	Design	Clinical Condition	Eyes (*n*)	DEX Injection	Follow up (Months)	Main Outcomes	Complications
Srour (2013) [111]	Retrospective case series	ME in RP	4	Single (2 eyes), Repeated (2 eyes, after 3 months)	6	Improved BCVA, Reduced CFT	None
Ahn (2014) [112]	Case report	ME in RP	2	Single	6	Improved BCVA, Reduced CFT	None
Ornek (2016) [113]	Case report	ME in RP	2	Single	6	Improved BCVA, Resolution of ME	None
Saatci (2013) [114]	Case report	ME in RP	2	Repeated after 3 months	7	Improved BCVA, Reduced CFT	None
Mansour (2018) [115]	Retrospective case series	ME in RP	45	Repeated (range 2–14 months)	Variable (15.5 ± 13.0)	Improved BCVA, Reduced CFT	Transient IOP elevation in 20 eyes, Cataract in 7 eyes

BCVA: Best corrected visual acuity, CFT: central foveal thickness, IOP: Intraocular pressure, ME: macular edema, RP: retinitis Pigmentosa.

Additionally, a couple of studies tried to elucidate the role of Dex implant in the treatment of CME secondary to RP [115,116]. Mansour et al., analyzed the outcomes of 45 eyes (34 patients) affected by CME secondary to RP treated with Ozurdex with a mean follow-up of 15.5 months [115]. The authors found that VA improved up to 4 months after the Dex implant in about 50% of cases.

Park et al., conducted a randomized, noncontrolled, paired-eye, single crossover clinical trial in which one eye of RP patients with bilateral CME was treated by Dex implant while the fellow eye was observed [116]. The authors treated 14 patients for 12 months and reported that Ozurdex could reduce the CME secondary to RP, but repeated injections were required in order to maintain the anatomical and functional results. In agreement with these results, Veritti and coauthors demonstrated that the Ozurdex implant produced better anatomic and functional outcomes in comparison to oral acetazolamide in patients affected by CME secondary to RP [117].

Based on these findings, intravitreal Dex implant seems to be a promising therapeutic option in patients with RP and CME. However, further prospective RCTs are warranted.

9. Dex Implant in Other Conditions

Evidence of the Efficacy of Dex in Other Conditions

The intravitreal DEX implant has been successfully employed in patients with infectious uveitis, though the presence of intraocular infection represents a formal contraindication (Table 3) [118–123].

Table 3. Characteristics of studies evaluating the efficacy and safety of DEX implant in Infectious Uveitis.

Author (Year)	Design	Etiology	Eyes (*n*)	DEX Injections	Follow up (Months)	Main Outcomes	Complications
Fonollosa (2016) [118]	Retrospective case series	Herpes simplex virus-type 1, Varicella-Zoster virus, Treponema Pallidum, Brucella Mellitensis, Borrelia Burgdorferi, Toxoplasma Gondii, Cytomegalovirus	8	Repeated (except 2 eyes)	6–31	Resolved ME, Improved BCVA, No reactivation of infectious disease	Transient IOP increase (1 eye)
Agarwal (2018) [119]	Retrospective case series	Mycobacterium tuberculosis	19	Single	3–4	Decreased ME, vitritis and progression of choroiditis lesions	Transient IOP increase (4 eyes), Cataract progression (2 eyes)
Jain (2018) [120]	Retrospective case series	Mycobacterium tuberculosis	9	Repeated	6–24	Stabilization of inflammatory lesions, Increased BCVA	IOP increase (2 eyes)
Lautredou (2018) [121]	Case report	Treponema pallidum and HIV	1	Repeated	15	Resolved ME, Improved BCVA	None
Majumder (2019) [122]	Case report	Treponema pallidum and HIV	1	Repeated	4	Resolved ME, Improved BCVA	Transient IOP increase
Majumder (2016) [123]	Retrospective case series	Herpes Virus	4	Repeated	6–24	Resolved ME, Improved BCVA, No reactivation of retinitis	None

DEX: Dexamethasone intravitreal implant, IOP: Intraocular pressure, BCVA: Best corrected visual acuity, HIV: Human immunodeficiency virus.

Table 4. Characteristics of studies evaluating efficacy and safety of DEX implant in miscellaneous conditions.

Author (Year)	Design	Clinical Condition	Eyes (*n*)	DEX Injection	Follow up (Months)	Main Outcomes	Complications
Frizziero (2017) [125]	Retrospective case series	Radiation Maculopathy following Iodine-125 brachytherapy	13	Single	6	Improved BCVA, Reduced CFT	None
Russo (2018) [126]	Retrospective case series	Radiation Maculopathy following plaque brachytherapy	8	Repeated	22	Improved BCVA, Reduced CFT	None
Seibel (2016) [124]	Retrospective case series	Radiation Maculopathy following proton beam therapy	5	Single	1	Stable BCVA in 80% of patients, Reduced CFT	None
Arrigo (2020) [127]	Case report	Combined CRVO and branch retinal artery occlusion	1	Single	24	Recovery of BCVA, Resolution of ME	None
Oztrurk (2015) [128]	Case report	Combined CRVO and branch retinal artery occlusion	1	Single	6	Improved BCVA, Resolution of ME	None
Fenicia (2013) [129]	Case report	CRAO associated with Waldenström's macroglobulinemia	1	Single	6	Resolution of ME	None
Georgakopoulos (2019) [130]	Case report	Bilateral CRAO associated with ImmunoglobulinA multiple myeloma	2	Single	9	Improved BCVA, Resolution of ME	None
Nuzzi (2017) [131]	Case report	Anterior Ischemic Optic Neuropathy	1	Single	1	Improved BCVA and visual field	None
Saatci (2018) [132]	Case report	Coats' disease	2	Single + Photocoagulation	50	Improved BCVA, Resolution of ME	None
Kumar (2019) [133]	Case report	Coats' disease	1	Single + Photocoagulation	4	Improved BCVA, Resolution of ME	None
Cebeci (2014) [134]	Case report	Coats' disease associated with vasoproliferative retinal tumor	1	Single + Photodynamic Therapy	12	Improved BCVA, Resolution of exudation	Subcapsular cataract
Kong (2019) [135]	Retrospective case series	Hypotony	15	Repeated	27	Increased intraocular pressure	Vitreous hemorrhage
Ahn (2018) [136]	Case report	Hydroxychloroquine Retinopathy	1	Single	2	Improvement of ME	None
Kim (2019) [137]	Case report	Cancer-associated retinopathy	2	Repeated (every 4 months)	48	Preservation of foveal photoreceptors	None
Mukhtar (2017) [138]	Case report	Subretinal fluid associated with X-linked retinoschisis	2	Single	6	Resolution of subretinal fluid	None
Bulut (2016) [139]	Case report	Accidental Foveal Photocoagulation by Alexandrite Laser	1	Single	3	Recovery of BCVA, Resolution of ME	Transient IOP elevation

BCVA: Best corrected visual acuity, CFT: central foveal thickness, CRAO: central retinal vein occlusion, DEX: Dexamethasone intravitreal implant, IOP: Intraocular pressure, ME: macular edema.

Intravitreal Dex should not be advocated as a primary treatment option in patients with infectious uveitis, however it could represent a useful and minimally invasive therapeutic resource in carefully selected cases. It can be considered a valuable adjunctive treatment, especially for patients presenting contraindication for systemic corticosteroids or requiring supplemental anti-inflammatory therapy. Several case reports and case series reported the use of the Dex implant in the management of various ocular disorders for which, at the present time, the device is not formally approved. Table 4 summarizes the characteristics and main outcomes of studies evaluating the efficacy and safety of the DEX implant in miscellaneous conditions [124–139].

10. Dex Implant in Ocular Surgery

10.1. Evidence of the Efficacy of Dex in Anterior Segment Surgery

Diabetic patients have an increased and independent risk of developing post-cataract ME, even after uncomplicated surgeries [140]. Ozurdex, combined with phacoemulsification in patients with cataract and DME, showed beneficial functional and anatomical effects for at least 3 months after surgery [141,142]. Additionally, intraoperative Dex implants performed at the time of surgery achieved the same long-term outcomes compared to a 1-month injection deferral in treating eyes with pre-existing DME [140].

Patients with NIUs have an increased risk for complications following eye surgery. These include a severe inflammatory response and unpredictably volatile postoperative IOP (ocular hypertension or hypotony).

Dex implant safely and effectively controlled postoperative inflammation in eyes with chronic recurrent NIU when concurrently implanted during anterior segment surgery, including cataract extraction or intraocular lens explantation [143]. The Ozurdex implant was also proven to be safe and effective in preventing and managing the postoperative inflammation in children with juvenile idiopathic arthritis-associated uveitic cataract [144]. Another possible application in the field of anterior segment surgery is related to immunological rejection occurring after keratoplasty. In fact, the Ozurdex implant has been shown to be an effective treatment option thanks to its potency and sustained therapeutic levels, even in cases of refractory to the standard topical and systemic therapy [145,146]. This option could be especially useful in patients with poor compliance to topical treatment, or with contraindications for the systemic therapy.

10.2. Evidence of the Efficacy of Dex in Vitreoretinal Surgery

Many of the pathologies requiring vitreoretinal (VR) surgery are accompanied by pro-inflammatory responses, which may result in vascular CME [147]. Retinal surgery itself may further enhance such inflammatory reactions, which may worsen or facilitate the onset of CME [148]. The use of Ozurdex as adjuvant to PPV may be useful, due to its long-lasting biological activity. This aspect may represent an advantage of Ozurdex over anti-VEGF agents, whose half-life is significantly reduced in a vitrectomized eye. Different reports have explored the safety and efficacy of Ozurdex as adjuvant to PPV in distinct retinal pathologies with a special focus on DR, rhegmatogenous and tractional retinal detachment (RD) and epiretinal membrane (ERM) [149–154].

Cakir et al., showed a prompt anatomical response to Dex implant over the first three months after PPV for CME associated with ERM [153]. With regard to surgical technique, the implant may be introduced through the same trocars used to perform PPV, at the end of the surgery. However, a 23-G trocar may be preferred as an injection through a 25-G trocar was shown to produce shattering with possible damage to the implant [155].

It may also be preferable to inject the implant when the eye is filled with balanced saline solution (BSS) rather than air, to avoid possible retinal trauma due to the implant's kinetic energy. If needed—i.e., in the case of RD repair—fluid-air exchange may be performed after this procedure [155].

One of the main issues when using Ozurdex as adjuvant to vitrectomy is a possible rise in IOP in the postoperative period. PPV has already been shown as an independent risk factor for the new-onset of open-angle glaucoma after surgery [156,157], and the use of Ozurdex may further boost such a risk. However, this hypothesis is speculative as there is no clear evidence on this matter in the published literature.

Surgical intervention with PPV may be required in the case of proliferative DR accompanied by vitreous hemorrhage, due to neovascularization, the presence of proliferative fibrovascular complexes causing tractional RD or a combination of these factors. PPV may be indicated even in the presence of tractional CME, normally associated with tractional ERMs or vitreomacular traction (VMT).

Kim et al., found the use of Ozurdex as adjuvant to PPV particularly effective in case of tractional CME if compared to the vascular subtype [152]. In such cases, the net benefit of Ozurdex is controversial, as the action of PPV alone may be sufficient to resolve tractional CME [148]. However, a purely tractional aetiology is rare in DME and often tractional and exudative components may overlap [148].

Comparable results were obtained by Pang et al., in a retrospective report analyzing functional and anatomical outcomes of an intraoperative Dex implant during PPV for DR [158]. Moreover, Jung and Lee found PPV plus internal limiting membrane peeling and the Dex implant to be effective in improving vision and reducing retinal thickness in eyes with persistent DME [154].

ERMs may be associated with CME, whose origin can be either tractional, exudative, or a combination of both [148]. In such contexts, the anti-inflammatory action of Ozurdex may be synergic with the mechanical release of tractional forces achieved with PPV.

Iovino et al., reported favorable anatomical and functional outcomes of the Dex implant as adjuvant to PPV in advanced stage ERMs with CME [150]. In this study, both visual recovery and reduction in macular thickness were higher in the Ozurdex-treated cohort up to 6 months after surgery, if compared to the non-Ozurdex treated control group. Similar results were illustrated by Hostovsky in a separate report [151].

Worthy of note, microcystoid ME does not respond to steroids as the pathophysiology of this condition is not inflammatory [159]. Further, as this entity may be found in eyes with advanced glaucoma, the use of Ozurdex may be contraindicated due to the risk of further increase in the IOP.

The use of the Dex implant in complex rhegmatogeneous and tractional RD associated with proliferative vitreoretinopathy (PVR) was explored by a few reports, and its use is controversial, as no consensus has been reached [149,160]. Based on the hypothesis that PVR pathophysiology is mainly inflammatory, steroids such as TA or Dex have been considered promising as prophylaxis and/or treatment options [147].

A prospective, RCT analyzing 140 patients undergoing PPV for PVR detachments did not find any difference in the postoperative anatomical and functional outcome between eyes with or without Ozurdex as adjuvant to PPV [149]. However, a reduction in CME rate was observed in eyes treated with Ozurdex. Conversely, Iglicki et al., described favorable outcomes in eyes with diabetic tractional RD treated with PPV and Ozurdex [160]. CME can complicate the postoperative recovery of RD repair with either PPV or scleral buckling (SB). Risk factors for postoperative CME in vitrectomized eyes include a greater number of surgeries, higher rates of PVR, and higher rates of retinectomies [161]. Few reports confirmed the efficacy of Ozurdex in post-surgery CME in patients receiving PPV [162], and SB surgeries [163].

11. Safety Profile of Dex Implant

Although IOP increase and cataract progression are known side effects of Ozurdex implant, some other less common events have been reported following the injection of this intravitreal drug. Hereafter, we summarize the safety profile and list the possible complications related to intravitreal Dex affecting either the anterior or the posterior segment of the eye and the adnexa.

11.1. Dex Implant and IOP

Dex, fluocinolone acetonide, and TA have been shown to activate different patterns of gene expression in human trabecular meshwork cell lines [164]. However, Dex differs from TA in pharmacologic activity, lipid solubility and delivery requirements. It is less lipophilic and does not accumulate to the same extent in the trabecular meshwork, with a lower risk of IOP increase [164]. Most commonly, the IOP increase after Ozurdex injection is typically noticed within the first 2 weeks, peaks roughly at day 60 and starts decreasing gradually to get to pre-injection values usually within 180 days [165]. No cumulative effect in IOP rise is reported, and no correlation is observed between glaucoma progression and number of DEX implants [165]. IOP rises greater than 10 mmHg were detected in 24–27% of the patients enrolled in the MEAD study and were managed with IOP-lowering medications [80]. During the follow-up period, only 1 patient needed filtration surgery to control the IOP.

On the other hand, the ARTES study group reported IOP values higher than 25 mmHg and 35 mmHg in 7.9% and 0.9% of the eyes with the Dex implant, respectively [166]. Again, all these cases were managed with anti-glaucoma medications, without the need of filtering surgery. Noticeably, glaucoma patients seem to be at higher risk of IOP spikes following Dex implant, supposedly because of an already impaired trabecular meshwork aqueous outflow before the Ozurdex injection. Nevertheless, the concomitant presence of glaucoma itself is not an absolute contraindication to Dex implant [167].

Similarly, previous history of IOP spikes after Dex implantation is a risk factor for future IOP rises following further injections. Therefore, patients with previous diagnoses of glaucoma or steroid-response after a Dex implant, need to be monitored more closely to detect IOP spikes [167]. Other significant risk factors for IOP increase after Dex implant were identified in young age, male sex, type I DM, with a previous history of uveitis or RVO [165]. Additionally, Latin American and South Asian ethnicities showed greater IOP rises as compared to Caucasians [168].

Of note, the temporary elevation of IOP after Dex implantation managed with IOP-lowering agents did not seem to cause a significant reduction in retinal nerve fiber layer (RNFL) thickness, measured by OCT [169,170].

11.2. Dex Implant and Anterior Segment Complications

The migration of the Dex implant into the anterior chamber (AC) was not described in multicenter clinical trials, such as the MEAD study [80], whereas it was documented in real life case series [171,172]. The major risk factors related to the AC migration are previous cataract extraction or PPV, reduced zonular or capsular bag integrity secondary to complicated cataract surgery, aphakia, sulcus intraocular lenses (IOLs), iris- or scleral-fixated IOLs and AC IOLs [171,172]. All these conditions create a communication between the posterior and the anterior segment of the eye facilitating the migration of the implant from the vitreous cavity to the AC. Corneal edema and endothelial damage due to mechanical and chemical toxicity may result from the AC migration of the Dex implant [171,172]. Urgent removal of the implant is suggested to avoid corneal decompensation, permanent visual loss and the need of subsequent corneal transplantation. Several surgical techniques have been described for this purpose [171,172].

With regard to cataract formation, it has been reported that repeated DEX implant injections increase the risk of cataract progression. The European DME registrar study (ARTES) registered 12.4% of patients treated with Ozurdex implant requiring cataract surgery during the follow-up [166].

Interestingly, sporadic errors in the intravitreal injection technique led to incomplete penetration of the device in the vitreous cavity. Although this complication should be avoided at any cost, the devices reabsorbed in a couple of months [173].

Similarly, Ozurdex can be inadvertently misplaced in the crystalline lens causing a cataract. This event could lead to subsequent complicated cataract surgery if the capsular bag was broken or severely impaired, requiring iris- or scleral-fixation IOL implants [174].

11.3. Dex Implant and Posterior Segment Complications

Because Dex implant is delivered in the vitreous cavity, some complications related to the posterior segment deserve to be mentioned.

Overall, endophthalmitis is a major complication related to intravitreal procedures [175]. Two cases of endophthalmitis over nearly 3000 DEX implants were reported in the MEAD trial [80], while no cases of endophthalmitis were reported in the GENEVA trial [19].

A large retrospective multicenter analysis reported an endophthalmitis rate of 0.07% (two cases over 6000 injections) [165], whereas the ARTES study group reported no cases of endophthalmitis [166]. Other reported uncommon ocular side effects following Ozurdex injection are vitreous haemorrhages, rarely requiring PPV, and RD [165].

The Dex implant is linked to a higher number of secondary ERMs compared to other intravitreal steroids, such as TA. A possible explanation may be found in the poly lactic-*co*-glycolic acid (PLGA) matrix drug delivery system of the Ozurdex implant, which is biodegradable [176]. It may be speculated that PLGA may induce liquefaction of the vitreous, posterior vitreous detachment, and subsequent epiretinal response with the formation of ERM.

However, it is still under debate whether the ERM limits drug penetration into the retina [167], or it rather provokes a tractional force onto the retina itself, limiting the decrease in CMT after the injection [176].

Two cases of retinal necrosis following Ozurdex injection were published in the past years [177,178]. Retinal necrosis was caused either by Herpes Simplex Virus [177], or Cytomegalovirus [178]. Systemic steroid sparing therapy (immunosuppressive) or systemic immunodepression were recognized as the main risk factors [177,178].

Other complications of the Dex implant affecting the posterior segment are quite unusual. A case of Dex implant, adherent to the retinal surface after the filling of the vitreous cavity with gas (sulfur hexafluoride 30%) at the end of PPV, was previously described [179]. As direct contact between the Ozurdex device and the retina could cause damage to the retinal layers, the implant was promptly removed without any persistent retinal defect [179].

Two cases of Ozurdex implant desegmentation were reported without any significant intraocular complications [180].

11.4. Dex Implant and Adnexa

A case of Periorbital Necrotizing Fasciitis (PNF), related to Ozurdex injection, was also described [181]. The surgical trauma associated with the Dex implant was hypothesized to act as a trigger for PNF. Nevertheless, the patient had multiple risk factors, such as diabetes, old age and immunosuppressive therapy. Proper evaluation of the patients' medical history and strict postoperative recommendations are mandatory, especially in fragile patients, to prevent such serious adverse events [181].

11.5. Dex Implant and Pregnancy

Anti-VEGF drugs for the treatment of retinal diseases are generally avoided during pregnancy, for the concerns related to the potential teratogen effect [182]. Steroids are considered generally safer than anti-VEGF medications in pregnant women, and they should be taken into consideration by retinal specialists. For instance, successful treatment of idiopathic and inflammatory choroidal neovascularization with Dex implant were previously reported [183].

Ozurdex may be a good option to manage the worsening of DME during pregnancy, due to the limited number of injections required to treat the condition. Published data reported both good anatomical and functional results with significant reduction in CMT and improvement of VA [184,185].

12. Conclusions

Intravitreal injection is the mainstream route of drug administration to treat diseases affecting the posterior segment of the eye. It is difficult to achieve and maintain significant levels of drugs into the vitreous cavity, and frequent injections are often needed [42].

Although anti-VEGFs have been largely indicated as a first-choice level, the Dex implant represents an important treatment option, especially for persistent DME, non-responders to anti-VEGF, vitrectomized eyes and in patients in whom anti-VEGF might be contraindicated (e.g., high cardiovascular risk, pregnancy) [78]. Additionally, the peculiar formulation and pharmacokinetic properties, which lead to less frequent retreatments, lower the costs and improve patient compliance, along with the satisfactory structural and functional outcomes, may allow to consider Ozurdex as a first-line approach in selected cases. Indeed, the role of DEX implant is crucial in chronic patients who often have comorbidities, requiring frequent visits to other health care professionals, since it reduces the healthcare burden both for patients and care-givers [78].

Of note, ophthalmologists should keep in mind that the type of drug, the particular design of the delivery system, and the long-lasting effect, could generate some major and minor complications. Notwithstanding, Ozurdex is still considered a safe procedure, as the most common complications reported are cataract progression and temporary IOP elevation.

In conclusion, the Dex implant is a very useful device for the management of a wide range of ocular diseases, but the choice of the best candidate to corticosteroid therapy is essential for a successful outcome.

Author Contributions: Conceptualization, C.I., and G.G.; methodology, C.I. and G.G.; writing—original draft preparation, C.I., R.M., M.L., D.B., M.P., F.B., E.B., R.S., A.C. (Adriano Carnevali), R.D., A.C. (Alessio Cerquaglia), L.F., A.G., S.E., G.T., A.D.Z., M.F., A.V. and G.G.; writing—review and editing, C.I., R.M., M.L., D.B., M.P., F.B., E.B., R.S., A.C. (Adriano Carnevali), R.D., A.C. (Alessio Cerquaglia), L.F., A.G., S.E., G.T., A.D.Z., M.F., A.V. and G.G.; supervision, C.I and G.G. All authors have read and agreed to the published version of the manuscript.

Funding: This research received no external funding.

Conflicts of Interest: The authors declare no conflict of interest.

References

1. Kuno, N.; Fujii, S. Biodegradable intraocular therapies for retinal disorders: Progress to date. *Drugs Aging* **2010**, *27*, 117–134. [CrossRef] [PubMed]
2. Lowder, C.; Belfort, R.; Lightman, S.; Foster, C.S.; Robinson, M.R.; Schiffman, R.M.; Li, X.Y.; Cui, H.; Whitcup, S.M. Dexamethasone intravitreal implant for noninfectious intermediate or posterior uveitis. *Arch. Ophthalmol.* **2011**, *129*, 545–553. [CrossRef] [PubMed]
3. Coscas, G.; Augustin, A.; Bandello, F.; De Smet, M.D.; Lanzetta, P.; Staurenghi, G.; Parravano, M.C.; Udaondo, P.; Moisseiev, E.; Soubrane, G.; et al. Retreatment with Ozurdex for macular edema secondary to retinal vein occlusion. *Eur. J. Ophthalmol.* **2013**, *24*, 1–9. [CrossRef] [PubMed]
4. Dugel, P.U.; Bandello, F.; Loewenstein, A. Dexamethasone intravitreal implant in the treatment of diabetic macular edema. *Clin. Ophthalmol.* **2015**, *9*, 1321–1335. [CrossRef]
5. Koronis, S.; Stavrakas, P.; Balidis, M.; Kozeis, N.; Tranos, P.G. Update in treatment of uveitic macular edema. *Drug Des. Devel. Ther.* **2019**, *13*, 667–680. [CrossRef]
6. He, Y.; Ren, X.J.; Hu, B.J.; Lam, W.C.; Li, X.R. A meta-analysis of the effect of a dexamethasone intravitreal implant versus intravitreal anti-vascular endothelial growth factor treatment for diabetic macular edema. *BMC Ophthalmol.* **2018**, *18*, 121. [CrossRef]
7. Campochiaro, P.A.; Hafiz, G.; Mir, T.A.; Scott, A.W.; Sophie, R.; Shah, S.M.; Ying, H.S.; Lu, L.; Chen, C.; Campbell, J.P.; et al. Pro-Permeability Factors after Dexamethasone Implant in Retinal Vein Occlusion; The Ozurdex for Retinal Vein Occlusion (ORVO) Study. *Am. J. Ophthalmol.* **2015**, *160*, 313–321. [CrossRef]
8. Chang-Lin, J.E.; Attar, M.; Acheampong, A.A.; Robinson, M.R.; Whitcup, S.M.; Kuppermann, B.D.; Welty, D. Pharmacokinetics and pharmacodynamics of a sustained-release dexamethasone intravitreal implant. *Investig. Ophthalmol. Vis. Sci.* **2011**, *52*, 80–86. [CrossRef]

9. Chin, E.K.; Almeida, D.R.; Velez, G.; Xu, K.; Peraire, M.; Corbella, M.; Elshatory, Y.M.; Kwon, Y.H.; Gehrs, K.M.; Culver Boldt, H.; et al. Ocular Hypertension after Intravitreal Dexamethasone (Ozurdex) Sustained-Release Implant. *Retina* **2017**, *37*, 1345–1351. [CrossRef]
10. Yau, J.W.Y.; Lee, P.; Wong, T.Y.; Best, J.; Jenkins, A. Retinal vein occlusion: An approach to diagnosis, systemic risk factors and management. *Intern. Med. J.* **2008**, *38*, 904–910. [CrossRef]
11. Campochiaro, P.A.; Choy, D.F.; Do, D.V.; Hafiz, G.; Shah, S.M.; Nguyen, Q.D.; Rubio, R.; Arron, J.R. Monitoring ocular drug therapy by analysis of aqueous samples. *Ophthalmology* **2009**, *116*, 2158–2164. [CrossRef] [PubMed]
12. Rehak, M.; Wiedemann, P. Retinal vein thrombosis: Pathogenesis and management. *J. Thromb. Haemost.* **2010**, *8*, 1886–1894. [CrossRef] [PubMed]
13. Au, A.; Hilely, A.; Scharf, J.; Gunnemann, F.; Wang, D.; Chehaibou, I.; Iovino, C.; Grondin, C.; Farecki, M.-L.; Falavarjani, K.G.; et al. Relationship between nerve fiber layer hemorrhages and outcomes in central retinal vein occlusion. *Investig. Ophthalmol. Vis. Sci.* **2020**, *61*, 54. [CrossRef] [PubMed]
14. Haller, J.A.; Bandello, F.; Belfort, R.; Blumenkranz, M.S.; Gillies, M.; Heier, J.; Loewenstein, A.; Yoon, Y.H.; Jiao, J.; Li, X.Y.; et al. Dexamethasone intravitreal implant in patients with macular edema related to branch or central retinal vein occlusion: Twelve-month study results. *Ophthalmology* **2011**, *118*, 2453–2460. [CrossRef]
15. Rezar-Dreindl, S.; Eibenberger, K.; Pollreisz, A.; Bühl, W.; Georgopoulos, M.; Krall, C.; Dunavölgyi, R.; Weigert, G.; Kroh, M.E.; Schmidt-Erfurth, U.; et al. Effect of intravitreal dexamethasone implant on intra-ocular cytokines and chemokines in eyes with retinal vein occlusion. *Acta Ophthalmol.* **2017**, *95*, e119–e127. [CrossRef]
16. Tadayoni, R.; Waldstein, S.M.; Boscia, F.; Gerding, H.; Gekkieva, M.; Barnes, E.; Das Gupta, A.; Wenzel, A.; Pearce, I. Sustained Benefits of Ranibizumab with or without Laser in Branch Retinal Vein Occlusion: 24-Month Results of the BRIGHTER Study. *Ophthalmology* **2017**, *124*, 1778–1787. [CrossRef]
17. Noma, H.; Funatsu, H.; Mimura, T.; Eguchi, S.; Hori, S. Soluble vascular endothelial growth factor receptor-2 and inflammatory factors in macular edema with branch retinal vein occlusion. *Am. J. Ophthalmol.* **2011**, *152*, 669–677. [CrossRef]
18. Campochiaro, P.A.; Heier, J.S.; Feiner, L.; Gray, S.; Saroj, N.; Rundle, A.C.; Murahashi, W.Y.; Rubio, R.G. Ranibizumab for Macular Edema following Branch Retinal Vein Occlusion. Six-Month Primary End Point Results of a Phase III Study. *Ophthalmology* **2010**, *117*, 1102–1112. [CrossRef]
19. Haller, J.A.; Bandello, F.; Belfort, R.; Blumenkranz, M.S.; Gillies, M.; Heier, J.; Loewenstein, A.; Yoon, Y.H.; Jacques, M.L.; Jiao, J.; et al. Randomized, Sham-Controlled Trial of Dexamethasone Intravitreal Implant in Patients with Macular Edema Due to Retinal Vein Occlusion. *Ophthalmology* **2010**, *117*, 1134–1146. [CrossRef]
20. Li, X.; Wang, N.; Liang, X.; Xu, G.; Li, X.Y.; Jiao, J.; Lou, J.; Hashad, Y. Safety and efficacy of dexamethasone intravitreal implant for treatment of macular edema secondary to retinal vein occlusion in Chinese patients: Randomized, sham-controlled, multicenter study. *Graefe's Arch. Clin. Exp. Ophthalmol.* **2018**, *256*, 59–69. [CrossRef]
21. Danis, R.P.; Sadda, S.; Jiao, J.; Li, X.Y.; Whitcup, S.M. Relationship between retinal thickness and visual acuity in eyes with retinal vein occlusion treated with dexamethasone implant. *Retina* **2016**, *36*, 1170–1176. [CrossRef] [PubMed]
22. Bezatis, A.; Spital, G.; Höhn, F.; Maier, M.; Clemens, C.R.; Wachtlin, J.; Lehmann, F.; Hattenbach, L.O.; Feltgen, N.; Meyer, C.H. Functional and anatomical results after a single intravitreal Ozurdex injection in retinal vein occlusion: A 6-month follow-up—The SOLO study. *Acta Ophthalmol.* **2013**, *91*, e340–e347. [CrossRef]
23. Kuppermann, B.D.; Haller, J.A.; Bandello, F.; Loewenstein, A.; Jiao, J.; Li, X.Y.; Whitcup, S.M. Onset and duration of visual acuity improvement after dexamethasone intravitreal implant in eyes with macular edema due to retinal vein occlusion. *Retina* **2014**, *34*, 1743–1749. [CrossRef]
24. Ferrini, W.; Ambresin, A. Intravitreal dexamethasone implant for the treatment of macular edema after retinal vein occlusion in a clinical setting. *Klin. Monbl. Augenheilkd.* **2013**, *230*, 423–426. [CrossRef] [PubMed]
25. Yeh, W.S.; Haller, J.A.; Lanzetta, P.; Kuppermann, B.D.; Wong, T.Y.; Mitchell, P.; Whitcup, S.M.; Kowalski, J.W. Effect of the duration of macular edema on clinical outcomes in retinal vein occlusion treated with dexamethasone intravitreal implant. *Ophthalmology* **2012**, *119*, 1190–1198. [CrossRef] [PubMed]

26. Singer, M.A.; Capone, A.; Dugel, P.U.; Dreyer, R.F.; Dodwell, D.G.; Roth, D.B.; Shi, R.; Walt, J.G.; Scott, L.C.; Hollander, D.A. Two or more dexamethasone intravitreal implants as monotherapy or in combination therapy for macular edema in retinal vein occlusion: Subgroup analysis of a retrospective chart review study retina. *BMC Ophthalmol.* **2015**, *15*, 33. [CrossRef]
27. Querques, L.; Querques, G.; Lattanzio, R.; Gigante, S.R.; Del Turco, C.; Corradetti, G.; Cascavilla, M.L.; Bandello, F. Repeated intravitreal dexamethasone implant (Ozurdex®) for retinal vein occlusion. *Ophthalmologica* **2012**, *229*, 21–25. [CrossRef] [PubMed]
28. Sadda, S.; Danis, R.P.; Pappuru, R.R.; Keane, P.A.; Jiao, J.; Li, X.Y.; Whitcup, S.M. Vascular changes in eyes treated with dexamethasone intravitreal implant for macular edema after retinal vein occlusion. *Ophthalmology* **2013**, *120*, 1423–1431. [CrossRef]
29. Campochiaro, P.A.; Sophie, R.; Pearlman, J.; Brown, D.M.; Boyer, D.S.; Heier, J.S.; Marcus, D.M.; Feiner, L.; Patel, A. Long-term outcomes in patients with retinal vein occlusion treated with ranibizumab: The RETAIN study. *Ophthalmology* **2014**, *121*, 209–219. [CrossRef] [PubMed]
30. Hoerauf, H.; Feltgen, N.; Weiss, C.; Paulus, E.M.; Schmitz-Valckenberg, S.; Pielen, A.; Puri, P.; Berk, H.; Eter, N.; Wiedemann, P.; et al. Clinical Efficacy and Safety of Ranibizumab Versus Dexamethasone for Central Retinal Vein Occlusion (COMRADE C): A European Label Study. *Am. J. Ophthalmol.* **2016**, *169*, 258–267. [CrossRef]
31. Hattenbach, L.O.; Feltgen, N.; Bertelmann, T.; Schmitz-Valckenberg, S.; Berk, H.; Eter, N.; Lang, G.E.; Rehak, M.; Taylor, S.R.; Wolf, A.; et al. Head-to-head comparison of ranibizumab PRN versus single-dose dexamethasone for branch retinal vein occlusion (COMRADE-B). *Acta Ophthalmol.* **2018**, *96*, e10–e18. [CrossRef] [PubMed]
32. Feltgen, N.; Hattenbach, L.O.; Bertelmann, T.; Callizo, J.; Rehak, M.; Wolf, A.; Berk, H.; Eter, N.; Lang, G.E.; Pielen, A.; et al. Comparison of ranibizumab versus dexamethasone for macular oedema following retinal vein occlusion: 1-year results of the COMRADE extension study. *Acta Ophthalmol.* **2018**, *96*, e933–e941. [CrossRef] [PubMed]
33. Eter, N.; Mohr, A.; Wachtlin, J.; Feltgen, N.; Shirlaw, A.; Leaback, R. Dexamethasone intravitreal implant in retinal vein occlusion: Real-life data from a prospective, multicenter clinical trial. *Graefe's Arch. Clin. Exp. Ophthalmol.* **2017**, *255*, 77–87. [CrossRef] [PubMed]
34. Yoon, Y.H.; Kim, J.W.; Lee, J.Y.; Kim, I.T.; Kang, S.W.; Yu, H.G.; Koh, H.J.; Kim, S.S.; Chang, D.J.; Simonyi, S. Dexamethasone intravitreal implant for early treatment and retreatment of macular edema related to branch retinal vein occlusion: The multicenter COBALT Study. *Ophthalmologica* **2018**, *240*, 81–89. [CrossRef] [PubMed]
35. Georgalas, L.; Tservakis, I.; Kiskira, E.E.; Petrou, P.; Papaconstantinou, D.; Kanakis, M. Efficacy and safety of dexamethasone intravitreal implant in patients with retinal vein occlusion resistant to anti-VEGF therapy: A 12-month prospective study. *Cutan. Ocul. Toxicol.* **2019**, *38*, 330–337. [CrossRef] [PubMed]
36. Bandello, F.; Augustin, A.; Tufail, A.; Leaback, R. A 12-month, multicenter, parallel group comparison of dexamethasone intravitreal implant versus ranibizumab in branch retinal vein occlusion. *Eur. J. Ophthalmol.* **2018**, *28*, 697–705. [CrossRef]
37. Kumar, P.; Sharma, Y.R.; Chandra, P.; Azad, R.; Meshram, G.G. Comparison of the Safety and Efficacy of Intravitreal Ranibizumab with or without Laser Photocoagulation Versus Dexamethasone Intravitreal Implant with or without Laser Photocoagulation for Macular Edema Secondary to Branch Retinal Vein Occlusion. *Folia Med. (Plovdiv.)* **2019**, *61*, 240–248. [CrossRef]
38. Chatziralli, I.; Theodossiadis, G.; Kabanarou, S.A.; Parikakis, E.; Xirou, T.; Mitropoulos, P.; Theodossiadis, P. Ranibizumab versus dexamethasone implant for central retinal vein occlusion: The RANIDEX study. *Graefe's Arch. Clin. Exp. Ophthalmol.* **2017**, *255*, 1899–1905. [CrossRef]
39. Gado, A.S.; Macky, T.A. Dexamethasone intravitreous implant versus bevacizumab for central retinal vein occlusion-related macular oedema: A prospective randomized comparison. *Clin. Exp. Ophthalmol.* **2014**, *42*, 650–655. [CrossRef]
40. Accorinti, M.; Okada, A.A.; Smith, J.R.; Gilardi, M. Epidemiology of Macular Edema in Uveitis. *Ocul. Immunol. Inflamm.* **2019**, *27*, 169–180. [CrossRef]
41. Carnahan, M.C.; Goldstein, D.A. Ocular complications of topical, peri-ocular, and systemic corticosteroids. *Curr. Opin. Ophthalmol.* **2000**, *11*, 478–483. [CrossRef] [PubMed]

42. Varela-Fernández, R.; Díaz-Tomé, V.; Luaces-Rodríguez, A.; Conde-Penedo, A.; García-Otero, X.; Luzardo-álvarez, A.; Fernández-Ferreiro, A.; Otero-Espinar, F.J. Drug delivery to the posterior segment of the eye: Biopharmaceutic and pharmacokinetic considerations. *Pharmaceutics* **2020**, *12*, 269. [CrossRef]
43. Lightman, S.; Belfort, R.; Naik, R.K.; Lowder, C.; Foster, C.S.; Rentz, A.M.; Cui, H.; Whitcup, S.M.; Kowalski, J.W.; Revicki, D.A. Vision-related functioning outcomes of dexamethasone intravitreal implant in noninfectious intermediate or posterior uveitis. *Investig. Ophthalmol. Vis. Sci.* **2013**, *54*, 4864–4870. [CrossRef] [PubMed]
44. Williams, G.A.; Haller, J.A.; Kuppermann, B.D.; Blumenkranz, M.S.; Weinberg, D.V.; Chou, C.; Whitcup, S.M. Dexamethasone Posterior-Segment Drug Delivery System in the Treatment of Macular Edema Resulting from Uveitis or Irvine-Gass Syndrome. *Am. J. Ophthalmol.* **2009**, *147*, 1048–1054. [CrossRef] [PubMed]
45. Myung, J.S.; Aaker, G.D.; Kiss, S. Treatment of noninfectious posterior uveitis with dexamethasone intravitreal implant. *Clin. Ophthalmol.* **2010**, *4*, 1423–1426. [PubMed]
46. Hasanreisoğlu, M.; Özdemir, H.B.; Özkan, K.; Yüksel, M.; Aktaş, Z.; Atalay, H.T.; Özdek, Ş.; Gürelik, G. Intravitreal Dexamethasone Implant in the Treatment of Non-infectious Uveitis. *Turkish J. Ophthalmol.* **2019**, *49*, 250–257. [CrossRef]
47. Pohlmann, D.; vom Brocke, G.A.; Winterhalter, S.; Steurer, T.; Thees, S.; Pleyer, U. Dexamethasone Inserts in Noninfectious Uveitis: A Single-Center Experience. *Ophthalmology* **2018**, *125*, 1088–1099. [CrossRef]
48. Tomkins-Netzer, O.; Taylor, S.R.J.; Bar, A.; Lula, A.; Yaganti, S.; Talat, L.; Lightman, S. Treatment with repeat dexamethasone implants results in long-term disease control in eyes with noninfectious uveitis. *Ophthalmology* **2014**, *121*, 1649–1654. [CrossRef]
49. Zarranz-Ventura, J.; Carreño, E.; Johnston, R.L.; Mohammed, Q.; Ross, A.H.; Barker, C.; Fonollosa, A.; Artaraz, J.; Pelegrin, L.; Adan, A.; et al. Multicenter study of intravitreal dexamethasone implant in noninfectious uveitis: Indications, outcomes, and reinjection frequency. *Am. J. Ophthalmol.* **2014**, *158*, 1136–1145. [CrossRef]
50. Saraiya, N.V.; Goldstein, D.A. Dexamethasone for ocular inflammation. *Expert Opin. Pharmacother.* **2011**, *12*, 1127–1131. [CrossRef]
51. Sallam, A.; Taylor, S.R.J.; Lightman, S. Review and update of intraocular therapy in noninfectious uveitis. *Curr. Opin. Ophthalmol.* **2011**, *22*, 517–522. [CrossRef] [PubMed]
52. Thorne, J.E.; Sugar, E.A.; Holbrook, J.T.; Burke, A.E.; Altaweel, M.M.; Vitale, A.T.; Acharya, N.R.; Kempen, J.H.; Jabs, D.A. Periocular Triamcinolone vs. Intravitreal Triamcinolone vs. Intravitreal Dexamethasone Implant for the Treatment of Uveitic Macular Edema: The PeriOcular vs. INTravitreal corticosteroids for uveitic macular edema (POINT) Trial. *Ophthalmology* **2019**, *126*, 283–295. [CrossRef] [PubMed]
53. Khurana, R.N.; Bansal, A.S.; Chang, L.K.; Palmer, J.D.; Wu, C.; Wieland, M.R. Prospective evaluation of a sustained-release dexamethasone intravitreal implant for cystoid macular edema in quiescent uveitis. *Retina* **2017**, *37*, 1692–1699. [CrossRef] [PubMed]
54. Cao, J.H.; Mulvahill, M.; Zhang, L.; Joondeph, B.C.; Dacey, M.S. Dexamethasone intravitreal implant in the treatment of persistent uveitic macular edema in the absence of active inflammation. *Ophthalmology* **2014**, *121*, 1871–1876. [CrossRef] [PubMed]
55. Miserocchi, E.; Modorati, G.; Pastore, M.R.; Bandello, F. Dexamethasone intravitreal implant: An effective adjunctive treatment for recalcitrant noninfectious uveitis. *Ophthalmologica* **2012**, *228*, 229–233. [CrossRef]
56. Fabiani, C.; Vitale, A.; Emmi, G.; Lopalco, G.; Vannozzi, L.; Bacherini, D.; Guerriero, S.; Favale, R.A.; Fusco, F.; Franceschini, R.; et al. Systemic Steroid Sparing Effect of Intravitreal Dexamethasone Implant in Chronic Noninfectious Uveitic Macular Edema. *J. Ocul. Pharmacol. Ther.* **2017**, *33*, 549–555. [CrossRef]
57. Ratra, D.; Barh, A.; Banerjee, M.; Ratra, V.; Biswas, J. Safety and Efficacy of Intravitreal Dexamethasone Implant for Refractory Uveitic Macular Edema in Adults and Children. *Ocul. Immunol. Inflamm.* **2018**, *26*, 1034–1040. [CrossRef]
58. Coşkun, E.; Celemler, P.; Kimyon, G.; Öner, V.; Kisacik, B.; Erbagci, I.; Onat, A.M. Intravitreal Dexamethasone Implant for Treatment of Refractory Behçet Posterior Uveitis: One-year Follow-up Results. *Ocul. Immunol. Inflamm.* **2015**, *23*, 437–443. [CrossRef]
59. Fabiani, C.; Emmi, G.; Lopalco, G.; Vannozzi, L.; Bacherini, D.; Guerriero, S.; Franceschini, R.; Frediani, B.; Iannone, F.; Marco Tosi, G.; et al. Intravitreal Dexamethasone Implant as an Adjunct Weapon for Severe and Refractory Uveitis in Behçet's Disease. *Isr. Med. Assoc. J.* **2017**, *19*, 415–419.

60. Kim, M.; Kim, S.A.; Park, W.; Kim, R.Y.; Park, Y.H. Intravitreal Dexamethasone Implant for Treatment of Sarcoidosis-Related Uveitis. *Adv. Ther.* **2019**, *36*, 2137–2146. [CrossRef]
61. Pelegrín, L.; De La Maza, M.S.; Molins, B.; Ríos, J.; Adán, A. Long-term evaluation of dexamethasone intravitreal implant in vitrectomized and non-vitrectomized eyes with macular edema secondary to non-infectious uveitis. *Eye* **2015**, *29*, 943–950. [CrossRef] [PubMed]
62. Kim, J.T.; Yoon, Y.H.; Lee, D.H.; Joe, S.G.; Kim, J.G. Dexamethasone intravitreal implant in the silicone oil-filled eye for the treatment for recurrent macular oedema associated with ankylosing spondylitis: A case report. *Acta Ophthalmol.* **2013**, *91*, e331–e332. [CrossRef] [PubMed]
63. Nguyen, T.; Kim, H.; Mielke, C.; Momont, A.C.; Brandt, J.D.; Liu, Y. Combined Dexamethasone Intravitreal Implant and Glaucoma Drainage Device Placement for Uveitic Glaucoma. *J. Glaucoma* **2020**, *29*, 252–257. [CrossRef] [PubMed]
64. Tomkins-Netzer, O.; Talat, L.; Seguin-Greenstein, S.; Bar, A.; Lightman, S. Outcome of Treating Pediatric Uveitis with Dexamethasone Implants. *Am. J. Ophthalmol.* **2016**, *161*, 110–115. [CrossRef] [PubMed]
65. Bratton, M.L.; He, Y.G.; Weakley, D.R. Dexamethasone intravitreal implant (Ozurdex) for the treatment of pediatric uveitis. *J. AAPOS* **2014**, *18*, 110–113. [CrossRef] [PubMed]
66. Pichi, F.; Nucci, P.; Baynes, K.; Lowder, C.Y.; Srivastava, S.K. Sustained-release dexamethasone intravitreal implant in juvenile idiopathic arthritis-related uveitis. *Int. Ophthalmol.* **2017**, *37*, 221–228. [CrossRef]
67. Sella, R.; Oray, M.; Friling, R.; Umar, L.; Tugal-Tutkun, I.; Kramer, M. Dexamethasone intravitreal implant (Ozurdex®) for pediatric uveitis. *Graefe's Arch. Clin. Exp. Ophthalmol.* **2015**, *253*, 1777–1782. [CrossRef]
68. Miserocchi, E.; Berchicci, L.; Iuliano, L.; Modorati, G.; Bandello, F. Dexamethasone intravitreal implant in serpiginous choroiditis. *Br. J. Ophthalmol.* **2017**, *101*, 327–332. [CrossRef]
69. Walsh, J.; Reddy, A.K. Intravitreal dexamethasone implantation for birdshot chorioretinopathy. *Retin. Cases Br. Rep.* **2017**, *11*, 51–55. [CrossRef]
70. Bajwa, A.; Peck, T.; Reddy, A.K.; Netland, P.A.; Shildkrot, Y. Dexamethasone implantation in birdshot chorioretinopathy—Long-term outcome. *Int. Med. Case Rep. J.* **2018**, *11*, 349–358. [CrossRef]
71. Barnes, A.C.; Lowder, C.Y.; Bessette, A.P.; Baynes, K.; Srivastava, S.K. Treatment of acute zonal occult outer retinopathy with intravitreal steroids. *Ophthalmic Surg. Lasers Imaging Retin.* **2018**, *49*, 504–509. [CrossRef] [PubMed]
72. Mora-Cantallops, A.; Pérez, M.D.; Revenga, M.; González-López, J.J. Ellipsoid layer restoration after Ozurdex® treatment in a patient with acute posterior multifocal placoid pigment epitheliopathy. *Eur. J. Ophthalmol.* **2019**. [CrossRef] [PubMed]
73. Empeslidis, T.; Banerjee, S.; Vardarinos, A.; Konstas, A.G.P. Dexamethasone intravitreal implant for idiopathic retinal vasculitis, aneurysms, and neuroretinitis. *Eur. J. Ophthalmol.* **2013**, *23*, 757–760. [CrossRef] [PubMed]
74. Saatci, A.O.; Ayhan, Z.; Takeş, Ö.; Yaman, A.; Söylev Bajin, F.M. Single bilateral dexamethasone implant in addition to panretinal photocoagulation and oral azathioprine treatment in IRVAN syndrome. *Case Rep. Ophthalmol.* **2015**, *6*, 56–62. [CrossRef]
75. Klein, R.; Klein, B.E.K.; Moss, S.E.; Davis, M.D.; DeMets, D.L. The Wisconsin Epidemiologic Study of Diabetic Retinopathy: IV. Diabetic Macular Edema. *Ophthalmology* **1984**, *91*, 1464–1474. [CrossRef]
76. Boyer, D.S.; Yoon, Y.H.; Belfort, R.; Bandello, F.; Maturi, R.K.; Augustin, A.J.; Li, X.Y.; Cui, H.; Hashad, Y.; Whitcup, S.M. Three-year, randomized, sham-controlled trial of dexamethasone intravitreal implant in patients with diabetic macular edema. *Ophthalmology* **2014**, *121*, 1904–1914. [CrossRef]
77. Schmidt-Erfurth, U.; Garcia-Arumi, J.; Bandello, F.; Berg, K.; Chakravarthy, U.; Gerendas, B.S.; Jonas, J.; Larsen, M.; Tadayoni, R.; Loewenstein, A. Guidelines for the management of diabetic macular edema by the European Society of Retina Specialists (EURETINA). *Ophthalmologica* **2017**, *237*, 185–222. [CrossRef]
78. Bandello, F.; Toni, D.; Porta, M.; Varano, M. Diabetic retinopathy, diabetic macular edema, and cardiovascular risk: The importance of a long-term perspective and a multidisciplinary approach to optimal intravitreal therapy. *Acta Diabetol.* **2020**, *57*, 513–526. [CrossRef]
79. Danis, R.P.; Sadda, S.; Li, X.Y.; Cui, H.; Hashad, Y.; Whitcup, S.M. Anatomical effects of dexamethasone intravitreal implant in diabetic macular oedema: A pooled analysis of 3-year phase III trials. *Br. J. Ophthalmol.* **2016**, *100*, 796–801. [CrossRef]
80. Maturi, R.K.; Pollack, A.; Uy, H.S.; Varano, M.; Gomes, A.M.V.; Li, X.Y.; Cui, H.; Lou, J.; Hashad, Y.; Whitcup, S.M. Intraocular pressure in patients with diabetic macular edema treated with dexamethasone intravitreal implant in the 3-year mead study. *Retina* **2016**, *36*, 1143–1152. [CrossRef]

81. Augustin, A.J.; Kuppermann, B.D.; Lanzetta, P.; Loewenstein, A.; Li, X.Y.; Cui, H.; Hashad, Y.; Whitcup, S.M.; Abujamra, S.; Acton, J.; et al. Dexamethasone intravitreal implant in previously treated patients with diabetic macular edema: Subgroup analysis of the MEAD study. *BMC Ophthalmol.* **2015**, *15*, 150. [CrossRef] [PubMed]
82. Mastropasqua, R.; Toto, L.; Borrelli, E.; Di Antonio, L.; De Nicola, C.; Mastrocola, A.; Di Nicola, M.; Carpineto, P. Morphology and function over a one-year follow up period after intravitreal dexamethasone implant (Ozurdex) in patients with diabetic macular edema. *PLoS ONE* **2015**, *10*, e0145663. [CrossRef] [PubMed]
83. Sarao, V.; Veritti, D.; Furino, C.; Giancipoli, E.; Alessio, G.; Boscia, F.; Lanzetta, P. Dexamethasone implant with fixed or individualized regimen in the treatment of diabetic macular oedema: Six-month outcomes of the UDBASA study. *Acta Ophthalmol.* **2017**, *95*, e255–e260. [CrossRef] [PubMed]
84. Lo Giudice, G.; Avarello, A.; Campana, G.; Galan, A. Rapid response to dexamethasone intravitreal implant in diabetic macular edema. *Eur. J. Ophthalmol.* **2018**, *28*, 74–79. [CrossRef] [PubMed]
85. Abdel-Hay, A.; Sivaprasad, S.; Subramanian, A.; Barbur, J.L. Acuity and colour vision changes post intravitreal dexamethasone implant injection in patients with diabetic macular oedema. *PLoS ONE* **2018**, *13*, e0199693. [CrossRef] [PubMed]
86. Gillies, M.C.; Lim, L.L.; Campain, A.; Quin, G.J.; Salem, W.; Li, J.; Goodwin, S.; Aroney, C.; McAllister, I.L.; Fraser-Bell, S. A randomized clinical trial of intravitreal bevacizumab versus intravitreal dexamethasone for diabetic macular edema: The BEVORDEX study. *Ophthalmology* **2014**, *121*, 2473–2481. [CrossRef]
87. Mehta, H.; Fraser-Bell, S.; Yeung, A.; Campain, A.; Lim, L.L.; Quin, G.J.; McAllister, I.L.; Keane, P.A.; Gillies, M.C. Efficacy of dexamethasone versus bevacizumab on regression of hard exudates in diabetic maculopathy: Data from the BEVORDEX randomised clinical trial. *Br. J. Ophthalmol.* **2016**, *100*, 1000–1004. [CrossRef]
88. Aroney, C.; Fraser-Bell, S.; Lamoureux, E.L.; Gillies, M.C.; Lim, L.L.; Fenwick, E.K. Vision-related quality of life outcomes in the BEVORDEX study: A clinical trial comparing ozurdex sustained release dexamethasone intravitreal implant and bevacizumab treatment for diabetic macular edema. *Investig. Ophthalmol. Vis. Sci.* **2016**, *57*, 5541–5546. [CrossRef]
89. Mehta, H.; Fraser-Bell, S.; Nguyen, V.; Lim, L.L.; Gillies, M.C. The Interval between Treatments of Bevacizumab and Dexamethasone Implants for Diabetic Macular Edema Increased over Time in the BEVORDEX Trial. *Ophthalmol. Retin.* **2018**, *2*, 231–234. [CrossRef]
90. Callanan, D.G.; Loewenstein, A.; Patel, S.S.; Massin, P.; Corcóstegui, B.; Li, X.Y.; Jiao, J.; Hashad, Y.; Whitcup, S.M. A multicenter, 12-month randomized study comparing dexamethasone intravitreal implant with ranibizumab in patients with diabetic macular edema. *Graefe's Arch. Clin. Exp. Ophthalmol.* **2017**, *255*, 463–473. [CrossRef]
91. Lazic, R.; Lukic, M.; Boras, I.; Draca, N.; Vlasic, M.; Gabric, N.; Tomic, Z. Treatment of anti-vascular endothelial growth factor-resistant diabetic macular edema with dexamethasone intravitreal implant. *Retina* **2014**, *34*, 719–724. [CrossRef] [PubMed]
92. Busch, C.; Zur, D.; Fraser-Bell, S.; Laíns, I.; Santos, A.R.; Lupidi, M.; Cagini, C.; Gabrielle, P.H.; Couturier, A.; Mané-Tauty, V.; et al. Shall we stay, or shall we switch? Continued anti-VEGF therapy versus early switch to dexamethasone implant in refractory diabetic macular edema. *Acta Diabetol.* **2018**, *55*, 789–796. [CrossRef] [PubMed]
93. Busch, C.; Fraser-Bell, S.; Iglicki, M.; Lupidi, M.; Couturier, A.; Chaikitmongkol, V.; Giancipoli, E.; Rodríguez-Valdés, P.J.; Gabrielle, P.H.; Laíns, I.; et al. Real-world outcomes of non-responding diabetic macular edema treated with continued anti-VEGF therapy versus early switch to dexamethasone implant: 2-year results. *Acta Diabetol.* **2019**, *56*, 1341–1350. [CrossRef] [PubMed]
94. Boyer, D.S.; Faber, D.; Gupta, S.; Patel, S.S.; Tabandeh, H.; Li, X.Y.; Liu, C.C.; Lou, J.; Whitcup, S.M. Dexamethasone intravitreal implant for treatment of diabetic macular edema in vitrectomized patients. *Retina* **2011**, *31*, 915–923. [CrossRef] [PubMed]
95. Maturi, R.K.; Bleau, L.; Saunders, J.; Mubasher, M.; Stewart, M.W. A 12-Month, Single-Masked, Randomized Controlled Study of Eyes with Persistent Diabetic Macular Edema after Multiple Anti-Vegf Injections to Assess the Efficacy of the Dexamethasone-Delayed Delivery System as an Adjunct to Bevacizumab Compared with Continued Bevacizumab Monotherapy. *Retina* **2015**, *35*, 1604–1614. [PubMed]

96. Maturi, R.K.; Glassman, A.R.; Liu, D.; Beck, R.W.; Bhavsar, A.R.; Bressler, N.M.; Jampol, L.M.; Melia, M.; Punjabi, O.S.; Salehi-Had, H.; et al. Effect of adding dexamethasone to continued ranibizumab treatment in patients with persistent diabetic macular edema: A DRCR network phase 2 randomized clinical trial. *JAMA Ophthalmol.* **2018**, *136*, 29–38. [CrossRef] [PubMed]
97. Callanan, D.G.; Gupta, S.; Boyer, D.S.; Ciulla, T.A.; Singer, M.A.; Kuppermann, B.D.; Liu, C.C.; Li, X.Y.; Hollander, D.A.; Schiffman, R.M.; et al. Dexamethasone intravitreal implant in combination with laser photocoagulation for the treatment of diffuse diabetic macular edema. *Ophthalmology* **2013**, *120*, 1843–1851. [CrossRef]
98. Podkowinski, D.; Orlowski-Wimmer, E.; Zlabinger, G.; Pollreisz, A.; Mursch-Edlmayr, A.S.; Mariacher, S.; Ring, M.; Bolz, M. Aqueous humour cytokine changes during a loading phase of intravitreal ranibizumab or dexamethasone implant in diabetic macular oedema. *Acta Ophthalmol.* **2020**, *98*, e407–e415. [CrossRef]
99. Borrelli, E.; Sarraf, D.; Freund, K.B.; Sadda, S.R. OCT angiography and evaluation of the choroid and choroidal vascular disorders. *Prog. Retin. Eye Res.* **2018**, *67*, 30–55. [CrossRef]
100. Ferris, F.L.; Wilkinson, C.P.; Bird, A.; Chakravarthy, U.; Chew, E.; Csaky, K.; Sadda, S.R. Clinical classification of age-related macular degeneration. *Ophthalmology* **2013**, *120*, 844–851. [CrossRef]
101. Kuppermann, B.D.; Goldstein, M.; Maturi, R.K.; Pollack, A.; Singer, M.; Tufail, A.; Weinberger, D.; Li, X.Y.; Liu, C.C.; Lou, J.; et al. Dexamethasone Intravitreal Implant as Adjunctive Therapy to Ranibizumab in Neovascular Age-Related Macular Degeneration: A Multicenter Randomized Controlled Trial. *Ophthalmologica* **2015**, *234*, 40–54. [CrossRef]
102. Chaudhary, V.; Barbosa, J.; Lam, W.C.; Mak, M.; Mavrikakis, E.; Mohaghegh, P.S.M. Ozurdex in age-related macular degeneration as adjunct to ranibizumab (The OARA Study). *Can. J. Ophthalmol.* **2016**, *51*, 302–305. [CrossRef] [PubMed]
103. Rezar-Dreindl, S.; Sacu, S.; Eibenberger, K.; Pollreisz, A.; Bühl, W.; Georgopoulos, M.; Krall, C.; Weigert, G.; Schmidt-Erfurth, U. The intraocular cytokine profile and therapeutic response in persistent neovascular age-related macular degeneration. *Investig. Ophthalmol. Vis. Sci.* **2016**, *57*, 4144–4150. [CrossRef] [PubMed]
104. Rezar-Dreindl, S.; Eibenberger, K.; Buehl, W.; Georgopoulos, M.; Weigert, G.; Krall, C.; Dunavoelgyi, R.; Schmidt-Erfurth, U.; Sacu, S. Role of additional dexamethasone for the management of persistent or recurrent neovascular agerelated macular degeneration under ranibizumab treatment. *Retina* **2017**, *37*, 962–970. [CrossRef] [PubMed]
105. Giancipoli, E.; Pinna, A.; Boscia, F.; Zasa, G.; Sotgiu, G.; Dore, S.; D'Amico Ricci, G. Intravitreal Dexamethasone in Patients with Wet Age-Related Macular Degeneration Resistant to Anti-VEGF: A Prospective Pilot Study. *J. Ophthalmol.* **2018**, *2018*, 5612342. [CrossRef] [PubMed]
106. Kaya, C.; Zandi, S.; Pfister, I.B.; Gerhardt, C.; Garweg, J.G. Adding a corticosteroid or switching to another anti-VEGF in insufficiently responsive wet age-related macular degeneration. *Clin. Ophthalmol.* **2019**, *13*, 2403–2409. [CrossRef]
107. Calvo, P.; Ferreras, A.; Al Adel, F.; Wang, Y.; Brent, M.H. Dexamethasone intravitreal implant as adjunct therapy for patients with wet age-related macular degeneration with incomplete response to ranibizumab. *Br. J. Ophthalmol.* **2015**, *99*, 723–726. [CrossRef]
108. Querques, G.; Rosenfeld, P.J.P.J.; Cavallero, E.; Borrelli, E.; Corvi, F.; Querques, L.; Bandello, F.M.F.M.; Zarbin, M.A.M.A. Treatment of dry age-related macular degeneration. *Ophthalmic Res.* **2014**, *52*, 107–115. [CrossRef]
109. Chung, H.; Hwang, J.-U.; Kim, J.-G.; Yoon, Y.H. Optical coherence tomography in the diagnosis and monitoring of cystoid macular edema in patients with retinitis pigmentosa. *Retina* **2006**, *26*, 922–927. [CrossRef]
110. Iovino, C.; Au, A.; Hilely, A.; Violanti, S.; Peiretti, E.; Gorin, M.B.; Sarraf, D. Evaluation of the Choroid in Eyes with Retinitis Pigmentosa and Cystoid Macular Edema. *Investig. Opthalmol. Vis. Sci.* **2019**, *60*, 5000. [CrossRef]
111. Srour, M.; Querques, G.; Leveziel, N.; Zerbib, J.; Tilleul, J.; Boulanger-Scemama, E.; Souied, E.H. Intravitreal dexamethasone implant (Ozurdex) for macular edema secondary to retinitis pigmentosa. *Graefe's Arch. Clin. Exp. Ophthalmol.* **2013**, *251*, 1501–1506. [CrossRef] [PubMed]
112. Ahn, S.J.; Kim, K.E.; Woo, S.J.; Park, K.H. The effect of an intravitreal dexamethasone implant for cystoid macular edema in retinitis pigmentosa: A case report and literature review. *Ophthalmic Surg. Lasers Imaging Retin.* **2014**, *45*, 160–164. [CrossRef] [PubMed]

113. Örnek, N.; Örnek, K.; Erbahçeci, İ.E. Intravitreal dexamethasone implant (Ozurdex) for refractory macular edema secondary to retinitis pigmentosa. *Turk Oftalmoloiji Derg.* **2016**, *46*, 179–181. [CrossRef] [PubMed]
114. Saatci, A.O.; Selver, O.B.; Seymenoglu, G.; Yaman, A. Bilateral Intravitreal Dexamethasone Implant for Retinitis Pigmentosa-Related Macular Edema. *Case Rep. Ophthalmol.* **2013**, *4*, 53–58. [CrossRef]
115. Mansour, A.M.; Sheheitli, H.; Kucukerdonmez, C.; Sisk, R.A.; Moura, R.; Moschos, M.M.; Lima, L.H.; Al-Shaar, L.; Arevalo, J.F.; Maia, M.; et al. Intravitreal Dexamethasone Implant in Retinitis Pigmentosa-related Cystoid Macular Edema. *Retina* **2018**, *38*, 416–423. [CrossRef]
116. Park, U.C.; Park, J.H.; Ma, D.J.; Cho, I.H.; Oh, B.-L.; Yu, H.G. A randomized paired-eye trial of intravitreal dexamethasone implant for cystoid macular edema in retinitis pigmentosa. *Retina* **2020**, *40*, 1359–1366. [CrossRef]
117. Veritti, D.; Sarao, V.; De Nadai, K.; Chizzolini, M.; Parmeggiani, F.; Perissin, L.; Lanzetta, P. Dexamethasone Implant Produces Better Outcomes than Oral Acetazolamide in Patients with Cystoid Macular Edema Secondary to Retinitis Pigmentosa. *J. Ocul. Pharmacol. Ther.* **2020**, *36*, 190–197. [CrossRef]
118. Fonollosa, A.; Llorenç, V.; Artaraz, J.; Jimenez, B.; Ruiz-Arruza, I.; Agirrebengoa, K.; Cordero-Coma, M.; Costales-Mier, F.; Adan, A. Safety and efficacy of intravitreal dexamethasone implants in the management of macular edema secondary to infectious uveitis. *Retina* **2016**, *36*, 1778–1785. [CrossRef]
119. Agarwal, A.; Handa, S.; Aggarwal, K.; Sharma, M.; Singh, R.; Sharma, A.; Agrawal, R.; Sharma, K.; Gupta, V. The Role of Dexamethasone Implant in the Management of Tubercular Uveitis. *Ocul. Immunol. Inflamm.* **2018**, *26*, 884–892. [CrossRef]
120. Jain, L.; Panda, K.G.; Basu, S. Clinical Outcomes of Adjunctive Sustained-Release Intravitreal Dexamethasone Implants in Tuberculosis-Associated Multifocal Serpigenoid Choroiditis. *Ocul. Immunol. Inflamm.* **2018**, *26*, 877–883. [CrossRef]
121. Lautredou, C.C.; Hardin, J.S.; Chancellor, J.R.; Uwaydat, S.H.; Ellabban, A.A.; Sallam, A.B. Repeat Intravitreal Dexamethasone Implant for Refractory Cystoid Macular Edema in Syphilitic Uveitis. *Case Rep. Ophthalmol. Med.* **2018**, *2018*, 7419823. [CrossRef] [PubMed]
122. Dutta Majumder, P.; Mayilvakanam, L.; Palker, A.; Sridharan, S.; Biswas, J. Intravitreal sustained-release dexamethasone implant for the treatment of persistent cystoid macular edema in ocular syphilis. *Indian J. Ophthalmol.* **2019**, *67*, 1487–1490. [PubMed]
123. Majumder, P.D.; Biswas, J.; Ambreen, A.; Amin, R.; Pannu, Z.R.; Bedda, A.M. Intravitreal dexamethasone implant for the treatment of cystoid macular oedema associated with acute retinal necrosis. *J. Ophthalmic Inflamm. Infect.* **2016**, *6*, 49. [CrossRef] [PubMed]
124. Seibel, I.; Hager, A.; Riechardt, A.I.; Davids, A.M.; Böker, A.; Joussen, A.M. Antiangiogenic or Corticosteroid Treatment in Patients with Radiation Maculopathy after Proton Beam Therapy for Uveal Melanoma. *Am. J. Ophthalmol.* **2016**, *168*, 31–39. [CrossRef]
125. Frizziero, L.; Parrozzani, R.; Trainiti, S.; Pilotto, E.; Miglionico, G.; Pulze, S.; Midena, E. Intravitreal dexamethasone implant in radiation-induced macular oedema. *Br. J. Ophthalmol.* **2017**, *101*, 1699–1703. [CrossRef]
126. Russo, A.; Reibaldi, M.; Avitabile, T.; Uva, M.G.; Franco, L.M.; Gagliano, C.; Bonfiglio, V.; Spatola, C.; Privitera, G.; Longo, A. Dexamethasone intravitreal implant vs. ranibizumab in the treatment of macular edema secondary to brachytherapy for choroidal melanoma. *Retina* **2018**, *38*, 788–794. [CrossRef]
127. Arrigo, A.; Knutsson, K.A.; Rajabjan, F.; Augustin, V.A.; Bandello, F.; Parodi, M.B. Combined central retinal vein occlusion and branch retinal artery occlusion treated with intravitreal dexamethasone implant: A case report. *Eur. J. Ophthalmol.* **2020**. [CrossRef]
128. Ozturk, T.; Takes, O.; Saatci, A.O. Dexamethasone implant (ozurdex) in a case with unilateral simultaneous central retinal vein and branch retinal artery occlusion. *Case Rep. Ophthalmol.* **2015**, *6*, 76–81. [CrossRef]
129. Fenicia, V.; Balestrieri, M.; Perdicchi, A.; Maraone, G.; Recupero, S.M. Intravitreal injection of dexamethasone implant in serous macular detachment associated with Waldenström's disease. *Case Rep. Ophthalmol.* **2013**, *4*, 64–69. [CrossRef]
130. Georgakopoulos, C.D.; Plotas, P.; Angelakis, A.; Kagkelaris, K.; Tzouvara, E.; Makri, O.E. Dexamethasone implant for immunogammopathy maculopathy associated with IgA multiple myeloma. *Ther. Adv. Ophthalmol.* **2019**, *11*, 251584141882044. [CrossRef]
131. Nuzzi, R.; Monteu, F. Use of Intravitreal Dexamethasone in a Case of Anterior Ischemic Optic Neuropathy. *Case Rep. Ophthalmol.* **2017**, *8*, 452–458. [CrossRef] [PubMed]

132. Saatci, A.O.; Ayhan, Z.; Yaman, A.; Bora, E.; Ulgenalp, A.; Kavukcu, S. A 12-Year-Old Girl with Bilateral Coats Disease and ABCA4 Gene Mutation. *Case Rep. Ophthalmol.* **2018**, *9*, 375–380. [CrossRef] [PubMed]
133. Kumar, K.; Raj, P.; Chandnani, N.; Agarwal, A. Intravitreal dexamethasone implant with retinal photocoagulation for adult-onset Coats' disease. *Int. Ophthalmol.* **2019**, *39*, 465–470. [CrossRef] [PubMed]
134. Cebeci, Z.; Oray, M.; Tuncer, S.; Tugal Tutkun, I.; Kir, N. Intravitreal dexamethasone implant (Ozurdex) and photodynamic therapy for vasoproliferative retinal tumours. *Can. J. Ophthalmol.* **2014**, *49*, e83–e84. [CrossRef] [PubMed]
135. Kong, X.; Psaras, C.; Stewart, J.M. Dexamethasone Intravitreal Implant Injection in Eyes with Comorbid Hypotony. *Ophthalmol. Retin.* **2019**, *3*, 993–997. [CrossRef] [PubMed]
136. Ahn, S.J.; Joung, J.; Lee, S.H.; Lee, B.R. Intravitreal dexamethasone implant therapy for the treatment of cystoid macular Oedema due to hydroxychloroquine retinopathy: A case report and literature review. *BMC Ophthalmol.* **2018**, *18*, 310. [CrossRef]
137. Kim, M.S.; Hong, H.K.; Park, K.H.; Woo, S.J. Intravitreal Dexamethasone Implant with Plasma Autoantibody Monitoring for Cancer-associated Retinopathy. *Korean J. Ophthalmol.* **2019**, *33*, 298. [CrossRef]
138. Mukhtar, S.; Potter, S.M.; Khurshid, S.G. Dexamethasone intravitreal implant for X-linked (juvenile) retinoschisis. *Retin. Cases Brief Rep.* **2019**, *13*, 18–20. [CrossRef]
139. Bulut, M.N.; Çalll, Ü.; Göktaş, E.; Bulut, K.; Kandemir, B.; Özertürk, Y. Use of an Intravitreal Dexamethasone Implant (Ozurdex) in a Case with Accidental Foveal Photocoagulation by Alexandrite Laser. *Case Rep. Ophthalmol.* **2016**, *7*, 130–134. [CrossRef]
140. Corbelli, E.; Fasce, F.; Iuliano, L.; Sacconi, R.; Lattanzio, R.; Bandello, F.; Querques, G. Cataract surgery with combined versus deferred intravitreal dexamethasone implant for diabetic macular edema: Long-term outcomes from a real-world setting. *Acta Diabetol.* **2020**. [CrossRef]
141. Panozzo, G.A.; Gusson, E.; Panozzo, G.; Dalla Mura, G. Dexamethasone intravitreal implant at the time of cataract surgery in eyes with diabetic macular edema. *Eur. J. Ophthalmol.* **2017**, *27*, 433–437. [CrossRef] [PubMed]
142. Furino, C.; Boscia, F.; Niro, A.; Giancipoli, E.; Grassi, M.O.; D'amico Ricci, G.; Blasetti, F.; Reibaldi, M.; Alessio, G. Combined Phacoemulsification and Intravitreal Dexamethasone Implant (Ozurdex®) in Diabetic Patients with Coexisting Cataract and Diabetic Macular Edema. *J. Ophthalmol.* **2017**, *2017*, 4896036. [CrossRef] [PubMed]
143. Ragam, A.P.; Kolomeyer, A.M.; Nayak, N.V.; Chu, D.S. The use of ozurdex (dexamethasone intravitreal implant) during anterior segment surgery in patients with chronic recurrent uveitis. *J. Ocul. Pharmacol. Ther.* **2015**, *31*, 344–349. [CrossRef] [PubMed]
144. Jinagal, J.; Gupta, G.; Agarwal, A.; Aggarwal, K.; Akella, M.; Gupta, V.; Suri, D.; Gupta, A.; Singh, S.; Ram, J. Safety and efficacy of dexamethasone implant along with phacoemulsification and intraocular lens implantation in children with juvenile idiopathic arthritis associated uveitis. *Indian J. Ophthalmol.* **2019**, *67*, 69–74. [PubMed]
145. Giannaccare, G.; Fresina, M.; Pazzaglia, A.; Versura, P. Long-lasting corneal endothelial graft rejection successfully reversed after dexamethasone intravitreal implant. *Int. Med. Case Rep. J.* **2016**, *9*, 187–191. [CrossRef] [PubMed]
146. Vinciguerra, P.; Albé, E.; Vinciguerra, R.; Romano, M.M.; Trazza, S.; Mastropasqua, L.; Epstein, D. Long-term resolution of immunological graft rejection after a dexamethasone intravitreal implant. *Cornea* **2015**, *34*, 471–474. [CrossRef]
147. Pastor, J.C.; Rojas, J.; Pastor-Idoate, S.; Di Lauro, S.; Gonzalez-Buendia, L.; Delgado-Tirado, S. Proliferative vitreoretinopathy: A new concept of disease pathogenesis and practical consequences. *Prog. Retin. Eye Res.* **2016**, *51*, 125–155. [CrossRef]
148. Govetto, A.; Sarraf, D.; Hubschman, J.P.; Tadayoni, R.; Couturier, A.; Chehaibou, I.; Au, A.; Grondin, C.; Virgili, G.; Romano, M.R. Distinctive Mechanisms and Patterns of Exudative Versus Tractional Intraretinal Cystoid Spaces as Seen with Multimodal Imaging. *Am. J. Ophthalmol.* **2020**, *212*, 43–56. [CrossRef]
149. Banerjee, P.J.; Quartilho, A.; Bunce, C.; Xing, W.; Zvobgo, T.M.; Harris, N.; Charteris, D.G. Slow-Release Dexamethasone in Proliferative Vitreoretinopathy: A Prospective, Randomized Controlled Clinical Trial. *Ophthalmology* **2017**, *124*, 757–767. [CrossRef]

150. Iovino, C.; Giannaccare, G.; Pellegrini, M.; Bernabei, F.; Braghiroli, M.; Caporossi, T.; Peiretti, E. Efficacy and safety of combined vitrectomy with intravitreal dexamethasone implant for advanced stage epiretinal membrane. *Drug Des. Devel. Ther.* **2019**, *13*, 4107–4114. [CrossRef]
151. Hostovsky, A.; Muni, R.H.; Eng, K.T.; Mulhall, D.; Leung, C.; Kertes, P.J. Intraoperative Dexamethasone Intravitreal Implant (Ozurdex) in Vitrectomy Surgery for Epiretinal Membrane. *Curr. Eye Res.* **2019**, *45*, 737–741. [CrossRef] [PubMed]
152. Kim, K.T.; Jang, J.W.; Kang, S.W.; Chae, J.B.; Cho, K.; Bae, K. Vitrectomy Combined with Intraoperative Dexamethasone Implant for the Management of Refractory Diabetic Macular Edema. *Korean J. Ophthalmol.* **2019**, *33*, 249. [CrossRef] [PubMed]
153. Cakir, A.; Erden, B.; Bolukbasi, S.; Aydin, A.; Yurttaser Ocak, S.; Maden, G.; Elcioglu, M.N. Comparison of the effect of ranibizumab and dexamethasone implant in diabetic macular edema with concurrent epiretinal membrane. *J. Fr. Ophtalmol.* **2019**, *42*, 683–689. [CrossRef] [PubMed]
154. Jung, Y.H.; Lee, Y. Efficacy of vitrectomy combined with an intraoperative dexamethasone implant in refractory diabetic macular edema. *Acta Diabetol.* **2019**, *56*, 691–696. [CrossRef]
155. Uwaydat, S.H.; Wang, H.; Sallam, A.B. Intraoperative Injection of Intravitreal Dexamethasone Implant Using a Vitrectomy Trocar-Assisted Technique. *Retina* **2019**, *39*, S123–S124. [CrossRef]
156. Miele, A.; Govetto, A.; Fumagalli, C.; Donati, S.; Biagini, I.; Azzolini, C.; Rizzo, S.; Virgili, G. Ocular hypertension and glaucoma following vitrectomy: A systematic review. *Retina* **2018**, *38*, 1–8. [CrossRef]
157. Govetto, A.; Domínguez, R.; Landaluce, M.L.; Álves, M.T.; Lorente, R. Prevalence of open angle glaucoma in vitrectomized eyes: A cross-sectional study. *Retina* **2014**, *34*, 1623–1629. [CrossRef]
158. Pang, J.P.; Son, G.; Yoon, Y.H.; Kim, J.-G.; Lee, J.Y. Combined vitrectomy with intravitreal dexamethasone implant for refractory macular edema secondary to diabetic retinopathy, retinal vein occlusion, and noninfectious posterior uveitis. *Retina* **2020**, *40*, 56–65. [CrossRef]
159. Govetto, A.; Su, D.; Farajzadeh, M.; Megerdichian, A.; Platner, E.; Ducournau, Y.; Virgili, G.; Hubschman, J.P. Microcystoid Macular Changes in Association with Idiopathic Epiretinal Membranes in Eyes With and Without Glaucoma: Clinical Insights. *Am. J. Ophthalmol.* **2017**, *181*, 156–165. [CrossRef]
160. Iglicki, M.; Zur, D.; Fung, A.; Gabrielle, P.H.; Lupidi, M.; Santos, R.; Busch, C.; Rehak, M.; Cebeci, Z.; Charles, M.; et al. TRActional DIabetic reTInal detachment surgery with co-adjuvant intravitreal dexamethasONe implant: The tradition study. *Acta Diabetol.* **2019**, *56*, 1141–1147. [CrossRef]
161. Tunc, M.; Lahey, J.M.; Kearney, J.J.; Lewis, J.M.; Francis, R. Cystoid macular oedema following pneumatic retinopexy vs. scleral buckling. *Eye* **2007**, *21*, 831–834. [CrossRef] [PubMed]
162. Bonfiglio, V.; Fallico, M.R.; Russo, A.; De Grande, V.; Longo, A.; Uva, M.G.; Reibaldi, M.; Avitabile, T. Intravitreal dexamethasone implant for cystoid macular edema and inflammation after scleral buckling. *Eur. J. Ophthalmol.* **2015**, *25*, e98–e100. [CrossRef] [PubMed]
163. Thanos, A.; Todorich, B.; Yonekawa, Y.; Papakostas, T.D.; Khundkar, T.; Eliott, D.; Dass, A.B.; Williams, G.A.; Capone, A.; Faia, L.J.; et al. Dexamethasone intravitreal implant for the treatment of recalcitrant macular edema after rhegmatogenous retinal detachment repair. *Retina* **2018**, *38*, 1084–1090. [CrossRef] [PubMed]
164. Nehmé, A.; Lobenhofer, E.K.; Stamer, W.D.; Edelman, J.L. Glucocorticoids with different chemical structures but similar glucocorticoid receptor potency regulate subsets of common and unique genes in human trabecular meshwork cells. *BMC Med. Genom.* **2009**. [CrossRef]
165. Rajesh, B.; Zarranz-Ventura, J.; Fung, A.T.; Busch, C.; Sahoo, N.K.; Rodriguez-Valdes, P.J.; Sarao, V.; Mishra, S.K.; Saatci, A.O.; Udaondo Mirete, P.; et al. Safety of 6000 intravitreal dexamethasone implants. *Br. J. Ophthalmol.* **2019**, *104*, 39–46. [CrossRef]
166. Rosenblatt, A.; Udaondo, P.; Cunha-Vaz, J.; Sivaprasad, S.; Bandello, F.; Lanzetta, P.; Kodjikian, L.; Goldstein, M.; Habot-Wilner, Z.; Loewenstein, A.; et al. A Collaborative Retrospective Study on the Efficacy and Safety of Intravitreal Dexamethasone Implant (Ozurdex) in Patients with Diabetic Macular Edema: The European DME Registry Study. *Ophthalmology* **2020**, *127*, 377–393. [CrossRef]
167. Srinivasan, R.; Sharma, U.; George, R.; Raman, R.; Sharma, T. Intraocular pressure changes after dexamethasone implant in patients with glaucoma and steroid responders. *Retina* **2019**, *39*, 157–162. [CrossRef]

168. Sharma, A.; Kuppermann, B.D.; Bandello, F.; Lanzetta, P.; Zur, D.; Park, S.W.; Yu, H.G.; Saravanan, V.R.; Zacharias, L.C.; Barreira, A.K.; et al. Intraocular pressure (IOP) after intravitreal dexamethasone implant (Ozurdex) amongst different geographic populations—GEODEX-IOP study. *Eye* **2019**, *34*, 1063–1068. [CrossRef]
169. Wannamaker, K.W.; Kenny, S.; Das, R.; Mendlovitz, A.; Comstock, J.M.; Chu, E.R.; Bahadorani, S.; Gresores, N.J.; Beck, K.D.; Krambeer, C.J.; et al. The effects of temporary intraocular pressure spikes after intravitreal dexamethasone implantation on the retinal nerve fiber layer. *Clin. Ophthalmol.* **2019**, *13*, 1079–1086. [CrossRef]
170. Ayar, O.; Alpay, A.; Koban, Y.; Akdemir, M.O.; Yazgan, S.; Canturk Ugurbas, S.; Ugurbas, S.H. The Effect of Dexamethasone Intravitreal Implant on Retinal Nerve Fiber Layer in Patients Diagnosed with Branch Retinal Vein Occlusion. *Curr. Eye Res.* **2017**, *42*, 1287–1292. [CrossRef]
171. Rahimy, E.; Khurana, R.N. Anterior segment migration of dexamethasone implant: Risk factors, complications, and management. *Curr. Opin. Ophthalmol.* **2017**, *28*, 246–251. [CrossRef] [PubMed]
172. Röck, D.; Bartz-Schmidt, K.U.; Röck, T. Risk factors for and management of anterior chamber intravitreal dexamethasone implant migration. *BMC Ophthalmol.* **2019**, *19*, 120. [CrossRef] [PubMed]
173. Sherman, T.; Raman, V. Incomplete scleral penetration of dexamethasone (Ozurdex) intravitreal implant. *BMJ Case Rep.* **2018**. [CrossRef] [PubMed]
174. Fasce, F.; Battaglia Parodi, M.; Knutsson, K.A.; Spinelli, A.; Mauceri, P.; Bolognesi, G.; Bandello, F. Accidental injection of dexamethasone intravitreal implant in the crystalline lens. *Acta Ophthalmol.* **2014**, *92*, e330–e331. [CrossRef]
175. Luaces-Rodríguez, A.; González-Barcia, M.; Blanco-Teijeiro, M.J.; Gil-Martínez, M.; Gonzalez, F.; Gómez-Ulla, F.; Lamas, M.J.; Otero-Espinar, F.J.; Fernández-Ferreiro, A. Review of intraocular pharmacokinetics of anti-infectives commonly used in the treatment of infectious endophthalmitis. *Pharmaceutics* **2018**, *10*, 66. [CrossRef]
176. Kang, Y.K.; Park, H.S.; Park, D.H.; Shin, J.P. Incidence and treatment outcomes of secondary epiretinal membrane following intravitreal injection for diabetic macular edema. *Sci. Rep.* **2020**, *10*, 528. [CrossRef]
177. Kucukevcilioglu, M.; Eren, M.; Yolcu, U.; Sobaci, G. Acute retinal necrosis following intravitreal dexamethasone (Ozurdex®) implant. *Arq. Bras. Oftalmol.* **2015**, *78*, 118–119. [CrossRef]
178. Thrane, A.S.; Hove, M.; Kjersem, B.; Krohn, J. Acute retinal necrosis and ocular neovascularization caused by cytomegalovirus following intravitreal dexamethasone implant (Ozurdex®) in an immunocompetent patient. *Acta Ophthalmol.* **2016**, *94*, e813–e814. [CrossRef]
179. Uwaydat, S.H.; Sallam, A.B.; Wang, H.; Goyal, S. Retinal indentation by a dexamethasone implant in a gas-filled eye: Report of an unusual complication. *JAMA Ophthalmol.* **2017**, *135*, 1125–1127. [CrossRef]
180. Agrawal, R.; Fernandez-Sanz, G.; Bala, S.; Addison, P.K.F. Desegmentation of Ozurdex implant in vitreous cavity: Report of two cases. *Br. J. Ophthalmol.* **2014**, *98*, 961–963. [CrossRef]
181. Danan, J.; Heitz, A.; Bourcier, T. Periorbital necrotizing fasciitis following dexamethasone intravitreal implant injection. *JAMA Ophthalmol.* **2016**, *134*, 110–111. [CrossRef] [PubMed]
182. Polizzi, S.; Mahajan, V.B. Intravitreal Anti-VEGF Injections in Pregnancy: Case Series and Review of Literature. *J. Ocul. Pharmacol. Ther.* **2015**, *31*, 605–610. [CrossRef] [PubMed]
183. Capuano, V.; Serra, R.; Oubraham, H.; Zambrowski, O.; Amana, D.; Zerbib, J.; Souied, E.H.; Querques, G. Dexamethasone intravitreal implant for choroidal neovascularization during pregnancy. *Retin. Cases Brief Rep.* **2019**, *13*, 300–307. [CrossRef] [PubMed]
184. Concillado, M.; Lund-Andersen, H.; Mathiesen, E.R.; Larsen, M. Dexamethasone Intravitreal Implant for Diabetic Macular Edema during Pregnancy. *Am. J. Ophthalmol.* **2016**, *165*, 7–15. [CrossRef] [PubMed]
185. Hodzic-Hadzibegovic, D.; Ba-Ali, S.; Valerius, M.; Lund-Andersen, H. Quantification of fluid resorption from diabetic macular oedema with foveal serous detachment after dexamethasone intravitreal implant (Ozurdex®) in a pregnant diabetic. *Acta Ophthalmol.* **2017**, *95*, 324–325. [CrossRef] [PubMed]

pharmaceutics

Pharmaceutics 2020, 12, 611

Article

Characterization, Stability, and In Vivo Efficacy Studies of Recombinant Human CNTF and Its Permeation into the Neural Retina in Ex Vivo Organotypic Retinal Explant Culture Models

Jaakko Itkonen [1,*], Ada Annala [2,3], Shirin Tavakoli [1], Blanca Arango-Gonzalez [4], Marius Ueffing [4], Elisa Toropainen [2], Marika Ruponen [2], Marco G. Casteleijn [1,5] and Arto Urtti [1,2,6,*]

1. Drug Research Program, Faculty of Pharmacy, University of Helsinki, Viikinkaari 5 E, 00790 Helsinki, Finland; shirin.tavakoli@helsinki.fi (S.T.); marco.casteleijn@vtt.fi (M.G.C.)
2. School of Pharmacy, University of Eastern Finland, Yliopistonranta 1, 70211 Kuopio, Finland; a.k.a.annala@uu.nl (A.A.); elisa.toropainen@uef.fi (E.T.); marika.ruponen@uef.fi (M.R.)
3. Utrecht Institute for Pharmaceutical Science, Utrecht University, David de Wiedgebouw, Universiteitsweg 99, 3584 CG Utrecht, The Netherlands
4. Institute for Ophthalmic Research, Centre for Ophthalmology, University of Tübingen, Elfriede-Aulhorn-Strasse 7, D-72076 Tübingen, Germany; blanca.arango-gonzalez@klinikum.uni-tuebingen.de (B.A.-G.); marius.ueffing@uni-tuebingen.de (M.U.)
5. VTT Technical Research Centre of Finland Ltd., Solutions for Natural Resources and Environment, Tietotie 2, Espoo, P.O. Box 1000, FI-02044 VTT, Finland
6. Laboratory of Biohybrid Technologies, Institute of Chemistry, St. Petersburg State University, Universitetskii pr. 26, Peterhoff, 198504 St. Petersburg, Russia

* Correspondence: jaakko.itkonen@helsinki.fi (J.I.); arto.urtti@helsinki.fi (A.U.)

Received: 10 June 2020; Accepted: 28 June 2020; Published: 30 June 2020

Abstract: Ciliary neurotrophic factor (CNTF) is one of the most studied neuroprotective agents with acknowledged potential in treating diseases of the posterior eye segment. Although its efficacy and mechanisms of action in the retina have been studied extensively, it is still not comprehensively understood which retinal cells mediate the therapeutic effects of CNTF. As with therapeutic proteins in general, it is poorly elucidated whether exogenous CNTF administered into the vitreous can enter and distribute into the retina and hence reach potentially responsive target cells. Here, we have characterized our purified recombinant human CNTF (rhCNTF), studied the protein's in vitro bioactivity in a cell-based assay, and evaluated the thermodynamic and oligomeric status of the protein during storage. Biological activity of rhCNTF was further evaluated in vivo in an animal model of retinal degeneration. The retinal penetration and distribution of rhCNTF after 24 h was studied utilizing two ex vivo retina models. Based on our characterization findings, our rhCNTF is correctly folded and biologically active. Moreover, based on initial screening and subsequent follow-up, we identified two buffers in which rhCNTF retains its stability during storage. Whereas rhCNTF did not show photoreceptor preservative effect or improve the function of photoreceptors in vivo, this could possibly be due to the used disease model or the short duration of action with a single intravitreal injection of rhCNTF. On the other hand, the lack of in vivo efficacy was shown to not be due to distribution limitations; permeation into the retina was observed in both retinal explant models as in 24 h rhCNTF penetrated the inner limiting membrane, and being mostly observed in the ganglion cell layer, distributed to different layers of the neural retina. As rhCNTF can reach deeper retinal layers, in general, having direct effects on resident CNTF-responsive target cells is plausible.

Keywords: retinal penetration; neuroprotection; protein aggregation; stability; intravitreal delivery; CNTF

1. Introduction

Progressive diseases of the posterior eye segment, and in particular those affecting the retina, are among the most common causes of visual impairment and blindness [1]. Cataract and glaucoma, for instance, are the two leading causes of blindness globally, whereas age-related macular degeneration (AMD) is the most common culprit for legal blindness in the aged population in high-income countries, affecting approximately 10% of the population over 60 years of age [2,3]. Degenerative diseases of the posterior eye segment, including conditions such as diabetic retinopathy and retinitis pigmentosa (RP), are often age-related, and their prevalence is growing in the aging populations.

Pharmaceuticals that target retinal disease pathogenesis are currently available only for the treatment of diabetic macular edema and the wet form of AMD, conditions that feature pathological angiogenesis in the retina, which is driven by the overexpression of pro-angiogenic factors [3]. Whereas other factors are involved, the vascular endothelial growth factors (VEGFs) are recognized as the main mediators responsible for the pathological neovascularization in the posterior eye segment [2]. Interfering with VEGFs' binding to their receptors (VEGFRs) inhibits the VEGF-triggered actions of these receptor tyrosine kinases. As such, VEGF-blocking as a treatment strategy is most commonly achieved with therapeutic proteins that bind and neutralize VEGF [1].

Although neovascular diseases result in retinal neurodegeneration in particular during advanced stages, anti-VEGF treatments rescue retinal neurons indirectly, and their ocular use is limited to treating neovascular diseases only. Effective treatments affecting retinal degeneration directly are still lacking [4]. As advanced posterior segment diseases in general feature degeneration and loss of retinal neurons, with photoreceptor loss ultimately accounting for the experienced loss of vision, targeting the involved pathways by means of direct neuroprotection is considered a more universal approach to combat retinal neurodegeneration [4,5]. Several growth factors and neurotrophic factors, e.g., brain-derived neurotrophic factor, fibroblast growth factors, glial cell-line derived factor, and nerve growth factor have been studied in preclinical animal models for their neuroprotective potential in oculo [6,7]. In addition to these, the ciliary neurotrophic factor (CNTF) is arguably the most studied and has progressed the furthest in clinical trials [4,8].

CNTF has an approximate molecular mass of 23 kDa and a four α-helix bundle tertiary structure [9,10]. It belongs to the interleukin-6 (IL-6) family of neuropoietic cytokines and exerts neurotrophic effects on a variety of neurons. Lacking a signal sequence for secretion, the mechanism by which CNTF gets released from cells is still unknown and postulated to occur upon cellular injury [8,11]. CNTF elicits its actions through a receptor complex consisting of the ligand-specific α-receptor CNTFRα, and β-receptors glycoprotein 130 (gp130) and leukemia inhibitory factor receptor β (LIFRβ) [9,11]. Lacking transmembrane and cytoplasmic domains, CNTFRα is anchored to the cell membrane by a glycosylphosphatidylinositol linker; cleavage of this linker can release soluble receptor, sCNTFRα, rendering cells expressing just gp130 and LIFRβ also capable of responding to CNTF [9].

In the retina, CNTF expression spans all layers and occurs in several cell types, such as retinal pigment epithelium (RPE), and particularly in glial cells such as astrocytes and Müller cells [8,12,13]. CNTF protein expression is upregulated in response to, e.g., stress and injury [12,14,15]. CNTFRα expressing retinal cells include astrocytes, Müller cells, retinal ganglion cells (RGC), rod and cone photoreceptors, and RPE [8,13,15–19]. Whereas both murine and rat central nervous system (CNS) microglia express CNTFRα [20–22], it is not fully clear whether local resident microglia do so in the retina, although they have nonetheless been shown to respond to CNTF [23].

Whereas CNTFRα expressing retinal cells are potentially responsive to CNTF, it is not established whether all of CNTF's effects on different cell types are, in fact, direct or mediated indirectly by specific cells [8]. Observations on species differences in retinal CNTFRα expression in part complicate interpreting and extrapolating findings from one species to another [16]. Additionally, non-CNTFRα expressing retinal cells expressing the common signal transduction components could nonetheless be conferred responsive to CNTF by sCNTFRα [8,24]. Currently, CNTF's neuroprotective effects on RGCs and photoreceptors are thought to take place (mostly) indirectly via Müller cells [8,12,25], which are postulated to respond to CNTF stimulation by expressing and releasing other cytokines and neurotrophic factors that relay CNTF's neuroprotective effects to other retinal cells [15,18,25–28].

Although the mechanisms and mediators of the biological effects of CNTF are still not fully resolved, its supportive and neuroprotective actions against retinal damage and degeneration have been demonstrated in various animal models of retinal disease [5,8]. The photoreceptor preservative effect related to upregulation of endogenous CNTF after mechanical or light-induced damage is well-reported in literature [14,29,30], and multiple teams working on viral-mediated gene therapies or sustained release delivery systems have demonstrated the protective effects of CNTF in different animal models of retinal degeneration [31–36]. While intravitreally administered CNTF has been shown to protect photoreceptors from light-induced damage, the preservative effect on photoreceptor degeneration caused by a genetic defect has not been as clear and seems, to some extent, to depend on the species and disease model [36–39]. In S334ter-3 rats, intravitreal (IVT) injection of CNTF improved the retinal morphology, and especially the cone photoreceptors seemed to benefit from the treatment [35,40]. In a Royal College of Surgeons (RCS) rat, single subretinal injection of recombinant CNTF showed a long-term photoreceptor preservative effect up to 36 days [33]. However, the efficacy of intravitreally administered CNTF has not been previously studied in this animal model.

Certain aspects of CNTF have been inadequately described in the literature. Whereas hCNTF variants with improved stability were in development for CNS delivery [41], publications reporting on the formulation and related stabilization efforts on CNTF are scarce. Previously, we reported on the optimized soluble expression and purification of our recombinant human CNTF (rhCNTF) [42]. Here, we describe further characterization and stability studies of rhCNTF. Although the Müller glia cells are considered the primary mediators of CNTF's actions in the retina, direct effects on other cells cannot be ruled out as CNTF-responsive as well as CNTFRα-expressing cells have been identified in several retinal layers [8]. However, little is known about the retinal penetration and distribution of exogenously administered CNTF, although the inner limiting membrane (ILM) at the vitreoretinal interface has been postulated to be the biggest limitation to CNTF's entry into the retina [27]. Here, we evaluate the efficacy of intravitreally administered rhCNTF in vivo in RCS rat and report on the retinal penetration and distribution of our rhCNTF in organotypic ex vivo retinal explant cultures.

2. Materials and Methods

2.1. Protein Production

The features and construction of the expression plasmid pOPINF-hCNTF as well as the expression and purification of soluble recombinant His_6-hCNTF, from now on referred to as rhCNTF, have been described earlier [42,43]. Aside from expression in Rosetta™ 2(DE3)pLysS (Novagen, Merck KGaA, Darmstadt, Germany) *E. coli* cells using the Overnight Express™ Instant TB auto-induction culture medium (Novagen, Merck) [44], rhCNTF was also expressed in the aforementioned cells using EnPresso® B growth system [45] (BioSilta Oy, Oulu, Finland) according to the manufacturer's specifications.

Protein purification was carried out as describer earlier [42] and is described in more detail in the Supplement. For further studies, the purified protein was kept on ice at 4 °C as well as snapfrozen with liquid N_2 for storage at −80 °C.

2.2. *rhCNTF In Vitro Bioactivity Study*

The correct function, and thus indirectly the proper folding of purified rhCNTF, was demonstrated earlier in an enzyme-linked immunosorbent assay (ELISA) binding study with the cognate receptor CNTFRα [42]. To ensure that rhCNTF can trigger downstream signaling and hence biological responses, an in vitro cell study was performed.

2.2.1. Cell Culture

TF-1-CN5a.1 (product CRL-2512™, American Type Culture Collection, ATCC®, Manassas, VA, USA) cells were obtained from LGC Standards (Teddington, UK). The cells were maintained in complete growth medium of Roswell Park Memorial Institute (RPMI) 1640 medium, 2 mM L-glutamine, 1.5 g/L sodium bicarbonate, 4.5 g/L glucose, 10 mM HEPES, and 1.0 mM sodium pyruvate (RPMI-1640, ATCC modification; Gibco™, Thermo Fisher Scientific, Waltham, MA, USA) supplemented with 10% fetal bovine serum (Gibco™, Thermo Fisher Scientific), 2 ng/mL human granulocyte macrophage colony-stimulating factor (hGM-CSF) (Sigma-Aldrich, St. Louis, MO, USA), 0.4 mg/mL G-418 (Calbiochem™, Merck), and 100 U/mL penicillin – 100 µg/mL streptomycin (Gibco™, Thermo Fisher Scientific). The cells were maintained as stationary suspension cultures in non-treated Nunc™ EasyFlask™ 75 cm^2 flasks (Thermo Fisher Scientific) in a fully humidified 5% CO_2 atmosphere at 37 °C. Cell number and viability were determined using trypan blue.

2.2.2. Cell Proliferation Assay

The bioactivity of the purified rhCNTF was verified by measuring cell proliferation in a 5-bromo-2′-deoxyuridine (BrdU) incorporation assay [46], using the Cell Proliferation ELISA BrdU kit (Roche Diagnostics, Mannheim, Germany) according to manufacturer's specifications. First, 50 µL of serial dilutions of purified rhCNTF in assay growth medium, i.e., complete growth medium without hGM-CSF and G-418, were prepared and added in triplicates to the wells of CELLSTAR® 96-well microplates for suspension cells (Greiner Bio-One GmbH, Kremsmünster, Austria). Cultured TF-1.CN5a.1 cells were first centrifuged and washed with RPMI-1640 to remove hGM-CSF, followed by resuspension in assay growth medium. Cells were then seeded at 1.0×10^4 cells in 50 µL/well (final rhCNTF concentrations 24 fg/mL–100 ng/mL). Cells cultured in assay growth medium with and without 2 ng/mL hGM-CSF were used as positive and negative controls, respectively. Treated cells were incubated at 37 °C, 5% CO_2 for 48 h.

After incubation, 10 µL of 100 µM BrdU labeling solution was added to the wells and the cells (were) incubated for an additional 2 h, allowing for the incorporation of BrdU into the synthesized DNA during cell proliferation. After labeling, the suspended cells were pelleted by centrifugation at 300× *g* for 10 min, the media removed from the wells gently by pipetting, and the cells dried at 60 °C for 60 min. Then, 200 µL of FixDenat was added to each well for cell fixation and DNA denaturation and removed by pipetting after 30 min incubation at room temperature. Incubation with a peroxidase-conjugated anti-BrdU antibody was carried out for 90 min at room temperature to allow for binding to the incorporated and now exposed BrdU. Antibody solutions were then aspirated, and the cells were washed 4 times with 200 µL/well washing solution. After incubation with the 3,3′,5,5′-tetramethylbenzidine substrate solution 15 min, the absorbances were determined at 370 nm and 492 nm on a microplate reader (Varioskan® Flash; Thermo Fisher Scientific).

2.3. *rhCNTF Characterization and Stability Studies*

Upon visual inspection, we had observed precipitation—likely due to protein aggregation—taking place upon freeze-thawing with previously purified rhCNTF stored in 100 mM NaH_2PO_4, 50 mM NaCl, pH 8.0, 1 mM dithiothreitol (DTT) buffer at −80 °C resulting in a loss of approximately a third of stored protein (not shown). There was, hence, a clear need to find a more suitable storage buffer to stabilize the protein.

To gain insight on the structure and stability of rhCNTF, the protein was subjected to experiments using circular dichroism, differential scanning fluorimetry, and dynamic light scattering to characterize, e.g., secondary structure, thermal unfolding, and oligomeric state.

2.3.1. Circular Dichroism

Circular Dichroism (CD) spectroscopy was utilized to study the secondary structure and folding of the purified rhCNTF. Far-UV CD spectra (190–260 nm) of rhCNTF (0.2 mg/mL) samples desalted with 5 mM phosphate buffer were obtained in a 0.1 cm quartz cuvette at 25 °C with a Chirascan^{TM}-Plus CD Spectrometer (Applied Photophysics Ltd., Leatherhead, Surrey, UK). Background spectrum of the buffer was recorded and subtracted from subsequent triplicate spectral scans with the rhCNTF samples, with the average spectrum plotted. Pro-Data Viewer (Applied Photophysics) was used for data collection and handling. Data were normalized to protein concentrations and expressed in units of mean residue molar ellipticity. The BeStSel algorithm was also used for secondary structure determination from CD spectra [47].

Thermal denaturation and unfolding of rhCNTF was studied during thermal ramping from 25 to 92 °C (1 °C/min) with far-UV CD (190–260 nm) measurements every 2 °C. Values for the onset (T_{onset}) and midpoint (T_m) of unfolding were determined by plotting measured ellipticity at 222 nm, a signal proportional to α-helical content, as a function of temperature.

2.3.2. ThermoFluor

Differential scanning fluorimetry, commonly known as ThermoFluor, is a thermal shift assay based on an increase in the fluorescence of several non-specific protein-binding dyes upon their binding to certain regions and residues that become accessible during protein unfolding [48,49]. From the recorded fluorescence signal, parameters such as the T_h—the temperature of hydrophobic exposure—and other information of the thermal unfolding of proteins can be extracted. Here, based on observations that higher T_h correlates with higher conformational stability in formulation, different conditions were tested for their effects on the T_h of rhCNTF to screen for suitable buffers to stabilize the protein.

Buffers were pipetted to semi-skirted qPCR 96-well plates (Agilent Technologies, Inc., Santa Clara, CA, USA) while rhCNTF protein samples and SYPRO® Orange (Thermo Fisher Scientific) were applied as droplets on opposing edges of the wells to prevent premature interactions. Wells were sealed with Bio-Seal 7 Transparent Adhesive Seals for PCR plates (BIOplastics, Landgraaf, The Netherlands), the plates were quickly centrifuged to bring all components together in a total reaction volume of 25 µL, mixed by gentle vortexing, and again centrifuged. The measurements were carried out in a Stratagene Mx3005P qPCR instrument (Agilent Technologies). Samples were heated from 25 to 95 °C at a rate of 1 °C per 30 s. Fluorescence readouts were taken at every °C step using 492 nm and 610 nm as the excitation and emission wavelengths, respectively. Measurements were analyzed and T_h values determined with MxPro qPCR software (Agilent Technologies).

ThermoFluor was first carried out on a grid of varying rhCNTF and dye concentrations as a pre-screening to optimize protein/dye concentrations [50], and the subsequent measurements carried out with the best match. To study the effects of buffer, ionic strength, and pH on rhCNTF thermostability, 94 different conditions were screened for increased rhCNTF T_h (Table S1). Arising trends in the T_h as a surrogate for conformational stability were then followed with rhCNTF stored in chosen buffers at 4 °C and −80 °C.

2.3.3. Dynamic Light Scattering

The formation and presence of protein aggregates was assessed using dynamic light scattering (DLS). DLS measurements were carried out using Zetasizer APS (Malvern Panalytical Ltd., Malvern, Worcestershire, UK) with a 830 nm laser source using the Zetasizer Software (Malvern Panalytical) for data acquisition and analysis. Purified rhCNTF samples in the chosen buffers were diluted to 1.0 mg/mL and filtered using 0.22 µm polyethersulfone (PES) membrane filters to remove large particulates. Each sample was measured in triplicate at 2 °C. The size and hydrodynamic radius (R_h) distributions of detected particles were obtained by measuring and integrating the intensity of the scattered light, whereas for follow-up and comparing measurements, parameters were derived both via intensity and volume analysis.

Samples kept on ice at 4 °C after purification as well as snap-frozen samples stored at −80 °C were measured at different time points to assess for changes and trends in the R_h. For the cryo-stored samples, measurements with thawed unmixed sample as well as with the supernatant from centrifuged (21,100× *g*, 30 min at 4 °C) thawed rhCNTF were carried out for comparison.

The thermal aggregation behavior of rhCNTF was also studied with DLS by carrying out R_h measurements with freshly purified rhCNTF in both buffers during thermal ramping. To determine the onset temperature (T_{agg}), i.e., the temperature at which proteins start to associate and aggregate and at which scattering from HMW species intensifies, samples were heated from 2 to 60 °C and particle size measurements taken at each °C step. The measured Z-average (in nm) was plotted as a function of temperature.

2.4. *rhCNTF In Vivo Efficacy Study*

2.4.1. Animals

The photoreceptor preservative effect of rhCNTF was assessed in vivo after an IVT bolus injection using Royal College of Surgeons (RCS) rat as an animal model of retinal degeneration. The animals were 18 or 21 days old, both male and female. Animals were kept in controlled conditions (12 h light/dark cycle, temperature 21 ± 2 °C, humidity 55 ± 15%, ventilation 15 times per hour), housed with a maximum of 5 animals per stainless-steel cage (28.5 cm × 48.5 cm × 20 cm) with food and water provided ad libitum. The cages were changed twice a week and provided with sufficient bedding, nesting material, and enrichment. All procedures were performed in accordance to the European and national legislation on the protection of animals used for scientific or educational purposes (Directive 2010/63/EU, Act 497/2013, Decree 564/2013; ESAVI/6791/04.10.07/2013).

2.4.2. Intravitreal Injections

Stock solution of rhCNTF protein in buffer M (100 mM MES, 500 mM NaCl, pH 7.0) was thawed on ice prior to purification from aggregates by centrifuging (13,000× *g*, 15 min, +2 °C, Heraeus Biofuge Fresco, Heraeus Instruments). The supernatant was diluted to 500 ng/mL with buffer M with 1 mM DTT, sterile filtered through 0.2 μm PTFE membrane (Acrodisc® Syringe Filter CR13; PALL Corporation, Port Washington, NY, USA), stored in 4 °C, and used within one week. The final concentrations used for experiments were diluted with buffer M prior to injection from the stock solution.

Animals were weighed and anaesthetized with intraperitoneal (i.p.) injection of 1 mg/kg of medetomidine (Domitor vet 1 mg/mL, Orion Corporation, Espoo, Finland) and 75 mg/kg of ketamine (Ketaminol vet 50 mg/mL, Intervet International B.V), diluted with 0.9% sodium chloride solution (Natriumklorid Braun, B.Braun, Germany). The pupils were dilated with tropicamide (Oftan Tropicamid 5 mg/mL, Santen Pharmaceutical Co., Ltd., Osaka, Japan), which was allowed to affect for 10 min to achieve full dilation of the pupils. Finally, carbomer eye gel (Viscotears, Novartis International GA, Basel, Switzerland) was added to the eyes to prevent corneal desiccation.

In the 1st study set, 21-day-old animals received single IVT injection (2 μL) of 1 μg rhCNTF (n = 4), 500 ng rhCNTF (n = 5) and 250 ng rhCNTF (n = 4) or buffer M (n = 4) into one eye, while the contralateral eye was left untreated and served as an internal control.

In the 2nd study set, 18-day-old animals received single IVT injection (2 μL) of 1 μg rhCNTF (n = 7), or buffer M (n = 6) to one eye, while the contralateral eye was left untreated and served as an internal control. Untreated naïve control animals, NControl (n = 7) served as external control.

Injection was performed with 5 μL Hamilton® syringe (Hamilton Company, Inc., Reno, NV, USA) using a sharp point 34-gauge needle. Incision was done approximately 1 mm from the limbus, at a 45-degree angle, towards the back of the vitreous. Eyes of the animals were treated with antibiotic ointment after injection (Dexamethasone 1 mg/g, chloramphenicol 2 mg/g, Oftan Dexa-Chlora, Santen Pharmaceutical Co.) to prevent inflammation and to minimize solution efflux from the vitreous. Anesthesia was reversed with i.p. injection of atipamezole (Antisedan vet 5 mg/mL, Orion Corporation.). The animals were monitored during anesthesia and recovery from procedure was ensured. Any animals with welfare issues, visible injuries to the injected eye, or other signs of unsuccessful operation were determined as outliers and eliminated from the experiment.

2.4.3. Electroretinogram (ERG) Recording

Full-field ERG was recorded 1- and 2-weeks post-treatment. Animals were weighed and dark-adapted overnight, for a minimum of 12 h. All procedures were carried out under dim red light. The animals were anesthetized, pupils dilated, and carbomer gel added to the eyes as previously described. The animals were placed on a heated surface during the measurements. Rod responses were stimulated in dark-adapted conditions with series of dim blue flashes with increasing intensities (0.003, 0.007, 0.03, and 0.5 cd $\times$ s/m^2, number of sweeps 3, inter-sweep delay 5000 ms), whereas cone responses were stimulated under light-adapted conditions with series of bright white flashes (0.1, 1, 3, 5, 10, and 20 cd $\times$ s/m^2, number of sweeps 12, inter-sweep delay 0 ms) using ColorDome D125 (Diagnosys LLC, Lowell, MA, USA). The retinal responses were detected from the cornea with custom-made circular golden electrodes and recorded using Espion Visual Electrophysiology System V6 (Diagnosys LLC). The resulting retinograms were analyzed using Espion V6 software. The recovery of the animals was monitored for two days after every recording.

2.4.4. Data-Analysis

ERG results were analyzed using non-parametric testing using Microsoft Excel, GraphPad Prism 8, and IBM SPSS software. The parameter distribution between all treatment groups at all flash intensities was analyzed with the Kruskal–Wallis test. The comparison between the treated and untreated contralateral eye, as well as the comparison between the ERG values recorded 1 week and 2 weeks post-injection, was achieved with the Wilcoxon signed-rank test.

2.4.5. Histology

Animals were euthanized at the age of 35 days (2nd study set) or 38 days (1st study set) with CO_2 overdose followed by perfusion through the heart with 9% sodium chloride. The ocular tissue was pre-fixed in situ by perfusion through the heart by 4% paraformaldehyde (PFA) followed by ocular enucleation and fixation overnight in 4% PFA in 12-well plates in 4 °C. Thereafter, the eyes were rinsed in phosphate-buffered saline (PBS) for 2 to 6 h and dehydrated in the processing machine as described in Table S2 (Shandon Citadel 2000 Tissue Processor, Thermo Fisher Scientific). The eyes were embedded in liquid paraffin (64 °C), cooled to ambient temperature, and 5 μm vertical cross sections were cut close to the papilla (Leica SM2000R, Leica instruments GmbH, Germany or HM 355S Rotary Microtome, Thermo Fisher Scientific). Sections were flattened on warm water bath and collected on microscope slides and treated with hematoxylin and eosin (H&E) staining procedure according to Table S3. Glass slides were covered with DPX plastic and allowed to dry for 18 to 30 h. Sections were imaged using a Zeiss light microscope (Axio Imager M2; Carl Zeiss AG, Oberkochen, Germany) with 20× magnification (EC Plan-NEOFLUAR 20X/0.5 objective, Carl Zeiss AG) using AxioCam MRm (Carl Zeiss AG).

2.5. Retinal Penetration of rhCNTF

2.5.1. rhCNTF Fluorescent Labeling

Purified rhCNTF was fluorescently labeled with Alexa Fluor™ 488 Microscale Protein Labeling Kit (Thermo Fisher Scientific) via tetrafluorophenyl ester linkage to free amines according to manufacturer's instructions. Unreacted dye was separated from labeled protein with provided spin filters and the degree of labeling analyzed with a DropSense16 spectrophotometer (Trinean NV, Gentbrugge, Belgium) according to manufacturer's instructions, with a calculated degree of labeling (DOL) of 1.16 indicating the average number of dye molecules conjugated to each protein molecule. Labeled rhCNTF was aliquoted and stored on ice until use on rat retinal explant cultures.

Similarly, rhCNTF was fluorescently labeled with NT-647 (NanoTemper Technologies, München, Germany) via *N*-hydroxysuccinimide ester linkage to free amines according to manufacturer's instructions. Unreacted dye was removed with provided columns and the DOL analyzed with Varian Cary® 50 spectrophotometer (Agilent Technologies) according to manufacturer's instructions, with a calculated DOL of 0.557 indicating the average number of dye molecules conjugated to each protein molecule. Labeled rhCNTF was aliquoted and stored at −80 °C until use on bovine retinal explant cultures.

2.5.2. Retinal Explant Culture Preparation and rhCNTF Treatment

Rat Retinal Explants

Eyes obtained from CD® (SD) IGS rats were used to prepare organotypic retinal explant cultures as described earlier [51,52]. In brief, 5-, 6-, or 8-day-old animals were killed and the eyes enucleated in an aseptic environment. After cleansing with 70% ethanol, the eyes were incubated in basal R16 medium (Invitrogen, Paisley, UK) for 5 min, followed by incubation in pre-warmed 0.12% proteinase K (MP Biomedicals™, Thermo Fisher Scientific) for 15 min at 37 °C. To inactivate proteinase K, the eyes were incubated in basal R16 medium containing 20% fetal bovine serum (Sigma-Aldrich) for 5 min, and finally washed in serum-free basal R16 medium. Dissections were carried out aseptically in a Petri dish containing basal R16 medium. The anterior segment, sclera, choroid, lens, and the vitreous body were carefully removed, leaving only the retina together with the attached RPE. Finally, four relaxing cuts were made, and the retinae flat-mounted with the photoreceptor-side down on culture membrane inserts (0.4 μm; Corning Incorporated, Corning, NY, USA; 3412). Complete R16 medium was placed in the lower compartments of 6-well culture dishes, and the cultures were incubated at 36.5 °C and 5% CO_2. No antibiotics or antimycotics were used.

Explants were left without treatment for 24 h to allow them to adapt to culture conditions, followed by rhCNTF treatments for the next 24 h; the experiment duration was kept at a minimum to minimize explant deterioration, i.e., to retain the structure of all the retinal layers as close to native as possible. Alexa Fluor™ 488-labeled rhCNTF was prepared in PBS, diluted in basal R16 medium, and sterilized with 0.22 μM PES membrane filter before use. To mimic dosing via IVT and e.g., subretinal injections, treatments were given either apically as 15 μL drops (200 ng dose) carefully applied directly on top of the explant cultures or basolaterally as 4.7 μg/mL in complete medium below the explant in the lower compartment, respectively. Untreated complete R16 medium was used as control.

Bovine Retinal Explants

Retinal explant cultures were prepared as described earlier [53]. Fresh bovine eyes obtained from a local slaughterhouse were first cleaned off extra-ocular connective tissues followed by dipping in 20% ethanol. The eye was bisected 10 mm below the limbus, the anterior segment discarded and the vitreous removed, with the remaining posterior eye cup filled with cold CO_2 independent medium (Gibco™, Thermo Fisher Scientific) and cut into 4 flaps. While submerged in the medium, two circular pieces of the retina were isolated using a biopsy punch and then gently transferred onto moisturized 75 mm Transwell® membrane with the photoreceptor-side down. Explant culture medium (Neurobasal™-A, 2% B-27™ supplement, 2% penicillin–streptomycin, 1% L-glutamine; all Gibco™, Thermo Fisher Scientific) was added below the insert and the explants incubated at 37 °C and 5% CO_2.

Treatments were given directly after explant preparation; 10 μL of NT-647-labeled rhCNTF (3 μg dose) was applied gently on top of each explant, followed by incubation for 24 h at 37 °C.

2.5.3. Tissue Culture Fixation and Sectioning

Rat Retinal Explants

Treated rat explants were fixed in 4% PFA (Polysciences, Inc., Warrington, PA, USA) at 4 °C for 40 min. The fixative was then changed to 1% PFA and incubated at 4 °C overnight. Retinae were then washed with PBS for 10 min and cryoprotected by incubation in graded sucrose solutions (10%, 20%, and 30%). Subsequently, tissues were embedded in Tissue-Tek® O.C.T.™ Compound (Science Services GmbH, Munich, Germany). Vertical sections (14 µm) were obtained on a Leica CM3050S Microtome (Leica Biosystems, Wetzlar, Germany), air-dried at 37 °C for 1 h, and stored at −20 °C until use.

Bovine Retinal Explants

Treated bovine explants were fixed by replacing the medium below the filter with 4% PFA (in PBS). After 2 h of incubation at 4 °C, PFA was discarded and replaced with 30% sucrose solution (in PBS) and incubated overnight at 4 °C. Explants were snap-frozen in Tissue-Tek® O.C.T Compound using liquid nitrogen and sections (16 µm) cut from four different region of the explant with cryostat (Leica CM3050s).

2.5.4. Culture Staining and Imaging

Rat Retinal Explants

To prepare tissue sections from retinal explants for imaging, frozen cryosections were first air-dried at 37 °C. Slides with fixed sections of retinal tissue were washed 3 times with PBS and then mounted in Vectashield® (Vector Laboratories, Inc., Burlingame, CA, USA). Immunofluorescence staining of the mounted sections was carried out as described in the Supplement.

Mounted sections were imaged using a Zeiss Axio Imager Z1 ApoTome microscope equipped with a Zeiss AxioCam digital camera and AxioVision 4.7 software (all ZEISS). To observe the penetration of labeled rhCNTF, acquired images from multiple explant areas were assessed manually for the presence of fluorescence.

Bovine Retinal Explants

Sections from retinal explants were incubated for 1 h at room temperature in blocking solution (5% goat serum) followed by overnight incubation at 4 °C with rabbit anti-Collagen IV antibody (1:200) (Abcam plc., Cambridge, UK). Next, sections were stained with Alexa Fluor™ 488-labeled goat anti-rabbit secondary antibody (1:500) (Thermo Fisher Scientific) and 10 µg/mL Hoechst 33,342 (Invitrogen™, Thermo Fisher Scientific) for 1 h at room temperature.

Sections were mounted with Vectashield® (Vector Laboratories) and prepared for imaging. Sections were imaged with a Leica TCS SP8 confocal microscope using 20x (HC PL APO 20x/0.75 IMM CORR CS2) and 93x (HC PL APO 93x/1.30 motCORR STED WHITE) objectives (all Leica Microsystems GmbH, Wetzlar, Germany). As before, the presence of fluorescence was assessed manually from multiple explant areas to observe penetration of labeled rhCNTF.

3. Results

3.1. Protein Production

After expression, harvesting, and lysis, expressed rhCNTF was found mostly in the lysate supernatant, indicating soluble protein overexpression. The soluble protein was purified from the lysate with immobilized metal-ion affinity chromatography (IMAC), and the eluted fractions analyzed with SDS-PAGE (not shown). Fractions containing rhCNTF were pooled, concentrated, and subjected to SEC purification, with rhCNTF eluting from the column as a mostly solitary major peak at 56 mL (Figure 1), corresponding to an estimated molecular weight of approximately 26 kDa and in accordance with published literature and earlier SDS-PAGE analysis [42], with void volume aggregates and smaller oligomers eluted as distinct minor peaks and readily discarded (data not shown). Four separate batches of rhCNTF were purified in high purity, on average yielding 70 mg of protein per liter of culture.

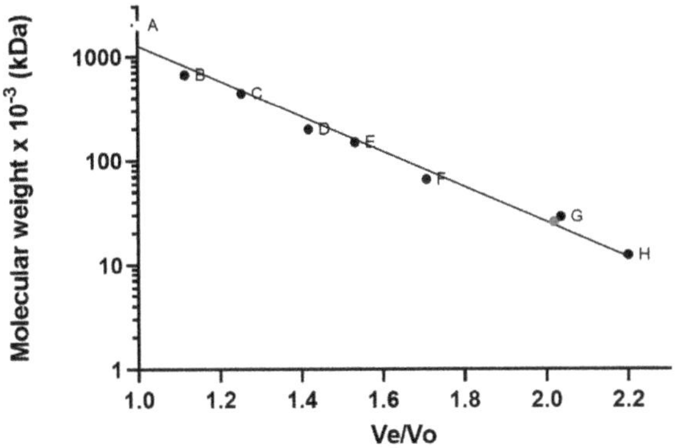

Figure 1. Size-exclusion chromatography of IMAC-purified recombinant human ciliary neurotrophic factor (rhCNTF). Pooled and concentrated eluates from IMAC batch-purification were subjected to SEC in a Superdex 200 prep grade packed C16/40 column with 100 mM NaH2PO4, 300 mM NaCl, pH 8.0, 1 mM DTT as the running buffer with a flow rate of 0.5 mL/min. The column was calibrated with blue dextran (A; 2000 kDa), thyroglobulin (B; 669 kDa), apoferritin (C; 443 kDa), β-amylase (D; 200 kDa), alcohol dehydrogenase (E; 150 kDa), bovine serum albumin (F; 66 kDa), carbonic anhydrase (G; 29 kDa), and cytochrome c (H; 12.4 kDa). rhCNTF eluted at 56 mL (shown in red), with an estimated molecular weight of 26 kDa.

3.2. *rhCNTF In Vitro Bioactivity*

Aside from previously confirmed binding to the cognate receptor CNTFRα [42], the in vitro activity of purified rhCNTF was assessed based on the proliferation of TF-1.CN5a.1. The cell-line is engineered to stably express CNTFRα, and CNTF-mediated stimulation can hence support the short-term proliferation of the cells. As illustrated in Figure 2, our purified rhCNTF supported the short-term proliferation of the cells, observed via BrdU incorporation, in a dose-dependent manner. An approximate EC_{50} of 19 pg/mL (0.8 pM) was estimated for this effect, indicating that our purified rhCNTF was biologically active.

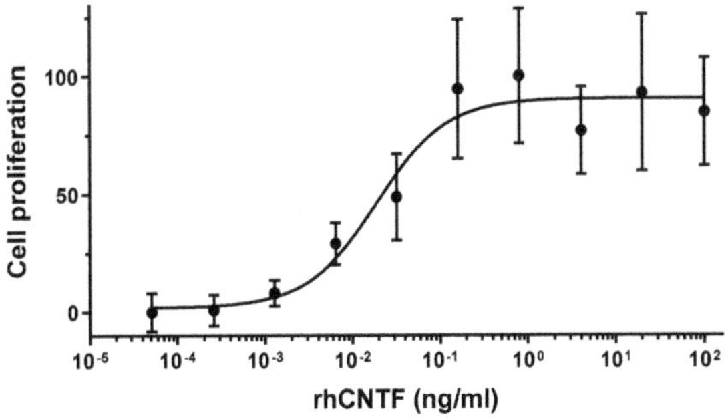

Figure 2. 5-bromo-2′-deoxyuridine (BrdU) incorporation assay analysis of the in vitro biological activity of rhCNTF to support the proliferation of TF-1.CN5a.1 cells. rhCNTF supports the short-term proliferation of TF-1.CN5a.1 cells, with BrdU incorporation into synthesized DNA observed as a proxy for cell proliferation. Each value shown as average mean of three biological replicates ± SD. Data were normalized to highest bioactivity of rhCNTF.

3.3. Characterization and Stability of rhCNTF

3.3.1. Circular Dichroism

To investigate the secondary structure and folding of purified rhCNTF, far-UV CD analysis was carried out. In the recorded spectrum, an intense maximum around 190 nm with minima at 208 and 220 nm were observed (Figure 3A), spectral features corresponding to a highly α-helical secondary structure [54]. The high estimated percentage of helicity (>50%), as obtained by spectral deconvolution with BeStSel, along with further comparison with published results, confirm the correct secondary structure and folding of purified rhCNTF [10,55–57]. Furthermore, CD analysis of the thermal denaturation of rhCNTF yielded a T_{onset} of 46 °C and a T_m of 53 °C (Figure 3B), in accordance with published literature [58].

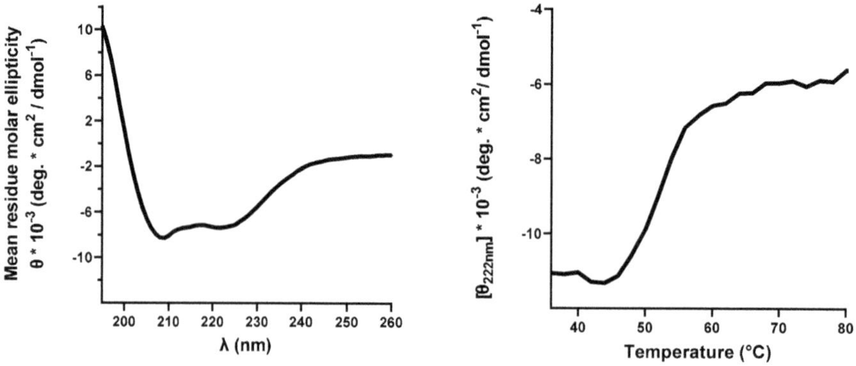

(a) (b)

Figure 3. Far-UV circular dichroism analysis of rhCNTF. (**a**) Analysis of rhCNTF secondary structure at 25 °C: characteristic maximum around 195 nm with minima at 208 and 220 nm point to a highly helical protein, reflecting the correct α-helical secondary structure and folding of purified rhCNTF. (**b**) Thermal denaturation of rhCNTF observed as changes in ellipticity at 222 nm, reporting α-helical unfolding.

3.3.2. ThermoFluor

First, a pre-screen was carried out to determine the optimal working concentrations of rhCNTF and SYPRO orange. The combination of 3.3 μM rhCNTF and 5X SYPRO Orange gave a maximal range of fluorescence and the best signal-to-noise ratio and was used for all subsequent measurements.

We screened 94 different buffers (Table S1) for optimal thermal stability of the purified rhCNTF. In general, poor thermal stability was observed at low pH, with highest thermal stability observed in slightly acidic to neutral pH; the presence of salt was observed to both increase and decrease thermal stability, depending strongly on the buffering component (Table S4). Two buffers yielding clear fluorescence responses and high T_h estimates were chosen for further use: 100 mM 2-(*N*-morpholino)ethanesulfonic acid (MES), 500 mM NaCl, pH 7.0 (buffer M), and 100 mM sodium citrate, pH 5.6 (buffer C); both buffers were supplemented with 1 mM dithiothreitol (DTT) to prevent covalent dimer formation via free cysteines in rhCNTF monomers. To gain insight on rhCNTF's stability during storage, ThermoFluor measurements were carried out with rhCNTF stored on ice at 4 °C as well as at −80 °C in these buffers. As the observed T_h showed only minor changes during the study, this was taken to reflect the retained conformational stability of rhCNTF (Figure 4A–C). Furthermore, protein loss due to precipitation was not observed upon visual inspection of rhCNTF cryo-stored in these buffers (data not shown).

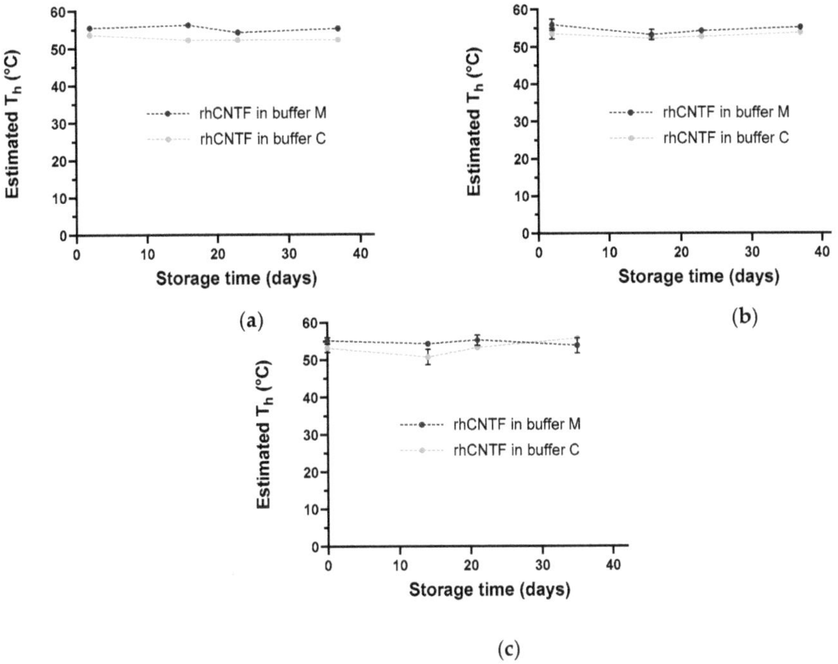

Figure 4. T_h estimation of rhCNTF during storage (**a**) on ice at 4 °C, (**b**) −80 °C, and (**c**) on ice at 4 °C post-thawing.

3.3.3. Dynamic Light Scattering

Hydrodynamic size estimation of rhCNTF was carried out with DLS. The mean estimated R_h of rhCNTF was 3.42 ± 0.50 nm and 2.95 ± 0.22 nm for protein stored on ice at 4 °C in buffers M and C, respectively (4 × 3 measurements). This peak likely reflects both monomeric and dimeric rhCNTF, as DLS often cannot distinguish between species of such similar sizes [59]. This peak had a slightly higher and more variable polydispersity index (PdI) of 0.06 ± 0.04 with rhCNTF stored in buffer M, whereas when stored in buffer C, the same peak was associated with a low PdI of 0.03 ± 0.01.

The size and oligomeric state of rhCNTF were monitored by following changes in the R_h of the monomer/dimer peak and volume distribution percentage of high molecular weight (HMW) species during storage on ice at 4 °C (Figure 5A,B and Table S5) as well as at −80 °C (Figure 5C,D and Table S6). To examine whether centrifugation affected sample quality and detecting HMW species, a comparison was made between thawed and (a) unmixed vs. (b) centrifuged samples (Figure 5C,D, Tables S5 and S6).

During storage at 4 °C, statistically significant differences were not observed in the (monomer/dimer) peak R_h of rhCNTF stored in buffer C (Figure 5B,D), whereas when stored in buffer M, statistically significant changes in the peak R_h were observed (Figure 5A,C). By intensity distribution, HMW species below, in, and occasionally above the sub-visible range (100–1000 nm) were detected (Table S5). However, as the scattering intensity is proportional to the sixth power of the particle radius, when expressed in intensity distribution, the observed intensities and population percentages are disproportionately biased towards the HMW species relative to dominant smaller particles [59]. When instead expressed in volume distribution, the contribution of HMW populations is significantly reduced. As observed from the volume distribution, HMW species were absent in buffer C, and as this remained unchanged (Table S5), and the protein was concluded not to cluster into aggregates during storage at 4 °C. When stored at −80 °C, detected aggregates were likewise negligible (less than 0.1%

of the total) or completely absent, and as removal by centrifugation had no effect, rhCNTF does not undergo aggregation during nor due to cryo-storage (Table S6).

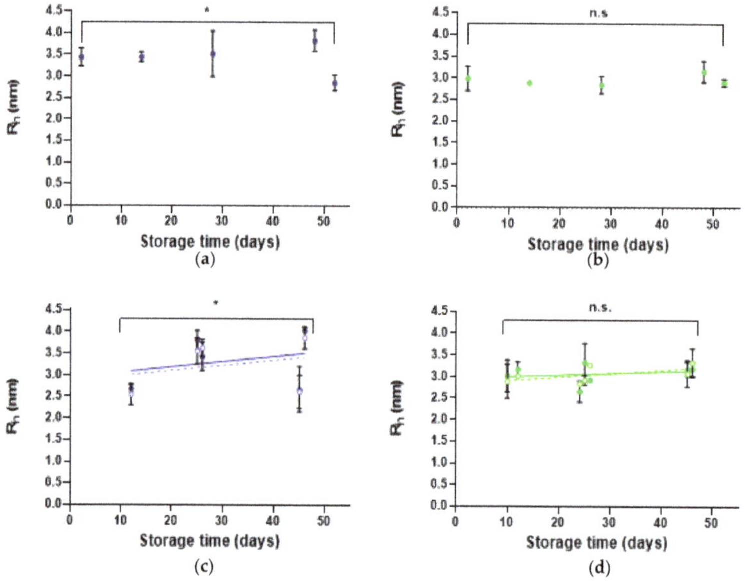

Figure 5. rhCNTF hydrodynamic radius estimates during storage on ice at 4 °C in (**a**) buffer M, and (**b**) buffer C, and at -80 °C in (**c**) buffer M, and (**d**) buffer C. Solid circles denote samples that were unmixed after thawing, and open circles denote centrifugally cleared thawed samples. Over time, more variations with the R_h of rhCNTF stored in buffer M were observed compared to only minor R_h variations with rhCNTF stored in buffer C. Each value shown as average mean ± SD (n = 3 technical replicates; one-way ANOVA, * $p < 0.05$, n.s. = no significance).

rhCNTF does, however, seem to undergo more aggregation in buffer M, as HMW particles were observed in both storage conditions also from volume distribution profiles/percentages, and as centrifugation was observed to influence the detection of aggregates (Tables S5 and S6).

The onset of rhCNTF aggregation was studied during thermal ramping. Thermal aggregation of rhCNTF started at a T_{agg} of 38 °C in both buffers as determined with the proprietary multi-parameter analysis (Figure 6); in volume distribution analysis, HMW species appear at temperatures above 40 °C.

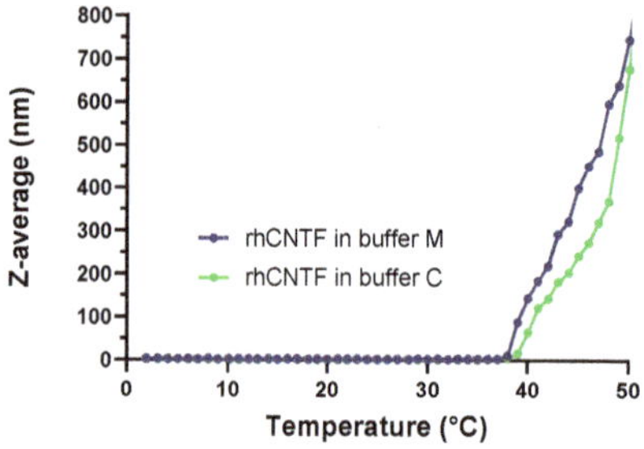

Figure 6. Thermal aggregation curve of freshly purified rhCNTF. Aggregation of purified rhCNTF was measured by following the estimated Z-average (nm) with dynamic light scattering (DLS) as a function of temperature. Appearance of high molecular weight (HMW) species is observed at temperatures above 38 °C in both buffers.

3.4. rhCNTF In Vivo Efficacy Study

3.4.1. ERG: First Study Set

Figure 7 presents individual scotopic ERG results for an animal in the 1 µg rhCNTF dosage group, one-week post-injection. The α and β wave amplitudes between the treated eye and the untreated contralateral eye do not substantially differ. Furthermore, the similarity of the graphs indicates equal visual capacity of the 1 µg rhCNTF treated and the untreated eye.

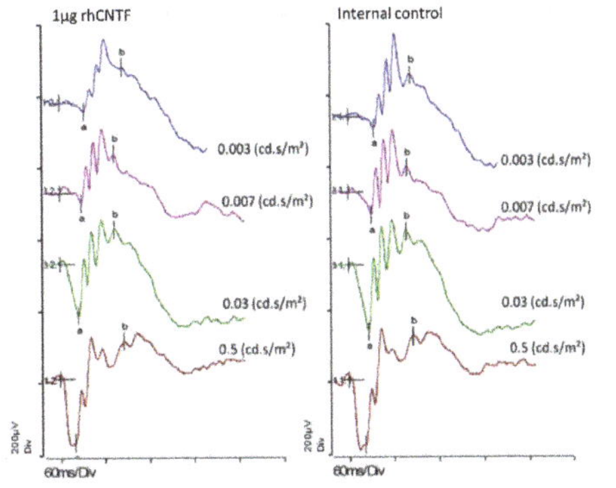

Figure 7. Scotopic Electroretinogram (ERG) recorded one week after 1 µg rhCNTF injection to the left eye. Equal visual acuity between the rhCNTF-treated eye and the contralateral untreated eye (internal control) was observed.

Figure 8 presents the recorded scotopic α and β wave amplitudes in different treatment groups one- and two-weeks post-injection (n = 3). Figure 9 presents the recorded photopic β wave value distribution at flash stimulus 1 cd × s/m^2 (n = 3). No statistically significant differences could be seen in the scotopic α and β wave values or photopic β wave values between the treated and untreated eyes in any treatment group at any flash intensity or timepoint (related samples Wilcoxon signed ranks test, significance level: $p < 0.05$). The differences in the parameter distribution across the different treatment groups were not statistically significant at any flash intensity in the scotopic or photopic ERG recorded 1 week or 2 weeks post-injection (Kruskal–Wallis test, significance level: $p < 0.05$). The large range in the observed values indicates a large within-group variation in the test population.

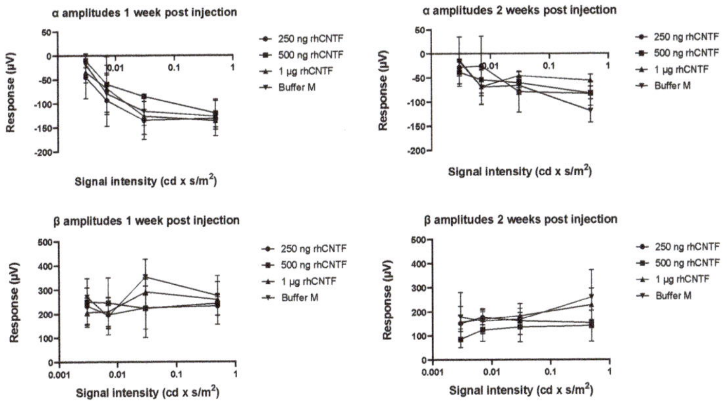

Figure 8. Scotopic α and β wave amplitudes one- and two-weeks post-injection. No statistically significant difference in the responses between any of the treatment groups could be detected.

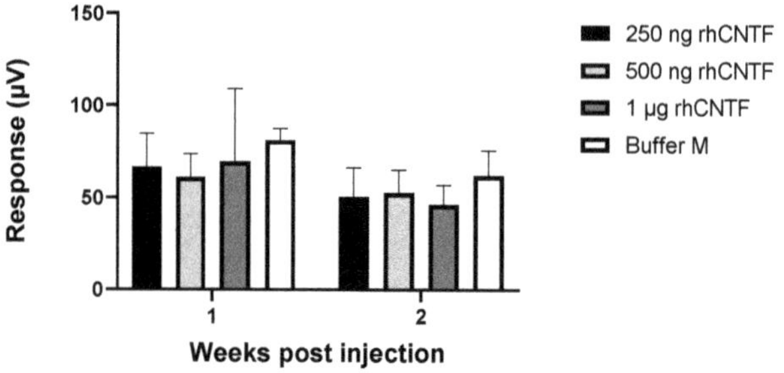

Figure 9. Photopic beta wave amplitudes at stimulus intensity 1 cd × s/m^2 one- and two-weeks post-injection. No statistically significant difference in the responses between any of the treatment groups at different timepoints could be detected.

3.4.2. ERG: Second Study Set

Mean values and standard error of the scotopic α and β wave amplitudes recorded one- and two-weeks post-injection are presented in Figure 10 (n = 6). Figure 11 presents the recorded photopic β wave value distribution at flash stimulus 1 cd × s/m^2 (n = 6). Only in the highest scotopic ERG stimulus intensity recorded two weeks post-injection, a statistically significantly steeper α wave was observed in the 1 μg rhCNTF-treated eyes than in the contralateral untreated eyes, used as internal control (related samples Wilcoxon signed ranks test, significance level: $p < 0.05$, $p = 0.043$). No statistically significant differences could be seen in the scotopic α and β wave values or photopic β wave values in other stimulus intensities or timepoints between the 1 μg rhCNTF-treated and internal control eyes. Comparison of the recorded scotopic α and β wave amplitudes in the 1 μg rhCNTF-treated eyes between the two time points showed no significant change at any flash intensity, indicating no change in visual acuity over time (Figures S1 and S2) (related samples Wilcoxon signed ranks test, significance level: $p < 0.05$). A comparison of parameter distribution between the treatment groups showed no statistically significant differences in parameter distribution between the treated and control eyes (Figures S3–S5) (Kruskal–Wallis test, significance level: $p < 0.05$).

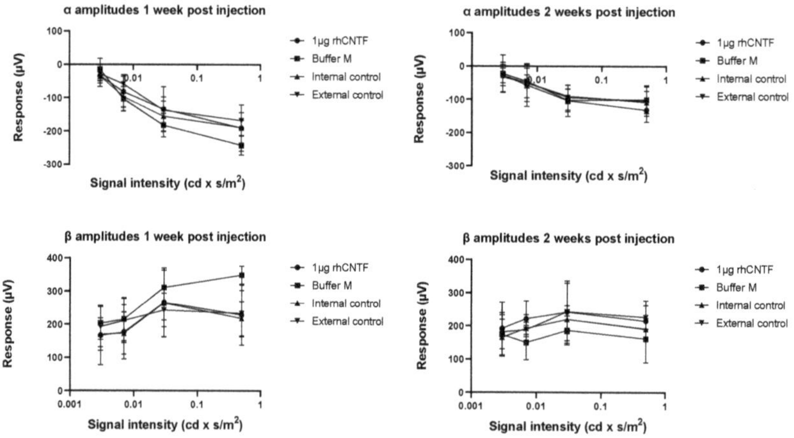

Figure 10. Mean and SD of scotopic alpha and beta wave amplitudes one and two-weeks post-injection. Scotopic 0.5 cd × s/m^2 β wave amplitudes recorded one-week post-injection were significantly higher in the 2-(*N*-morpholino)ethanesulfonic acid (MES)-treated group than in 1 μg rhCNTF-treated group (Kruskal–Wallis test, $p = 0.018$) and NControl group ($p = 0.025$). However, the 1 μg CNTF-treated group and the NControl group did not show any statistically significant difference between their mean values ($p = 0.831$) (n = 6).

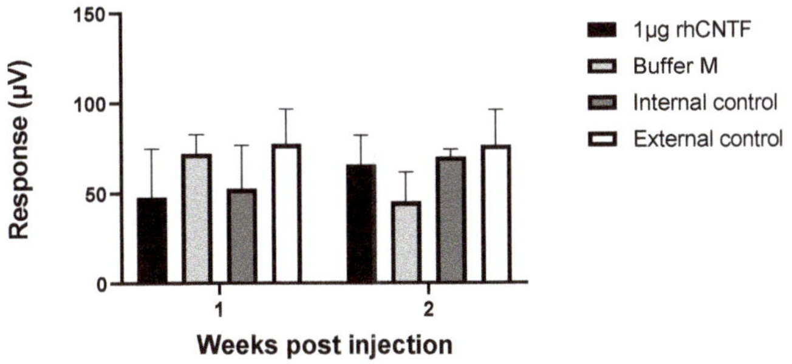

Figure 11. Mean and SD of photopic beta wave amplitudes at stimulus intensity 1 cd × s/m^2 one and two-weeks post-injection. No statistically significant difference in the responses between any of the treatment groups at different time points could be detected (n = 6).

3.4.3. Histology

The effect of rhCNTF treatment on the morphology of the animals in the second study set was evaluated by the thickness and density of the outer nuclear layer (ONL) of the retina. Representative histological samples prepared of MES (n = 2) NControl (n = 3) and 1 µg CNTF (n = 4) treated animals are presented in Figure 12. One animal in the 1 µg CNTF-treated group seemed to have denser and thicker ONL in the treated eye (A) than in the contralateral eye (B), however, this effect could not be seen in any other animals of the same treatment group. There was also variation in the progress of photoreceptor degeneration between individual animals at the same time-point.

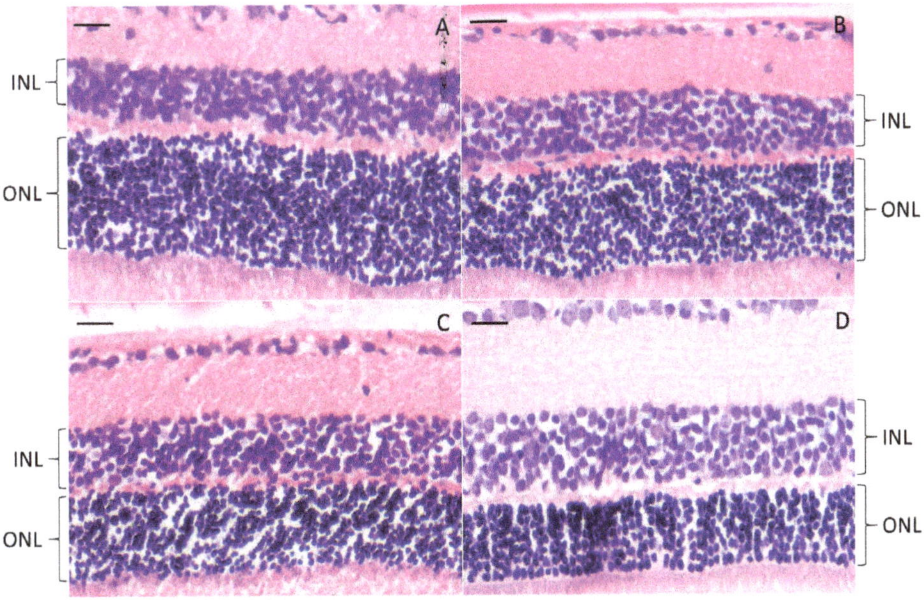

Figure 12. Effect of rhCNTF treatment on the morphology of the retina. Histological analysis of retinal sections did not show clear benefit of treatment with 1 µg rhCNTF (**a**) compared to internal control (**b**), Buffer M control (**c**), and Ncontrol (**d**). Scale bar 20 µm. INL, inner nuclear layer; ONL, outer nuclear layer.

3.5. Retinal Penetration of Labeled rhCNTF

In vivo, rhCNTF did not show any observable effect on photoreceptor function nor survival. Since this raised concerns on whether the IVT injected protein permeates the retina to reach CNTF-responsive target cells, this was studied with fluorescently labeled rhCNTF in an ex vivo setting with retinal explants.

In the rat retinal explants, fluorescence from labeled rhCNTF was observed mainly in the ganglion cell layer (GCL) but also deeper, for example in the inner nuclear layer (INL), 24 h after apical application, as illustrated in Figure 13A–E,G–K. No evident fluorescence from labeled rhCNTF was observed 24 h after basolateral application, as shown in Figure 13F,L.

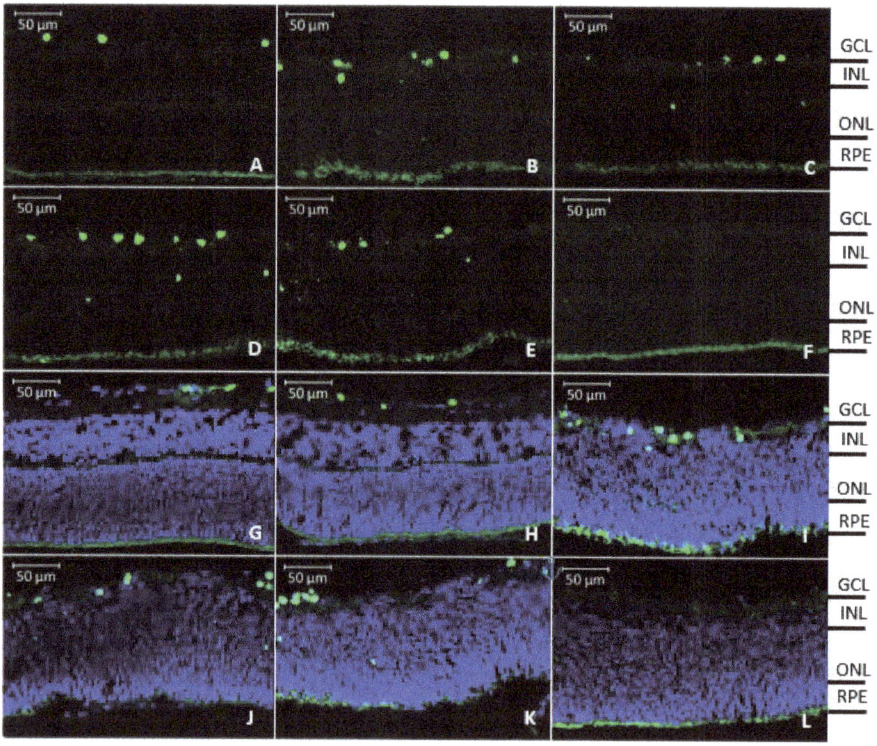

Figure 13. rhCNTF penetration in rat retinal explants as visualized without (**A–F**) and with DAPI counterstaining (**G–L**). Alexa Fluor™ 488 labeled rhCNTF (green) penetrates and distributes in the retina after apical administration, with rhCNTF-positive cells observed in the neural retina in layers ranging from the GCL to the INL (**A–E**,**G–K**). No rhCNTF penetration is seen with basolaterally applied protein (**F**,**L**). GCL, ganglion cell layer; INL, inner nuclear layer; ONL, outer nuclear layer; RPE, retinal pigment epithelium.

Since fluorescence from labeled rhCNTF was observed mostly in the GCL, and as retinal cells expressing CNTFRα include e.g., retinal ganglion cells and Müller glia in this layer, staining to visualize Iba-1 immunoreactivity was carried out to identify microglial cells. Upon closer inspection, rhCNTF was observed to co-localize with microglia in the rat explants, as illustrated in Figure 14.

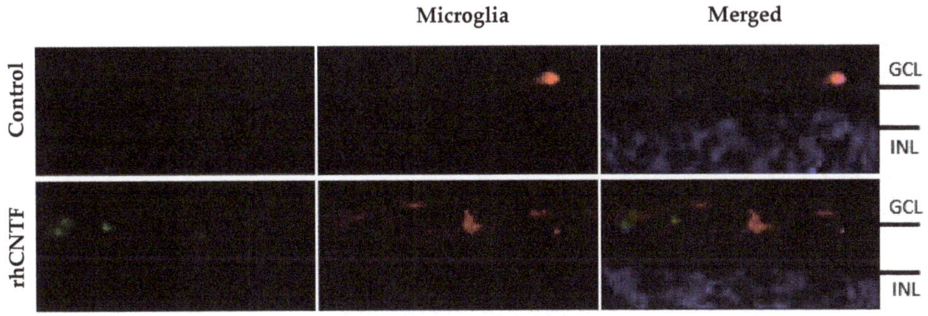

Figure 14. rhCNTF co-localizes with microglia in the ganglion cell layer. Fluorescence from Alexa Fluor™ 488 labeled rhCNTF (green) co-localizes with Iba-1 immunopositivity (red). GCL, ganglion cell layer; INL, inner nuclear layer.

24 h after apical application, fluorescence from the labeled rhCNTF was observed in most retinal layers in the bovine retinal explants, as shown in Figure 15 and Figure S6. Whereas fluorescence can be observed mostly at the ILM and GCL, rhCNTF-positivity is also observed in the outer plexiform layer (OPL) and the ONL.

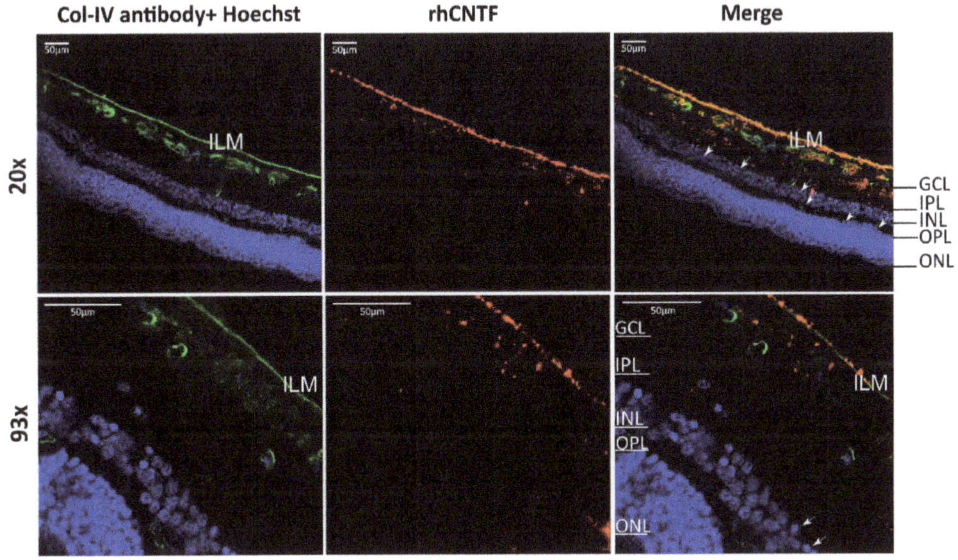

Figure 15. rhCNTF penetration in bovine retinal explant. NT-647 labeled rhCNTF (red) readily penetrates across inner limiting membrane (ILM) and distributes in the retina after apical administration, with evident fluorescence observed in the neural retina in layers ranging from ganglion cell layer (GCL) to outer plexiform layer (OPL). ILM, inner limiting membrane; GCL, ganglion cell layer; IPL, Inner plexiform layer; INL, inner nuclear layer; OPL, outer plexiform layer; ONL, outer nuclear layer.

4. Discussion

Pharmacotherapeutic intervention affecting the disease mechanisms and causes is often limited to specific pathologies. For example, using anti-VEGF biologicals is restricted to treating posterior eye segment conditions featuring pathological neovascularization. Instead of blocking pathways ultimately leading to neurodegeneration, directly supporting the function and survival of neurons—for example with different neurotrophic factors—is an attractive strategy to alter the course of pathology, and a potentially more universal approach in treating neurodegenerative diseases of diverse etiologies. The cytokine CNTF is of great interest as the protein's neuroprotective effects on various retinal neurons have been demonstrated in numerous retinal disease models, subsequently ushering clinical evaluation in treating various retinal conditions in humans.

In vitro bioactivity in a cell-based assay was used to verify the biological activity of purified rhCNTF by assessing its effects on the proliferation of a CNTF-responsive cell line. It is known that the lymphoblastoid cell line TF-1 responds to multiple cytokines, e.g., GM-CSF, IL-3, and erythropoietin by proliferating [60]. As TF-1 cells express IL-6Rα, another receptor subunit for CTNF [11], they can respond to exogenous CNTF. However, this binding is of markedly lower affinity compared to that with CNTFRα, resulting in a less pronounced proliferative response; simultaneous addition of soluble CNTFRα makes the TF-1 considerably more responsive to exogenous CNTF [61]. To circumvent the need to add exogenous CNTFRα to cultured TF-1 cells, we used TF-1.CN5a.1, a TF-1 derived cell line transfected to stably express CNTFRα. The cells are thus capable of proliferating in response to much lower CNTF concentrations, and the cell line can be used to assess, e.g., the activity and potency of CNTF and its variants. Here, we demonstrated that aside from binding to its cognate receptor, our rhCNTF has the correct α-helical structure (Figure 3A) and is biologically active as it supported the short-term proliferation of TF-1.CN5a.1 cells with an estimated EC_{50} of 19 pg/mL (0.8 pM).

4.1. Buffer Screening and Stability Studies

We investigated the stability of rhCNTF in various buffers. Although widely used in formulations for therapeutic proteins, sodium phosphate buffer has been reported to be unsuitable for the cryo-storage of many proteins, as the buffer undergoes so-called freeze acidification [62,63]. Particularly, the dibasic phosphate salt undergoes a selective crystallization process during cooling, leading to a decrease of up to 3 pH units during freezing [62,64]. Furthermore, low temperature, freeze-concentration of solutes, and the formation of ice-aqueous interfaces are but some examples of the physicochemical changes and potentially destabilizing stresses that proteins may experience during freezing [62]. Destabilization of the protein structure may lead to (partial) denaturation of the protein structure, and further to protein aggregation. Indeed, we observed major loss of purified protein when rhCNTF was stored in a sodium phosphate buffer at -80 °C. Thus, a more suitable buffer was required for the protein.

Here, different buffer, salt, and pH conditions were screened with ThermoFluor to assess their effects on the conformational stability and T_h of rhCNTF. Although high T_h estimates were seen with several buffers, the observed fluorescence responses were low and the negative peaks in the first derivative plots were poorly discernible with certain buffers and the T_h was therefore challenging to estimate reliably. Among the screened buffers, two with clear fluorescence responses and high T_h estimates reflecting high thermal stability of rhCNTF (100 mM MES, 500 mM NaCl, pH 7.0, and 100 mM sodium citrate, pH 5.6; both supplemented with 1 mM DTT) were chosen and further tested. Although the number of screened conditions is arguably limited, and as replications could admittedly reinforce our confidence in the obtained results, they, along with the DLS results, nonetheless provide information on suitable buffers that can serve as a basis of further formulation development for rhCNTF. Moreover, our results indicate useful starting points around which 'fine' screening, i.e., buffer optimization with different additives (e.g., glycerol, surfactants, polyols, and reducing agents) is advisable to further increase the stability of rhCNTF [65]. As the T_h estimates remained fairly consistent during the follow-up measurements (Figure 4), despite being insufficient for rigorous statistical analysis, this led us to draw the conclusion that the conformational stability of our rhCNTF was retained during the study and in our experimental setup.

Although thermal aggregation of rhCNTF initiates at temperatures above 38 °C in both buffers, this is not concomitant with heat-induced unfolding. As measured with CD and ThermoFluor, rhCNTF starts to unfold at temperatures above 46 °C (T_{onset}; Figure 3B). The onset of aggregation at 38 °C is, however, not necessarily due to association via exposed hydrophobic patches, as can be expected to occur later at higher temperatures. Further elucidation is warranted to gain a more comprehensive understanding of the protein's aggregation behavior. Moreover, upon administration, the protein gets exposed to the vastly different, complex, and potentially hostile in vivo environment that has been postulated to influence the formation and nature of aggregates [66,67]. Therefore, as the T_{agg} is close to normal body temperature, it cannot be ruled out that rhCNTF could not undergo aggregation to some degree in oculo after administration at 35 °C in the vitreous. Although engineered CNTF variants with improved chemical and physical properties were originally developed for CNS delivery [41], it would be of interest to investigate whether they are more stable in the eye as well.

Particle sizing results suggest that oligomerization of rhCNTF differs in the two buffers. Overall, the slightly larger R_h estimate with rhCNTF in buffer M is likely due to the composition of the solvent. The presence of high salt concentration – in this case, 500 mM NaCl – can shield the charge-mediated protein-protein repulsive forces, decreasing the diffusivity of macromolecules in solution and appearing as an increase in measured hydrodynamic size [68,69]. When stored in this buffer, appearance of HMW species is detectable, whereas no dramatic oligomerization takes place in buffer C in either storage condition (Tables S3 and S4). In intensity distributions, HMW particles were detected in both buffers, but when expressed in volume distribution, larger particles were evident only in buffer M (Table S4). Although based on volume distribution profiles, the amount of HMW species is negligible in buffer C; further development of a therapeutic rhCNTF lead molecule and its formulation may still require additional engineering and optimization to prevent the formation of even trace aggregates detected only in intensity distributions here.

Even though DLS is a powerful method for the detection and rate determination of oligomer and larger aggregate formation, the underlying mechanism(s) of aggregation cannot be determined with this method. Our studies were not set up for uncovering whether trace oligomers and HMW aggregates present in storage and induced during thermal ramping are irreversible, covalent, insoluble, etc., and this would require further studies with orthogonal methods, such as SEC with multi-angle laser light scattering (MALLS), analytical ultracentrifugation (AUC), and nanoparticle tracking analysis (NTA) [70,71]. Such studies could also yield results to corroborate the findings presented here. Lastly, although not feasible during our study, we realize that assessing rhCNTF's binding to CNTFRα and/or effect on cell proliferation during our stability studies could provide even more concrete proof of the stability and retention of rhCNTF function during storage.

Finally, the intraocular stability of therapeutic proteins is of immense importance; even though the eye is often considered an immune-privileged site, it is possible that therapeutic protein aggregates in the vitreous would induce immune responses [67] that could affect the efficacy and safety of these drugs. Studies on therapeutic protein stability, aggregation, and immunogenicity after intravitreal administration are still, however, scarce. Although not studied here, in situ stability concerns are equally pertinent with IVT CNTF, warranting further investigations that could, for example, be carried out by adopting recently described ex vivo approaches [72,73] to study these aspects with rhCNTF.

4.2. In Vivo Bioactivity of rhCNTF

Based on the results from the first study set, the rhCNTF treatment did not have a dose-dependent positive or negative effect on the recorded ERG values, and the photoreceptors in the rhCNTF-treated eyes did not seem to benefit from the treatment compared to the control eyes. As there was no significant reduction in the photoreceptor function over time, it is possible that the photoreceptor degeneration did not progress dramatically between the recordings, or that the photoreceptor degeneration was already rather extensive in the animals aged 28 days, when the ERG was recorded for the first time. Therefore, in the second study set, the animals were treated at an earlier time point, around the onset of photoreceptor degeneration. In the second study set, the group treated with 1 μg rhCNTF was the only group that showed no significant reduction in the scotopic ERG values over time; however, this finding alone was not substantial enough to prove any therapeutic effect of CNTF treatment on photoreceptor degeneration.

While ERG has proven to be an effective method in evaluation of retinal function in RCS rats, it appears that the reduction of the ERG response might not always correlate well with the anatomical loss of photoreceptors [74]. There has also been some scientific debate whether CNTF is, in fact, detrimental to the rod photoreceptors as in some in vivo studies intraocular CNTF therapy has paradoxically reduced the scotopic ERG responses. A dose-dependent transient reduction in ERG responses has been observed in normal Long-Evans rats after IVT injection of CNTF that corresponded with a morphological reduction in ROS length with full recovery observed by three weeks post-injection [75]. Multiple teams using viral-mediated gene therapy have also reported diminished ERG amplitudes in treatment groups or no observable improvement in ERG, whilst the number of preserved photoreceptors has been higher in treatment groups [18,31,32,76]. Some teams, however, have been able to improve the scotopic or photopic ERG values with viral CNTF treatments or CNTF secreting devices in different animal models [33,35,36,40]. There is evidence that CNTF can reduce the rhodopsin levels and other proteins important in the phototransduction cascade [25]. Therefore, the photoreceptor preservative effect of CNTF could be counteracted by the negative effect it presents on the functionality of the preserved photoreceptor in the retina. However, in our experiments, rhCNTF did not affect the retinal morphology, nor the function.

RCS rat has a mutation in the gene encoding tyrosine kinase receptor Mer, affecting the ability of RPE cells to phagocytise rod outer segment (ROS) debris [74,77,78]. With time, the ROS debris accumulates, eventually forming a layer between the RPE cells and photoreceptors, leading to gradual photoreceptor degeneration and full blindness by the age of two to three months [74]. The gradual decrease in the scotopic ERG responses in RCS rats is presented in Figure 16. Even though CNTF related photoreceptor preservative effect has been observed in RCS rat [14,30,33], it is possible that halting the rapid progression of photoreceptor generation in this animal model is challenging with a single bolus injection of therapeutic protein, making sustained delivery systems more feasible options.

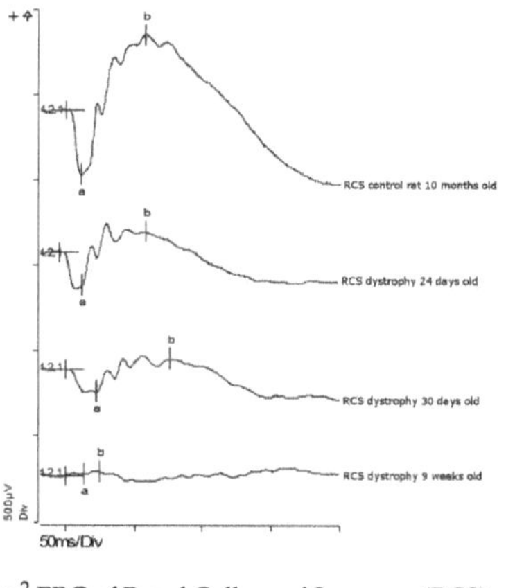

Figure 16. Scotopic 0.5 cd x s/m^2 ERG of Royal College of Surgeons (RCS) control animal at the age of 10 months, RCS dystrophic rat at the age of 24 days, 30 days, and 9 weeks. The progressive photoreceptor degeneration and loss of photoreceptor functionality can be seen as the α and β wave (marked as a and b in the graph) amplitudes decrease in magnitude rather rapidly between 24 and 30 days in the RCS dystrophic rat, whilst the 10-month old RCS control animal exhibits distinct α and β wave responses. The fully blind nine-week-old RCS dystrophy rat has no measurable α or β wave amplitudes.

The pharmacokinetics (PK) of CNTF have so far been studied in rats only with systemic CNTF, reporting a short systemic half-life of 2.9 min; when discussing the ocular PK of CNTF, the 1994 papers by Dittrich et al. [79] and Sendtner et al. [80] and subsequent publications citing these are commonly referred to. Although the early papers discuss the PK of systemically administered CNTF in rats, in the citing literature the results are often straightforwardly extrapolated to represent the in vivo PK of CNTF in general, and it has been assumed that CNTF would lose its therapeutic effect quickly also in the vitreous after IVT injection due to rapid clearance [36,81]. Regrettably, claiming the ocular half-life of CNTF to be in the same time-scale—of mere minutes—as in the circulation, is a gross and lamentable misinterpretation of the publications' results.

Studies on the intravitreal pharmacokinetics of macromolecules carried out in rabbits have shown that macromolecules can have a half-life of several days, and that the half-life of the macromolecule in the vitreous is greatly dependent on the intravitreal clearance, which in turn is small for those macromolecules that cannot pass the BRB, as is thought to be the case with CNTF [6,82]. Biologicals are eliminated from the vitreous predominantly via the anterior route [83], with the hydrodynamic size considered as the major determinant in the ocular half-life of a given biological [84,85]. Although experimental data on the vitreal half-life of CNTF is as of writing scarcely published, in a study with rat CNTF injected in mouse vitreous—although owing to practical limitations the vitreal CNTF levels were not assessed with total retinal levels reported instead [17]—we doubt that the levels would be as high as reported if the protein truly had a rapid vitreal elimination. Based on hydrodynamic radius estimations presented here, the calculated intravitreal half-life of rhCNTF are 4.67 days (R_h 2.95 nm) and 4.96 days (R_h 3.32 nm) (see Supplement), estimates that do not differ drastically from experimentally determined half-lives of other IVT administered macromolecules [86–88] and definitely not in the order of minutes. Even so, the vitreal half-life of CNTF is nevertheless finite and sustained intraocular release, and retinal delivery of CNTF has been explored utilizing various strategies: for example, an intravitreally injected hydrogel [58], cell-based systems [89], and several gene therapy approaches [18,90–94]. The most clinically advanced, Renexus® (NT-501; Neurotech Pharmaceuticals, Inc., Cumberland, RI, USA) is an implant with encapsulated, genetically engineered ARPE-19 cells, that secrete and maintain low concentrations of human CNTF in the vitreous over several years [19]. Its neuroprotective effects have been evaluated in patients with dry AMD [95,96], CNGB3-achromatopsia [97], glaucoma [98], retinitis pigmentosa [5,19,99], and macular telangiectasia type 2 (MacTel 2) [100]. No efficacy was evident in CNGB3-achromatopsia patients [97], and only moderate efficacy was observed in RP patients and patients with geographic atrophy secondary to dry AMD [95,96]. However, after some therapeutic efficacy was observed in a recent phase 2 study in MacTel 2 patients [100], two phase 3 studies are now recruiting patients for evaluating the safety and efficacy of Renexus® in treating MacTel 2 (NCT03316300, NCT03319849), whereas the results of a recent phase 2 study in glaucoma patients (NCT02862938) are currently expected.

4.3. Retinal Penetration and Effects of rhCNTF

As no apparent neuroprotective effects were observed with IVT administered rhCNTF in vivo, in case this was related to the protein's ability to permeate into the retina, the postulated target cells were evaluated. Here, we demonstrate that after apical administration, our labeled rhCNTF—a small (26 kDa) protein—permeates into the neural retina in both explant models in 24 h. Consistent with findings with intravitreally administered antibody fragments [101], crossing the RPE was not observed with basolaterally applied rhCNTF as the protein did not permeate to the neural retina.

Given that the half-lives of intravitreally administered protein therapeutics are in the range of several days [102], we realize that in this context, the time scale of the given rhCNTF treatments is short. However, we chose to limit the treatments to 24 h in order to ensure the structural and physiological integrity of the explants, and on the other hand, that the stability of the protein–fluorophore conjugates was also retained during the experiments. Whilst not studied with the rat explants, and although based on collagen staining, the ILM appears intact in our experiments with the bovine explant (Figure 15 and Figure S6), adapting a recently described bovine explant model developed to ensure the integrity of the ILM and vitreoretinal interface [53] could be used to complement our findings, and to further define the contribution of these primary barriers in the retinal permeation of biologicals in general. It should also be noted that as the ILM in the rodent eye is poorly representative of human physiology compared to larger species, information obtained with bovine models may better reflect the in vivo situation in the human eye [53,101]. Even though the ILM is considered the primary barrier to retinal entry from the vitreous [53], e.g., the size-cutoffs remain undetermined [83], whereas the porosity of the ILM meshwork in human and animal eyes is still not fully clear [103]. Likewise, how recognized species differences relate to the applicability of different animals' eyes in evaluating the retinal penetration of vastly different particles remains to be comprehensively elucidated. Whilst reports on the retinal permeation of biomacromolecules is by and large qualitative with sparse truly quantitative estimates published [83], as several full-sized mAbs [86–88] and even large particles such as nanocarriers have nonetheless been reported to penetrate into the retina [103], the ILM could, in fact, be an insignificant barrier to the retinal entry of biologicals, and in particular small proteins as seen with rhCNTF here.

As our retinal penetration experiments were not set up for studying the neuroprotective effects of our rhCNTF, conclusions thereof cannot be drawn here. Nonetheless, as labeled rhCNTF penetrated the ILM and permeated to retinal layers with CNTFRα-expressing cells, our results indicate that CNTF's availability to the target cells should not be a limitation for its direct effects in the retina. Although published results suggest that the retinal microglia respond to CNTF in rats [23] and our labeled rhCNTF did indeed co-localize with local microglia in the GCL, it is not clear if these cells express CNTFRα and whether they are responsive to CNTF directly or indirectly. Therefore, verifying the microglial expression of the cognate receptor is pertinent to further corroborate our findings. The experiments could straightforwardly be expanded to assess the activation of the identified downstream signaling pathways of CNTF, such as JAK/STAT3, ras-MAPK, and PI3K/AKT [11,23]. Similarly, since the neurotrophic effects of CNTF are in part mediated by glial cells in the eye, mass spectrometry for example could be utilized to analyze microglial expression and secretion of other growth factors in response to stimulation with rhCNTF. Lastly, application of conditioned medium of microglial cells treated with rhCNTF to retinal explants and explant models of retinal degeneration and pathologies may also be carried out to assess e.g., protection of photoreceptors as well as to investigate the stimulation and secretory responses of Müller glia.

Although the bovine explants are viable only for a short duration [53], rodent explants can in comparison be maintained in culture for several weeks; explants exhibiting retinal pathologies and degeneration can also be induced, or, as eyes from preclinical animal disease models are available, prepared thereof [51,104]. As aging and diseases can affect the structures and the integrity of drug delivery barriers such as the BRB and the ILM [83,105], we see such rodent explant models potentially applicable in comparing how such changes in the retinal physiology influence the retinal permeation and distribution of protein therapeutics. In order to ensure that meaningful information is extracted in such studies, it is obviously essential to confirm that the explants retain their physiological integrity and truthfully reflect the physiological situation [106].

Even though the relevance of the retinal permeation of protein therapeutics is underlined in several publications [88,103,107,108], it is still an incompletely understood area of the intravitreal pharmacokinetics thereof. Aside from presented studies with rhCNTF, we envision the retinal explant models utilized in studying the retinal penetration and distribution of various other proteins of therapeutic interest, e.g., mAbs, Fab fragments, and Fc-fusion proteins. In particular, the explants could prove invaluable in systematically elucidating how different factors, such as protein hydrodynamic radius, charge, and FcRn-binding act as determinants in this regard. As it is possible that protein therapeutics with differing characteristics permeate into the retina at different rates, study designs naturally require robustness. On one hand, it has been proposed that retinal penetration might not be a universal requisite with all modalities [83]. On the other hand, there is support for opposing views; although current anti-VEGF therapeutics have extracellular targets, their permeation into the retina to bind free retinal VEGF is necessary for maximal VEGF inhibition based on a recent in silico study [109]. Even though posterior clearance is considered to play only a minor role in the vitreal clearance of protein therapeutics, it is indeed unclear whether penetrating into the retina interplays with the pharmacological effects of protein therapeutics in vivo. It is thus of great importance to investigate how retinal permeation of proteins, especially with different modes of action, is connected to their therapeutic efficacies in the eye and whether this can be influenced by protein engineering for example. Such studies could potentially provide explanations on why many proteins developed for ocular conditions have failed in clinical trials. Ultimately, they might offer valuable clues on overcoming recognized ocular barriers and thus help in bringing novel treatments to the clinic. Here, utilizing both in vivo as well as ex vivo methods, such as the described retinal explants, are essential [105].

5. Conclusions

Here, we focused first on verifying the bioactivity of rhCNTF, and subsequently on the characterization and stability studies of the protein. Whereas the protein's activity was demonstrated in an in vitro cell proliferation assay, screening identified buffers in which the physicochemical stability of rhCNTF was retained during storage, providing a basis for further rhCNTF development and formulation efforts. Even though here rhCNTF showed no photoreceptor preservative effects in vivo, using ex vivo organotypic retinal explants we demonstrated, to the best of our knowledge, for the first time the permeation of labeled rhCNTF to the neural retina and additionally the exogenous cytokine's co-localization with outer retinal macrophages. Whilst the lack of in vivo effects could, for example, be due to the extent of degeneration in the used disease model or the limited duration of action achievable with a single bolus injection, as the cytokine was observed to distribute to the neural retina, we conclude that this was not due to rhCNTF failing to reach responsive cells.

As the factors affecting retinal penetration of protein therapeutics are still unclear, there is a need for methods with which such information can be acquired. To improve the knowledge in this area, further studies are clearly necessary. As such, complementing the in vivo and in silico work carried out and described in recent literature, we hope our findings give impetus to—among other applications—explore the further use of retinal explant models to systematically elucidate the retinal permeation of protein therapeutics.

Supplementary Materials: The following are available online at http://www.mdpi.com/1999-4923/12/7/611/s1, Figure S1: Mean and SD of recorded scotopic α and β wave amplitudes in the 2nd study set 1 week after intravitreal injection; Figure S2: Mean and SD of recorded scotopic α and β wave amplitudes in the 2nd study set 2 weeks after intravitreal injection; Figure S3: Left eye α wave distribution 1 week post-injection; Figure S4: Left eye β wave distribution 1 week post-injection; Figure S5: Left eye β wave distribution 2 weeks post-injection; Figure S6: rhCNTF penetration in bovine retinal explant; Table S1: Layout of the ThermoFluor buffer, salt, and pH screen; Table S2: Tissue processing procedure; Table S3: H&E staining protocol; Table S4: Heat map of rhCNTF T_h measured in ThermoFluor screen; Table S5: R_h estimation of rhCNTF stored on ice at 4 °C; Table S6: R_h estimation of rhCNTF stored at −80 °C.

Author Contributions: J.I. planned experiments, and carried out expression and purification of rhCNTF, in vitro activity studies, characterization, buffer optimization, and stability studies of purified rhCNTF, as well as the retinal penetration studies in rat retinal explant cultures. He also analyzed the experimental data and composed the first draft of the manuscript. A.A. and E.T. planned and carried out the in vivo experiments and prepared, stained, and imaged the histological samples. A.A. analyzed the experimental data related to in vivo activity of rhCNTF. S.T. carried out the retinal penetration studies in bovine retinal explant cultures. B.A.-G. carried out retinal penetration studies in rat retinal explant cultures and contributed to study planning therein. M.U., M.R., M.G.C., and A.U. helped in planning the experiments, funded the studies, and provided feedback on the results and written manuscript. All authors have read and agreed to the published version of the manuscript.

Funding: J.I. was funded by The Finnish Cultural Foundation, The Paulo Foundation, Evald and Hilda Nissi Foundation, and Päivikki and Sakari Sohlberg Foundation. S.T. was funded by the European Union's Horizon 2020 research and innovation programme Marie Skłodowska-Curie ITN (NANOMED, grant 676137). B.A.-G. was funded by FFB Grant PPA-0717-0719-RAD, Kerstan Foundation and ProRetina Foundation. M.U. was funded by Land Baden-Württemberg and Kerstan Foundation. A.A., E.T. and M.R. were funded by The University of Eastern Finland. M.G.C. was funded by the Academy of Finland Key-project (303884). A.U. was funded by Academy of Finland (project 311122).

Acknowledgments: Biocenter Finland Crystallisation Facility and the Institute of Biotechnology are gratefully acknowledged for access to and assistance with the ThermoFluor instrument and software. The use of the facilities and expertise of the Biocenter Oulu biophysical protein analysis core facility, a member of Biocenter Finland, is gratefully acknowledged. The personnel of Kuopio Lab Animal Centre, as well as Leena Pietilä, Lea Pirskanen, Aija Kekkonen, Sylvia Bolz, and Christine Henes are acknowledged for their skilled technical assistance with the experiments. Eva del Amo is gratefully acknowledged for her calculations on the intravitreal half-life of CNTF.

Conflicts of Interest: The authors declare no conflict of interest. The funders had no role in the design of the study; in the collection, analyses, or interpretation of data; in the writing of the manuscript, or in the decision to publish the results.

References

1. Mandal, A.; Pal, D.; Agrahari, V.; Trinh, H.M.; Joseph, M.; Mitra, A.K. Ocular delivery of proteins and peptides: Challenges and novel formulation approaches. *Adv. Drug Deliv. Rev.* **2018**, *126*, 67–95. [CrossRef] [PubMed]
2. Awwad, S.; Ahmed, A.H.M.; Sharma, G.; Heng, J.S.; Khaw, P.T.; Brocchini, S.; Lockwood, A. Principles of pharmacology in the eye. *Br. J. Pharmacol.* **2017**, *174*, 4205–4223. [CrossRef] [PubMed]
3. Delplace, V.; Payne, S.; Shoichet, M. Delivery strategies for treatment of age-related ocular diseases: From a biological understanding to biomaterial solutions. *J. Control. Release* **2015**, *219*, 652–668. [CrossRef] [PubMed]
4. Pardue, M.T.; Allen, R.S. Neuroprotective strategies for retinal disease. *Prog. Retin. Eye Res.* **2018**, *65*, 50–76. [CrossRef] [PubMed]
5. MacDonald, I.M.; Sauvé, Y.; Sieving, P.A. Preventing blindness in retinal disease: Ciliary neurotrophic factor intraocular implants. *Can. J. Ophthal.* **2007**, *42*, 399–402. [CrossRef]
6. Kimura, A.; Namekata, K.; Guo, X.; Harada, C.; Harada, T. Neuroprotection, growth factors and BDNF-TrkB signalling in retinal degeneration. *Int. J. Mol. Sci.* **2016**, *17*, 1584. [CrossRef]
7. Unsicker, K. Neurotrophic molecules in the treatment of neurodegenerative disease with focus on the retina: Status and perspectives. *Cell Tissue Res.* **2013**, *353*, 205–218. [CrossRef]
8. Wen, R.; Tao, W.; Li, Y.; Sieving, P.A. CNTF and retina. *Prog. Retin. Eye Res.* **2012**, *31*, 136–151. [CrossRef]
9. Sleeman, M.W.; Anderson, K.D.; Lambert, P.D.; Yancopoulos, G.D.; Wiegand, S.J. The ciliary neurotrophic factor and its receptor, CNTFRα. *Pharm. Acta Helv.* **2000**, *74*, 265–272. [CrossRef]
10. Wagener, E.M.; Aurich, M.; Aparicio-Siegmund, S.; Floss, D.M.; Garbers, C.; Breusing, K.; Rabe, B.; Schwanbeck, R.; Grotzinger, J.; Rose-John, S. The amino acid exchange R28E in ciliary neurotrophic factor (CNTF) abrogates interleukin-6 receptor-dependent but retains CNTF receptor-dependent signaling via glycoprotein 130 (gp130)/leukemia inhibitory factor receptor (LIFR). *J. Biol. Chem.* **2014**, *289*, 18442–18450. [CrossRef]
11. Schuster, B.; Kovaleva, M.; Sun, Y.; Regenhard, P.; Matthews, V.; Grotzinger, J.; Rose-John, S.; Kallen, K.J. Signaling of human ciliary neurotrophic factor (CNTF) revisited. The interleukin-6 receptor can serve as an alpha-receptor for CTNF. *J. Biol. Chem.* **2003**, *278*, 9528–9535. [CrossRef] [PubMed]
12. Li, R.; Wen, R.; Banzon, T.; Maminishkis, A.; Miller, S.S. CNTF mediates neurotrophic factor secretion and fluid absorption in human retinal pigment epithelium. *PLoS ONE* **2011**, *6*, e23148. [CrossRef] [PubMed]
13. Li, S.; Sato, K.; Gordon, W.C.; Sendtner, M.; Bazan, N.G.; Jin, M. Ciliary neurotrophic factor (CNTF) protects retinal cone and rod photoreceptors by suppressing excessive formation of the visual pigments. *J. Biol. Chem.* **2018**, *293*, 15256–15268. [CrossRef] [PubMed]
14. Heiduschka, P.; Renninger, D.; Fischer, D.; Müller, A.; Hofmeister, S.; Schraermeyer, U. Lens injury has a protective effect on photoreceptors in the RCS rat. *ISRN Ophthalmol.* **2013**, *2013*, 814814. [CrossRef] [PubMed]
15. Peterson, W.M.; Wang, Q.; Tzekova, R.; Wiegand, S.J. Ciliary neurotrophic factor and stress stimuli activate the Jak-STAT pathway in retinal neurons and glia. *J. Neurosci.* **2000**, *20*, 4081–4090. [CrossRef]
16. Beltran, W.; Rohrer, H.; Aguirre, G.D. Immunolocalization of ciliary neurotrophic factor receptor α (CNTFRα) in mammalian photoreceptor cells. *Mol. Vis.* **2005**, *11*, 232–244.
17. Bucher, F.; Walz, J.M.; Bühler, A.; Aguilar, E.; Lange, C.; Diaz-Aguilar, S.; Martin, G.; Schlunck, G.; Agostini, H.; Friedlander, M. CNTF attenuates vasoproliferative changes through upregulation of SOCS3 in a mouse-model of oxygen-induced retinopathy. *Investig. Ophthalmol. Vis. Sci.* **2016**, *57*, 4017–4026. [CrossRef]
18. Rhee, K.D.; Nusinowitz, S.; Chao, K.; Yu, F.; Bok, D.; Yang, X.J. CNTF-mediated protection of photoreceptors requires initial activation of the cytokine receptor gp130 in Müller glial cells. *Proc. Natl. Acad. Sci. USA* **2013**, *110*, E4520–E4529. [CrossRef]
19. Sieving, P.A.; Caruso, R.C.; Tao, W.; Coleman, H.R.; Thompson, D.J.S.; Fullmer, K.R.; Bush, R.A. Ciliary neurotrophic factor (CNTF) for human retinal degeneration: Phase I trial of CNTF delivered by encapsulated cell intraocular implants. *Proc. Natl. Acad. Sci. USA* **2006**, *103*, 3896–3901. [CrossRef]

20. Krady, J.K.; Lin, H.; Liberto, C.M.; Basu, A.; Kremlev, S.G.; Levison, S.W. Ciliary neurotrophic factor and interleukin-6 differentially activate microglia. *J. Neurosci. Res.* **2008**, *86*, 1538–1547. [CrossRef]
21. Baek, J.; Jeong, J.; Kim, K.; Won, S.; Chung, Y.; Nam, J.; Cho, E.; Ahn, T.; Bok, E.; Shin, W. Inhibition of microglia-derived oxidative stress by ciliary neurotrophic factor protects dopamine neurons in vivo from MPP neurotoxicity. *Int. J. Mol. Sci.* **2018**, *19*, 3543. [CrossRef] [PubMed]
22. Lin, H.; Jain, M.R.; Li, H.; Levison, S.W. Ciliary neurotrophic factor (CNTF) plus soluble CNTF receptor α increases cyclooxygenase-2 expression, PGE 2 release and interferon-γ-induced CD40 in murine microglia. *J. Neuroinflammation* **2009**, *6*, 7. [CrossRef] [PubMed]
23. Cen, L.; Luo, J.; Zhang, C.; Fan, Y.; Song, Y.; So, K.; van Rooijen, N.; Pang, C.P.; Lam, D.S.; Cui, Q. Chemotactic effect of ciliary neurotrophic factor on macrophages in retinal ganglion cell survival and axonal regeneration. *Investig. Ophthalmol. Vis. Sci.* **2007**, *48*, 4257–4266. [CrossRef] [PubMed]
24. Van Adel, B.; Arnold, J.; Phipps, J.; Doering, L.; Ball, A. Ciliary neurotrophic factor protects retinal ganglion cells from axotomy-induced apoptosis via modulation of retinal glia *in vivo*. *J. Neurobiol.* **2005**, *63*, 215–234. [CrossRef]
25. Wen, R.; Song, Y.; Kjellstrom, S.; Tanikawa, A.; Liu, Y.; Li, Y.; Zhao, L.; Bush, R.A.; Laties, A.M.; Sieving, P.A. Regulation of rod phototransduction machinery by ciliary neurotrophic factor. *J. Neurosci.* **2006**, *26*, 13523–13530. [CrossRef]
26. Harada, T.; Harada, C.; Kohsaka, S.; Wada, E.; Yoshida, K.; Ohno, S.; Mamada, H.; Tanaka, K.; Parada, L.F.; Wada, K. Microglia-Müller glia cell interactions control neurotrophic factor production during light-induced retinal degeneration. *J. Neurosci.* **2002**, *22*, 9228–9236. [CrossRef]
27. Müller, A.; Hauk, T.G.; Leibinger, M.; Marienfeld, R.; Fischer, D. Exogenous CNTF stimulates axon regeneration of retinal ganglion cells partially via endogenous CNTF. *Mol. Cell Neurosci.* **2009**, *41*, 233–246. [CrossRef]
28. Wahlin, K.J.; Campochiaro, P.A.; Zack, D.J.; Adler, R. Neurotrophic factors cause activation of intracellular signaling pathways in Müller cells and other cells of the inner retina, but not photoreceptors. *Investig. Ophthalmol. Vis. Sci.* **2000**, *41*, 927–936.
29. Wen, R.; Song, Y.; Cheng, T.; Matthes, M.T.; Yasumura, D.; LaVail, M.M.; Steinberg, R.H. Injury-induced upregulation of bFGF and CNTF mRNAs in the rat retina. *J. Neurosci.* **1995**, *15*, 7377–7385. [CrossRef]
30. Nir, I.; Liu, C.; Wen, R. Light treatment enhances photoreceptor survival in dystrophic retinas of Royal College of Surgeons rats. *Investig. Ophthalmol. Vis. Sci.* **1999**, *40*, 2383–2390.
31. Schlichtenbrede, F.; MacNeil, A.; Bainbridge, J.; Tschernutter, M.; Thrasher, A.; Smith, A.; Ali, R. Intraocular gene delivery of ciliary neurotrophic factor results in significant loss of retinal function in normal mice and in the Prph2 Rd2/Rd2 model of retinal degeneration. *Gene Ther.* **2003**, *10*, 523–527. [CrossRef] [PubMed]
32. Bok, D.; Yasumura, D.; Matthes, M.T.; Ruiz, A.; Duncan, J.L.; Chappelow, A.V.; Zolutukhin, S.; Hauswirth, W.; LaVail, M.M. Effects of adeno-associated virus-vectored ciliary neurotrophic factor on retinal structure and function in mice with a P216L Rds/peripherin mutation. *Exp. Eye Res.* **2002**, *74*, 719–735. [CrossRef] [PubMed]
33. Huang, S.; Lin, P.; Liu, J.; Khor, C.; Lee, Y. Intraocular gene transfer of ciliary neurotrophic factor rescues photoreceptor degeneration in RCS rats. *J. Biomed. Sci.* **2004**, *11*, 37–48. [CrossRef] [PubMed]
34. Bush, R.A.; Lei, B.; Tao, W.; Raz, D.; Chan, C.; Cox, T.A.; Santos-Muffley, M.; Sieving, P.A. Encapsulated cell-based intraocular delivery of ciliary neurotrophic factor in normal rabbit: Dose-dependent effects on ERG and retinal histology. *Investig. Ophthalmol. Vis. Sci.* **2004**, *45*, 2420–2430. [CrossRef]
35. Li, Y.; Tao, W.; Luo, L.; Huang, D.; Kauper, K.; Stabila, P.; LaVail, M.M.; Laties, A.M.; Wen, R. CNTF induces regeneration of cone outer segments in a rat model of retinal degeneration. *PLoS ONE* **2010**, *5*, e9495. [CrossRef]
36. Cayouette, M.; Behn, D.; Sendtner, M.; Lachapelle, P.; Gravel, C. Intraocular gene transfer of ciliary neurotrophic factor prevents death and increases responsiveness of rod photoreceptors in the retinal degeneration slow mouse. *J. Neurosci.* **1998**, *18*, 9282–9293. [CrossRef]
37. LaVail, M.M.; Yasumura, D.; Matthes, M.T.; Lau-Villacorta, C.; Unoki, K.; Sung, C.; Steinberg, R.H. Protection of mouse photoreceptors by survival factors in retinal degenerations. *Investig. Ophthalmol. Vis. Sci.* **1998**, *39*, 592–602.

38. Beltran, W.A.; Wen, R.; Acland, G.M.; Aguirre, G.D. Intravitreal injection of ciliary neurotrophic factor (CNTF) causes peripheral remodeling and does not prevent photoreceptor loss in canine RPGR mutant Retina. *Exp. Eye Res.* **2007**, *84*, 753–771. [CrossRef]
39. LaVail, M.M.; Unoki, K.; Yasumura, D.; Matthes, M.T.; Yancopoulos, G.D.; Steinberg, R.H. Multiple growth factors, cytokines, and neurotrophins rescue photoreceptors from the damaging effects of constant light. *Proc. Natl. Acad. Sci. USA* **1992**, *89*, 11249–11253. [CrossRef]
40. Wen, R.; Tao, W.; Luo, L.; Huang, D.; Kauper, K.; Stabila, P.; LaVail, M.M.; Laties, A.M.; Li, Y. Regeneration of cone outer segments induced by CNTF. *Adv. Exp. Med. Biol.* **2012**, *723*, 93–99.
41. Fandl, J.P.; Stahl, N.E.; Wiegand, S.J. Modified Ciliary Neurotrophic Factor (CNTF). U.S. Patent 7119066B2, 10 October 2006.
42. Itkonen, J.M.; Urtti, A.; Bird, L.E.; Sarkhel, S. Codon optimization and factorial screening for enhanced soluble expression of human ciliary neurotrophic factor in *Escherichia coli*. *BMC Biotechnol.* **2014**, *14*, 92. [CrossRef] [PubMed]
43. Berrow, N.S.; Alderton, D.; Owens, R.J. The precise engineering of expression vectors using high-throughput in-Fusion PCR cloning. *Methods Mol. Biol.* **2009**, *498*, 75–90.
44. Studier, F.W. Protein production by auto-induction in high-density shaking cultures. *Protein Expr. Purif.* **2005**, *41*, 207–234. [CrossRef] [PubMed]
45. Panula-Perälä, J.; Šiurkus, J.; Vasala, A.; Wilmanowski, R.; Casteleijn, M.G.; Neubauer, P. Enzyme controlled glucose auto-delivery for high cell density cultivations in microplates and shake flasks. *Microb. Cell Fact.* **2008**, *7*, 31. [CrossRef]
46. Porstmann, T.; Ternynck, T.; Avrameas, S. Quantitation of 5-bromo-2-deoxyuridine incorporation into DNA: An enzyme immunoassay for the assessment of the lymphoid cell proliferative response. *J. Immunol. Methods* **1985**, *82*, 169–179. [CrossRef]
47. Micsonai, A.; Wien, F.; Kernya, L.; Lee, Y.H.; Goto, Y.; Refregiers, M.; Kardos, J. Accurate secondary structure prediction and fold recognition for circular dichroism spectroscopy. *Proc. Natl. Acad. Sci. USA* **2015**, *112*, E3095–E3103. [CrossRef] [PubMed]
48. Sviben, D.; Bertoša, B.; Hloušek-Kasun, A.; Forcic, D.; Halassy, B.; Brgles, M. Investigation of the thermal shift assay and its power to predict protein and virus stabilizing conditions. *J. Pharm. Biomed. Anal.* **2018**, *161*, 73–82. [CrossRef] [PubMed]
49. Kopec, J.; Schneider, G. Comparison of fluorescence and light scattering based methods to assess formation and stability of protein–protein complexes. *J. Struct. Biol.* **2011**, *175*, 216–223. [CrossRef] [PubMed]
50. Boivin, S.; Kozak, S.; Meijers, R. Optimization of protein purification and characterization using Thermofluor screens. *Protein Expr. Purif.* **2013**, *91*, 192–206. [CrossRef]
51. Caffe, A.; Ahuja, P.; Holmqvist, B.; Azadi, S.; Forsell, J.; Holmqvist, I.; Söderpalm, A.; Van Veen, T. Mouse retina explants after long-term culture in serum free medium. *J. Chem. Neuroanat.* **2002**, *22*, 263–273. [CrossRef]
52. Arango-Gonzalez, B.; Szabó, A.; Pinzon-Duarte, G.; Lukáts, Á.; Guenther, E.; Kohler, K. In vivo and in vitro development of S-and M-cones in rat retina. *Investig. Ophthalmol. Vis. Sci.* **2010**, *51*, 5320–5327. [CrossRef] [PubMed]
53. Peynshaert, K.; Devoldere, J.; Forster, V.; Picaud, S.; Vanhove, C.; De Smedt, S.C.; Remaut, K. Toward smart design of retinal drug carriers: A novel bovine retinal explant model to study the barrier role of the vitreoretinal interface. *Drug Deliv.* **2017**, *24*, 1384–1394. [CrossRef] [PubMed]
54. Greenfield, N.J. Using circular dichroism spectra to estimate protein secondary structure. *Nat. Protoc.* **2006**, *1*, 2876–2890. [CrossRef]
55. Xu, L.; Zhang, C.; Liu, L.; Zhang, Y.; Wang, Q.; Wang, J.; Liu, Y.; Su, Z. Purification and characterization of a long-acting ciliary neurotrophic factor via genetically fused with an albumin-binding domain. *Protein Expr. Purif.* **2017**, *139*, 14–20. [CrossRef] [PubMed]
56. Wang, Q.; Liu, Y.; Zhang, C.; Guo, F.; Feng, C.; Li, X.; Shi, H.; Su, Z. High hydrostatic pressure enables almost 100% refolding of recombinant human ciliary neurotrophic factor from inclusion bodies at high concentration. *Protein Expr. Purif.* **2017**, *133*, 152–159. [CrossRef]
57. Negro, A.; Grassato, L.; Polverino De Laureto, P.; Skaper, S.D. Genetic construction, properties and application of a green fluorescent protein-tagged ciliary neurotrophic factor. *Protein Eng.* **1997**, *10*, 1077–1083. [CrossRef]

58. Delplace, V.; Ortin-Martinez, A.; Tsai, E.L.S.; Amin, A.N.; Wallace, V.; Shoichet, M.S. Controlled release strategy designed for intravitreal protein delivery to the retina. *J. Control. Release* **2019**, *293*, 10–20. [CrossRef]
59. Stetefeld, J.; McKenna, S.A.; Patel, T.R. Dynamic light scattering: A practical guide and applications in biomedical sciences. *Biophys. Rev.* **2016**, *8*, 409–427. [CrossRef]
60. Kitamura, T.; Tange, T.; Terasawa, T.; Chiba, S.; Kuwaki, T.; Miyagawa, K.; Piao, Y.; Miyazono, K.; Urabe, A.; Takaku, F. Establishment and characterization of a unique human cell line that proliferates dependently on GM-CSF, IL-3, or erythropoietin. *J. Cell. Physiol.* **1989**, *140*, 323–334. [CrossRef]
61. Auguste, P.; Robledo, O.; Olivier, C.; Froger, J.; Praloran, V.; Pouplard-Barthelaix, A.; Gascan, H. Alanine substitution for Thr268 and Asp269 of soluble ciliary neurotrophic factor (CNTF) receptor alpha component defines a specific antagonist for the CNTF response. *J. Biol. Chem.* **1996**, *271*, 26049–26056. [CrossRef]
62. Bhatnagar, B.S.; Bogner, R.H.; Pikal, M.J. Protein stability during freezing: Separation of stresses and mechanisms of protein stabilization. *Pharm. Dev. Technol.* **2007**, *12*, 505–523. [CrossRef] [PubMed]
63. Zbacnik, T.J.; Holcomb, R.E.; Katayama, D.S.; Murphy, B.M.; Payne, R.W.; Coccaro, R.C.; Evans, G.J.; Matsuura, J.E.; Henry, C.S.; Manning, M.C. Role of buffers in protein formulations. *J. Pharm. Sci.* **2017**, *106*, 713–733. [CrossRef] [PubMed]
64. Szkudlarek, B.A. Selective Crystallization of Phosphate Buffer Components and pH Changes during Freezing: Implications to Protein Stability. Ph.D. Thesis, University of Michigan, Ann Arbor, MI, USA, 1997.
65. Seabrook, S.A.; Newman, J. High-throughput thermal scanning for protein stability: Making a good technique more robust. *ACS Comb. Sci.* **2013**, *15*, 387–392. [CrossRef]
66. Jiskoot, W.; Randolph, T.W.; Volkin, D.B.; Middaugh, C.R.; Schöneich, C.; Winter, G.; Friess, W.; Crommelin, D.J.; Carpenter, J.F. Protein instability and immunogenicity: Roadblocks to clinical application of injectable protein delivery systems for sustained release. *J. Pharm. Sci.* **2012**, *101*, 946–954. [CrossRef]
67. Wakshull, E.; Quarmby, V.; Mahler, H.; Rivers, H.; Jere, D.; Ramos, M.; Szczesny, P.; Bechtold-Peters, K.; Masli, S.; Gupta, S. Advancements in understanding immunogenicity of biotherapeutics in the intraocular space. *AAPS J.* **2017**, *19*, 1656–1668. [CrossRef] [PubMed]
68. Lorber, B.; Fischer, F.; Bailly, M.; Roy, H.; Kern, D. Protein analysis by dynamic light scattering: Methods and techniques for students. *Biochem. Mol. Biol. Educ.* **2012**, *40*, 372–382. [CrossRef]
69. Parmar, A.S.; Muschol, M. Hydration and hydrodynamic interactions of lysozyme: Effects of chaotropic versus kosmotropic ions. *Biophys. J.* **2009**, *97*, 590–598. [CrossRef]
70. Amin, S.; Barnett, G.V.; Pathak, J.A.; Roberts, C.J.; Sarangapani, P.S. Protein aggregation, particle formation, characterization & rheology. *Curr. Opin. Colloid Interface Sci.* **2014**, *19*, 438–449.
71. Filipe, V.; Hawe, A.; Carpenter, J.F.; Jiskoot, W. Analytical approaches to assess the degradation of therapeutic proteins. *Trends Anal. Chem.* **2013**, *49*, 118–125. [CrossRef]
72. Patel, S.; Müller, G.; Stracke, J.O.; Altenburger, U.; Mahler, H.; Jere, D. Evaluation of protein drug stability with vitreous humor in a novel *ex-vivo* intraocular model. *Eur. J. Pharm. Biopharm.* **2015**, *95*, 407–417. [CrossRef]
73. Patel, S.; Stracke, J.O.; Altenburger, U.; Mahler, H.; Metzger, P.; Shende, P.; Jere, D. Prediction of intraocular antibody drug stability using *ex-vivo* ocular model. *Eur. J. Pharm. Biopharm.* **2017**, *112*, 177–186. [CrossRef] [PubMed]
74. Rösch, S.; Aretzweiler, C.; Müller, F.; Walter, P. Evaluation of retinal function and morphology of the pink-eyed Royal College of Surgeons (RCS) rat: A comparative study of in vivo and in vitro methods. *Curr. Eye Res.* **2017**, *42*, 273–281. [CrossRef] [PubMed]
75. McGill, T.J.; Prusky, G.T.; Douglas, R.M.; Yasumura, D.; Matthes, M.T.; Nune, G.; Donohue-Rolfe, K.; Yang, H.; Niculescu, D.; Hauswirth, W.W. Intraocular CNTF reduces vision in normal rats in a dose-dependent manner. *Investig. Ophthalmol. Vis. Sci.* **2007**, *48*, 5756–5766. [CrossRef] [PubMed]
76. Do Rhee, K.; Ruiz, A.; Duncan, J.L.; Hauswirth, W.W.; LaVail, M.M.; Bok, D.; Yang, X. Molecular and cellular alterations induced by sustained expression of ciliary neurotrophic factor in a mouse model of retinitis pigmentosa. *Investig. Ophthalmol. Vis. Sci.* **2007**, *48*, 1389–1400. [CrossRef] [PubMed]
77. Chaitin, M.; Hall, M.O. Defective ingestion of rod outer segments by cultured dystrophic rat pigment epithelial cells. *Investig. Ophthalmol. Vis. Sci.* **1983**, *24*, 812–820. [PubMed]
78. D'Cruz, P.M.; Yasumura, D.; Weir, J.; Matthes, M.T.; Abderrahim, H.; LaVail, M.M.; Vollrath, D. Mutation of the receptor tyrosine kinase gene Mertk in the retinal dystrophic RCS rat. *Hum. Mol. Genet.* **2000**, *9*, 645–651. [CrossRef]

79. Dittrich, F.; Theonen, H.; Sendtner, M. Ciliary neurotrophic factor: Pharmacokinetics and acute-phase response in rat. *Ann. Neurol.* **1994**, *35*, 151–163. [CrossRef]
80. Sendtner, M.; Dittrich, F.; Hughes, R.A.; Thoenen, H. Actions of CNTF and neurotrophins on degenerating motoneurons: Preclinical studies and clinical implications. *J. Neurol. Sci.* **1994**, *124*, 77–83. [CrossRef]
81. Pasquin, S.; Sharma, M.; Gauchat, J. Ciliary neurotrophic factor (CNTF): New facets of an old molecule for treating neurodegenerative and metabolic syndrome pathologies. *Cytokine Growth Factor Rev.* **2015**, *26*, 507–515. [CrossRef]
82. del Amo, E.M.; Vellonen, K.; Kidron, H.; Urtti, A. Intravitreal clearance and volume of distribution of compounds in rabbits: In silico prediction and pharmacokinetic simulations for drug development. *Eur. J. Pharm. Biopharm.* **2015**, *95*, 215–226. [CrossRef]
83. del Amo, E.M.; Rimpelä, A.; Heikkinen, E.; Kari, O.K.; Ramsay, E.; Lajunen, T.; Schmitt, M.; Pelkonen, L.; Bhattacharya, M.; Richardson, D. Pharmacokinetic aspects of retinal drug delivery. *Prog. Retin. Eye Res.* **2017**, *57*, 134–185. [CrossRef] [PubMed]
84. Shatz, W.; Hass, P.E.; Mathieu, M.; Kim, H.S.; Leach, K.; Zhou, M.; Crawford, Y.; Shen, A.; Wang, K.; Chang, D.P. Contribution of antibody hydrodynamic size to vitreal clearance revealed through rabbit studies using a species-matched Fab. *Mol. Pharm.* **2016**, *13*, 2996–3003. [CrossRef] [PubMed]
85. Crowell, S.R.; Wang, K.; Famili, A.; Shatz, W.; Loyet, K.M.; Chang, V.; Liu, Y.; Prabhu, S.; Kamath, A.V.; Kelley, R.F. Influence of charge, hydrophobicity, and size on vitreous pharmacokinetics of large molecules. *Transl. Visc. Sci. Technol.* **2019**, *8*, 1. [CrossRef] [PubMed]
86. Ekdawi, N.S.; Pulido, J.S.; Itty, S.; Marler, R.J.; Herman, D.C.; Hardwig, P.; Mohney, B.G.; Valyi-Nagy, T.; Shukla, D. Intravitreal alemtuzumab penetrates full-thickness retina in rabbit eyes. *Retina* **2009**, *29*, 1532–1534. [CrossRef] [PubMed]
87. Melo, G.B.; Moraes Filho, M.N.; Rodrigues, E.B.; Regatieri, C.V.; Dreyfuss, J.L.; Penha, F.M.; Pinheiro, M.M.; Coimbra, R.C.; Haapalainen, E.F.; Farah, M.E. Toxicity and retinal penetration of infliximab in primates. *Retina* **2012**, *32*, 606–612. [CrossRef]
88. Heiduschka, P.; Fietz, H.; Hofmeister, S.; Schultheiss, S.; Mack, A.F.; Peters, S.; Ziemssen, F.; Niggemann, B.; Julien, S.; Bartz-Schmidt, K.U. Penetration of bevacizumab through the retina after intravitreal injection in the monkey. *Investig. Ophthalmol. Vis. Sci.* **2007**, *48*, 2814–2823. [CrossRef]
89. Jankowiak, W.; Kruszewski, K.; Flachsbarth, K.; Skevas, C.; Richard, G.; Rüther, K.; Braulke, T.; Bartsch, U. Sustained neural stem cell-based intraocular delivery of CNTF attenuates photoreceptor loss in the Nclf mouse model of neuronal ceroid lipofuscinosis. *PLoS ONE* **2015**, *10*, e0127204. [CrossRef]
90. Leaver, S.G.; Cui, Q.; Plant, G.W.; Arulpragasam, A.; Hisheh, S.; Verhaagen, J.; Harvey, A.R. AAV-mediated expression of CNTF promotes long-term survival and regeneration of adult rat retinal ganglion cells. *Gene Ther.* **2006**, *13*, 1328. [CrossRef]
91. Pease, M.E.; Zack, D.J.; Berlinicke, C.; Bloom, K.; Cone, F.; Wang, Y.; Klein, R.L.; Hauswirth, W.W.; Quigley, H.A. Effect of CNTF on retinal ganglion cell survival in experimental glaucoma. *Investig. Ophthalmol. Vis. Sci.* **2009**, *50*, 2194–2200. [CrossRef]
92. LeVaillant, C.J.; Sharma, A.; Muhling, J.; Wheeler, L.P.; Cozens, G.S.; Hellström, M.; Rodger, J.; Harvey, A.R. Significant changes in endogenous retinal gene expression assessed 1 year after a single intraocular injection of AAV-CNTF or AAV-BDNF. *Mol. Ther. Methods Clin. Dev.* **2016**, *3*, 16078. [CrossRef]
93. Lipinski, D.M.; Barnard, A.R.; Singh, M.S.; Martin, C.; Lee, E.J.; Davies, W.I.; MacLaren, R.E. CNTF gene therapy confers lifelong neuroprotection in a mouse model of human retinitis pigmentosa. *Mol. Ther.* **2015**, *23*, 1308–1319. [CrossRef] [PubMed]
94. Liang, F.; Dejneka, N.S.; Cohen, D.R.; Krasnoperova, N.V.; Lem, J.; Maguire, A.M.; Dudus, L.; Fisher, K.J.; Bennett, J. AAV-mediated delivery of ciliary neurotrophic factor prolongs photoreceptor survival in the rhodopsin knockout mouse. *Mol. Ther.* **2001**, *3*, 241–248. [CrossRef]
95. Kauper, K.; McGovern, C.; Sherman, S.; Heatherton, P.; Rapoza, R.; Stabila, P.; Dean, B.; Lee, A.; Borges, S.; Bouchard, B. Two-year intraocular delivery of ciliary neurotrophic factor by encapsulated cell technology implants in patients with chronic retinal degenerative diseases. *Investig. Ophthalmol. Vis. Sci.* **2012**, *53*, 7484–7491. [CrossRef]

96. Zhang, K.; Hopkins, J.J.; Heier, J.S.; Birch, D.G.; Halperin, L.S.; Albini, T.A.; Brown, D.M.; Jaffe, G.J.; Tao, W.; Williams, G.A. Ciliary neurotrophic factor delivered by encapsulated cell intraocular implants for treatment of geographic atrophy in age-related macular degeneration. *Proc. Natl. Acad. Sci. USA* **2011**, *108*, 6241–6245. [CrossRef] [PubMed]
97. Zein, W.M.; Jeffrey, B.G.; Wiley, H.E.; Turriff, A.E.; Tumminia, S.J.; Tao, W.; Bush, R.A.; Marangoni, D.; Wen, R.; Wei, L.L. CNGB3-achromatopsia clinical trial with CNTF: Diminished rod pathway responses with no evidence of improvement in cone function. *Investig. Ophthalmol. Vis. Sci.* **2014**, *55*, 6301–6308. [CrossRef] [PubMed]
98. Ghasemi, M.; Alizadeh, E.; Saei Arezoumand, K.; Fallahi Motlagh, B.; Zarghami, N. Ciliary neurotrophic factor (CNTF) delivery to retina: An overview of current research advancements. *Artif. Cells Nanomed. Biotechnol.* **2018**, *46*, 1694–1707. [CrossRef]
99. Talcott, K.E.; Ratnam, K.; Sundquist, S.M.; Lucero, A.S.; Lujan, B.J.; Tao, W.; Porco, T.C.; Roorda, A.; Duncan, J.L. Longitudinal study of cone photoreceptors during retinal degeneration and in response to ciliary neurotrophic factor treatment. *Investig. Ophthalmol. Vis. Sci.* **2011**, *52*, 2219–2226. [CrossRef]
100. Chew, E.Y.; Clemons, T.E.; Jaffe, G.J.; Johnson, C.A.; Farsiu, S.; Lad, E.M.; Guymer, R.; Rosenfeld, P.; Hubschman, J.; Constable, I.; et al. Effect of ciliary neurotrophic factor on retinal neurodegeneration in patients with macular telangiectasia type 2: A randomized clinical trial. *Ophthalmology* **2019**, *126*, 540–549. [CrossRef]
101. El Sanharawi, M.; Kowalczuk, L.; Touchard, E.; Omri, S.; De Kozak, Y.; Behar-Cohen, F. Protein delivery for retinal diseases: From basic considerations to clinical applications. *Prog. Retin. Eye Res.* **2010**, *29*, 443–465. [CrossRef]
102. Lau, C.M.L.; Yu, Y.; Jahanmir, G.; Chau, Y. Controlled release technology for anti-angiogenesis treatment of posterior eye diseases: Current status and challenges. *Adv. Drug Deliv. Rev.* **2018**, *126*, 145–161. [CrossRef]
103. Peynshaert, K.; Devoldere, J.; Minnaert, A.; De Smedt, S.C.; Remaut, K. Morphology and composition of the inner limiting membrane: Species-specific variations and relevance toward drug delivery research. *Curr. Eye Res.* **2019**, *44*, 465–475. [CrossRef] [PubMed]
104. Valdés, J.; Trachsel-Moncho, L.; Sahaboglu, A.; Trifunović, D.; Miranda, M.; Ueffing, M.; Paquet-Durand, F.; Schmachtenberg, O. Organotypic retinal explant cultures as in vitro alternative for diabetic retinopathy studies. *ALTEX* **2016**, *33*, 459–464. [CrossRef] [PubMed]
105. Peynshaert, K.; Devoldere, J.; De Smedt, S.C.; Remaut, K. In vitro and ex vivo models to study drug delivery barriers in the posterior segment of the eye. *Adv. Drug Deliv. Rev.* **2018**, *126*, 44–57. [CrossRef] [PubMed]
106. Alarautalahti, V.; Ragauskas, S.; Hakkarainen, J.J.; Uusitalo-Järvinen, H.; Uusitalo, H.; Hyttinen, J.; Kalesnykas, G.; Nymark, S. Viability of mouse retinal explant cultures assessed by preservation of functionality and morphology. *Investig. Ophthalmol. Vis. Sci.* **2019**, *60*, 1914–1927. [CrossRef]
107. Shahar, J.; Avery, R.L.; Heilweil, G.; Barak, A.; Zemel, E.; Lewis, G.P.; Johnson, P.T.; Fisher, S.K.; Perlman, I.; Loewenstein, A. Electrophysiologic and retinal penetration studies following intravitreal injection of bevacizumab (Avastin). *Retina* **2006**, *26*, 262–269. [CrossRef]
108. Hutton-Smith, L.A.; Gaffney, E.A.; Byrne, H.M.; Maini, P.K.; Gadkar, K.; Mazer, N.A. Ocular pharmacokinetics of therapeutic antibodies given by intravitreal injection: Estimation of retinal permeabilities using a 3-Compartment semi-mechanistic model. *Mol. Pharm.* **2017**, *14*, 2690–2696. [CrossRef]
109. Hutton-Smith, L.A.; Gaffney, E.A.; Byrne, H.M.; Caruso, A.; Maini, P.K.; Mazer, N.A. Theoretical insights into the retinal dynamics of vascular endothelial growth factor in patients treated with ranibizumab, based on an ocular pharmacokinetic/pharmacodynamic model. *Mol. Pharm.* **2018**, *15*, 2770–2784. [CrossRef]

Pharmaceutics 2020, 12, 404

Article

Topical Application of Hyaluronic Acid-RGD Peptide-Coated Gelatin/Epigallocatechin-3 Gallate (EGCG) Nanoparticles Inhibits Corneal Neovascularization via Inhibition of VEGF Production

Takuya Miyagawa [1,2], Zhi-Yu Chen [1], Che-Yi Chang [1], Ko-Hua Chen [3,4], Yang-Kao Wang [5], Guei-Sheung Liu [1,6,7,*] and Ching-Li Tseng [1,8,9,10,*]

1 Graduate Institute of Biomedical Materials and Tissue Engineering, College of Biomedical Engineering, Taipei Medical University, Taipei City 110, Taiwan; takuya.miyagawa@tu-dresden.de or michael_idea@hotmail.com (T.M.); D05548017@ntu.edu.tw or d79010340217@gmail.com (Z.-Y.C.); D825107002@tmu.edu.tw or orzdinoqoo1@gmail.com (C.-Y.C.)
2 B CUBE, Center for Molecular Bioengineering, Technische Universität Dresden, Tatzberg 41, 01307 Dresden, Germany
3 Department of Ophthalmology, Taipei Veterans General Hospital, Taipei City 112, Taiwan; Khchen@vghtpe.gov.tw or khchen7637@gmail.com
4 Department of Ophthalmology, School of Medicine, College of Medicine, Taipei Medical University, Taipei 11031, Taiwan
5 Department of Cell Biology and Anatomy, College of Medicine, National Cheng Kung University, Tainan City 701, Taiwan; humwang@ncku.edu.tw
6 Menzies Institute for Medical Research, University of Tasmania, Hobart, TAS 7000, Australia
7 Ophthalmology, Department of Surgery, University of Melbourne, East Melbourne, VIC 3002, Australia
8 International Ph. D. Program in Biomedical Engineering, College of Biomedical Engineering, Taipei Medical University, Taipei city 110, Taiwan
9 Research Center of Biomedical Device, College of Biomedical Engineering, Taipei Medical University, Taipei City 110, Taiwan
10 International Ph. D. Program in Cell Therapy and Regenerative Medicine, College of Medicine, Taipei Medical University, Taipei City 110, Taiwan
* Correspondence: gueisheung.liu@utas.edu.au or rickliu0817@gmail.com (G.-S.L.); chingli@tmu.edu.tw (C.-L.T.); Tel.: +61-03-62264250 (G.-S.L.); +886-2736-1661 (ext. 5214) (C.-L.T.)

Received: 28 March 2020; Accepted: 26 April 2020; Published: 28 April 2020

Abstract: Neovascularization (NV) of the cornea disrupts vision which leads to blindness. Investigation of antiangiogenic, slow-release and biocompatible approaches for treating corneal NV is of great importance. We designed an eye drop formulation containing gelatin/epigallocatechin-3-gallate (EGCG) nanoparticles (NPs) for targeted therapy in corneal NV. Gelatin-EGCG self-assembled NPs with hyaluronic acid (HA) coating on its surface (named GEH) and hyaluronic acid conjugated with arginine-glycine-aspartic acid (RGD) (GEH-RGD) were synthesized. Human umbilical vein endothelial cells (HUVECs) were used to evaluate the antiangiogenic effect of GEH-RGD NPs in vitro. Moreover, a mouse model of chemical corneal cauterization was employed to evaluate the antiangiogenic effects of GEH-RGD NPs in vivo. GEH-RGD NP treatment significantly reduced endothelial cell tube formation and inhibited metalloproteinase (MMP)-2 and MMP-9 activity in HUVECs in vitro. Topical application of GEH-RGD NPs (once daily for a week) significantly attenuated the formation of pathological vessels in the mouse cornea after chemical cauterization. Reduction in both vascular endothelial growth factor (VEGF) and MMP-9 protein in the GEH-RGD NP-treated cauterized corneas was observed. These results confirm the molecular mechanism of the antiangiogenic effect of GEH-RGD NPs in suppressing pathological corneal NV.

Keywords: anti-angiogenesis; corneal neovascularization (NV); epigallocatechin gallate (EGCG); gelatin; hyaluronic acid (HA), nanoparticles; RGD peptide; eye drops

1. Introduction

Corneal neovascularization (NV) is the formation of new vessels from pre-existing vascular structures in the transparent cornea, resulting from a variety of ocular pathologic conditions which are detrimental to vision [1–4]. These newly-formed vessels sprouting from the capillaries of the pericorneal plexus may block light, compromise visual acuity, cause inflammation and corneal scarring, and may eventually result in blindness [2,5–8]. Etiologies of corneal NV include infection, injury, surgery, autoimmune disease, inflammation, neoplasm, dystrophy, deficiency of limbal barrier function, corneal hypoxia, and improper use of contact lenses [9–12]. There were over 150 million people worldwide wearing contact lenses in 2019, implying a large population is at risk of developing corneal NV due to corneal hypoxia [13–18]. To combat this, vascular endothelial growth factor (VEGF) targeting antigen-binding fragment has been developed to treat NV; it demonstrates great promise for the treatment of corneal NV [2]. New drug/compounds for inhibiting vessel formation have also been developed to effectively treat NV-related pathological corneal conditions [19].

Green tea is one of the most popular beverages in the world. Early studies have indicated that the consumption of green tea can inhibit inflammation and angiogenesis [19]. The major active component of green tea is a catechin-derived polyphenol, including (–)-epigallocatechin gallate (EGCG), which has been shown to inhibit angiogenesis via inhibition of vascular endothelial cell growth [19–25]. The EGCG has also been shown to effectively limit the upregulation of metalloproteinase (MMP)-9 and VEGF in a mouse model of corneal NV treated by subconjunctival injection of EGCG [23]. Therefore, EGCG was chosen to treat corneal NV in this study. During vascular remodeling and formation in damaged and regenerated tissues, several integrins are found to be expressed in vascular endothelial cells [26–29]. Among them, $\alpha v\beta 3$ integrins are involved in ocular angiogenesis [27]. The adhesion molecule integrins, $\alpha v\beta 3$, plays an important role in angiogenesis, and several studies have shown that arginine-glycine-aspartic acid (RGD) peptides particularly recognize $\alpha v\beta 3$ integrins on the tumoral endothelial cell membrane and newly-formed blood vessels during angiogenesis [27–31]. In a previous study, we reported that RGD peptide modified nanoparticles (NPs) can specifically deliver EGCG to human umbilical vein endothelial cells (HUVEC) [20]. Therefore, RGD-based targeting strategy could be used to enhance biomaterial-endothelial cell interaction [29,30,32] to target pathological angiogenesis.

Conventional methods of ocular drug delivery include topical administration, intravitreal injection, and intraocular implant [17,33–35]. The topical application with an eye drop formulation represents a common, noninvasive approach for ocular drug delivery. The major drawbacks of eye drops include poor ocular drug bioavailability, nasolacrimal duct drainage, and poor penetration to the posterior segments of the eye [17,34,35]. Therefore, seeking a next-generation delivery material/strategy becomes an urgent issue in the context of eye drop delivery. Recently, biodegradable NPs have been applied to ophthalmic research for less invasive and cheaper intervention alternatives [3,34–36]. The application of NPs on ocular diseases allows targeted delivery, slow-release, and enhanced pharmacokinetics, thereby improving the bioavailability of drugs in the eyes [35,36]. However, the detailed therapeutic mechanism and performance for this nanomedicine for corneal NV have not yet been elucidated.

In this study, we applied RGD-modified NPs containing EGCG as an eye drop formula for the treatment of corneal NV. We conducted an in vitro functional assay using HUVECs as our cellular model system. In addition to in vitro study, we also employed a mouse model of chemical cauterization-induced corneal NV to investigate the antiangiogenic effect of RGD-modified NPs and their underlying molecular mechanisms in corneal NV inhibition in vivo. This topical nanomedicine could be a potential therapeutic alternative for the treatment of corneal NV (a schematic of this study is shown in Figure 1).

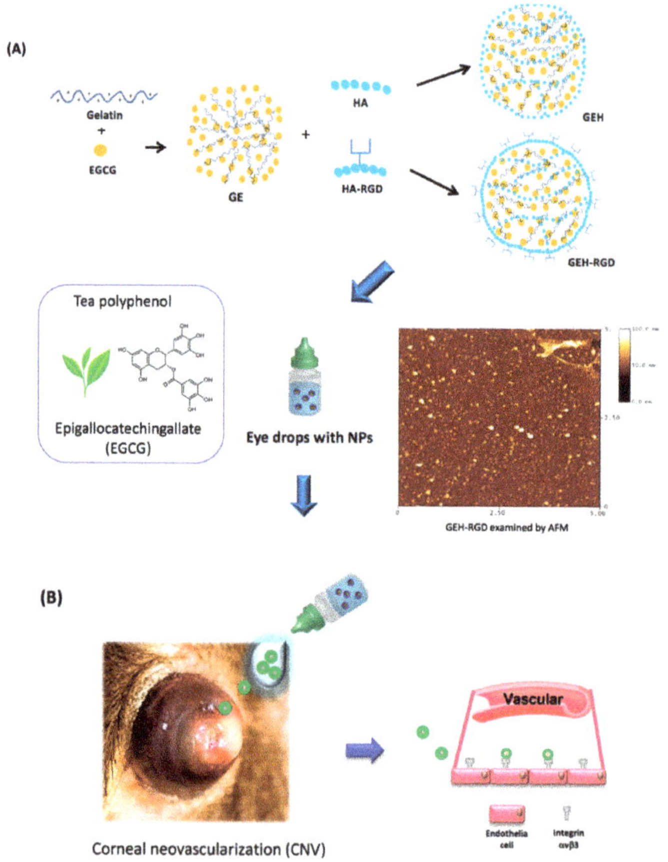

Figure 1. Schematic illustration of this study. (**A**) Synthesis of GEH-RGD NPs with EGCG loading and (**B**) application in corneal NV treatment as an eye drop formulation. Abbreviation: EGCG: epigallocatechin-3 gallate, HA: hyaluronic acid, NPs: nanoparticles, RGD: arginine-glycine-aspartic acid, GE: Gelatin/EGCG self-assembling NPs, GEH: GE NPs with HA surface coating, GEH-RGD: GE NPs with HA-RGD surface decoration, AFM: atomic force microscope.

2. Materials and Methods

2.1. Reagents and Chemicals

HUVECs were purchased from Bioresource Collection and Research Center (Hsinchu, Taiwan) and grown in Medium 199 containing 10% fetal bovine serum (Thermo Fisher Scientific, Waltham, MA, USA) as well as Penicillin-Streptomycin (Life technologies, Eugene, OR, USA) and endothelial cell growth supplement (ECGS) (Merck Millipore, Darmstadt, Germany) at 37 °C under 5% CO_2 in a humidified incubator. Upon reaching 90% confluence, cells were trypsinized with 0.25% (*w/v*) trypsin/1 mM EDTA (Gibco BRL, Gaithersburg, MD, USA) and split for further use. Gelatin type A (bloom 110, from porcine skin), EGCG (≥95%), 1-Ethyl-3-(3-dimethyllaminopropyl) carbodiimide hydrochloride (EDC), and N-Hydroxysuccinimide (NHS) were purchased from Sigma-Aldrich (St. Louis, MO, USA). One percent highly purified sodium hyaluronate (defined molecular weight 600~1200 kDa) in 3 mL was obtained from Maxigen (ArtiAid®, Maxigen Co. Ltd., Wu-gu district, New Taipei City, Taiwan). H-Gly-Arg-Asp-Ser-Pro-Lys-OH (GRGDSPK) was acquired from MDBio, Inc. (Shandong, China). Succinimidyl ester (TAMRA-SE) mixed isomers (a fluorescence dye) and 5(6)Carboxytetramethyl rhodamine were acquired from Thermo Fisher Scientific (Waltham, MA, USA). The topical anesthesia solution (0.5% Alcaine®) was from Alcon-Couvreur (Puurs, Belgium). Grafco®Silver Nitrate Applicators were purchased from Medline Industries Inc. (Mundelein, IL, USA). All other reagent-grade chemicals were from Sigma-Aldrich.

2.2. *Preparation of Gelatin/EGCG NPs with Surface HA-RGD-Conjugation (GEH-RGD)*

The HA solution (5 mg/mL, 2mL) was added to the EDC solution (38 mg/mL, 1mL) and mixed at room temperature (RT) for 1 h. Then, 1μL of GRGDSPK peptide in 0.1 M $NaHCO_3$ (10 mg/mL) solution was added for peptide-HA conjugation [20]. This reaction was kept at 4 °C for 72 h. Nonreacting residues were removed by centrifugation, the purified solution finally was lyophilized, and the dried power of HA-RGD conjugation was obtained. The identification of conjugation by ^{1}H-nuclear magnetic resonance (NMR) and Fourier-transform infrared spectroscopy (FTIR) was described in a previous study [20]. An equal volume of gelatin and EGCG solution (both in 0.44 *w/v* %) was mixed gently to form the self-assembly NPs under stirring, named GE hereafter [20,37]. Surface-modified NPs were then prepared, and 100 μL of HA or HA-RGD was separately added into the GE NP suspension (final HA concentration, 0.25 *w/v* %). GE with HA coating on the surface is referred to as GEH hereafter, and GEH-RGD is the abbreviation for GE with HA-RGD peptide modifications on the surface. A schematic representation of the preparation process is shown in Figure 1A. The synthesized NPs were then characterized by dynamic light scattering (DLS) for particle size and zeta potential measurement. Similar to our previous study [20], the ζ-potential of GE is positive (+18 mV). After applying the HA coating (GEH), the ζ-potential of GEH became negative (−13 mV) due to the HA possessing carboxyl groups ($-COO^-$). When HA-RGD was added to the particle surface, a positive ζ-potential of GEH-RGD (+12.9 mV) was acquired, since the side chain of GRGDSPK peptide present many amide ($-NH_3^+$) groups on HA-RGD. This is one way to confirm the RGD on the particle surface. The encapsulation efficiency of EGCG was determined by reacting with cation-radicals of 2,2′-azino-bis (3-ethylbenz -othiazoline-6-sulfonic acid) diammonium salt (ABTS) (ABTS+, Sigma-Aldrich, St Louis, MO, USA; Supplemental-1 in Appendix A) [37,38]. The EGCG loading rate in GEH or GEH-RHD NPs was around 95%. The EGCG loaded NPs prepared from three batches ($n = 6$) were used in this test. The morphology of nanoparticles was examined by an MFP-3D atomic force microscope (AFM, Asylum Research, Santa Barbara, CA, USA) using tapping-mode. GEH-RGD NPs with EGCG and free-form EGCG were freshly prepared for the experiments.

2.3. *Functional Evaluation of GEH-RGD NPs on HUVECs*

2.3.1. Tube Formation Assay

HUVECs were treated with EGCG, GEH, and GEH-RGD NP solution (EGCG: 20 μg/mL), and then seeded on a Matrigel®-coated 96-well plate (Corning, Corning, NY, USA). The morphology of tube formation was observed and images in each treatment were taken at 9 and 24 h ($n = 3$). Images were acquired using an inverted fluorescence microscope (Olympus, IX81, Tokyo, Japan). The branch points and tubule length were quantified by ImageJ (http://imagej.nih.gov/ij/; provided in the public domain by the National Institutes of Health, Bethesda, MD, USA).

2.3.2. Gelatin Zymography

HUVECs were treated with EGCG, GEH, and GEH-RGD (20 μg/mL) containing media for 24 h, and then the media was harvested. Preparation of separating gel included gelatin type A solution, (20 mg/mL, 1% *w/v* SDS), followed by sample loading and gel running. After gel electrophoresis, separating gel was incubated in 2.5% Triton X-100-containing incubation buffer for 20 h in an incubator at 37 °C. The gel was then stained 0.05% Coomassie Brilliant Blue G-250 for an hour. After gel destaining, the gel was photographed, and the gelatinolytic area of each image was quantified by ImageJ ($n = 3$).

2.4. *Topical Delivery of NPs in a Mouse Model of Corneal NV*

C57BL/6J male mice aged from 8 to 10 weeks were used in this study. The experimental procedure was performed following the ARVO Statement for the Use of Animals in Ophthalmic and Vision Research and approved by the Institutional Animal Care and Use Committee (IACUC) of the Taipei Medical University (IACUC approval no. LAC-10-0289, 9 May 2013). Briefly, mice were anesthetized, followed by pressing the tip of an applicator containing silver nitrate to the center of the cornea to generate chemical cauterization. Each mouse only suffered one eye cauterization. The nanoparticles containing eye drops (GEH or GEH-RGD NPs) were diluted in PBS to adjust the EGCG concentration to 30 μg/mL for use in this test (Figure 1B). The free drug (EGCG solution) was also prepared in the same EGCG concentration. Five microliters of tested eye drops were applied to the eye of the mice once a day for seven days, and PBS topical application was used as vehicle control (n = 6/group). The burn response and the severity of NV were assessed by a hand-held portable slit lamp (SL-17, Kowa Company Ltd., Torrance, CA, USA) on anesthetized mice. Four batches of the animal experiment were performed in this study. Seven days after cauterization, the extent of NV was assessed in the anaesthetized mice by an ophthalmologist masked to the treatments under a slit-lamp and dissecting microscope. The cauterized cornea was observed under a hand-hold portable slit lamp and each quadrant was photographed. The image of the cauterized cornea was then processed using ImageJ software (http://imagej.nih.gov/ij/) to quantify the NV area through the following steps: 1) remove the eyeball background and retain the corneal area; 2) use the RGB function to remove a nonred color area (nonvessel area); 3) calculate the vascular area (in red) among the total corneal area and present it as a percentage. The area of corneal NV was calculated by averaging the four quadrants of the cornea.

2.4.1. Histopathology Examination of Corneal Sections

Mouse eyes were harvested and fixed in 10% formaldehyde. The extracted eyeballs were embedded in paraffin and cut into 5-μm-thick sections, deparaffinized and hydrated, and stained with hematoxylin and eosin (H&E stain). The sections were reviewed and evaluated under a light microscope.

2.4.2. Quantification of VEGF and MMP-9 in Cornea Extraction

Corneal tissues (6 eyeballs/group from two batches) were harvested and homogenized with protein extraction buffer (Thermo Fisher Scientific). The mixture from each sample was then centrifuged, and the supernatant was collected. Total protein of cornea lysate was quantified by Bradford assay (p010, GeneCopoeia, Rockville, MD, USA). An equal amount of total protein (15 μg in 100 μL) from each sample was used to quantify the VEGF and MMP-9 by ELISA (Quantikine ELISA kits, R&D system, Minneapolis, MN, USA). This experiment was conducted according to the manufacturer's protocol.

2.5. *Statistical Analysis*

All data are shown as mean ± standard deviation (SD) from three independent experiments. Statistical differences between groups were tested by Student's t-test or one-way ANOVA using SPSS 17.0 (SPSS, Inc., Chicago, IL, USA). A probability (p) value less than 0.05 was considered statistically significant.

3. Results

3.1. *Characterization of EGCG-Loaded GEH-RGD NPs*

The gelatin/EGCG NPs (GE) were first formed by self-assembling. The surface of NPs was then decorated with HA or HA-RGD, termed GEH and GEH-RGD, respectively (Figure 1A). The particle size of GE, GEH, and GEH-RGD was 91.90 ± 44.53, 277.40 ± 73.00, and 158.10 ± 11.06 nm, respectively (Table 1). The GE presented a positive surface with a zeta (ζ) potential value at 18.4 ± 4.4 mV. The ζ potential of GEH and GEH-RGD were the opposite. GEH was −13.2 ± 4.1 mV, and GEH-RGD was

12.9 ± 4.1 mV. All NPs with low PDI value presented as monodispersed colloidal systems with narrow size distribution. An image of GEH-RGD acquired from AFM examination (in Figure 1A) revealed round particle deposition on the surface with no aggregation and proper dispersion.

Table 1. Characterization of variant NPs.

NP's Group	Particle Size (nm)	Zeta Potential (mV)	PDI
GE	91.90 ± 44.53	18.4 ± 4.4	0.30 ± 0.20
GEH	277.40 ± 73.00	−13.2 ± 4.1	0.38 ± 0.18
GEH-RGD	158.10 ± 11.06	12.9 ± 4.1	± 0.03

Values represent: mean ± standard division ($n = 6$); PDI: Poly dispersive index; EGCG: epigallocatechin-3-gallate; NPs: nanoparticles; RGD: arginine-glycine-aspartic acid; GE: Gelatin/EGCG self-assembling NPs; GEH: GE NPs with hyaluronic acid (HA) surface coating; GEH-RGD: GE NPs with HA-RGD surface decoration.

3.2. GEH-RGD NPs Inhibit In Vitro Angiogenetic Activity

The in vitro tube formation assay was performed to evaluate the effect of EGCG NPs on angiogenesis. When HUVECs were cultured on Matrigel, they gradually formed capillary-like tubular structures which connected to each other, arranging themselves in a mesh-like network (Figure 2A, control). The network gradually disappeared with time and less capillary structure was observed when cocultured with variant EGCG formula addition (Figure 2A, EGCG/GEH/GEH-RGD). Almost no mesh-like structure was found in the GEH-RGD NP-treated cells (Figure 2A). The GEH-RGD-treated group has a smaller number of branch points (25.3 ± 2.5, Figure 2B) and the shortest tubule length (5284.3 ± 54.6, Figure 2C) compared with the control group (60.7 ± 4.9; 7896.7 ± 437.6) at 24-hour time points (*$p < 0.05$) (Figure 2B,C). Together, these results demonstrate that GEH-RGD NPs can effectively inhibit angiogenic activity in vitro.

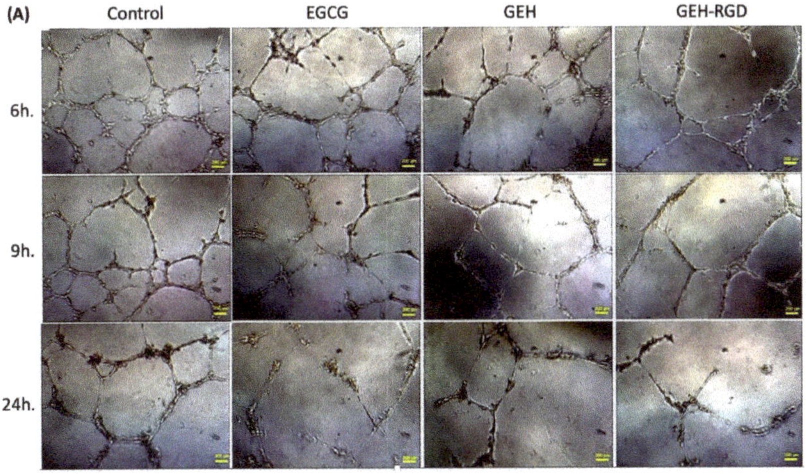

Figure 2. *Cont.*

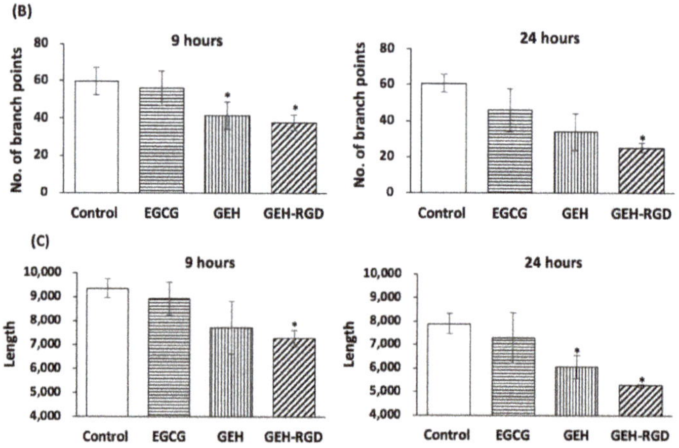

Figure 2. EGCG NPs inhibit endothelial tube formation. (**A**) Representative images of HUVECs cultured on Matrigel at a different time point (EGCG: 20 µg/mL, 100×). The images in each treatment were taken at 9 and 24 h, and (**B**) the number of branch points and (**C**) total length of tubing cells were quantified (n = 3). *p < 0.05 compared with control. Abbreviation: PBS: Phosphate buffer saline, EGCG: epigallocatechin-3 gallate, HA: hyaluronic acid, RGD: arginine-glycine-aspartic acid, GE: Gelatin/EGCG self-assembling.

3.3. GEH-RGD NPs Inhibit MMP-2 and MMP-9 Activities

The formation of corneal NV is closely associated with the activity of MMPs, such as MMP-2 and MMP-9. We examined the effect of EGCG NPs on the activity of MMPs secreted from the treated HUVECs via gelatin zymography (Figure 3A,B). The gelatinolytic of the control group (only culture medium) was normalized as 100%. Cells treated by EGCG revealed the gelatinolytic activity of MMP-2 at 90.1 ± 1.6% and MMP-9 at 71.4 ± 2.4%. Conditioned media harvested from GEH-RGD-treated cells had a lower gelatinolytic activity of both MMP-2 (81.1 ± 1.5%) and MMP-9 (61.1 ± 1%) compared to cells treated with other groups (*p < 0.05 for control, #p < 0.05 for EGCG). Our results indicate that GEH-RGD NPs inhibit the activity of MMPs, which contributes to the inhibition of angiogenesis.

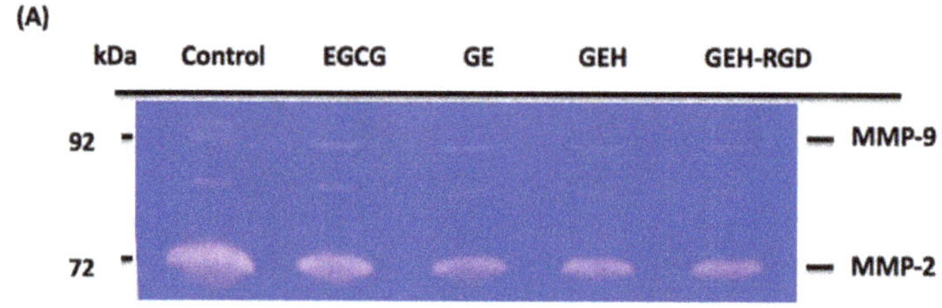

Figure 3. *Cont.*

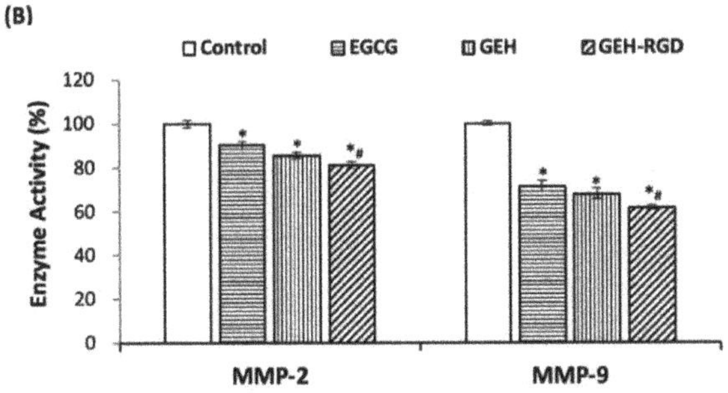

Figure 3. EGCG NPs inhibit activity of MMPs in endothelial cells. (**A**) Results of gelatin zymography from culture medium after 24 h incubation with a variant formulation for confirm the MMPs activity. (**B**) Quantification of MMP-2 and MMP-9 activities compared with the control group ($n = 3$). $^{*}p < 0.05$ compared with control, $^{\#}p < 0.05$ compared with EGCG. Abbreviation: EGCG: epigallocatechin-3 gallate, HA: hyaluronic acid, RGD: arginine-glycine-aspartic acid, GE: Gelatin/EGCG self-assembling nanoparticles (NPs), GEH: GE NPs with HA surface coating, GEH-RGD: GE NPs with HA-RGD surface decoration, MMP: metalloproteinase.

3.4. Topical Application of GEH-RGD NPs Suppresses the Corneal NV in a Mouse Model of Chemical Cauterization

To further investigate whether the above in vitro findings were applicable in vivo, we then tested the antiangiogenic effect of EGCG, GEH and GEH-RGD NPs in a mouse model of chemical cauterization-induced corneal NV. The normal cornea was in a transparent and smooth surface, as seen in Figure 4A. A white or cloudy patch on the center of the cornea accompanied by swelling was observed immediately after chemical cauterization (Figure 4A, cauterization). Chemical cauterization results in a growth of new blood vessels from limbus toward the burn scar. Dense ingrown vessels surrounding the entire eyeball were observed from the corneal limbus to the burning edge in the PBS (Figure 4A) and EGCG-treated groups acquired on day 7 (Figure 4A, EGCG). In contrast, fewer and thinner visible NVs were observed in both GEH and GEH-RGD-treated groups (Figure 4A). Moreover, better corneal transparency with the least amount of vessel formation was found in the GEH-RGD-treated group compared to other treatment groups.

The quantification of NV areas in the cornea is shown in Figure 4B. The pathological blood vessels absent in healthy cornea tissue was normalized as 0%. Our results indicate a good therapeutic potential of GEH-RGD NPs, which shows the lowest NV area (20.7 ± 2.2%. $^{*}p < 0.05$) compared with PBS (53.2 ± 4.5%), while the EGCG- and GEH-treated group had a higher NV area (37.0 ± 10.5% and 40.1 ± 7.1%, $^{\#}p < 0.05$) (Figure 4G).

We then evaluated the microstructure of corneas after treatment with GEH-RGD NPs. The outer part of normal mouse cornea is composed of 3–5 layers of epithelium cells, bowman's membrane, and stroma (Figure 5A). After chemical cauterization, a thinner corneal epithelium was found in the PBS, EGCG, GEH and GEH-RGD-treated groups (Figure 5B–E). We observed relatively loose and irregular structures of stroma and more newly-formed blood vessels in the PBS, EGCG, and GEH-treated groups (Figure 5B–D). In contrast, the GEH-RGD-treated group showed a relatively normal stroma and reduced newly-formed vessel formation (Figure 5E). Therefore, these results demonstrate that GEH-RGD NPs can effectively prevent the development of NV in the cornea after chemical cauterization.

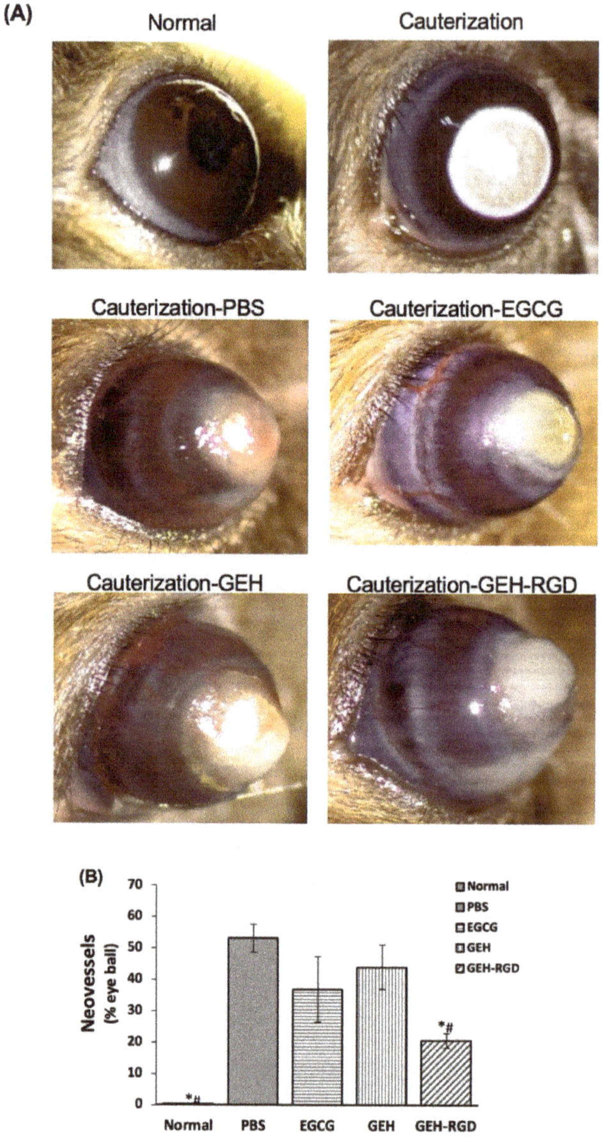

Figure 4. EGCG NPs inhibit neovessels formation in chemical cauterization-induced corneal neovascularization (NV). (**A**) Representative images of normal cornea, cauterized cornea and PBS-, EGCG-, GEH-, or GEH-RGD-treated cornea on day 7 following chemical cauterization. (**B**) The area of blood vessels in the cornea was quantified ($n = 6$). $^{*}p < 0.05$ compared with PBS, $^{\#}p < 0.05$ compared with EGCG and GEH. Abbreviation: PBS: Phosphate buffer saline, EGCG: epigallocatechin-3 gallate, HA: hyaluronic acid, RGD: arginine-glycine-aspartic acid, GE: Gelatin/EGCG self-assembling nanoparticles (NPs), GEH: GE NPs with HA surface coating, GEH-RGD: GE NPs with HA-RGD surface decoration.

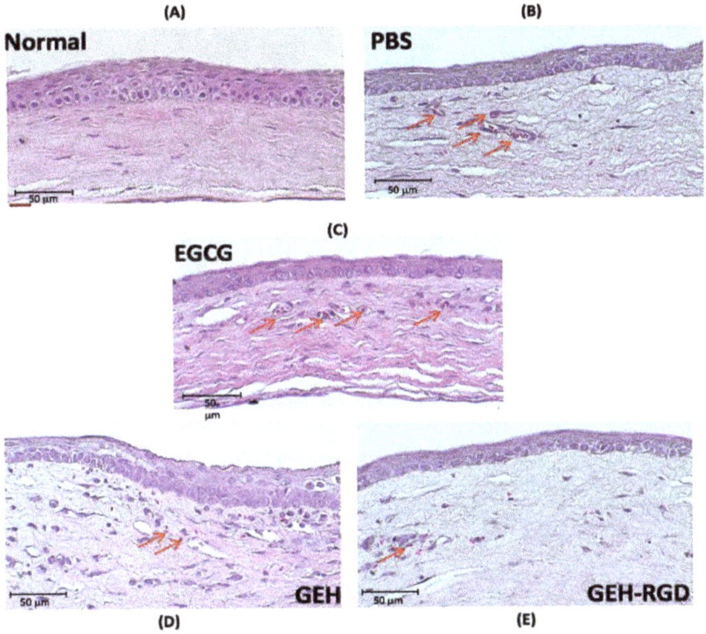

Figure 5. Histological assessment of corneal sections after treatment. Representative images of the central corneal section were depicted on day 7 following chemical cauterization. The development of fibrovascular proliferation was observed (red arrows). Groups: (**A**) normal, (**B**) PBS, (**C**) EGCG, (**D**) GEH, (**E**) GEH-RGD. Abbreviation: PBS: Phosphate buffer saline, EGCG: epigallocatechin-3 gallate, HA: hyaluronic acid, RGD: arginine-glycine-aspartic acid, GE: Gelatin/EGCG self-assembling nanoparticles (NPs), GEH: GE NPs with HA surface coating, GEH-RGD: GE NPs with HA-RGD surface decoration.

3.5. Topical Application of GEH-RGD NPs Attenuates the Expression of VEGF and MMP-9 in the Chemical Cauterized Corneas

To further elucidate the factors that contribute to the GEH-RGD NP-mediated angiogenesis inhibition in the cauterized corneas, the protein level of VEGF and MMP-9 protein in the cauterized corneas were measured by ELISA. Normal corneas showed a concentration of (74.3 ± 4.0 pg/mL) for VEGF, while the amount of MMP-9 was almost undetectable in corneal tissues. The PBS-treated corneas showed the highest concentration of VEGF (124.6 ± 3.8 pg/mL) and MMP-9 (7554 ± 1678 pg/mL) compared to all other treated groups after chemical cauterization (Figure 6A,B). The VEGF level was significantly reduced in the EGCG- (100.8 ± 0.8 pg/mL), GEH- (98.1 ± 1.8 pg/mL) and GEH-RGD-treated cauterized corneas (79.9 ± 5.0 pg/mL). The VEGF protein in the cauterized corneas with GEH-RGD NPs treatment was reduced to the level similar to normal corneas ($^{*}p < 0.05$ compared with control, $^{\&}p < 0.05$ compared with PBS, $^{\#}p < 0.05$ compared with EGCG, $^{>}p < 0.05$ compared with GEH; Figure 6A). Moreover, the MMP-9 level in the cauterized cornea treated with GEH NPs and GEH-RGD NPs were 4762 ± 680 pg/mL and 2800 ± 2326 pg/mL, respectively. In contrast, EGCG solution had no effect still representing high MMP-9 concentration (7295 ± 1630 pg/mL), similar to the PBS-treated corneas (Figure 6B). These results indicate that GEH-RGD NPs inhibit corneal NV by inhibiting the production of VEGF and MMP-9 in chemical-cauterized corneal tissue.

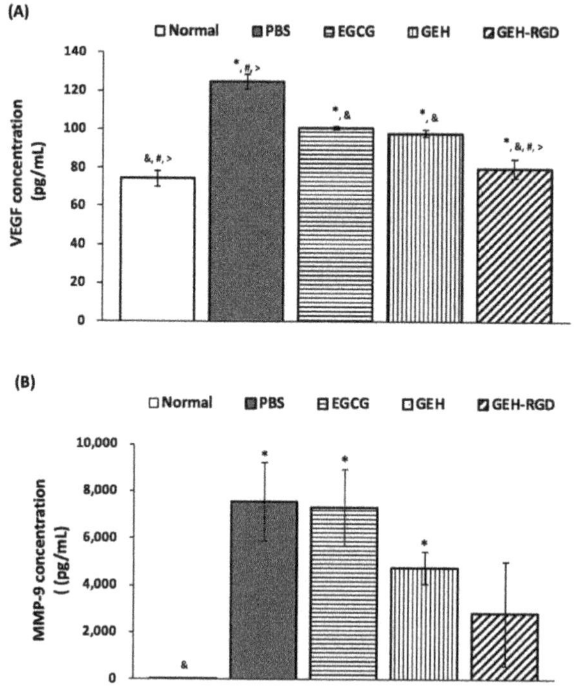

Figure 6. GEH-RGD NPs inhibit the expression of angiogenic factors in the cauterized cornea. Mice received chemical cauterization and were treated with PBS, EGCG, GEH NPs, GEH-RGD NPs-contained eye drops once daily for 7 days. The corneas were harvested and homogenized, and the protein level of (**A**) VEGF or (**B**) MMP-9 were assayed by ELISA (6 eyeballs/group from two batches). (*$p < 0.05$ compared with control, $^{\&}p < 0.05$ compared with PBS, $^{\#}p < 0.05$ compared with EGCG, $^{>}p < 0.05$ compared with GEH). Abbreviation: PBS: Phosphate buffer saline, EGCG: epigallocatechin-3 gallate, HA: hyaluronic acid, RGD: arginine-glycine-aspartic acid, GE: Gelatin/EGCG self-assembling nanoparticles (NPs), GEH: GE NPs with HA surface coating, GEH-RGD: GE NPs with HA-RGD surface decoration. MMP: metalloproteinase, VEGF: vascularization endothelium growth factor, ELISA: enzyme-linked immunosorbent assay.

4. Discussion

The importance of this study lies in the demonstration that RGD-HA conjugation on the gelatin/EGCG NP surface to target integrin can decrease the angiogenic activity in human endothelial cells. Our data also suggest that the GEH-RGD NP eye drop formulation is superior to EGCG free drug and nontargetable GEH NPs, as it can effectively inhibit corneal NV in a mouse model of chemical injury.

EGCG is a dual-functional agent which has both antiangiogenic and anti-inflammatory capacity [25,37–41]. EGCG has also been shown to inhibit angiogenesis by regulating endothelial cell growth, thereby reducing pathological corneal NV [18]. Green tea extract inhibits the angiogenesis of human endothelial cells through the reduction of expression of VEGFR [42]. Sánchez-Huerta et al. revealed that the administration of EGCG to the ocular surface can suppress corneal NV due to its ability to mediate a variety of inflammatory and angiogenic factors such as interleukin-1β, cyclooxygenase 2 (COX2), VEGF, and MMPs [43]. Our previous study (Chang C.Y et al. 2017, [20]) and current data suggest that EGCG, GEH, and GEH-RGD NPs can suppress the angiogenesis activity of HUVECs, especially the GEH-RGD NPs.

Many eye diseases can be treated by eye drops. The major disadvantages of eye drop dosage include tear screening, nasolacrimal duct drainage, and corneal tight junction as a barrier that reduces drug bioavailability in the eyes [33]. The application of a nanoformulation for ocular drug delivery allows targeted transportation and slow drug release, as well as enhancing drug retention in the eye, thereby improving the bioavailability of drugs. Positively-charged nanoparticles with a diameter of 250 nm consisting of EGCG with surface decoration by HA resulted in increased tear volume, reduced inflammatory gene expression, and the restoration of a normal corneal architecture with improving associated clinical signs [37]. The HA-RGD conjugated gelatin/EGCG NPs were around 160 nm in size, and the ζ-potential presented a positive value at 12.9 mV (Table 1), which was in a similar range to what was observed in our previous study, indicating that the synthetic quality for producing GEH-RGD NPs is stable [20].

Under normal conditions, VEGF promotes endothelial migration and proliferation, which helps to maintain normal vasculatures by preventing the apoptosis of endothelial cells [43]. Our results have also demonstrated that EGCG NPs inhibit endothelial cell migration (Supplemental-2 in Appendix A). However, overexpression of VEGF is associated with several vascular eye diseases such as diabetic retinopathy [44], corneal NV [2,3], and choroidal NV [45]. For endothelial targeting, cell surface markers such as P-selectin, E-selectin, vascular cell adhesion molecule-1, and integrin are considered potential target moieties [46–49]. One of integrin with subunit in $\alpha v\beta 3$ type is important in mediating angiogenesis, blocking $\alpha v\beta 3$ function which reduces the blood flow to certain tumors [29–31]. Moreover, normal epidermis and corneal epithelium lack expression of $\alpha 5\beta 1$ and $\alpha v\beta 3$ integrins [27]. Therefore, targeting RGD would not misrecognize the integrin expression on vascular endothelial cells on the cornea. According to the specific targeting capacity of RGD [20], our designed GEH-RGD NPs can be specifically uptaken by human endothelial cells and modulate the angiogenic activities with a long-lasting effect due to the slow release of EGCG from GEH-RGD [20].

The antiangiogenic effect of GEH-RGD and its underlying molecular mechanism was confirmed by employing a chemical cauterized mouse model. Chemical injury is a prevalent cause of corneal NV clinically due to easy vessel observation [50]. In this study, corneal NV was induced by silver nitrate cauterization to obtain a robust in vivo model for mimicking the clinical condition of corneal injury. Considering that topical application is the most accessible and least invasive delivery route to the ocular surface, a GEH-RGD NPs eye drop formulation was designed and manufactured. In this study, EGCG concentration for the treatment of corneal NV was 30 μg/mL, given once a day for 7 days. Due to the slow release of EGCG from GEH-RGD NPs, only one dose per day can achieve the therapeutic effect, i.e., inhibiting the formation of new blood vessels. The GEH/GEH-RGD NPs were synthesized from biocompatible materials, i.e., gelatin and hyaluronic acid; these materials possess good biocompatibility and prolonged ocular retention time [20,51].

Angiogenesis requires MMPs to dissolve the basement membrane to initial endothelial sprouting. EGCG was found to decrease VEGF receptor phosphorylation and inhibit the secretion of MMP-2 and MMP-9 in human endothelial cells [52]. Lee, H.S. et al. reported that EGCG could be an inhibitor of ocular angiogenesis. They reported that EGCG can attenuate the expression of pro-angiogenic factors (such as MMP-9 and VEGF) by inhibiting the generation of reactive oxygen species in human retinal pigment epithelial cells, and block angiogenic activity in human retinal microvascular endothelial cells [23]. In this study, our results show that GEH-RGD NPs blocked the activity of MMP-2 and MMP-9 in HUVECs in vitro and reduced the MMP-9 and VEGF proteins in chemical cauterized corneas in vivo. Interestingly, we did not observe a significant difference in MMP-9 activity between GEH and GEH-RGD NPs. Since MMP-9 is secreted by a range of cell types, including immune cells and fibroblasts, GEH NPs can interact with corneal cells and block the MMP-9 activity of the surrounding cells by releasing EGCG. This noncell type-specific effect of EGCG may also be found in cornea treated with GEH-RGD NPs. Overall, these data indicate that the mechanism underlying the inhibitory effects of GEH-RGD NPs was, at least, through the reduction of MMPs and VEGF expression, and that further antiangiogenesis effect in the damaged cornea was achieved.

Koh CH et al. evaluated the topical delivery of 0.1% EGCG eye drops 4 times daily for 2 weeks in a rabbit model of silk suture-stimulated corneal NV [53]. They reported that topical administration of EGCG effectively inhibits corneal vessel formation in rabbits via suppression of VEGF and COX-2 [53]. In our study, a chemical cauterized mouse model was used and the targetable nanoformulation, GEH-RGD, as eye drops can effectively inhibit corneal NV with one dosage per day at a very lower concentration (30 μg/mL, 0.03% *w/v*). One study using curcumin-loaded polyethylene glycol-block-polycaprolactone (PEG-PCL) NPs to treat corneal NV in mice with alkaline burned reveals that this treatment can also successfully decrease vessel formation in the cornea using nano-curcumin once daily up to 2 weeks [54]. These results suggest that using these specific nanoparticle-encapsulated drug releasing systems as eye drops can reduce the dosing frequency thanks to the advantages of nanoparticle interaction with the ocular surface to achieve higher drug bioavailability to effectively inhibit the formation of vessels.

5. Conclusions

In conclusion, our study confirms the antiangiogenic effects of GEH-RGD NPs in vitro by inhibiting vascular endothelial cells function. Our data evidence that an eye drop formulation with GEH-RGD NPs can effectively target corneal vessels and thereby inhibit chemical cauterized-induced corneal NV by a once-daily treatment. These findings suggest that the topical application of GEH-RGD NPs is a potential therapeutic approach for the management of corneal NV.

Author Contributions: Conceptualization: K.-H.C., Y.-K.W., G.-S.L., and C.-L.T.; Methodology: T.M., Z.-Y.C., C.-Y.C., Y.-K.W., G.-S.L., and C.L.T.; Formal Analysis: T.M., Z.-Y.C., Y.-K.W., G.-S.L., and C.-L.T.; Investigation: T.M., Z.-Y.C., C.-Y.C., G.-S.L., and C.-L.T.; Resources: K.-H.C., Y.-K.W., G.-S.L., and C.-L.T.; Data Curation: T.M., Z.-Y.C., Y.-K.W., G.-S.L. and C.-L.T.; Writing—Original Draft Preparation: T.M., Y.-K.W.; Writing—Review and Editing: K.-H.C., Y.-K.W., G.-S.L. and C.-L.T.; Project Administration: K.-H.C., G.-S.L. and C.-L.T.; Funding Acquisition: G.-S.L. and C.-L.T. All authors have read and agreed to the published version of the manuscript.

Funding: This work was supported by grants from the integrated research grant in health and medical sciences from National Health Research Institute, Taiwan (NHRI-EX105-10334EI), the Ministry of Science and Technology, Taiwan (MOST 106-2628-E-038-001-MY3) and the National Health and Medical Research Council of Australia (GNT1185600).

Acknowledgments: The authors would also like to thank Feng-Huei Lin (National Health Research Institute, Taiwan) for constructive discussions and suggestions. We also would like to acknowledge the Laboratory Animal Center at TMU for technical support in histological experiment.

Conflicts of Interest: The authors declare no conflict of interest.

Appendix A.

Appendix A.1. Supplement 1—The Protocol for EGCG Quantification by ABST+ Method

The supernatant with EGCG after centrifugation was assayed by determining unloaded EGCG content with ABTS+ method. Added 88 μL $K_2S_2O_8$ solution (0.14 M) into 5 mL of ABTS stock solution (7×10^{-3} M), this mixture was kept overnight at room temperature for working solution (ABTS+) preparation. Two microliter EGCG contained sample was added into the 800 μL ABTS+ working solution reacted for 24 h., then measured the absorbance at 734 nm by Varioskan Flash spectral scanning multimode reader (Thermo Fisher Scientific, Waltham, MA, USA). The OD value of sample was compared with the EGCG standard curve to calculate the concentration [38]. The EGCG encapsulation efficiency (EE) was counted by calculated as the following equation: EE % = (Total amount of EGCG − Free EGCG)/(Total amount of EGCG) × 100.

Appendix A.2. Supplement 2—Transwell Migration Assay

HUVECs (1.2× 10^4 cells/well) were seeded in the Transwell®(Corning, Corning, NY, USA) then putting in a 24-well plate. In the upper chamber, HUVEC cells were incubated with EGCG, GEH NPs, and GEH-RGD NPs (EGCG: 20 μg/mL) overnight. After migration, cells on top of the transwell membrane were removed and the remaining cells pass through the transwell membrane were fixed with 10% formaldehyde. Nuclei were stained with 4′,6-diamidino-2-phenylindole (DAPI, Thermo Fisher Scientific, Waltham, MA, USA). Images were acquired using an inverted fluorescence microscope (Olympus, IX81, Tokyo, Japan) and the number of migrated cells was quantified using ImageJ ($n = 3$). Here, it is suggested that GEH-RGD NPs significantly inhibit endothelial migration through the transwell membrane, less cells nuclei were observed (Figure A1A–D) and counted (Figure A1E, $^*p < 0.05$ compared with control).

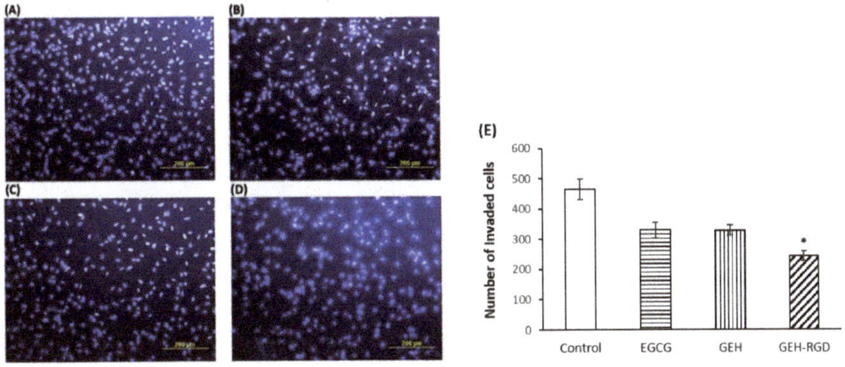

Figure A1. EGCG NPs inhibit endothelial cell migration. Representative images of HUVECs invaded across the membrane treated by (**A**) culture medium as control, (**B**) EGCG solution, (**C**) GEH NPs, and (**D**) GEH-RGD NPs at EGCG concentration of 20 μg/mL ($n = 3$). (**E**) Numbers of invaded cells were calculated using ImageJ. $^*p < 0.05$ compared with control, $^{\#}p < 0.05$ compared with GEH. Abbreviation: EGCG: epigallocatechin-3 gallate, HA: hyaluronic acid, RGD: arginine-glycine-aspartic acid, GE: Gelatin/EGCG self-assembling nanoparticles (NPs), GEH: GE NPs with HA surface coating, GEH-RGD: GE NPs with HA-RGD surface decoration, HUVECs: human umbilical vein endothelial cells.

References

1. Menzel-Severing, J. Emerging techniques to treat corneal neovascularisation. *Eye* **2012**, *26*, 2–12. [CrossRef] [PubMed]
2. Stevenson, W.; Cheng, S.F.; Dastjerdi, M.H.; Ferrari, G.; Dana, R.; Cheng, S.F.; Dastjerdi, M.H.; Ferrari, G.; Dana, R. Corneal neovascularization and the utility of topical VEGF inhibition: Ranibizumab (Lucentis) vs. bevacizumab (Avastin). *Ocul. Surf.* **2012**, *10*, 67–83. [CrossRef] [PubMed]
3. Gonzalez, L.; Loza, R.J.; Han, K.Y.; Sunoqrot, S.; Cunningham, C.; Purta, P.; Drake, J.; Jain, S.; Hong, S.; Chang, J.-H. Nanotechnology in Corneal Neovascularization Therapy—A Review. *J. Ocular Pharmacol. Ther.* **2013**, *29*, 1–10. [CrossRef]
4. Chang, J.H.; Garg, N.K.; Lunde, E.; Han, K.Y.; Jain, S.; Azar, D.T. Corneal neovascularization: An anti-VEGF therapy review. *Surv. Ophthalmol.* **2012**, *57*, 415–429. [CrossRef] [PubMed]
5. Shakiba, Y.; Mansouri, K.; Arshadi, D.; Rezaei, N. Corneal neovascularization: Molecular events and therapeutic options. *Recent Pat. Inflamm. Allergy Drug Discov.* **2009**, *3*, 221–231. [CrossRef] [PubMed]
6. Whitcher, J.P.; Srinivasan, M.; Upadhyay, M.P. Corneal blindness: A global perspective. *Bull. World Health Organ.* **2001**, *79*, 214–221. [PubMed]
7. Bachmann, B.O.; Bock, F.; Wiegand, S.J.; Maruyama, K.; Dana, M.R.; Kruse, F.E.; Luetjen-Drecoll, E.; Cursiefen, C. Promotion of graft survival by vascular endothelial growth factor a neutralization after high-risk corneal transplantation. *Arch. Ophthalmol.* **2008**, *126*, 71–77. [CrossRef] [PubMed]
8. Feizi, S.; Azari, A.A.; Safapour, S. Therapeutic approaches for corneal neovascularization. *Eye Vis. (Lond.)* **2017**, *4*, 1–10. [CrossRef]
9. Abdelfattah, N.S.; Amgad, M.; Zayed, A.A.; Salem, H.; Elkhanany, A.E.; Hussein, H.; El-Baky, N.A. Clinical correlates of common corneal neovascular diseases: A literature review. *Int. J. Ophthalmol.* **2015**, *8*, 182–193.

10. Cope, J.R.; Collier, S.A.; Rao, M.M.; Chalmers, R.; Mitchell, L.; Richdale, K.; Wagner, H.; Kinoshita, B.T.; Lam, D.Y.; Sorbara, L.; et al. Contact lens wearer demographics and risk behaviors for contact lens-related eye infections—United States, 2014. *MMWR Morb. Mortal Wkly Rep.* **2015**, *64*, 865–870. [CrossRef]
11. Ang, J.H.; Efron, N. Corneal hypoxia and hypercapnia during contact lens wear. *Optom. Vis. Sci.* **1990**, *67*, 512–521. [PubMed]
12. Singh, N.; Amin, S.; Richter, E.; Rashid, S.; Scoglietti, V.; Jani, P.D.; Wang, J.; Kaur, R.; Ambati, J.; Dong, Z.; et al. Flt-1 intraceptors inhibit hypoxia-induced VEGF expression in vitro and corneal neovascularization in vivo. *Investig. Ophthalmol. Vis. Sci.* **2005**, *46*, 1647–1652. [CrossRef] [PubMed]
13. Moreddu, R.; Vigolo, D.; Yetisen, A.K. Contact Lens Technology: From fundamentals to Applications. *Adv. Healthc. Mater.* **2019**, *8*, 1900368. [CrossRef] [PubMed]
14. Walker, M.K.; Bergmanson, J.P.; Miller, W.L.; Marsack, J.D.; Johnson, L.A. Complications and fitting challenges associated with scleral contact lenses: A review. *Cont. Lens. Anterior Eye* **2016**, *39*, 88–96. [CrossRef] [PubMed]
15. Alipour, F.; Khaheshi, S.; Soleimanzadeh, M.; Heidarzadeh, S.; Heydarzadeh, S. Contact lens-related complications: A review. *J. Ophthalmic. Vis. Res.* **2017**, *12*, 193–204. [PubMed]
16. Lee, P.; Wang, C.C.; Adamis, A.P. Ocular neovascularization: An epidemiologic review. *Surv. Ophthalmol.* **1998**, *43*, 245–269. [CrossRef]
17. Lau, C.M.L.; Yu, Y.; Jahanmir, G.; Chau, Y. Controlled release technology for anti-angiogenesis treatment of posterior eye diseases: Current status and challenges. *Adv. Drug Deliv. Rev.* **2018**, *126*, 145–161. [CrossRef]
18. Ferrari, G.; Dastjerdi, M.H.; Okanobo, A.; Cheng, S.-F.; Amparo, F.; Nallasamy, N.; Dana, R. Topical 4anibizumab as a treatment of corneal neovascularization. *Cornea* **2013**, *32*, 992–997. [CrossRef]
19. Sánchez-Huerta, V.; Gutiérrez-Sánchez, L.; Flores-Estrada, J. (-)-Epigallocatechin 3-gallate (EGCG) at the ocular surface inhibits corneal neovascularization. *Med. Hypotheses* **2011**, *76*, 311–313. [CrossRef]
20. Chang, C.Y.; Wang, M.C.; Miyagawa, T.; Chen, Z.Y.; Lin, F.H.; Chen, K.H.; Liu, G.S.; Tseng, C.L. Preparation of RGD modified biopolymeric nanoparticles contained epigalloccatechin-3-gallate for targeting vascular endothelium cells applied in corneal angiogenesis inhibition. *Int. J. Nanomed.* **2017**, *12*, 279–294. [CrossRef]
21. Chen, Y.C.; Yu, S.H.; Tsai, G.J.; Tang, D.W.; Mi, F.L.; Peng, Y.P. Novel technology for the preparation of self-assembled catechin/gelatin nanoparticles and their characterization. *J. Agric. Food Chem.* **2010**, *58*, 6728–6734. [CrossRef] [PubMed]
22. Rodriguez, S.K.; Guo, W.; Liu, L.; Band, M.A.; Paulson, E.K.; Meydani, M. Green tea catechin, epigallocatechin-3-gallate, inhibits vascular endothelial growth factor angiogenic signaling by disrupting the formation of a receptor complex. *Int. J. Cancer* **2006**, *118*, 1635–1644. [CrossRef] [PubMed]
23. Lee, H.S.; Jun, J.-H.; Jung, E.-H.; Koo, B.A.; Kim, Y.S. Epigalloccatechin-3-gallate inhibits ocular neovascularization and vascular permeability in human retinal pigment epithelial and human retinal microvascular endothelial cells via suppression of MMP-9 and VEGF activation. *Molecules* **2014**, *19*, 12150–12172. [CrossRef] [PubMed]
24. Carter, R.T.; Kambampati, R.; Murphy, C.J.; Bentley, E. Expression of matrix metalloproteinase 2 and 9 in experimentally wounded canine corneas and spontaneous chronic corneal epithelial defects. *Cornea* **2007**, *26*, 1213–1219. [CrossRef] [PubMed]
25. Cavet, M.E.; Harrington, K.L.; Vollmer, T.R.; Ward, K.W.; Zhang, J.Z. Anti-inflammatory and anti-oxidative effects of the green tea polyphenol epigallocatechin gallate in human corneal epithelial cells. *Mol. Vis.* **2011**, *17*, 533–542. [PubMed]
26. Friedlander, M.; Theesfeld, C.L.; Sugita, M.; Fruttiger, M.; Thomas, M.A. Involvement of integrins alpha v beta 3 and alpha v beta 5 in ocular neovascular diseases. *Proc. Natl. Acad. Sci. USA* **1996**, *93*, 9764–9769. [CrossRef]
27. Stepp, M.A. Corneal integrins and their functions. *Exp. Eye Res.* **2006**, *83*, 3–15. [CrossRef]
28. Fan, T.P.; Yeh, J.C.; Leung, K.W.; Yue, P.Y.; Wong, R.N. Angiogenesis: From plants to blood vessels. *Trends Pharmacol. Sci.* **2006**, *27*, 297–309. [CrossRef]
29. Danhier, F.; Breton, A.L.; Préat, V. RGD-based strategies to target alpha(v) beta(3) integrin in cancer therapy and diagnosis. *Mol. Pharm.* **2012**, *9*, 2961–2973. [CrossRef]
30. Guo, Z.; He, B.; Jin, H.; Zhang, H.; Dai, W.; Zhang, L.; Zhang, H.; Wang, X.; Wang, J.; Zhang, X.; et al. Targeting efficiency of RGD-modified nanocarriers with different ligand intervals in response to integrin $\alpha v\beta 3$ clustering. *Biomaterials* **2014**, *35*, 6106–6117. [CrossRef]

31. Tucker, G.C. Alpha v integrin inhibitors and cancer therapy. *Curr. Opin. Investig. Drugs* **2003**, *4*, 722–731. [PubMed]
32. Bellis, S.L. Advantages of RGD peptides for directing cell association with biomaterials. *Biomaterials* **2011**, *32*, 4205–4210. [CrossRef] [PubMed]
33. Davies, N.M. Biopharmaceutical considerations in topical ocular drug delivery. *Clin. Exp. Pharmacol. Physiol.* **2000**, *27*, 558–562. [CrossRef] [PubMed]
34. Davis, J.; Gilger, B.; Robinson, M. Novel approaches to ocular drug delivery. *Curr. Opin. Mol. Ther.* **2004**, *6*, 195–205.
35. Gaudana, R.; Ananthula, H.K.; Parenky, A.; Mitra, A.K. Ocular drug delivery. *AAPS J.* **2010**, *12*, 348–360. [CrossRef]
36. Tsai, C.H.; Wang, P.Y.; Lin, I.C.; Huang, H.; Liu, G.S.; Tseng, C.L. Ocular Drug Delivery: Role of Degradable Polymeric Nanocarriers for Ophthalmic Application. *Int. J. Mol. Sci.* **2018**, *19*, 2830. [CrossRef]
37. Huang, H.Y.; Wang, M.C.; Chen, Z.Y.; Chiu, W.Y.; Chen, K.H.; Lin, I.C.; Yang, W.C.V.; Wu, C.C.; Tseng, C.L. Gelatin–epigallocatechin gallate nanoparticles with hyaluronic acid decoration as eye drops can treat rabbit dry-eye syndrome effectively via inflammatory relief. *Int. J. Nanomed.* **2018**, *13*, 7251–7273. [CrossRef]
38. Shutava, T.G.; Balkundi, S.S.; Lvov, Y.M. (-)-Epigallocatechin gallate/gelatin layer-by-layer assembled films and microcapsules. *J. Colloid Interface Sci.* **2009**, *330*, 276–283. [CrossRef]
39. Yang, C.S.; Lambert, J.D.; Ju, J.; Lu, G.; Sang, S. Tea and cancer prevention: Molecular mechanisms and human relevance. *Toxicol. Appl. Pharmacol.* **2007**, *224*, 265–273. [CrossRef]
40. Li, Z.; Gu, L. Fabrication of self-assembled (-)-epigallocatechin gallate (EGCG) ovalbumin-dextran conjugate nanoparticles and their transport across monolayers of human intestinal epithelial Caco-2 cells. *J. Agric. Food Chem.* **2014**, *62*, 1301–1309. [CrossRef]
41. Sanna, V.P.G.; Roggio, A.M.; Punzoni, S.; Posadino, A.M.; Arca, A.M.S.; Bandiera, P.; Uzzau, S.; Sechi, M. Targeted biocompatible nanoparticles for the delivery of (−)-epigallocatechin 3-gallate to prostate cancer cells. *J. Med. Chem.* **2011**, *54*, 1321–1332. [CrossRef] [PubMed]
42. Kojima-Yuasa, A.; Hua, J.J.; Kennedy, D.O.; Matsui-Yuas, I. Green tea extract inhibits angiogenesis of human umbilical vein endothelial cells through reduction of expression of VEGF receptors. *Life Sci.* **2003**, *73*, 1299–1313. [CrossRef]
43. Ferrara, N.; Gerber, H.-P.; LeCouter, J. The biology of VEGF and its receptors. *Nat. Med.* **2003**, *9*, 669–676. [CrossRef] [PubMed]
44. Salam, A.; Mathew, R.; Sivaprasad, S. Treatment of proliferative diabetic retinopathy with anti-VEGF agents. *Acta Ophthalmol.* **2011**, *89*, 405–411. [CrossRef] [PubMed]
45. Kwak, N.; Okamoto, N.; Wood, J.M.; Campochiaro, P.A. VEGF is major stimulator in model of choroidal neovascularization. *Investig. Ophthalmol. Vis. Sci.* **2000**, *41*, 3158–3164.
46. Spragg, D.D.; Alford, D.R.; Greferath, R.; Larsen, C.E.; Lee, K.-D.; Gurtner, G.C.; Cybulsky, M.I.; Tosi, P.F.; Nicolau, C.; Michael, A.; et al. Immunotargeting of liposomes to activated vascular endothelial cells: A strategy for site-selective delivery in the cardiovascular system. *Proc. Natl. Acad. Sci. USA* **1997**, *94*, 8795–8800. [CrossRef]
47. Kelly, K.A.; Allport, J.R.; Tsourkas, A.; Shinde-Patil, V.R.; Josephson, L.; Weissleder, R. Detection of vascular adhesion molecule-1 expression using a novel multimodal nanoparticle. *Circ. Res.* **2005**, *96*, 327–336. [CrossRef]
48. Tsourkas, A.; Shinde-Patil, V.R.; Kelly, K.A.; Patel, P.; Wolley, A.; Allport, J.R.; Weissleder, R. In vivo imaging of activated endothelium using an anti-VCAM-1 magnetooptical probe. *Bioconjug. Chem.* **2005**, *16*, 576–581. [CrossRef]
49. Runnels, J.M.; Zamiri, P.; Spencer, J.A.; Veilleux, I.; Wei, X.; Bogdanov, A.; Lin, C.P. Imaging molecular expression on vascular endothelial cells by in vivo immunofluorescence microscopy. *Mol. Imaging* **2006**, *5*, 31–40. [CrossRef]
50. Eslani, M.; Baradaran-Rafii, A.; Movahedan, A.; Djalilian, A.R. The ocular surface chemical burns. *J Ophthalmol.* **2014**, *2014*, 1–9. [CrossRef]
51. Tseng, C.L.; Chen, K.H.; Su, W.Y.; Lee, Y.H.; ChangWu, C.; Lin, F.H. Cationic gelatin nanoparticles for drug delivery to the ocular surface: In vitro and In vivo evaluation. *J. Nanomater.* **2013**, *2013*, 1–11.

52. Neuhaus, T.; Pabst, S.; Stier, S.; Weber, A.-A.; Schrör, K.; Sachinidis, A.; Vetter, H.D.; Ko, Y. Inhibition of the vascular-endothelial growth factor-induced itracellualr signaling and mitogenesis of human endothelial cells by epigallocatechin-3 gallate. *Eur. J. Pharmacol.* **2004**, *483*, 223–227. [CrossRef] [PubMed]
53. Koh, C.H.; Lee, H.S.; Chung, S.K. Effect of topical epigallocatechin gallate on corneal neovascularization in rabbits. *Cornea* **2014**, *33*, 527–532. [CrossRef] [PubMed]
54. Pradhan, N.; Guha, R.; Chowdhury, S.; Nandi, S.; Konar, A.; Hazra, S. Curcumin nanoparticles inhibit corneal neovascularization. *J. Mol. Med.* **2015**, *93*, 1095–1106. [CrossRef]

pharmaceutics

MDPI

Review

Drug Delivery to the Posterior Segment of the Eye: Biopharmaceutic and Pharmacokinetic Considerations

Rubén Varela-Fernández [1,2,†], Victoria Díaz-Tomé [1,3,†], Andrea Luaces-Rodríguez [1,3,†], Andrea Conde-Penedo [1,4,†], Xurxo García-Otero [1,5,†], Asteria Luzardo-Álvarez [1,4], Anxo Fernández-Ferreiro [1,3,*] and Francisco J. Otero-Espinar [1,4,*]

1 Department of Pharmacology, Pharmacy and Pharmaceutical Technology, University of Santiago de Compostela (USC), Campus vida, 15782 Santiago de Compostela, Spain; rubenvf1@gmail.com (R.V.-F.); victoriadiaztome@gmail.com (V.D.-T.); andrealuaces21@gmail.com (A.L.-R.); andrea.conde.penedo@rai.usc.es (A.C.-P.); xurxo.garcia.otero@gmail.com (X.G.-O.); asteriam.luzardo@usc.es (A.L.-Á.)

2 Clinical Neurosciences Group, University Clinical Hospital, Health Research Institute of Santiago de Compostela (IDIS), Travesía da Choupana s/n, 15706 Santiago de Compostela, Spain

3 Clinical Pharmacology Group, University Clinical Hospital, Health Research Institute of Santiago de Compostela (IDIS), Travesía da Choupana s/n, 15706 Santiago de Compostela, Spain

4 Paraquasil Group, Health Research Institute of Santiago de Compostela (IDIS), Travesía da Choupana s/n, 15706 Santiago de Compostela, Spain

5 Molecular Imaging Group. University Clinical Hospital, Health Research Institute of Santiago de Compostela (IDIS), Travesía da Choupana s/n, 15706 Santiago de Compostela, Spain

* Correspondence: anxordes@gmail.com (A.F.-F.); francisco.otero@usc.es (F.J.O.-E.)

† These authors contributed equally to this work.

Received: 2 February 2020; Accepted: 11 March 2020; Published: 16 March 2020

Abstract: The treatment of the posterior-segment ocular diseases, such as age-related eye diseases (AMD) or diabetic retinopathy (DR), present a challenge for ophthalmologists due to the complex anatomy and physiology of the eye. This specialized organ is composed of various static and dynamic barriers that restrict drug delivery into the target site of action. Despite numerous efforts, effective intraocular drug delivery remains unresolved and, therefore, it is highly desirable to improve the current treatments of diseases affecting the posterior cavity. This review article gives an overview of pharmacokinetic and biopharmaceutics aspects for the most commonly-used ocular administration routes (intravitreal, topical, systemic, and periocular), including information of the absorption, distribution, and elimination, as well as the benefits and limitations of each one. This article also encompasses different conventional and novel drug delivery systems designed and developed to improve drug pharmacokinetics intended for the posterior ocular segment treatment.

Keywords: ocular pharmacokinetics; ocular drug delivery systems; ocular routes of drug administration; intravitreal administration; topical administration

1. Introduction

The posterior segment of the eye comprises the back two-thirds of the eye, including the vitreous humor, the retina, the choroid and the optic nerve. Posterior Segment Eye Diseases (PSEDs) are then defined as the disorders that affect these tissues with the common main outcome of varying degrees of visual impartment and blindness. The most prevalent diseases are glaucoma, age-related macular degeneration (AMD) and diabetic retinopathy (DR) (see Figure 1). Nowadays, millions of people are suffering from retinal and choroid diseases and the number is increasing every year, as the incidence significantly increases with age. Both disorders are characterized by their severity and difficulty of treating. Despite numerous efforts, effective intraocular drug delivery remains unresolved and therefore, it is highly desirable to improve the current treatments of diseases affecting the vitreous cavity.

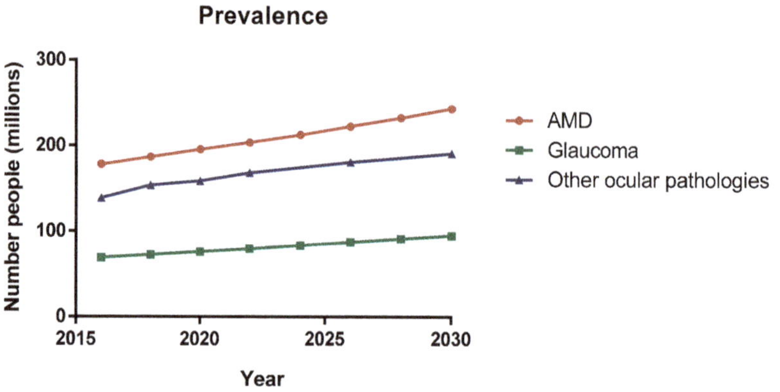

Figure 1. Prevalence of the main ocular pathologies. Data from the world report on vision published by the World Health Organization (WHO), 2019 [1].

In clinical practice, the standard procedure in treating these disorders is the intravitreal administration of injected drugs, although topical and systemic administration have also been addressed with limited results. Thus, other approaches have been developed for the treatment of posterior segment diseases such as periocular, suprachoroidal, and subretinal administration (Figure 2). All these routes of drug administration consist of the drug/system injection in the surroundings of the target site. Periocular administration includes subconjunctival, sub-Tenon's, peribulbar, retro bulbar, and posterior juxtascleral injection. However, these injections might not result in therapeutic drug levels in the target site due to the necessity of crossing several barriers to reach the intended site of action. This limitation could be overcome by using more effective drug delivery systems, where improved therapies may also be achieved.

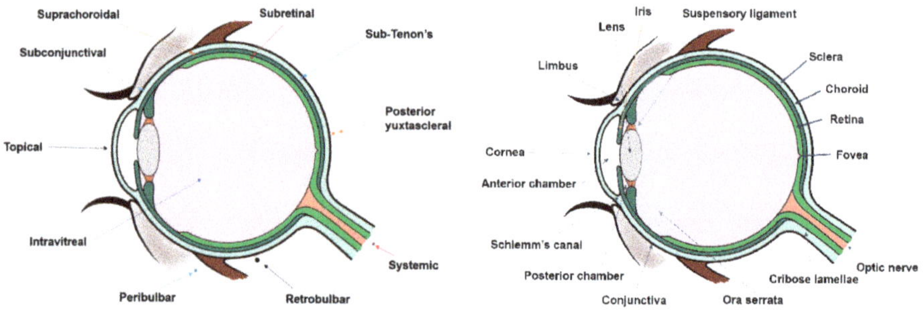

Figure 2. The first image represents a scheme of the different routes of drug administration to the posterior segment (dots symbolize the injection site of each route), while second image exemplifies the anatomy of the eye.

One of the main drawbacks of drug delivery to the back of the eye is the narrow interval dosing because of the low effectiveness and bioavailability of the administered drug. Also, it should be taken into consideration that intravitreal and periocular routes are highly invasive, being associated to discomfort and patient compliance. Intraocularly, a prolonged drug release not only entails the patient acceptability by increasing their quality of life, but also, a notable reduction in the economic costs associated to the hospital stays due to the frequently repeated injections that are necessary to complete the treatment.

Drug delivery to the posterior segment of the eye still remains a great challenge in the pharmaceutical industry due to the complexity and particularity of the anatomy and physiology of the eye. Some advances have been made with the purpose of maintaining constant drug levels in the site of action. The anatomical ocular barriers have a great impact on drug pharmacokinetics and, subsequently, on the pharmacological effect. For this reason, understanding pharmacokinetics plays a critical role in the design of effective pharmaceutical forms.

The aim of this review is to show an overview of the main aspects involved in ocular drug pharmacokinetics intended to treat PSEDs. A discussion of the different factors that are involved in the ocular drug delivery is first made, encompassing the different routes towards the posterior segment of the eye. Physiological barriers and drug transport pathways are described and the advantages and drawbacks of different administration routes to the eye are also discussed.

2. Routes of Drug Delivery to the Posterior Segment of the Eye

2.1. *Intravitreal Administration*

Intravitreal injection is the mainstream route of administration to treat diseases affecting the posterior segment of the eye. The drug is placed directly into the vitreous humor, though it is a highly targeted drug route. It has the inconvenience of being an invasive route. However, intravitreal drug administration is always selected to deliver to the posterior ocular segment due to the possibility of overcoming systemic exposure and obtaining high drug levels into the vitreous chamber.

2.1.1. Vitreous and Posterior Compartment Barriers to Drug Delivery

Vitreous

The vitreous body shows a transparent jelly-like structure mostly composed of types II, IX, and V/XI collagen fibers, whose spaces are filled with glycosaminoglycans, mainly hyaluronic acid. This structure acts as both a static and dynamic barrier. The static barrier is the vitreous structure by itself, although it is not a very restrictive barrier in terms of molecular mobility. The so-called dynamic barrier consists of the flow and clearance processes.

Initially, the superficial charge becomes vitally important for positively charged particles due to interactions with the components of the vitreous network such as hyaluronic acid (negatively charged), while negatively charged particles diffuse without any problem. Likewise, particle size may also impact on drug permeation, even though this parameter seems to be less clear. Certainly, several studies showed the distribution of same-sized particles (1 μm) through the vitreous is charge-dependent [2].

The convective flow from the anterior to the posterior segment of the eye should be taken into consideration for drug uptake due to the difference in pressure of the vitreous. This natural fact influences the drug distribution, having more impact on large molecules.

The drug particle size also plays a role in the type of clearance that drugs undergo, since smaller and more lipophilic drugs are mainly cleared in the posterior segment of the eye because of their ability of crossing the blood–retinal barrier (BRB), while larger and hydrophilic molecules are removed through anterior segment due to the aqueous humor outflow [2,3].

Posterior Compartment Barriers to Drug Delivery

1. Inner Limiting Membrane

The inner limiting membrane is a mechanical and electrostatic barrier located between the vitreous and the retina composed of collagen, laminin, and fibronectin. Its composition and thickness (~4 μm) may be variable along its structure, showing a 10 nm pore size.

Both drug charge and size can play an important role in the passage of molecules through this membrane, being the charge the most critical factor. Thus, positively charged nanoparticles seem to present more difficulty than neutral and negatively charged ones because of the negative charge of the membrane [3,4].

2. Neural Retina

The neural retina is the innermost layer of the eye and consists of a multi-layered structure which is responsible for transmitting the light to the brain by means of photoreceptors, neurons, and glial cells (Figure 3). These layers are: The outer limiting barrier, the outer nuclear layer, the outer plexiform layer, the inner nuclear layer, the inner plexiform layer, the ganglion cell layer, and the nerve fiber layer. It also must be taken into account that molecules cannot freely diffuse through the retina due to Muller glial cells presence between the inner and the outer limiting membranes. Furthermore, certain components of the retina can interact with some molecules, hindering their diffusion [2,3].

3. Blood–Retinal Barrier (BRB)

The BRB is composed of two types of cells: The retinal capillary endothelial cells (which make up the inner BRB) and the retinal pigment epithelial cells (RPE) (which form the outer BRB) [5]. Both are considered an important impediment to retinal drug delivery as it restricts the drug transport between neural retina and circulating blood [4]. In the RPE, drug permeability is determined by physicochemical factors (e.g., molecular weight, lipophilicity, protein binding), as well as drug concentration gradient and their affinity with the existing transporters at that level, which can increase or decrease drug transfer through RPE [6].

The BRB limits the drug diffusion from the vitreous humor to inner parts of the retina. It is composed of the inner BRB, which contacts with the vitreous humor and it is formed by capillary endothelial cells connected by tight junctions, and the outer BRB, also called the RPE, which exhibits a high amount of melanin, being surrounded by choroidal capillaries [3,7,8].

Paracellular transport through retinal capillaries is limited by the tight junctions (about 2 nm), although certain larger-size molecules can transcellularly permeate by passive diffusion and/or active transport (e.g., ganciclovir or dexamethasone) [9,10]. Nevertheless, both processes are also restricted due to the absence of fenestrations and the lack of transport vesicles in the endothelial cells.

The outer BRB located between the photoreceptors and the choriocapillaris, is composed of tight, gap and adherent junctions that can be removed by molecules via passive diffusion. Also, the pump proteins that are in the layer and the invagination vesicles allow active transport (e.g., Na^+/K^+-ATPase, P-glycoprotein, Multidrug Resistance Proteins -MRP1-) [11].

Molecules permeation is restricted depending on their size, charge, and/or lipophilicity. Thus, hydrophilic compounds follow the paracellular route through tight junctions while lipophilic molecules can cross the epithelium by the transcellular route. It has been demonstrated that only small lipophilic molecules can easily diffuse from bloodstream to the vitreous and vice versa [2,3,12].

4. Choroid

The choroid is a highly vascularized barrier that lies between the RPE and the sclera (Figure 3). This layer supplies oxygen and nutrients to the retina. It has a 200 μm thickness and it is divided into five layers: The Bruch's membrane, the choriocapillaris layer, two vascular layers, and the suprachoroidal layer [2].

The Brunch´s membrane presents a 2–4 μm thickness, whose structure is composed of collagen and elastin fibers. The choriocapillaris layer is formed by highly fenestrated capillaries with a 6–12 nm pore size, allowing the passage of large molecules [13]. The suprachoroid is located between the sclera and the choroid and it is composed of collagen fibers, melanocytes, and fibroblasts.

In terms of drug delivery, it must be taken into consideration that choroid shows two different behaviors: (1) It acts as a static barrier due to suprachoroid structure and (2) it provides a dynamic barrier as a consequence of a high choriocapillaris-layer blood flow. Both actions prevent the passage of hydrophilic compounds while positively charged lipophilic drugs can stabilize bindings with the tissue, leading to slow-release depots. The molecular size of the drug also determines the diffusivity into the posterior segment [2,12].

5. Sclera

The sclera is the outer opaque layer of the eye (Figure 3), which provides support to this structure. It shows a 0.5–1 mm average thickness, although it varies along the eye. It is composed of collagen fibers, proteoglycans, and glycoproteins, creating a network in an aqueous medium [14,15]. The organization of the collagen fibers gives rise to different regions, such as: Tenon's capsule, episcleral layer, the scleral stroma tissue and the lamina fusca, melding into the underlying choroid.

Drug permeability through the sclera depends on molecular weight, molecular radius, charge and lipophilicity, although it is usually more permeable than the cornea and conjunctiva [2,12]. Large molecules, up to 150 kDa, find harder to get through the sclera and their clearance is lower than smaller molecules. Transscleral diffusion consists of the permeation through porous spaces within a collagen aqueous network. Likewise, the hydrophilic molecules (e.g., methazolamide) are able to go through the sclera [16,17]. Matrix structure of proteoglycans is negatively charged at physiological pH and, consequently, the passage of negatively charged solutes across the sclera is facilitated [18].

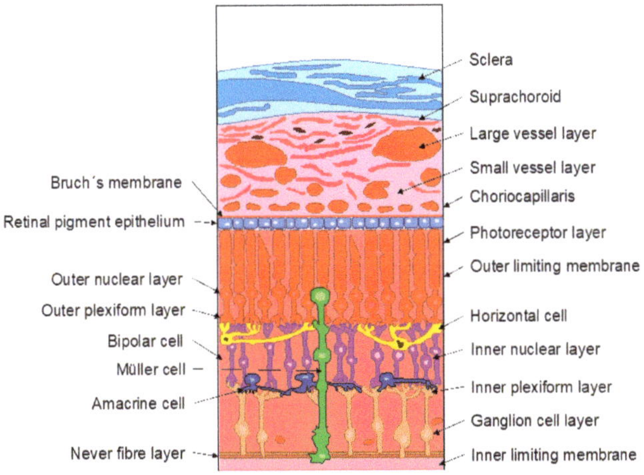

Figure 3. Schematic drawing of the sclera, choroid, and retina.

2.1.2. Advantages and Limitations

Intravitreal administration is performed by injecting a drug solution, suspension, and even intraocular implants into the vitreous cavity. In recent years, the intravitreal injection has become the mainstream of the treatment of ocular diseases affecting the posterior segment. Direct intravitreal injection has the obvious advantage of achieving immediate therapeutic concentrations in the vitreous humor. However, sites of action are normally the retina or the choroid, so the drug is injected in the surroundings of the site of action, but it has yet to overcome some barriers in order to achieve its target site. Therefore, drug delivery into the vitreous humor does not necessarily implies that the drug will be able to exert the pharmacological effect [19]. Nevertheless, intravitreal administration has proved to be the best administration route to achieve high and effective drug concentrations in the posterior segment of the eye.

Additionally, intravitreal administration has the advantage that largely avoids the systemic exposure; hence, the systemic adverse effects are limited. However, not all side effects are completely eliminated, being the most common ones: Endophthalmitis, vitreous detachment, retinal hemorrhage, inflammation, increased intraocular pressure, conjunctival hemorrhage, retinal toxicity, and cataracts, among others [19]. As an invasive procedure, the injection itself may cause a patient's discomfort and eye pain, mainly where repeated injections are needed. The need to treat the posterior segment of the eye increases interest in getting available novel controlled release formulations to maintain the therapeutic drug concentration in the vitreous as well as minimizing the number of injections.

The vitreous humor is composed of a polysaccharide aqueous meshwork. Apparently, it would seem that it acts itself as a retention compartment against drug distribution [7]. Nevertheless, drugs are quickly removed from the vitreous via the anterior route to the aqueous humor, hampering prolonged release phenomena [20]. In addition, the relatively high volume of the vitreous chamber allows administering drug delivery systems of different size and form (implants and inserts).

In clinical practice, intravitreal injections are directly administered into the vitreous cavity and the procedure is performed by a trained specialist. As an invasive procedure, some risks may be taken into account and several precautions should be taken during the intravitreal administration, such as avoiding touching the retina or the lens [19]; the vision line must be left untouched (the vision field can be blocked); and the injection incision should be as small as possible since it can prevent the development of eye infections and the leakage of vitreous [19]. Other major risks after intravitreal injection (although uncommon) are eye infections or vitreous hemorrhage. Depending on the disease being treated, a follow-up visit to the specialist should be scheduled for the administration of repeated intravitreal injections, always needed in chronic disorders such as DP or AMD [21].

Despite the associated complications to the injection procedure and discomfort after administration, repeated intravitreal injections are the only alternative to administer drugs as anti-VEGF, steroids, and antibiotics to treat pathologies affecting the posterior segment of the eye.

2.1.3. Pharmacokinetics

Nowadays, the pharmacokinetics and pharmacodynamics of pharmacological agents after intravitreal administration remain relatively unexplored and poorly understood. The vitreous-humor clearance mechanisms of intraocular-administered drugs limit the duration of their effect and injection's repeated administration. Nevertheless, there remains a real need to develop novel drug delivery systems intended to sustain release and more effective therapy.

Pharmacokinetics studies of intravitreal injection have demonstrated the drawbacks of an invasive administration route and the difficulty of acquiring direct samples. Most of the in vivo studies have been performed in rabbits as an experimental animal model [22]. Vitreous humor samples collection may require animal sacrifice, even though novel techniques such as micro-dialysis can be applied for continuous sample collections without animal detriment [23]. According to the 3Rs regulatory frameworks, the alternative is to extract aqueous humor or blood samples and then make a correlation with the drug concentration in the vitreous humor.

The drug concentration at any certain time after injection depends on the drug distribution volume, the initial injected dose and the elimination rate. Therefore, the two factors that predominantly affect the pharmacokinetics of injected drugs into the vitreous are their vitreous humor distribution and their clearance.

Drug Distribution in the Vitreous Humor

Drug distribution in the posterior segment of the eye is a crucial step in ocular pathologies treatment in order to obtain a pharmacological effect at the right target site. The factors that affect the drug distribution in the vitreous humor are predominantly its diffusion through the vitreous, the effect of the convective flow and the possible drug interactions with the vitreous humor elements. Moreover, other ocular barriers may limit the drug passage depending on the target site within the vitreous cavity [24].

Another aspect that should be taken into consideration is the effect of the injection itself, as the needle creates a channel through the vitreous humor. After the needle is being removed, it leaves behind a low resistance pathway for the passage of the drugs due to a change of the integrity of the vitreous humor [25].

The impact of both diffusion and convection flow in the drug pharmacokinetics within the vitreous humor has been studied based on different experimental data and mathematical models [7,26–29].

1. Diffusion

Once the drug is injected into the vitreous humor, it will diffuse through the vitreous humor until reaching its target tissue. The diffusion speed of this process depends on the drug physiochemical properties and the vitreous retention effect. The mesh size of the bovine vitreous humor was calculated to be approximately 500 nm [30]. Also, the different structural components presented in the vitreous constitute a barrier to the diffusion of the drugs depending of the characteristics on the drug.

Drug diffusion through the vitreous humor is created as drug concentration gradients from the injection site, which provides the moving force for the drug-particles' movement until a concentration balance is reached, where not more diffusion occurs. Regarding the drug physicochemical properties, the molecular weight and the drug net's charge are the parameters that most influence in the diffusion speed through the vitreous humor.

Generally, low molecular-weight drugs (e.g., fluorescein, glycerol, mannitol) exhibit high diffusion coefficients as they do not have the diffusion restriction through the vitreous meshwork [31,32]. In fact, the diffusivity in an aqueous solution could be a specific representation of this parameter in the vitreous humor. Diffusion of high molecular-weight molecules (e.g., FITC dextran) can be limited by the vitreous structure [33].

On the other hand, the drug net's charge could affect its diffusion since the vitreous humor is a negatively charged polymer network. Anionic and neutral molecules will not show any type of restriction in the vitreous humor considering their charge. However, cationic drugs could electrostatically interact with the negative charges of the vitreous humor [30,34]. This will lead to a decrease in the drug diffusion due to its retention in the vitreous humor.

2. Convection

Convection is the process of moving a fraction of volume of the aqueous humor produced by the ciliary processes throughout the vitreous humor towards the retina [7,26,28,29]. This process takes place due to the differences in pressure and temperature between the anterior chamber and the retinal surface [7].

The significance of the vitreous outflow effect on drug distribution depends on drug diffusivity in the vitreous [28]. It has been seen that drugs with high diffusivity values within the vitreous are not affected by the convective flow due to the high net movement through the vitreous humor, while low molecular weight drugs do not suffer any type of restriction through the vitreous. On the other hand, the relevance of the convective flow in the movement of drugs with low diffusivity values is quite unclear, even though it is generally accepted that the convective flow has a major effect when the diffusivity is lower and the flow is increased.

Park et al. have calculated the drug diffusivity values that could be affected by the convective flow, using a mathematical model. The convection does not affect the drug distribution with high diffusivity values within the vitreous (1×10^{-5} cm^2/s) but it starts to become relevant in the case of drugs with low diffusivity values (1×10^{-5} cm^2/s), particularly if the flow is increased [26,28]. Moreover, Xu et al. predicted that convection could be responsible for the 30% of the drug movement through the vitreous humor [27]. In the light of these results, it can be concluded that the convection is not a major contributing factor in the drug distribution through the vitreous humor [3].

Since the intravitreal convective flow depends on pressure, it seems obvious that an increase in the intraocular pressure could change flow values in the vitreous humor. As an example, in some pathologies such as glaucoma and retinal detachment, where higher intraocular pressure values are noticed, an increase in the convection has been observed [26,29].

3. Drug Interaction with Vitreous Humor

Hyaluronic acid, as one of the main vitreous components (65–400 mg/mL concentration range), may establish charge interactions with intraocularly administered drugs that are positively charged [35]. This binding could importantly decrease the cationic-drug diffusion through the vitreous humor (e.g., poly-L-lysine) [3]. However, up to now, the effect of this binding on drug pharmacokinetics remains to be elucidated.

4. Drug Interaction with Proteins

Protein concentration in the vitreous humor was estimated to be 4.7 ± 1.2 μg/μL in human samples [36], being the albumin the most abundant one (60–70% of the total protein) [37]. Between 1000 and 2500 different proteins have been identified in the vitreous cavity [36,38]. Although their concentration is very low in comparison with plasma concentration, the interaction between drugs and vitreous proteins can occur in the same way with plasma proteins. This interaction will lead to a free drug decrease to exert a pharmacological effect. Furthermore, the drug binding to a protein could slow down its diffusion through the vitreous humor increasing the residence time in the vitreous.

In some vitreoretinal pathologies, such as diabetic vitreoretinopathy, an increment in protein concentration in the vitreous humor is observed, as well as new proteins are expressed and linked to inflammation and immunity processes [36]. However, there is no available data regarding the impact of the increased protein concentration in the drug interaction with the proteins in these chronic diseases.

5. Liquefaction

One factor influencing both drug diffusion and convection processes in the vitreous humor is its own liquefaction, that is, the degeneration process of the vitreous humor associated with aging. The vitreous humor is observed in both liquid and jelly forms at the same time in the vitreous cavity [39]. Nevertheless, the proportion between these two forms gets modified with age, being observed as an increase in the liquid proportion and a decrease in the gel one [7], due to the disruption of the fibers mesh composing the vitreous humor. Vitreous liquefaction could cause an increase in the drug diffusivity, particularly in those that showed a limited diffusion, since the fibers mesh presents less movement restriction of molecules in its interior. This expanded diffusion can lead to an elimination increase, although the liquefaction itself does not directly affect the drug elimination from the posterior segment of the eye. The vitreous humor higher liquefaction, the more closely the diffusivity of the molecules in it approximates to their diffusion in water [3]. On the other hand, liquefaction and the vitreous homogeneity loss through aging are also associated with an increase in the convection flow [40].

Such data entails that the treatment of different-age-group patients with the same dosing scheme might be inappropriate, leading to overdose or insufficient dosage situations. Even though, so far it is not clear whether the vitreous liquefaction can affect the intravitreal pharmacokinetics or not [41,42].

It is also worthwhile to mention that the injection position during the administration and the injected volume may have an influence on the distribution of molecules in the vitreous humor. Different injection sites affect the drug distribution and permeability through the retina [43], whereas the injected volume could affect the drug elimination in different degree, depending of the injection position [43].

On the other hand, special patient situations, such as vitrectomy (procedure where the vitreous humor is removed), also determine the drug behavior into the vitreous. The motivations to perform a vitrectomy are varied, where the most common ones are: (1) Removal of infection, (2) obtention of a better access to the retina, (3) removal of scar tissue, and (4) correction of retinal detachment.

After the vitrectomy procedure, the drug elimination is greatly increased, regardless of the elimination pathway. In different animal studies, the half-life reduction of intravitreal drugs has been detected after a vitrectomy was performed, including: Amikacin [44], amphotericin B [45,46], cefazolin [47], ceftazidime [48], ciprofloxacin [49], and vancomycin [50], as well as some biologics, such as bevacizumab [51,52], ranibizumab [51,53], and aflibercept [53]. It also must be taken into account that these studies were performed in animal models and that its extrapolation to humans lacks of enough knowledge. However, it seems to be a general decrease in the half-life in humans and might affect the efficacy of the intravitreal drug, although this aspect is still under investigation [54].

Moreover, a higher risk of retinal toxicity is expected in vitrectomized eyes. The anti-infective is supposed to be placed in contact to the retinal surface on a high concentration, instead of being distributed all over the vitreous humor, consequently causing the retinal toxicity [55]. This is extremely important in drugs as amikacin since it has proven to produce retinal toxicity [56].

Surgical vitrectomy is normally followed by the filling of the vitreous chamber with silicone oil, which acts as a long-term buffer in the management of vitreous detachment. Injected silicone oil can also behave as a slow-release reservoir for some drugs [7], although it must be taken into consideration that most anti-inflammatory drugs are not soluble in the silicone oils. Several studies confirmed the drug injection into silicone oil-filled eyes led to its migration to the aqueous interface, resulting in an increase in the local concentration and the ulterior precipitation. This may cause retinal toxicity [57,58], supposedly caused by a decrease on the preretinal-space, which can also affect the drug distribution and half-life.

Therefore, the drug pharmacokinetics in silicone oil-filled eyes is still not well defined, although some authors recommend a substantial reduction of the drug dose (1/4–1/10 of the standard dose) to prevent these phenomena [59].

Drug Distribution to Surrounding Tissues

Depending on the type of disease, the target site could be located in the vitreous humor itself (e.g., infections), the retina (e.g., AMD, diabetic macular degeneration), or the choroid (e.g., serpiginous choroiditis). Therefore, the drug distribution to the surrounding tissues could be considered as part of the elimination process if the site of action is in the vitreous humor or as part of the drug distribution in order to achieve its target site. Nevertheless, studies performed in rabbit eyes have shown that the distribution volume is close to the anatomical volume of the vitreous chamber which implies that the surrounding tissues do not contribute too much to the distribution process [3].

The vitreous body is limited by the anterior blood–aqueous barrier (BAB) and posterior BRB. The inner BRB allows for the permeation of small molecules, where molecules with a size higher than 2 nm are prevented from their diffusion. Likewise, the RPE is a tight cellular layer between the photoreceptors and the choroid, which its permeability depends on the molecule's size and lipophilicity [3]. Once the drug reaches to the choroid, the drug diffusion is quite rapid, because of the higher permeability of the choroid and, subsequently, the drug is quickly removed to the blood circulation [3].

There is evidence of BRB influx-and-efflux carriers that ensure the retina is constantly supplied of nutrients and ions [7,8,60]. The evidence of efflux transporters at the BRB has been recently investigated, as the studies performed in animal models might not correlate with the results that could be obtained in humans. MDR1, BCRP, some MRP, and OATP are some of the main carrier families that have been detected in the BRB [61].

It should be noted that some drugs can be substrates of the BRB active transporters, but their contribution to the drug pharmacokinetics is still unclear. Firstly, it is needed to be addressed that the presence of active transport at the BRB could be an advantage if the drug target is in the choroid, as it will help the drug to reach the target site or even ensure that some drugs, that normally are not able to cross the BRB, can achieve the choroid. Conversely, this fact could be a disadvantage if the target site is prior to the retina or in the retina itself, the active transport will act as an elimination pathway.

Overall, the active transport contribution on the drug movement through the BRB is quite low, the effect being also reduced over the time. As the drug concentration at the vitreous humor is usually very high after administration, the transporters are prone to be saturated [61].

The drug elimination from the vitreous humor involves the drug possible metabolism in the ocular tissues and the removal from the ocular compartments to the systemic blood flow.

Drug metabolism in the vitreous humor has not been deeply investigated. Mainly, studies have aimed at the enzyme identification in the vitreous humor, but not at analyzing its impact of drug pharmacokinetics [45]. For example, the presence of enzymes such as esterases or peptidases in rabbits´ vitreous humor should be mentioned here [62]. The drug in situ metabolism have been exploited for the development of prodrugs, such as ganciclovir esters (prodrugs with no pharmacological activity) which are biotransformed into ganciclovir (drug with pharmacological activity) once injected into the vitreous humor [62].

Metabolic enzymes have been detected in other ocular tissues posterior to the elimination of the drug from the vitreous humor, such as retina, ciliary body, and iris [63].

There are two major routes of drug elimination from the vitreous: Anterior and posterior clearance (Figure 4).

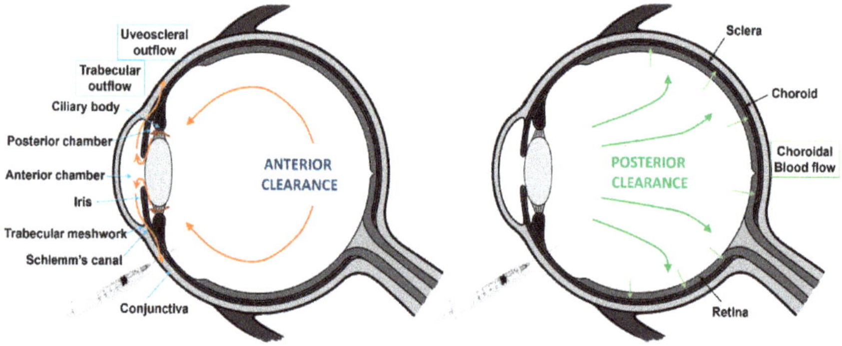

Figure 4. Schematic representation of the anterior and posterior clearance from the vitreous humor.

1. Anterior Route

After intravitreal injection, the drugs will be eliminated following the anterior route from the vitreous by a diffusion process across the lens and the ciliary body, to enter afterwards into the posterior chamber. From there, drugs are removed through the aqueous humor turnover to the anterior chamber, where they are subsequently removed along with aqueous humor by the trabecular and uveoscleral outflow [8]. The rapid turnover of the aqueous humor into the anterior chamber is the main force for the anterior clearance [7].

This elimination route is accessible for all type of drugs as they can freely move across the hyaloid membrane, avoiding the lens. However, drugs that are typically removed from this pathway are hydrophilic and large molecules that are not able to cross the retina [7]. The elimination of high molecular-weight compounds by the anterior route has been widely studied [40,42,64] (see Table 1). In fact, there is an inverse relationship between the molecular weight and the elimination rate from the vitreous.

Experimental data have determined that drugs which are removed from the anterior pathway exhibit higher half-lives than the ones that are removed from the posterior route. The relationship between vitreous half-life and aqueous humor/vitreous humor ratio is not broadly clarified. However, it is known that the presence of the drug is higher in the aqueous humor, i.e., it is removed by the anterior route, as the half-life is higher [65].

Table 1. Vitreous half-life times for intravitreally administered drugs with different pharmacokinetic characteristics.

Pharmacologic Group	Drug	Characteristics	Half-Life Time (h)	Ref.
Corticosteroids	Dexamethasone	Low molecular weight Water insoluble	3.48	[66]
Antibiotics	Ceftizoxime	Low molecular weight Water soluble	5.70	[67]
Somatostatin analogues	Octreotide acetate	High molecular weight Water soluble	16.00	[68]
Antiviral	ISIS 2922	High molecular weight Water soluble	62.00	[69]

2. Posterior Route

In the posterior route, administered drugs permeate through the retina and subsequently are cleared by the choroidal blood flow. Drugs that are removed by the posterior route exhibit short half-lives due to the large surface area available for permeation and the presence of active transport mechanisms [65].

In posterior elimination processes, a relationship between the drug physicochemical properties and their half-lives within the vitreous humor has been identified. Durairaj et al. established that the drug molecular weight, its lipophilia, and the dose/solubility ratio at pH 7.4 are the major parameters that affect the drug half-life in the vitreous [70].

Therefore, the posterior route is the main elimination pathway for small and lipophilic molecules since they can easily cross the retina. The diffusion process could take place via the paracellular and/or transcellular route.

As can be seen in Table 2, some important differences are shown between the parameters affecting the anterior and posterior elimination route of drugs from the vitreous humor.

Table 2. Comparison of the anterior and posterior route of drug elimination from the vitreous humor [65,70].

Features	Anterior Route	Posterior Route
Tissue involved	BAB	BRB
Elimination pathway	Aqueous humor outflow	Choroidal flow
Molecule characteristics	Hydrophilic High molecular weight	Lipophilic Small molecular weight

2.1.4. Drug Delivery Systems

Several reviews about the development of drug delivery systems have been published previously [71–74]. For this reason, in this article is not going to be treated in depth.

Biodegradable implants [75], non-biodegradable implants [76], biodegradable microspheres [71], nanoparticles [77], dendrimers [78], and hydrogels [79] have been used for intravitreal drug administration. Moreover, some sophisticated systems have been developed for the treatment of chronic and refractory ocular diseases, such as a microelectromechanical systems (MicroPump) [80] and a port delivery systems (PDS) [81].

In addition, to the current research on new systems of intravitreal release [82], there are already commercialized formulations such as Lucentis®, Ozurdex®, Eylea®, Avastyn®, among others (see Table 3).

Table 3. Summary of the main key pharmacokinetic parameters for different intravitreally administered drugs.

Pharmacologic Group	Subgroup/Drug	Half-Life Time (h)	MRT (h)	C_{max} (μg/mL)	Ref.
Nonsteroidal anti-inflammatory drugs	Ketorolac	4.3	6.16	175	[83]
	Diclofenac	2.05	2.95	65	[83]
Antibiotics	Penicillines	10–20	5–25	1000–5000	[84–86]
	Cephalosporines	5–15	5–30	1000–2250	[48,85,87]
	Tetracyclines	10–20	NA	125–400	[86,88]
	Fluoroquinolones	3.5–5.5	0.25–5	100–500	[49,89,90]
	Monobactams	7.5	NA	1000	[91]
	Carbapenems	2.5–10	NA	50–100	[92,93]
	Macrolides	40–60	NA	100–200	[85,94,95]
Antibodies	Bevacizumab	4.32	5.92	400	[96]
	Ranibizumab	2.88	4.03	162	[97]

2.2. *Topical Administration*

Ophthalmic topical administration by eye drops is commonly used for the treatment of anterior-segment diseases [98,99]. Most of the topically applied drugs are intended for the treatment of diseases that affect different layers of the cornea, the conjunctiva, iris, or the ciliary body [5]. However, topical administration for the treatment of posterior ocular diseases is considered an ineffective pharmacological strategy since therapeutic drug concentrations are not reached in the posterior segment of the eye due to low drug penetration.

2.2.1. Ocular Barriers for the Entry of Drugs: Precorneal Factors

After topical eye-drops administration, the first tissue barrier that drug molecules must overcome to access the target is the tear drainage of the excess volume through the nasolacrimal duct. In normal conditions, this drainage occurs at 1.45 $\mu L \cdot min^{-1}$ and it results in a drug loss into systemic circulation, especially related to hydrophilic molecules [100]. In fact, the loss of eye drop solution occurs until the tear volume returns to a normal range (7–9 μL).

Likewise, the thin precorneal tear film secreted by different glands and the Globet cells, which is about 8 μm thickness and with a 7 μL volume, also acts as a barrier in terms of drug absorption. It is composed of three layers: mucin, an aqueous and a lipid layer. The rate of drug elimination from the tear fluid is in the range of 0.5–1.0 $\mu L \cdot min^{-1}$ [101,102]. As a result of these facts and the systemic absorption through the conjunctiva, the ocular drug absorption is limited to less than 5% (<5%) when this delivery method is used [102].

2.2.2. Corneal and Anterior Compartment Barriers

Cornea

The cornea is the transparent portion surrounding the sixth anterior part of the eyeball with a 0.5 mm thickness and a 12 mm diameter. Tear film and aqueous humor provide nourishment and oxygen as it lacks blood vessels. The cornea consists of a collagen structure organized in six layers: Epithelium, Bowman's membrane, stroma, Dua´s layer, Descemet's membrane, and endothelium (Figure 5). The stratified, squamous and non-keratinized epithelium is the most critical barrier to penetration with a 10^{-7}–10^{-5} cm^{-1} drug permeability rate because of the fact that tight junctions impair the permeation of low lipophilic molecules [12,100,103].

Drug absorption depends on their physicochemical characteristics. In consequence, only hydrophilic molecules can diffuse through the stroma due to the hydrophilic nature of the hydrated collagen. Only small molecules with a log D value between 2 and 3 can penetrate through all the layers. The paracellular route allows molecules with a 500 Da molecular weight or a <5.5 Å size penetrate across tight junctions. The solute charge is also an important factor, as the cornea decreases the absorption of negatively charged molecules because of the negatively charged corneal surface [12].

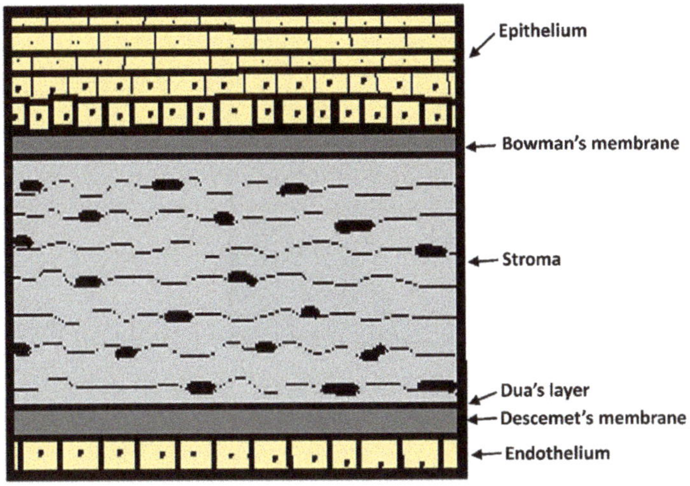

Figure 5. Schematic representation of the human corneal layers.

Conjunctiva

1. Conjunctiva

The conjunctiva is a thin vascularized stratified cylindrical epithelium with its underlying stroma covering the exposed sclera and the eyelids. This membrane shows a 17-times higher surface area than the cornea [104], although conjunctiva is less permeable for lipophilic molecules. Hydrophilic compounds absorption is also reduced because of tight junctions in the corneal epithelium. Despite this fact, the conjunctival absorption is higher than the corneal's due to the wider intercellular spacing allowing the passage of molecules up to 10 kDa. Furthermore, through the corneal route, via the conjunctiva, drugs are removed into the systemic circulation because of the presence of blood and lymphatic capillaries in the conjunctiva [12].

2. Blood–Aqueous Barrier (BAB)

The BAB is formed by the iris and ciliary muscle vasculature endothelium and by the posterior iris and non-pigmented ciliary epithelium (Figure 6). This barrier is poorly permeable due to the tight intercellular junctions, which limit the passage of substances with high molecular weight or high hydrophilicity. This biological barrier is also responsible for the selective diffusion of ions and small solutes through space between cells. There are active transporters that alters drug permeation, depending their activity on the passive diffusion rate. However, their significance in drug absorption is still unclear and requires elucidation.

For systemically delivered drug, the tight junctions of the iris vasculature limit the passage of substances from the plasma to the iris stroma. The non-pigmented ciliary epithelium tight junctions restrict the passage of substances from ciliary body stroma to the posterior chamber [12,105]. Overall, this barrier modulates the passage of molecules between the anterior and posterior segment, as well as from plasma to aqueous humor. The drainage of aqueous humor (2.0 to 3.0 mL/min) also hinders the passage of drugs [106].

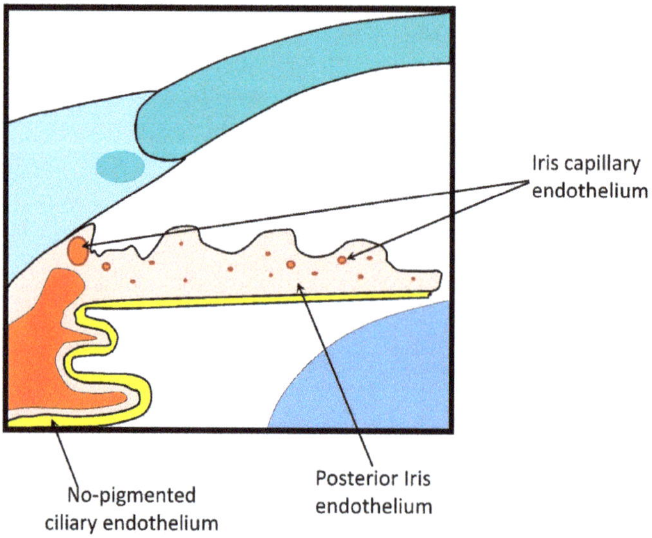

Figure 6. Blood–aqueous barrier (BAB) structure.

2.2.3. Advantages and Limitations

Topical administration is the most challenging administration route for drugs intended to treat pathologies that are affecting the posterior segment of the eye. Once administered onto the ocular external surface, the drug absorption is restricted by the different barriers, these being: Static (cornea and the BAB), dynamic (conjunctival and lymphatic conjunctival lymphatic and lacrimal drainage), and metabolic (carriers and receptors) barriers [99]. Nevertheless, it is considered the least invasive method of ophthalmic application due to patient compliance and ease of administration. Moreover, it is not required the ophthalmologist intervention since eye drops can be instilled by the patients themselves [5]. However, significant disadvantages have been found using this administration route to the posterior segment, such as the significantly low bioavailability (1–5%) and ocular penetration (less than 0.001%) in the intraocular tissues (aqueous humor among others) [107]. The main reasons are that the drug applied topically is quickly removed by ocular protective mechanisms such as nasolacrimal drainage, blinking (6 to 15 times/minute), tear renewal (0.5–2.2 μL/min) and high lacrimal clearance [108,109]. Besides, the unproductive absorption to the systemic circulation through the conjunctiva, choroid, uveal tract and internal retina also limits the drug access to the posterior segment. Significant efforts towards the development of new drug delivery systems to the posterior segment of the eye have been carried out to overcome the obvious limitations of topical ocular administration.

2.2.4. Pharmacokinetics

Drug topical absorption into the posterior segment of the eye strictly depends on the route through which the drug is distributed (Figure 7). Thus, the drug corneal exposure will allow for its concentration to be higher in the aqueous humor, whereas higher drug concentrations in the back of the eye will be reached after direct exposure on the conjunctival surface.

For example, the drug loss in the precorneal segment is because of the tear fluid. The administered drug will be released from the vehicle to the tear film, where tear fluid dynamics accelerate its elimination due to the complete replacement of the tear film every 2–3 min [99]. Furthermore, different enzymes and lacrimal proteins can influence the drug metabolism in the precorneal surface [107].

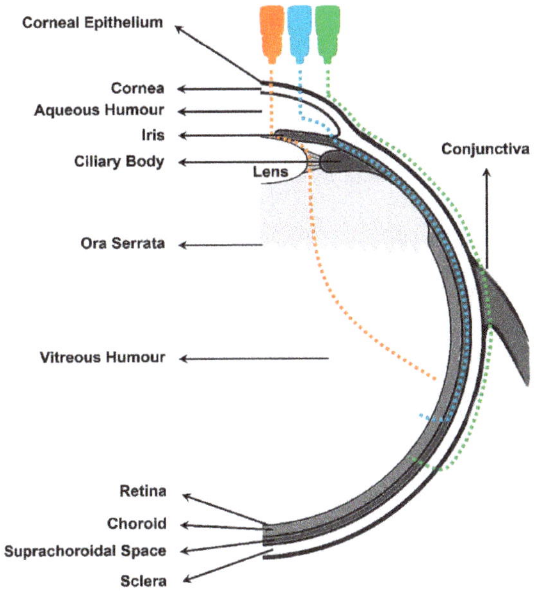

Figure 7. Different topical routes of drug absorption from the cornea/conjunctiva to the vitreous humor: Periocular route marked in green. Uvea-scleral route in blue. Transvitreal route marked in orange.

When administered topically, the low amount of drug that has been able to be absorbed will permeate from the cornea/conjunctiva surface to the retina across three different routes [98]: transvitreal route, uvea–scleral route and periocular route, being all of them conditioned by the nature of the drug, the pharmaceutical form and the anatomical characteristics of the eye.

The transvitreal pathway of absorption is the one followed by the drug via the transcorneal diffusion until it reaches the vitreous humor. The passage of molecules through the cornea depends on their lipophilicity, molecular weight, charge and ionization degree [110,111]. Once the drug is applied to the ocular surface by eye drops, the passage to the anterior chamber is driven by a diffusion process passing through the corneal epithelium via the paracellular or transcellular route. The penetration through these routes always depends on the drug concentration in the tear film and the drug retention time on the ocular surface. Hydrophilic drugs cross the corneal epithelium via the paracellular route while lipophilic drugs cross the epithelial barrier along the transcellular route. Once the drug crosses the cornea and reaches the aqueous humor, it is distributed to the surrounding tissues (ciliary, iris, crystalline body) and to the vitreous humor by diffusion process [98].

The aqueous humor is mainly drained (75–85%) through the Schlemm's canal (tubular conduct with thin and porous walls that allows the absorption of large protein molecules). The rest of the elimination process is carried out through the iris and the connective tissue of the ciliary and suprachoroidal muscles, leading to the uvea towards the extraocular connective tissue. The drug removed from aqueous humor contributes to a decrease in the amount of drug that could be able to reach the posterior segment of the eye.

The iris is one of the two ocular tissues that contain melanin, a pigment responsible for its color. Melanin can interact with some drugs, causing its retention in the iris. This retentive effect is more pronounced in case of lipophilic drugs, resulting in a drug sustained action [112] but decreases its pharmacological activity [5]. Overall, the drug bioavailability in the aqueous humor through this route has been determined to be less than 5% of the applied dose [113].

The uveal-scleral route followed by the administered drug after topical administration corresponds to the transcorneal diffusion to the anterior chamber and its drainage through the aqueous humor to the uvea–scleral tissue towards the posterior tissues.

This route follows the same absorption process through the cornea until reaching the aqueous humor as the transvitreal one. Once in the aqueous humor, the drug diffuses through the suprachoroidal space to the choroid causing an unproductive absorption. To a large extent, this is due to the drug partial elimination to the systemic circulation through the BAB capillary fenestrations, giving rise to the appearance of side effects. The drug is transported towards the systemic circulation through the choriocapillaris, which can cause side effects systemically. However, some other external factors, such as prostaglandins (drug penetration improvement to the back of the eye when they are co-administered via the uveo–scleral route) can affect the process [114,115]. The periocular drug absorption comprises the drug diffusion through the conjunctiva to the Tenon's capsule and its diffusion through the sclera, choroid, and retina.

It also must be taken into account that between 34% and 79% of the administered dose on the ocular surface is primarily removed by this way into the systemic circulation due to the high degree of conjunctival vascularization and its large surface area (16–18 cm^2) [113]. Therefore, for a drug to penetrate must have a molecular weight no greater than 70 kDa [116]. In addition, it should be considered that the drug transport through the conjunctiva, sclera, choroids and retina can occur by passive (paracellular or transcellular) or active routes (membrane carriers) [114,117]. Some lipophilic drugs can passively penetrate throughout the RPE by directly accessing the posterior segment through lateral scleral diffusion followed by penetration through the Bruch's membrane and the RPE.

2.2.5. Drug Delivery Systems

Currently, there are few commercial topical formulations specifically intended for the treatment of ocular posterior segment diseases. Even so, in recent years, new advanced topically drug release systems have been developed in order to improve the drug access to the back of the eye, such as nanoparticles [99,118], emulsions [119], nanostructured lipid carriers [120], liposomes [121], and nanosuspensions [122].

Despite the enormous efforts to develop efficient topical formulations intended to reach therapeutic drug concentrations in the posterior segment of the eye, the most relevant results have been obtained by using eye drops. In an ex vivo assays using cow eyes, the topical application of a memantine hydrochloride ring that functioned as a reservoir on the corneal surface demonstrated the efficient drug distribution of the into the choroid and retina [123]. Currently, memantine is in phase III studies in humans as a neuroprotector and neuroreparative drug in ophthalmic diseases. Another approach has been made by investigating the topical application of a brimonidine ocular solution in monkeys, rats, and rabbits. Results have shown that the formulation administered repeatedly reached an enough drug concentration to provide neuroprotection in the retina [124]. In the AMD treatment, promising results have been obtained in rabbit retina by the dexamethasone-cyclodextrin complexes topical application [125,126].

2.3. Systemic Administration

Systemic administration route constitutes an alternative route in the treatment of eye's posterior segment pathologies. It is normally used as a coadjutant treatment or as a second choice after the failure of intravitreal or subconjunctival injections treatment. It is based on drug administration by conventional routes (e.g., oral, intravenous, or intramuscular). Once the drug reaches the bloodstream, the absorption will take place through conjunctival, episcleral and/or choroidal vessels to get the vitreous cavity, although most of the drugs do not pass the main blood–ocular barriers [6].

2.3.1. Advantages and Limitations

Systemic drug administration shows a series of advantages and disadvantages compared to other administration routes to treat posterior segment diseases. Firstly, systemic administration is very effective in the case of concomitant ocular and systemic diseases as they can both be treated with only one treatment. Although ocular effects slowly appear with the systemic administration compared to other routes, the duration of the effect is more prolonged [127].

The oral administration to treat ocular diseases presents some positive features: Non-invasive, no need to use strict sterile conditions, high patient compliance, and adherence to treatment and width availability of pharmaceutical forms that provide great drug stability [5,103,128]. Oral administration is usually combined with topical ocular administration [5].

However, the systemic route presents certain drawbacks [5,103]. The presence of physiological barriers (BAB and BRB mainly) prevents the drug passage to the eye, leading to a drug bioavailability of less than 2% [5]. This low bioavailability forces the administration of high doses of the drug to obtain therapeutic concentrations into the vitreous which may lead to systemic toxicity and severe side effects. In addition, a lag time occurs between the drug administration and onset of pharmacological effect. An important prerequisite for a drug to be administered by oral route (for ocular applications) is to have a high drug oral bioavailability [5]. Even though, the limited access to the posterior segment of the eye implies the administration of high doses of drug or an increased administration frequency to obtain a significant therapeutic response [103,116,129]. However, these procedures can exacerbate drug toxicity as a consequence of the drug non-specific absorption to other organs [116,130,131]. Trained personnel are also required in case of intravenous or intramuscular administration.

Likewise, parenteral administration is also a systemic administration route used as an alternative pathway in posterior ocular pathologies. Ocular drugs can be administered by intravenous injection, although its use is less frequent than oral administration route [132].

2.3.2. Pharmacokinetics

Absorption to Ocular Tissues

Systemically administered drugs can easily reach the choroid due to the high vascularization of this tissue, as more than 85% of the ocular blood flow takes place in this layer, with a value of 43 mL/h [133], and choriocapillaris fenestrations [5,130].

Drug transport from blood circulation to the ocular cavity is strictly regulated by two anatomical and physiological barriers: The BAB and the BRB [8,134]. These barriers limit drug bioavailability by restricting its intercellular permeation to the anterior and posterior segment of the eye. This barrier effect is mainly due to the presence of highly complex tight junctions among epithelial and endothelial cells, which are located on the interface between blood flow and intraocular tissue. Moreover, it was observed that the drug passage improves during inflammatory conditions [135]. This is due to an increase in vascular permeability that leads to greater extravasation of components from the bloodstream to extravascular tissue [136].

Drug entry into posterior ocular tissues is mainly governed by the BRB. Thus, the relationship between drug permeability and physicochemical factors has been demonstrated, concluding that drug permeability increases with decreasing molecular weight and/or protein binding but improves with increasing lipophilicity [127]. As a result, small and lipophilic compounds can easily cross eye barriers (RPE, non-pigmented internal ciliary epithelium and retinal blood vessels), while hydrophilic and large compounds penetration is restricted [133]. However, hydrophobicity and high molecular weight tend to increase drug's half-life time in the posterior segment of the eye [137]. Therefore, RPE presents a selective permeability to highly hydrophobic drugs, whereas the penetration of hydrophilic and/or large substances being much more limited.

The type (influx or output flow) and/or location (vitreous or blood side) of the ocular transporters also condition the drug absorption and its concentration in the intraocular cavity [138].

Recently, many drug efflux pumps were identified in the ocular barriers. Among transporters with the greatest influence on the drug´s arrival to the posterior segment of the eye are the efflux transporters, these being a part of the ATP-binding cassette (ABC) protein family located in the RPE [139]. Specifically, two efflux pumps related to the development of chemoresistance were described, these being: P-glycoprotein (ABCB1) and the multidrug-resistance associated protein (MRP1) (ABCC1).

P-glycoprotein is an efflux protein located in the iris, cornea and ciliary muscle, as well as in conjunctival epithelium, non-pigmented ciliary epithelium and RPE. It is a 170 KDa membrane protein that is expressed on the apical surface of the aforementioned cells [139]. It actively promotes drug molecules' exit from retinal endothelial cells, reducing drugs accumulation within them [139].

For its part, MRP1 is a 190 KDa efflux protein encoded by the MRP1 gene on chromosome 16p13.1 and bounded to the choroidal side of the retinal barrier. It is an atypical ABC transporter with two cytosolic nucleotide-binding domains (NBD) and seventeen membrane-spanning domains (MSD) [140]. It functions as a multispecific organic anion transporter, mediating an ATP-dependent transport of drugs and other xenobiotics [141]. In any case, molecular mechanisms of these drug transporters are not completely known.

Distribution to Ocular Tissues

In general, systemically administered drugs reach the target tissues from the blood. Drug plasma transport is protein-binding dependent, giving rise to (1) free drug fraction, which is active and susceptible of excretion/metabolism and (2) protein-bound fraction that acts as a drug inactive reservoir. Only the free drug fraction can cross biological membranes and, consequently, reach the ocular tissues.

Specifically, drug distribution through blood–ocular barriers is a key factor in the achievement of an effective ocular treatment with systemically administered drugs. Before mentioned ocular barriers regulate drug transfer between blood circulation and the eye in both directions. Drugs whose transport is predominantly carried out by passive diffusion, distribution and clearance are independent of the drug transport direction, although mediated permeation by transporters could lead to a drug preferred transport direction (inward or outward) [3,128].

In any case, it must be taken into account that, although the eye barriers structure and main permeability trends have been known for some time, the distribution process from the blood circulation to the posterior segment of the eye is not yet fully elucidated. However, pharmacokinetic simulation models have been created for the drug concentrations prediction in the vitreous humor, depending on the free drug concentration and the blood flow between the general circulation and the posterior segment of the eye [133].

Once drugs reach the vitreous humor, their distribution and elimination follow the same pattern as the followed after an intravitreal administration. The parameters that affect the drug pharmacokinetics within vitreous humor have been discussed in the section of intravitreal administration.

1. Proteins and Biological Binding

The free drug may accumulate more than expected in any posterior ocular layers if it binds to cellular components or if it acts as a substrate for a significant active transport process. Specifically, drugs binding to ocular tissues' proteins and pigments, mainly melanin, significantly affects their transport to the posterior segment of the eye [6,130,142,143].

Melanin is a polyanionic biological pigment located in the uvea and the RPE in the ocular tissues as melanosomes or pigment granules, which are melanoprotein complexes where melanin is bound to a protein matrix [142]. Menon et al. determined the existence of 6–8 mg melanin at the ocular level [6,144].

Drug binding to melanin and proteins in ocular tissues is an important factor in drugs administration by systemic route since they can modify the drug bioavailability in the target site and, consequently, reduce its pharmacological activity [5,145].

Specifically, ocular melanin has a significant influence on drug pharmacokinetics and permeation through the retina [5,146] due to its capacity to bind (mainly reversible binding) free radicals and chemicals, especially basic (pKa values above 7) and lipophilic drugs by electrostatic, charge transfer, and van der Waals forces [5,147]. Main pharmacological consequences of the drug-melanin complexes are drug accumulation and retinal toxicity, besides the fact that larger doses are needed to obtain a therapeutic response due to the bound-to-melanin drug inactivation (e.g., betaxolol, metoprolol, and phosphodiesther oligonucleotides) [142]. Nevertheless, this drug depot may act as a reservoir over a long time, prolonging drug effects [145,146].

Drug Elimination

Regarding drug elimination process by this route, it must be taken into account that the administered drug not only faces passive barriers but also active barriers, such as clearance through the choroidal blood flow, which is extremely high, and the number and size of the choriocapillaris fenestrations that make up this system [6,148], by presenting a 70–80 nm pore size and a number between 30–50 fenestrations/μm^2 [149,150].

In general, drug elimination from the posterior segment of the eye can be carried out by two different ways, anterior and/or posterior pathways [103], following the same pattern described for the intravitreal administration route.

2.3.3. Drug Delivery Systems

The design of ophthalmic drugs systemic administration forms is aimed at achieving therapeutic concentrations in the posterior segment of the eye without causing undesired side effects. Drug targeted administration to these tissues from the systemic circulation has only been studied in preclinical animal models. Studies were carried out based on qualitative investigations performance and assessed by microscopy, immunohistochemistry, and/or angiography techniques [3]. Some of the novel systemic targeting systems studied for drug transport through the choroid to the posterior segment of the eye include [137]: 20 nm gold nanoparticles [151], polyethylene glycol (PEG) conjugated immunoliposomes [103], PLGA nanoparticles or Visudyne®. Currently, none of them is commercialized except for Visudyne®, an intravenous administration formulation used in photodynamic therapy for age-related wet macular degradation treatment [151].

Even so, several strategies related to the design of advanced delivery systems are currently under study, such as: (1) Structurally modified drugs that can effectively avoid MRP1 efflux transporter to improve ocular penetration, (2) hydrophilic drug administration through advanced delivery systems directed by transporter/receiver (superficially marked systems with an ocular-receptor specific substrate and/or vehicles attached to substrates that show a high affinity for ocular tissues) [139], and (3) drug affinity improvement to BRB transporters, such as amino acid, oligopeptides or cation and anion transporters, in order to increase drug transport to the posterior segment of the eye [152].

2.3.4. Systemic Drugs for Posterior Segment Eye Diseases

Drug systemic administration is not the preferable route in the treatment of posterior ocular segment pathologies, although it is still useful in many cases, being an administration pathway carried out by different routes (e.g., oral, intravenous, intramuscular). Thus, some drugs are administered orally (see Table 4).

Table 4. Summary of orally administered drugs for the treatment of posterior segment ocular diseases.

Pharmacologic Group	Drug	Pathology	Administration Route	Reference
Analgesics	Paracetamol	Ocular trauma treatment-associated pain	Oral	[153]
	NSAIDs (Flurbiprofen, Ketorolac, Diclofenac, Bromfenac and Nepafenac)	Ocular trauma treatment-associated pain	Oral	[153]
Antibiotics	Doxycycline	Neovascularization	Oral	[110,154]
	Tetracycline	Ocular rosacea	Oral	[111,155]
	Erythromycin	Orbital cellulitis	Oral	[111]
	Minomycline	Ocular rosacea	Oral	[110]
Corticosteroids	Dexamethasone	Giant cell arteritis	Oral	[153]
Immunosuppressants	Cyclosporine	Idiopathy or related-to-Behçet's-disease uveitis	Oral	[156]
Carbonic anhydrase inhibitors	Acetazolamide (Diamox sequel®)	Glaucoma	Oral	[113,157]
	Etoxolamide	Glaucoma	Oral	[114,158]

Apart from these, orally administration formulations with antineoplastic and antiviral agents have also been studied [103]. In relation to the latter one, it must be considered that the most frequent ocular posterior segment pathologies with viral etiology are associated with immunosuppression states (e.g., AIDS or transplants). These include: Cytomegalovirus retinitis, whose treatment is based on the antivirals intravenous administration (valganciclovir, ganciclovir, foscarnet, and/or cidofovir) as well as acute retinal necrosis and progressive external retinal necrosis, whose etiology is broad (varicella-zoster, herpes simplex, cytomegalovirus, or Epstein-Bar virus) and whose treatment is based on the acyclovir (very effective), ganciclovir or foscarnet administration [159].

Similarly, parenteral administration formulations have also been developed for the same purpose, including different intramuscular and intravenous preparations. These encompass: Parenteral antibodies for the uveitis treatment [3] and hydroxocobalamin intramuscular injections (B12 vitamin, Alpha Redisol) for the treatment of B12 vitamin deficiency states, as well as certain antibiotics (e.g., penicillin, gentamicin, ceftazidime, or amikacin) used in the subsequent ocular infections treatment (uveitis, scleritis, and/or pseudoscleritis) (see Table 5).

Likewise, the antibiotic combinations administration by continuous perfusion for the serious-eye-diseases treatment, such as endophthalmitis, is quite frequent [127,160]. As an example, ceftazidime is the best studied cephalosporine due to its activity spectrum against Gram-negative bacilli (including *Pseudomonas aeruginosa*). It is more frequently used as a first election treatment in this pathology, in monotherapy or combined with other antibiotics, since it allows reaching ocular concentrations in the order of 35.4 mg/l after intravenous administration of a 100 mg/kg antibiotic dose [161].

Table 5. Summary of systemically administered drugs for the treatment of posterior segment ocular diseases.

Pharmacologic Group	Drug	Pathology	Target	Route	Reference
Antibodies	Secukinumab Tocilizumab Ustekinumab Abatacept Rituximab	Uveitis	Inflammatory cytokines T-cell activation B-cell targeting	Intravenous Subcutaneous Subcutaneous	[162,163]
Vitamins	B12	Vitamin B12 Deficiency Optic Neuropathy	Folate receptor	Intramuscular	[164]
Antibiotics	Penicillin Gentamicin Ceftazidime Amikacin	Uveitis Scleritis Pseudoscleritis Endophtalmitis	Bacteria	Intravenous	[165–167]

In addition to these, different intravenous drug delivery strategies have been tested for drug arrival to the posterior segment of the eye [168]. Specifically, photodynamic therapy with verteporfin has been practiced, being a choroidal neovascularization effective treatment by stopping the neovascular membrane growth. Apart from this, ocular posterior segment diagnostic intravenous techniques have also been developed, being the most prominent the fluorescein digital angiography, an exploratory technique for the retinal vasculature visualization by means of the sodium fluorescein injection (vegetable origin orange dye).

In order to point out, eyes can be also exposed to systemic drugs (as a kind of side effects) and xenobiotics not intended for ophthalmic treatment, such as bisphosphonates (whose action mechanism is based on the bone-resorption inhibition, being used in the osteoporosis prevention and treatment), which can cause ocular inflammatory reactions (uveitis, neuritis, iritis, scleritis, or pseudoscleritis) [169]. Reformulation studies have also been carried out on these drugs in order to reduce their passage from the blood to the eye, making them more selective in order to decrease associated ocular side effects [169].

2.4. Periocular Administration

The periocular route has been considered as a promising drug administration route for the posterior ocular segment diseases treatment due to the high concentrations obtained with this kind of formulations' inoculation. This route allows the drug deposition on the scleral external surface and includes the following administration routes: subconjunctival, subTenon´s, retrobulbar, peribulbar and posterior juxtascleral. These pathways differ from one another in the location and/or injection direction in the proximity of the sclera.

2.4.1. Advantages and Limitations

Periocular injections are associated with greater adherence to treatment by patients compared to intravitreal injections [139] since it is considered a less invasive administration route and capable of providing a relatively great drug bioavailability in the posterior ocular segment [150,170].

The sclera provides a relatively large area for the drug absorption (approximately 17 cm^2) [171] compared to other ocular surfaces, like the cornea. Moreover, periocular administration takes advantage of the high scleral permeability. These two factors contribute to the potential effectiveness of the periocular administration compared to other ocular routes.

On the other hand, the main drawback is that the drug needs to diffuse from the site injection to the target site, with the possibility of drug losses.

2.4.2. Pharmacokinetics

In general, although this type of administration avoids the corneal-conjunctive barrier, the drug must cross several barriers to reach the target sites in the choroid, the RPE, or the neural retina [65,150]. To do this, it must overcome several dynamic, static, and metabolic barriers that limit drug access to the posterior segment of the eye. Two different types of barriers should be mentioned: (1) Physical barriers, which include sclera, choroid (its high blood flow can remove a significant fraction of drug before it can reach neural retina), and RPE, and (2) physiological barriers, as occurs with conjunctival, episcleral, and choroidal lymphatic flow [150], whose drug elimination ability is relatively fast [3,65,103]. In any case, episcleral blood and lymphatic flows are seen as the main limiting factors in drug periocular distribution, while anatomical barriers and choroidal blood flow are less important [116,150,170].

As a result, drug is removed into the systemic circulation, decreasing ocular bioavailability thereof. However, molecules that escape from the conjunctival vasculature can penetrate through the sclera and choroid to reach the neural retina and photoreceptor cells. In addition, permeability through sclera is lipophilicity-independent (e.g., inulin, methazolamide, pilocarpine, hydrocortisone) [172], unlike corneal and conjunctival layers, being dependent on molecular radio [4,42,137,148].

Drug reflux after periocular administration is the initial loss factor and contributes to its low bioavailability in the posterior segment of the eye [116,173]. It was demonstrated that the use of an adequate injection technique, volume and/or formulation type can improve drug bioavailability and ocular penetration [116,173–175].

Absorption

Drugs administered by periocular injections can reach its target site in the posterior segment of the eye through three different routes: Transscleral or direct penetration route, systemic circulation route, and anterior route [6,176]. In the anterior route, the drug diffuses directly through the sclera and the ciliary body, or indirectly through the lacrimal fluid and the cornea because of the conjunctival circulation reflux. In the systemic circulation route, the drug goes to systemic circulation through conjunctival, episcleral and/or choroidal vessels, where it is diluted, and then it returns to the eye by the blood flow. In the direct penetration route, drug reaches the vitreous humor through the underlying tissues; it represents the most important absorption route in terms of drug penetration and distribution to the posterior chamber of the eye.

In any case, it should be taken into consideration that the scleral permeability depends on the molecular radio, scleral hydration, and intraocular pressure [176,177] instead of molecular lipophilia [17]. Although the latter improves permeability through the RPE, it also increases drug loss from the choroidal and subconjunctival space to the bloodstream [3]. Regardless of the absorption route, only a small portion of the drug reaches the posterior segment of the eye [116,178] mainly due to the drug loss through periocular space, BRB, choroidal circulation, efflux transporters, and drug binding to ocular tissue proteins [116].

Elimination

Once the drug reached its target site, small molecules are rapidly removed from the administration site, presumably through conjunctival and episcleral blood and lymphatic flow [103,139,150], whereas larger molecules have much slower elimination kinetics, around 10 times lower [150], so that their residence time is much greater.

2.4.3. Subconjunctival Route

Subconjunctival injection has been used to administer drugs in the anterior segment of the eye, achieving higher concentrations in the anterior chamber compared to the topical administration. However, this route has also been investigated as an alternative pathway to intravitreal injection for the drug administration of retinal diseases treatment [6] due to the fact that it is considered a less invasive technique, comparing it with the intravitreal administration route [116,179]. It also minimizes the side effects, mainly endophthalmitis, cataracts, and retinal damage [116].

The drug is injected under the conjunctival membrane that covers the sclera, avoiding the conjunctival epithelial barrier. In this way, direct access to the transscleral route is achieved [116], increasing its bioavailability in aqueous humor in comparison with the topical route, which presents the corneal barrier as an impediment.

Advantages and Limitations

Subconjunctival administration shows two effective types of sustained drug delivery to the retina, both the topical and intravitreal administration. Moreover, it is an alternative route in order to allow easy and better accessibility and reduce the side effects caused by the intravitreal injection procedure (e.g., intraocular pressure and cataracts) [3].

The injection volume with the same drug concentration could be higher in this route in comparison with the intravitreal injection [3], enabling a wide dose range. In addition, the enzyme absence in the injection area is an important advantage due to the low enzymatic drug degradation.

The availability of pharmacokinetic and pharmacodynamic data about this route is limited. However, the drug delivery to the back of the eye through this route is better compared with topical and systemic administration routes [150].

This pathway also has some limitations regarding the concentration that can cross to the retina. The elimination via systemic circulation and to the tear cause a reduced bioavailability. Nevertheless, the permeability is modified by the age, according to the patient get older, the permeation through the sclera is less prevented so the amount of drug that can reach the retina is higher.

Pharmacokinetics

The permeation speed through the sclera is drug size-dependent [17], where the small molecules movement is constant. Macromolecules permeation is slower [3,150,172,180], although up to 70 kDa size molecules can easily penetrate the sclera [17,33,116,181–183]. Once the sclera is crossed, a rapid elimination caused by the choroidal blood flow takes place due to its large choriocapillaris fenestrations. Molecules that pass through this barrier faster and better are the small lipophilic ones compared to macromolecules [3,33,172,184]. However, small molecules are also quickly removed.

Likewise, lymphatic flow plays an important role in the drug elimination since conjunctival lymphatic vessels represent 50% of the surface [185]. Once drug crosses the sclera, it must break through the choroid and the RPE to reach the vitreous humor. For all these reasons, between 80–95% of small molecules drain into the systemic circulation [150]. Approximately, 10% of the drug is available for the anterior segment of the eye and only about 0.1% reaches the retina [3]. Thus, high initial drug concentrations are needed in order to achieve effective levels in the posterior segment due to the deficient bioavailability observed.

The injection volume is an important factor in the subconjunctivally administered drug pharmacokinetics as the drug reflux from the injection site is the initial loss factor that contributes to its low bioavailability [116,173]. Adequate volumes should be used in order to achieve high drug levels in the back of the eye. If large volumes are administered (over 200 μL), the reflux of drug solution out of the injection site increases and a greater drug permeation to the aqueous humor is obtained.

Drug Delivery Systems

Different techniques have been developed in order to increase the subconjunctival administered drug penetration through the sclera. One of these is the transscleral iontophoresis, an electrodynamic technique that may improve the periocular injections efficacy in some ophthalmic drugs (see Table 6), such as corticosteroids, antibiotics, NSAIDs, and immunosuppressants [186,187].

Nano- and microparticles are interesting sustained drug delivery systems for treating posterior segment diseases. These types of systems were tested, obtaining promising results for the VEGF inhibition with corticosteroids (budesonide and dexamethasone) and selective COX2 inhibitors (celecoxib) [188–192].

Table 6. Summary of subconjunctival administered drugs for the treatment of posterior segment ocular diseases.

Pharmacologic Group	Drug	Pathology	Reference
Antidiabetics	Insulin	Diabetic retinopathy	[193]
Chemotherapeutics	Carboplatin	Retinoblastoma	[194]
	Topotecan		
Folic acid analogues	Methotrexate	Granulomatous panuveitis	[195]
Corticosteroids	Dexamethasone	Uveitis	[196]

Thermo-responsive hydrogels are also systems that can be used to facilitate a sustained drug delivery. This pharmaceutical form turns into a gel when contacting with the injection area due to a temperature difference. These systems are employed as an alternative to the classic intravitreal route mainly because of its minimally invasive procedure. Subconjunctival placement of insulin-impregnated hydrogels has presented advantages over topical and intravitreal injection in DR treatment [197,198].

2.4.4. SubTenon's Route

SubTenon's route is one of the most promising routes to reach the eye posterior segment due to the possibility of obtaining better pharmacokinetic profiles of the administered drugs [116,130,199]. SubTenon's injection is placed in an avascular area between Tenon´s capsule and sclera, around the upper portion of the eye and into the belly of the superior rectus muscle [179,200]. It is divided into anterior and posterior segments at the insertions of extraocular muscles and their associated fasciae [179,201].

Advantages and Limitations

As a general idea, subconjunctival injections show a better drug efficacy in the anterior segment, while subTenon's injections lead to an increased penetration to the posterior segment of the eye [202,203].

Drug passage to systemic circulation is reduced and the contact time with the sclera is prolonged as a consequence of the pharmaceutical form injection. Nevertheless, drug elimination caused by the choroidal circulation can produce a shortened duration of action [130].

Besides that, it should bear in mind that Tenon´s capsule degeneration is age-related, which leads to an easier drug diffusion towards the retrobulbar cone. As a result, better drug levels are achieved in the posterior segment of the eye [130].

Pharmacokinetics

A 2.5 cm long blunt-tipped cannula needle is usually employed in the injection procedure into the Tenon´s capsule after a surgical incision. This is a widely used technique for local anesthesia during ocular surgery because the cannula approach avoids sharp-needle complications [103,179]. The formulation volume is up to 4 mL and is injected around the muscle belly, behind the equator [179]. The possibility to inject a large volume into the subTenon's space causes a lower and slower clearance and a more readily transscleral drug delivery [199].

Some of the most employed applications by using subTenon's administration route are: corticosteroid injections (triamcinolone acetonide (TA)) for chronic posterior uveitis [204] and cystoid macular edema treatment (see Table 7) [205].

Comparing the intravitreal effects versus subTenon's TA administration for diabetic macular edema (DMA), results showed that intravitreal TA injection had greater clinical effects than the subTenon's injection [206,207]. Nevertheless, a lower incidence of serious complications has been shown with subTenon's injections than the intravitreal ones [206,208].

Table 7. Vitreous pharmacokinetic parameters for long-acting triamcinolone acetonide subTenon's injection.

Pharmacologic Group	Drug	Half-Life Time (days)	MRT (days)	C_{max} (ng/mL)	T_{max} (h)	Reference
Corticosteroids	Triamcinolone acetonide	17.1	23.1	22	24	[209]

2.4.5. Retrobulbar Route

Retrobulbar administration arises as an alternative route to the drug targeting the posterior ocular pathologies treatment where the optic nerve or retrobulbar spaces are involved. Injection procedure is based on drug inoculation into the space between the orbital rim and the balloon edge [176], the retrobulbar space, which lies inside the extraocular muscle cone, behind the globe, being a deeper injection and uses less volume (comparing it with the peribulbar one). The usual procedure for the retrobulbar injection implies a 3 mm insertion beyond the posterior surface of the eyeball and the maximum volumes of injections are 3–4 mL.

Advantages and Limitations

Complications associated with retrobulbar injections, although potentially severe, are uncommon. Possible complications of retrobulbar injection include retrobulbar hemorrhage, globe perforation, optic nerve damage, respiratory arrest, optic atrophy, retinal vascular occlusion, and extraocular muscle myopathy [210]. This route has serious risks of causing ocular damage due to the proximity of the optic, motor and sensory nerves [151].

As retrobulbar injections are performed outside the ocular globe, there is little or no influence on intraocular pressure, in contrast to the intravitreal injections [179]. Compared to peribulbar injections, retrobulbar administration is a deeper injection and uses less volume.

Moreover, an injection up to 5 mL may be made, which is a considerably higher volume compared to the other types of administration to treat the ocular posterior segment diseases. This means that higher amounts of drug can be administered.

Retrobulbar administration is mainly used for corticosteroids administration as an alternative treatment to reduce the posterior segment inflammation. It is also used for local anesthesia injection in certain intraocular surgeries, where drugs are directly administered into the muscular cone, an area located among four eye muscles in the back of the globe.

2.4.6. Peribulbar Route

Peribulbar administration enables drug injection into the muscular extraconal compartment of the eye, also called peribulbar space, which is externally localized to the rectus muscles.

Advantages and Limitations

It is frequently preferred for its ocular complications' low rate, theoretical safety and ease of application comparing it with the retrobulbar route. Although both routes showed to be useful in anesthesia or akinesia, their use is limited due to the procedure associated complications (e.g., eyeball perforation, oculomotor reflex stimulation, optic nerve trauma, and orbital hemorrhage) [160]. Moreover, the peribulbar administration is less effective for anesthetizing the eye than the retrobulbar route, although a higher volume, up to 8–10 mL, may be injected [181]. However, this technique is slower and less efficient than retrobulbar injection, besides the fact that it requires multiple injections and larger volume of the injected formulation. It also carries a higher risk of potential chemosis and an intraocular pressure increase [211].

Currently, the peribulbar approach is a widely used method for the local anesthesia administration. The injection procedure has been briefly described for the administration of lidocaine and bupivacaine mixture as a local anesthesia pre-treatment in modern intraocular surgery [160]. A mixture of peribulbar bupivacaine combined with TA and cefazolin was also studied as a prophylactic treatment to reduce pain and possible inflammation and/or infection associated with vitreoretinal surgery [212].

2.4.7. Posterior Juxtascleral Route

The posterior juxtascleral injection, recently developed by Alcon Laboratories®, is an alternative administration route based on the therapeutic agent deposition directly in the closest area to the macula, without puncturing the eyeball [116]. It allows achieving higher drug concentrations in the target site due to the fact that the scleral thickness decreases near the equatorial region, an aspect that promotes a greater drug penetration towards the posterior segment of the eye [3,65].

This novel technique requires inserting a blunt-curved cannula after a conjunctival incision. The curved cannula follows the scleral surface without puncturing the ocular globe and drug is injected into the juxtascleral space overlying the macula. Besides, no clinically significant safety and efficacy issues related to this administration pathway were reported [213].

In addition, this route reaches a drug therapeutic dose for up to 6 months in the macular region [174], avoiding the risk of intraocular damage and reducing side effects, such as endophthalmitis, retinal detachment and glaucoma, among others [116,174]. Besides, drug reflux, which occurs when the drug flows back out of the incision made at the insertion site, may affect drug efficacy, although Alcon Laboratories® have developed a counter pressure device to deal with this side effect. There is an increased risk of systemic drug exposure due to the drug contact with the orbital tissue when compared with intravitreal injections, though there is much less systemic exposure than occurs with either topical or systemic therapy.

Currently, there are few commercial formulations which are administrated by using this administration route, such as anecortave acetate (Retaane®) [214], a cortisol synthetic analogue used for AMD treatment and prevention, or TA for DMA treatment unresponsive to laser photocoagulation [213].

2.4.8. Suprachoroidal Route

Suprachoroidal injection was introduced as a potential drug administration route to the posterior segment of the eye although it is not clinically used at present [150]. Drug is injected into the suprachoroidal space below the sclera inner surface using microneedles (micron-dimensions needles that can infuse fluid into tissue with excellent spatial targeting), up to 50 μL maximum volume. Formulation is distributed throughout the suprachoroidal space as a consequence of the pressure exerted by the injection process itself [215].

The suprachoroidal space circumferentially goes around the eye and is located between the sclera and choroid, leading to reach the macular area [216,217]. This administration route was tested for drug delivery into the posterior segment of the eye employing surgical procedures (by introducing catheters into this space) and gave rise to a long-term therapy, where drugs could be targeted towards the choroid and retina by direct contact with the administration site [218,219].

Advantages and Limitations

Suprachoroidal delivery route theoretically presents several key advantages compared to the standard intravitreal injections [220], such as that this space does not interfere with the optical pathways and it is a good pathway to target diseases at the outer retina, photoreceptors, RPE and choroid. Moreover, its diffusional pathways and pharmacokinetics are completely different from the intravitreal one, being a possible resourceful way to target drugs to the posterior segment of the eye. In comparison to other periocular administration routes, drug diffusion from the suprachoroidal space avoids several ocular barriers (e.g., cornea, conjunctiva and sclera). Additionally, the suprachoroidal space could act as a potential reservoir inside the eye and sustained release formulations or devices could optimize diffusional kinetics from this space. Finally, this space provides a safer way with larger biologic and/or immunogenic agents [220]. There are also disadvantages involved, such as suprachoroidal hemorrhage and choroidal detachment [221].

However, the access to the suprachoroidal space is complicated and the methods used were usually invasive and too complex to be performed as a simple office procedure [218,219]. Pre- and post-injection histology demonstrated that the potential space of the suprachoroidal region returns to a normal configuration after a brief time period [220]. Also, using die-casting methods, the suprachoroidal space is rather extensive and has the capacity to expand and accommodate a relatively large volume of material [220]. Delivery device parameters' optimization showed that microneedle length, pressure and particle size played an important role in determining a successful delivery into the suprachoroidal space. 800–1000 μm needle lengths, and 250–300 kPa applied pressures provided the most reliable delivery [215]. The usual injection volume for the suprachoroidal administration has been determined to be 25 μL [220].

Pharmacokinetics

Suprachoroidal administration leads to greater vitreous bioavailability for small lipophilic (1.5%) and hydrophilic (0.19%) molecules, while macromolecules (4.2%) show a 6–23 times improvement in terms of ocular bioavailability compared to the drug administration by subconjunctival route [150].

Compared with small molecules, macromolecules have a much longer half-life time in ocular tissues where steady state is slowly reached. Drug levels in the vitreous humor are generally reached 15 h for small lipophilic drugs, 70 h later for small hydrophilic drugs and 500 h later for larger molecules. Therefore, it was seen steady-state drug levels are quickly reached for small molecules, becoming 100–1000 times slower for macromolecules [150].

Several studies showed a significant fraction of the drug administered by the suprachoroidal route was removed through conjunctival and regional lymphatic nodes, including those of high molecular weight [6,175]. In addition, it should be taken into account that choroidal blood flow also removes a huge part of the inoculated drug (96–99%) in the case of low molecular weight compounds, whereas high molecular weight drugs will be removed from the tissue almost equally through the choriocapillaris (54%) and the subconjunctival space (41%) [150].

Drug Delivery Systems

Currently, there are no pharmaceutical forms commercialized to be administered by suprachoroidal injections. Nevertheless, this type of administration was widely studied by using fluorescein and fluorescently tagged dextrans (40 and 250 kDa), bevacizumab and polymeric particles (20 nm to 10 μm in diameter). Sulforhodamine B microneedle injection was also studied as well as nanoparticle and microparticle suspensions into the suprachoroidal space [215,222]. TA formulations were also researched as a way of DMA alternative treatment, as well as ranibizumab and bevacizumab injections, although recent studies showed these large biologic proteins are quickly removed from the suprachoroidal space [220].

2.4.9. Subretinal Route

Drug subretinal route has emerged as an alternative administration route to intravitreal administration due to its side effects and lower adherence to treatment by patients derived from the latter [223,224]. Thus, subretinal administration involves drug inoculation into the subretinal space [224], an ocular space located between RPE cells and photoreceptors [224,225].

Advantages and Limitations

Subretinal injection is an especially useful route for the posterior ocular pathologies treatment by providing a direct route with a very precise location through a minimally invasive injection. A typical volume of around 150 μL is injected, leading to a transient detachment between these two layers [2]. A lower drug dose is needed to accurately reach subretinal-space cells.

Compared to intravitreal administration, subretinal injection has a direct effect on subretinal space cells. Unlike vitreous cavity, subretinal space is an isolated closed anatomical area, which also has a greater immunological defense mechanism providing a safer route of administration in case of entry of bacteria [178,224].

Basically, three subretinal injection techniques have been studied, these being: (1) A transcorneal route through the pupil, surrounding the lens, and passing the vitreous humor and the retina [226], (2) a transscleral route through pars plana or limbus, crossing the vitreous humor and the opposite side of the retina into the subretinal space [227], and (3) a transscleral route through the choroid and Bruch's membrane without penetrating the retina [224]. All routes were equally effective regardless of the chosen one. The administration procedure is performed under direct visualization by using a surgical microscope and where blister formation should be observed as a sign of the procedure success.

Drug Delivery Systems

Subretinal administration has been considered as one of the best strategies for gene therapy using viral vectors, a carried-out treatment effectively achieved for pigmentary retinitis (PR) and Leber's congenital amaurosis (LCA) [225,227]. Gene expression is however limited to the injection site, suggesting that the primary barrier for efficient therapy following subretinal injection is the retina itself [2]. In addition, it was reported macrophages subretinal injection leads to pathological fibrosis, which could be used for the advanced AMD evaluation [224]. Subretinal delivery can also be used for stem cell transplantation in ocular degenerative diseases, which was reported in vivo studies and aimed at clinical applications [224].

3. Conclusions

The eye is one of the most inaccessible organs in terms of obtaining therapeutic drug concentrations, especially in the treatment of posterior segment ocular pathologies. Conventional administration pathways, such as topical or systemic routes, usually show important limitations, either by low ocular penetration or by the appearance of side effects linked to the posology, among others.

New drug delivery systems (DDS) are needed to prolong the administration intervals for posterior segment ocular pathologies, even though the development of novel DDS is particularly complicated due to several aspects must be considered, such as pharmacokinetics, immunogenicity, biodegradation, tolerability and toxicity, among others. Apart from these, different technological requirements must be taken into account, including reproducible manufacturing, clinical performance and sterility.

In the last few decades, an exponential increase in the design and development of novel DDS intended for the treatment of posterior segment ocular pathologies was observed. Biodegradable and non-biodegradable implants, microparticles, nanoparticles, microneedles, and microelectromechanical systems are the most innovative ones. Unfortunately, knowledge about drug targeting to the posterior segment of the eye is still sparse and, thus, there is not many DDS in clinical trials. Even so, memantine ophthalmic formulations as neuroprotective are in III phase studies at the moment, inter alia.

Likewise, huge advances were made in terms of research and development of new alternative administration routes to the posterior segment of the eye, including intravitreal and periocular pathways as the most relevant ones, as well as their subtypes. All of them, including a conventional administration routes (topical and systemic) show a series of specific pharmacokinetic characteristics, making them useful for the treatment of certain posterior segment ocular pathologies. However, these pathways have shown several advantages and limitations, where the election of one or another is dependent on, not just the pathology itself, but the pharmaceutical form, the drug used and the patient´s adherence to treatment, among others.

Author Contributions: R.V.-F., V.D.-T., A.L.-R., A.C.-P., and X.G.-O. contribute equally to the elaboration of the article and realized formal analysis and writing—original draft preparation. A.L.-Á., writing—review and editing. A.F.-F. and F.J.O.-E., conceptualization, funding acquisition, supervised the project, and writing—review and editing. All authors have read and agreed to the published version of the manuscript.

Funding: This work was partially supported by the Spanish Ministry of Science, Innovation and Universities (RTI2018-099597-B-100), the ISCIII (PI17/00940, RETICS Oftared, RD16/0008/0003 and RD12/0034/0017) and by Xunta de Galicia grant number GRC2013/015 and GPC2017/015.

Acknowledgments: X.G.-O. and R.V.-F. acknowledge the financial support of the IDIS (Health Research Institute of Santiago de Compostela) (predoctoral research fellowships), A.L.-R. acknowledges the financial support of the Xunta de Galicia and the European Union (European Social Fund ESF) (predoctoral research fellowship). A.F.-F. acknowledges the support obtained from the Instituto de Salud Carlos III (ISCIII) through its research grants (JR18/00014).

Conflicts of Interest: The authors have declared no potential conflicts of interest, financial or otherwise.

References

1. WHO Team. *World Report on Vision*; WHO: Geneva, Switzerland, 2019; p. 180. ISBN 978-92-4-151657-0.
2. Peynshaert, K.; Devoldere, J.; De Smedt, S.C.; Remaut, K. In vitro and ex vivo models to study drug delivery barriers in the posterior segment of the eye. *Adv. Drug Deliv. Rev.* **2018**, *126*, 44–57. [CrossRef] [PubMed]
3. Del Amo, E.M.; Rimpelä, A.-K.; Heikkinen, E.; Kari, O.K.; Ramsay, E.; Lajunen, T.; Schmitt, M.; Pelkonen, L.; Bhattacharya, M.; Richardson, D.; et al. Pharmacokinetic aspects of retinal drug delivery. *Prog. Retin. Eye Res.* **2017**, *57*, 134–185. [CrossRef]
4. Hosoya, K.; Tachikawa, M. Inner Blood-Retinal Barrier Transporters: Role of Retinal Drug Delivery. *Pharm. Res.* **2009**, *26*, 2055–2065. [CrossRef] [PubMed]
5. Gaudana, R.; Ananthula, H.K.; Parenky, A.; Mitra, A.K. Ocular drug delivery. *AAPS J.* **2010**, *12*, 348–360. [CrossRef] [PubMed]
6. Ranta, V.-P.; Urtti, A. Transscleral drug delivery to the posterior eye: Prospects of pharmacokinetic modeling. *Adv. Drug Deliv. Rev.* **2006**, *58*, 1164–1181. [CrossRef] [PubMed]
7. Wilson, C.G.; Tan, L.E.; Mains, J. Principles of Retinal Drug Delivery from Within the Vitreous. In *Drug Product Development for the Back of the Eye*; Springer Science & Business Media: Berlin/Heidelberg, Germany, 2011; pp. 125–158. ISBN 978-1-4419-9920-7.
8. Cunha-Vaz, J.G. The blood–retinal barriers system. Basic concept sand clinical evaluation. *Exp. Eye Res.* **2004**, *78*, 715–721. [CrossRef]
9. Gunda, S.; Hariharan, S.; Mitra, A.K. Corneal absorption and anterior chamber pharmacokinetics of dipeptide monoester prodrugs of ganciclovir (GCV): In vivo comparative evaluation of these prodrugs with Val-GCV and GCV in rabbits. *J. Ocul. Pharmacol. Ther. Off. J. Assoc. Ocul. Pharmacol. Ther.* **2006**, *22*, 465–476. [CrossRef] [PubMed]
10. Zambito, Y.; Zaino, C.; Di Colo, G. Effects of N-trimethylchitosan on transcellular and paracellular transcorneal drug transport. *Eur. J. Pharm. Biopharm.* **2006**, *64*, 16–25. [CrossRef]
11. Dey, S.; Mitra, A.K. Transporters and receptors in ocular drug delivery: Opportunities and challenges. *Expert Opin. Drug Deliv.* **2005**, *2*, 201–204. [CrossRef]
12. Huang, D.; Chen, Y.-S.; Rupenthal, I.D. Overcoming ocular drug delivery barriers through the use of physical forces. *Adv. Drug Deliv. Rev.* **2018**, *126*, 96–112. [CrossRef]
13. Hussain, A.A.; Starita, C.; Hodgetts, A.; Marshall, J. Macromolecular diffusion characteristics of ageing human Bruch's membrane: Implications for age-related macular degeneration (AMD). *Exp. Eye Res.* **2010**, *90*, 703–710. [CrossRef] [PubMed]
14. Cruysberg, L.P.J.; Nuijts, R.M.M.A.; Geroski, D.H.; Koole, L.H.; Hendrikse, F.; Edelhauser, H.F. In vitro human scleral permeability of fluorescein, dexamethasone-fluorescein, methotrexate-fluorescein and rhodamine 6G and the use of a coated coil as a new drug delivery system. *J. Ocul. Pharmacol. Ther.* **2002**, *18*, 559–569. [CrossRef] [PubMed]

15. Watson, P.G.; Young, R.D. Scleral structure, organisation and disease: A review. *Exp. Eye Res.* **2004**, *78*, 609–623. [CrossRef]
16. Jaffe, G.J.; Ashton, P.; Andrew, P. *Intraocular Drug Delivery*, 1st ed.; CRC Press: Boca Raton, FL, USA, 2006; ISBN 978-0-8247-2860-1.
17. Ambati, J.; Canakis, C.S.; Miller, J.W.; Gragoudas, E.S.; Edwards, A.; Weissgold, D.J.; Kim, I.; Delori, F.C.; Adamis, A.P. Diffusion of high molecular weight compounds through sclera. Invest. *Ophthalmol. Vis. Sci.* **2000**, *41*, 1181–1185.
18. Cheruvu, N.P.S.; Kompella, U.B. Bovine and Porcine Transscleral Solute Transport: Influence of Lipophilicity and the Choroid–Bruch's Layer. *Invest. Ophthalmol. Vis. Sci.* **2006**, *47*, 4513–4522. [CrossRef]
19. Marsh, D.A. Selection of Drug Delivery Approaches for the Back of the Eye: Opportunities and Unmet Needs. In *Drug Product Development for the Back of the Eye*; Springer Science & Business Media: Berlin/Heidelberg, Germany, 2011; pp. 125–158. ISBN 978-1-4419-9920-7.
20. Ashton, P. Retinal Drug Delivery. In *Intraocular Drug Delivery*; Taylor & Francis Group: New York, NY, USA, 2006; pp. 1–25. ISBN 978-1-4200-1650-5.
21. Maroñas, O.; García-Quintanilla, L.; Luaces-Rodríguez, A.; Fernández-Ferreiro, A.; Latorre-Pellicer, A.; Abraldes, M.J.; Lamas, M.J.; Carracedo, Á. Anti-VEGF treatment and response in Age-related Macular Degeneration: Disease´s susceptibility, pharmacogenetics and pharmacokinetics. *Curr. Med. Chem.* **2019**. [CrossRef]
22. García-Quintanilla, L.; Luaces-Rodríguez, A.; Gil-Martínez, M.; Mondelo-García, C.; Maroñas, O.; Mangas-Sanjuan, V.; González-Barcia, M.; Zarra-Ferro, I.; Aguiar, P.; Otero-Espinar, F.J.; et al. Pharmacokinetics of Intravitreal Anti-VEGF Drugs in Age-Related Macular Degeneration. *Pharmaceutics* **2019**, *11*, 365. [CrossRef]
23. Macha, S.; Mitra, A.K. Ocular pharmacokinetics in rabbits using a novel dual probe microdialysis technique. *Exp. Eye Res.* **2001**, *72*, 289–299. [CrossRef]
24. Castro-Balado, A.; Mondelo-García, C.; González-Barcia, M.; Zarra-Ferro, I.; Otero-Espinar, F.J.; Ruibal-Morell, Á.; Aguiar-Fernández, P.; Fernández-Ferreiro, A. Ocular Biodistribution Studies using Molecular Imaging. *Pharmaceutics* **2019**, *11*, 237. [CrossRef]
25. Maurice, D.M. The Regurgitation of Large Vitreous Injections. *J. Ocul. Pharmacol. Ther.* **1997**, *13*, 461–463. [CrossRef]
26. Stay, M.S.; Xu, J.; Randolph, T.W.; Barocas, V.H. Computer simulation of convective and diffusive transport of controlled-release drugs in the vitreous humor. *Pharm. Res.* **2003**, *20*, 96–102. [CrossRef] [PubMed]
27. Xu, J.; Heys, J.J.; Barocas, V.H.; Randolph, T.W. Permeability and diffusion in vitreous humor: Implications for drug delivery. *Pharm. Res.* **2000**, *17*, 664–669. [CrossRef] [PubMed]
28. Park, J.; Bungay, P.M.; Lutz, R.J.; Augsburger, J.J.; Millard, R.W.; Sinha Roy, A.; Banerjee, R.K. Evaluation of coupled convective-diffusive transport of drugs administered by intravitreal injection and controlled release implant. *J. Control. Release* **2005**, *105*, 279–295. [CrossRef] [PubMed]
29. Krishnamoorthy, M.K.; Park, J.; Augsburger, J.J.; Banerjee, R.K. Effect of retinal permeability, diffusivity, and aqueous humor hydrodynamics on pharmacokinetics of drugs in the eye. *J. Ocul. Pharmacol. Ther.* **2008**, *24*, 255–267. [CrossRef]
30. Xu, Q.; Boylan, N.J.; Suk, J.S.; Wang, Y.-Y.; Nance, E.A.; Yang, J.-C.; McDonnell, P.J.; Cone, R.A.; Duh, E.J.; Hanes, J. Nanoparticle diffusion in, and microrheology of, the bovine vitreous ex vivo. *J. Control. Release* **2013**, *167*, 76–84. [CrossRef]
31. Cunha-Vaz, J.; Maurice, D. Fluorescein dynamics in the eye. *Doc. Ophthalmol.* **1969**, *26*, 61–72. [CrossRef]
32. Thornit, D.N.; Vinten, C.M.; Sander, B.; Lund-Andersen, H.; la Cour, M. Blood-retinal barrier glycerol permeability in diabetic macular edema and healthy eyes: Estimations from macular volume changes after peroral glycerol. *Invest. Ophthalmol. Vis. Sci.* **2010**, *51*, 2827–2834. [CrossRef]
33. Pitkänen, L.; Ranta, V.-P.; Moilanen, H.; Urtti, A. Permeability of Retinal Pigment Epithelium: Effects of Permeant Molecular Weight and Lipophilicity. *Investig. Opthalmology Vis. Sci.* **2005**, *46*, 641. [CrossRef]
34. Käsdorf, B.T.; Arends, F.; Lieleg, O. Diffusion Regulation in the Vitreous Humor. *Biophys. J.* **2015**, *109*, 2171–2181. [CrossRef]
35. Lee, B.; Litt, M.; Buchsbaum, G. Rheology of the vitreous body: Part 3. Concentration of electrolytes, collagen and hyaluronic acid. *Biorheology* **1994**, *31*, 339–351. [CrossRef]

36. Loukovaara, S.; Nurkkala, H.; Tamene, F.; Gucciardo, E.; Liu, X.; Repo, P.; Lehti, K.; Varjosalo, M. Quantitative Proteomics Analysis of Vitreous Humor from Diabetic Retinopathy Patients. *J. Proteome Res.* **2015**, *14*, 5131–5143. [CrossRef] [PubMed]
37. Angi, M.; Kalirai, H.; Coupland, S.E.; Damato, B.E.; Semeraro, F.; Romano, M.R. Proteomic Analyses of the Vitreous Humour. *Mediat. Inflamm.* **2012**, *2012*, e148039. [CrossRef] [PubMed]
38. Murthy, K.R.; Goel, R.; Subbannayya, Y.; Jacob, H.K.; Murthy, P.R.; Manda, S.S.; Patil, A.H.; Sharma, R.; Sahasrabuddhe, N.A.; Parashar, A.; et al. Proteomic analysis of human vitreous humor. *Clin. Proteom.* **2014**, *11*, 29. [CrossRef] [PubMed]
39. Chirila, T.V.; Hong, Y. Chapter C2 The Vitreous Humor. In *Handbook of Biomaterial Properties*; Springer Nature: Basel, Switzerland, 2016; pp. 125–134.
40. Maurice, D.M. Mishima Ocular Pharmacokinetics. In *Pharmacology of the Eye*; Springer Science & Business Media: Berlin/Heidelberg, Germany, 2012; pp. 19–116. ISBN 978-3-642-69222-2.
41. Del Amo, E.M.; Urtti, A. Rabbit as an animal model for intravitreal pharmacokinetics: Clinical predictability and quality of the published data. *Exp. Eye Res.* **2015**, *137*, 111–124. [CrossRef] [PubMed]
42. Maurice, D. Review: Practical issues in intravitreal drug delivery. *J. Ocul. Pharmacol. Ther.* **2001**, *17*, 393–401. [CrossRef] [PubMed]
43. Friedrich, S.; Cheng, Y.L.; Saville, B. Drug distribution in the vitreous humor of the human eye: The effects of intravitreal injection position and volume. *Curr. Eye Res.* **1997**, *16*, 663–669. [CrossRef]
44. Mandell, B.A.; Meredith, T.A.; Aguilar, E.; el-Massry, A.; Sawant, A.; Gardner, S. Effects of inflammation and surgery on amikacin levels in the vitreous cavity. *Am. J. Ophthalmol.* **1993**, *115*, 770–774. [CrossRef]
45. Doft, B.H.; Weiskopf, J.; Nilsson-Ehle, I.; Wingard, L.B. Amphotericin clearance in vitrectomized versus nonvitrectomized eyes. *Ophthalmology* **1985**, *92*, 1601–1605. [CrossRef]
46. Wingard, L.B.; Zuravleff, J.J.; Doft, B.H.; Berk, L.; Rinkoff, J. Intraocular distribution of intravitreally administered amphotericin B in normal and vitrectomized eyes. *Invest. Ophthalmol. Vis. Sci.* **1989**, *30*, 2184–2189.
47. Ficker, L.; Meredith, T.A.; Gardner, S.; Wilson, L.A. Cefazolin levels after intravitreal injection. Effects of inflammation and surgery. *Invest. Ophthalmol. Vis. Sci.* **1990**, *31*, 502–505.
48. Shaarawy, A.; Meredith, T.A.; Kincaid, M.; Dick, J.; Aguilar, E.; Ritchie, D.J.; Reichley, R.M. Intraocular injection of ceftazidime. Effects of inflammation and surgery. *Retina* **1995**, *15*, 433–438. [CrossRef] [PubMed]
49. Pearson, P.A.; Hainsworth, D.P.; Ashton, P. Clearance and distribution of ciprofloxacin after intravitreal injection. *Retina* **1993**, *13*, 326–330. [CrossRef] [PubMed]
50. Aguilar, H.E.; Meredith, T.A.; el-Massry, A.; Shaarawy, A.; Kincaid, M.; Dick, J.; Ritchie, D.J.; Reichley, R.M.; Neisman, M.K. Vancomycin levels after intravitreal injection. Effects of inflammation and surgery. *Retina* **1995**, *15*, 428–432. [CrossRef] [PubMed]
51. Christoforidis, J.B.; Williams, M.M.; Wang, J.; Jiang, A.; Pratt, C.; Abdel-Rasoul, M.; Hinkle, G.H.; Knopp, M.V. Anatomic and pharmacokinetic properties of intravitreal bevacizumab and ranibizumab after vitrectomy and lensectomy. *Retina* **2013**, *33*, 946–952. [CrossRef] [PubMed]
52. Kakinoki, M.; Sawada, O.; Sawada, T.; Saishin, Y.; Kawamura, H.; Ohji, M. Effect of vitrectomy on aqueous VEGF concentration and pharmacokinetics of bevacizumab in macaque monkeys. *Investig. Ophthalmol. Vis. Sci.* **2012**, *53*, 5877–5880. [CrossRef]
53. Niwa, Y.; Kakinoki, M.; Sawada, T.; Wang, X.; Ohji, M. Ranibizumab and Aflibercept: Intraocular Pharmacokinetics and Their Effects on Aqueous VEGF Level in Vitrectomized and Nonvitrectomized Macaque Eyes. *Investig. Ophthalmol. Vis. Sci.* **2015**, *56*, 6501–6505. [CrossRef]
54. Edington, M.; Connolly, J.; Chong, N.V. Pharmacokinetics of intravitreal anti-VEGF drugs in vitrectomized versus non-vitrectomized eyes. *Expert Opin. Drug Metab. Toxicol.* **2017**, *13*, 1217–1224. [CrossRef]
55. Peyman, G.A.; Vastine, D.W.; Raichand, M. Experimental Aspects and Their Clinical Application. *Ophthalmology* **1978**, *85*, 374–385. [CrossRef]
56. Campochiaro, P.A.; Lim, J.I. Aminoglycoside toxicity in the treatment of endophthalmitis. *Arch. Ophthalmol.* **1994**, *112*, 48–53. [CrossRef] [PubMed]
57. Da, M.; Li, K.K.W.; Chan, K.C.; Wu, E.X.; Wong, D.S.H. Distribution of Triamcinolone Acetonide after Intravitreal Injection into Silicone Oil-Filled Eye. *BioMed Res. Int.* **2016**, *2016*, 5485467. [CrossRef]

58. Spitzer, M.S.; Kaczmarek, R.T.; Yoeruek, E.; Petermeier, K.; Wong, D.; Heimann, H.; Jaissle, G.B.; Bartz-Schmidt, K.U.; Szurman, P. The distribution, release kinetics, and biocompatibility of triamcinolone injected and dispersed in silicone oil. *Investig. Ophthalmol. Vis. Sci.* **2009**, *50*, 2337–2343. [CrossRef]
59. Aras, C.; Ozdamar, A.; Karacorlu, M.; Ozkan, S. Silicone oil in the surgical treatment of endophthalmitis associated with retinal detachment. *Int. Ophthalmol.* **2001**, *24*, 147–150. [CrossRef]
60. Mannermaa, E.; Vellonen, K.-S.; Urtti, A. Drug transport in corneal epithelium and blood-retina barrier: Emerging role of transporters in ocular pharmacokinetics. *Adv. Drug Deliv. Rev.* **2006**, *58*, 1136–1163. [CrossRef] [PubMed]
61. Vellonen, K.-S.; Hellinen, L.; Mannermaa, E.; Ruponen, M.; Urtti, A.; Kidron, H. Expression, activity and pharmacokinetic impact of ocular transporters. *Adv. Drug Deliv. Rev.* **2018**, *126*, 3–22. [CrossRef] [PubMed]
62. Dias, C.S.; Anand, B.S.; Mitra, A.K. Effect of mono- and di-acylation on the ocular disposition of ganciclovir: Physicochemical properties, ocular bioreversion, and antiviral activity of short chain ester prodrugs. *J. Pharm. Sci.* **2002**, *91*, 660–668. [CrossRef] [PubMed]
63. Duvvuri, S.; Majumdar, S.; Mitra, A.K. Role of metabolism in ocular drug delivery. *Curr. Drug Metab.* **2004**, *5*, 507–515. [CrossRef] [PubMed]
64. Dias, C.S.; Mitra, A.K. Vitreal elimination kinetics of large molecular weight FITC-labeled dextrans in albino rabbits using a novel microsampling technique. *J. Pharm. Sci.* **2000**, *89*, 572–578. [CrossRef]
65. Durairaj, C. Ocular Pharmacokinetics. In *Pharmacologic Therapy of Ocular Disease*; Handbook of Experimental Pharmacology; Springer: Cham, Switzerland, 2016; pp. 31–55. ISBN 978-3-319-58288-7.
66. Kwak, H.W.; D'Amico, D.J. Evaluation of the retinal toxicity and pharmacokinetics of dexamethasone after intravitreal injection. *Arch. Ophthalmol.* **1992**, *110*, 259–266. [CrossRef]
67. Barza, M.; Lynch, E.; Baum, J.L. Pharmacokinetics of newer cephalosporins after subconjunctival and intravitreal injection in rabbits. *Arch. Ophthalmol.* **1993**, *111*, 121–125. [CrossRef]
68. Robertson, J.E.; Westra, I.; Woltering, E.A.; Winthrop, K.L.; Barrie, R.; O'Dorisio, T.M.; Holmes, D. Intravitreal injection of octreotide acetate. *J. Ocul. Pharmacol. Ther.* **1997**, *13*, 171–177. [CrossRef]
69. Leeds, J.M.; Henry, S.P.; Truong, L.; Zutshi, A.; Levin, A.A.; Kornbrust, D. Pharmacokinetics of a potential human cytomegalovirus therapeutic, a phosphorothioate oligonucleotide, after intravitreal injection in the rabbit. *Drug Metab. Dispos. Biol. Fate Chem.* **1997**, *25*, 921–926.
70. Durairaj, C.; Shah, J.C.; Senapati, S.; Kompella, U.B. Prediction of vitreal half-life based on drug physicochemical properties: Quantitative structure-pharmacokinetic relationships (QSPKR). *Pharm. Res.* **2009**, *26*, 1236–1260. [CrossRef] [PubMed]
71. Christoforidis, J.B.; Chang, S.; Jiang, A.; Wang, J.; Cebulla, C.M. Intravitreal devices for the treatment of vitreous inflammation. *Mediat. Inflamm.* **2012**, *2012*, 126463. [CrossRef] [PubMed]
72. Sides Media, www sidesmedia com Retina Today—Ocular Drug Delivery Systems for the Posterior Segment: A Review. Available online: http://retinatoday.com/2012/05/ocular-drug-delivery-systems-for-the-posterior-segment-a-review/ (accessed on 23 April 2019).
73. Shikari, H.; Samant, P.M. Intravitreal injections: A review of pharmacological agents and techniques. *J. Clin. Ophthalmol. Res.* **2016**, *4*, 51. [CrossRef]
74. Wang, J.; Jiang, A.; Joshi, M.; Christoforidis, J. Drug Delivery Implants in the Treatment of Vitreous Inflammation. *Mediators Inflamm.* **2013**, *2013*, 780634. [CrossRef]
75. Lee, S.S.; Hughes, P.; Ross, A.D.; Robinson, M.R. Biodegradable implants for sustained drug release in the eye. *Pharm. Res.* **2010**, *27*, 2043–2053. [CrossRef]
76. Smith, T.J.; Pearson, P.A.; Blandford, D.L.; Brown, J.D.; Goins, K.A.; Hollins, J.L.; Schmeisser, E.T.; Glavinos, P.; Baldwin, L.B.; Ashton, P. Intravitreal sustained-release ganciclovir. *Arch. Ophthalmol.* **1992**, *110*, 255–258. [CrossRef]
77. Abrishami, M.; Abrishami, M.; Mahmoudi, A.; Mosallaei, N.; Vakili Ahrari Roodi, M.; Malaekeh-Nikouei, B. Solid Lipid Nanoparticles Improve the Diclofenac Availability in Vitreous after Intraocular Injection. *J. Drug Deliv.* **2016**, *2016*, 1368481. [CrossRef]
78. Kambhampati, S.P.; Clunies-Ross, A.J.M.; Bhutto, I.; Mishra, M.K.; Edwards, M.; McLeod, D.S.; Kannan, R.M.; Lutty, G. Systemic and Intravitreal Delivery of Dendrimers to Activated Microglia/Macrophage in Ischemia/Reperfusion Mouse Retina. *Investig. Ophthalmol. Vis. Sci.* **2015**, *56*, 4413–4424. [CrossRef]

79. Pachis, K.; Blazaki, S.; Tzatzarakis, M.; Klepetsanis, P.; Naoumidi, E.; Tsilimbaris, M.; Antimisiaris, S.G. Sustained release of intravitreal flurbiprofen from a novel drug-in-liposome-in-hydrogel formulation. *Eur. J. Pharm. Sci.* **2017**, *109*, 324–333. [CrossRef]
80. Wang, C.; Seo, S.-J.; Kim, J.-S.; Lee, S.-H.; Jeon, J.-K.; Kim, J.-W.; Kim, K.-H.; Kim, J.-K.; Park, J. Intravitreal implantable magnetic micropump for on-demand VEGFR-targeted drug delivery. *J. Control. Release* **2018**, *283*, 105–112. [CrossRef] [PubMed]
81. Genentech: Press Releases. 2018. Available online: https://www.gene.com/media/press-releases/14739/2018-07-25/genentech-unveils-positive-phase-ii-resu (accessed on 22 April 2019).
82. Luaces-Rodríguez, A.; Mondelo-García, C.; Zarra-Ferro, I.; González-Barcia, M.; Aguiar, P.; Fernández-Ferreiro, A.; Otero-Espinar, F.J. Intravitreal anti-VEGF drug delivery systems for age-related macular degeneration. *Int. J. Pharm.* **2020**, *573*, 118767. [CrossRef] [PubMed]
83. Barañano, D.E.; Kim, S.J.; Edelhauser, H.F.; Durairaj, C.; Kompella, U.B.; Handa, J.T. Efficacy and pharmacokinetics of intravitreal non-steroidal anti-inflammatory drugs for intraocular inflammation. *Br. J. Ophthalmol.* **2009**, *93*, 1387–1390. [CrossRef] [PubMed]
84. Von Sallmann, L.; Meyer, K.; Grandi, J.D. Experimental study on penicillin treatment of ectogenous infection of vitreous. *Arch. Ophthalmol.* **1944**, *32*, 179–189. [CrossRef]
85. Radhika, M.; Mithal, K.; Bawdekar, A.; Dave, V.; Jindal, A.; Relhan, N.; Albini, T.; Pathengay, A.; Flynn, H.W. Pharmacokinetics of intravitreal antibiotics in endophthalmitis. *J. Ophthalmic Inflamm. Infect.* **2014**, *4*, 22. [CrossRef]
86. Barza, M.; Kane, A.; Baum, J. Pharmacokinetics of intravitreal carbenicillin, cefazolin, and gentamicin in rhesus monkeys. *Investig. Ophthalmol. Vis. Sci.* **1983**, *24*, 1602–1606.
87. Doft, B.H.; Barza, M. Ceftazidime or Amikacin: Choice of Intravitreal Antimicrobials in the Treatment of Postoperative Endophthalmitis. *Arch. Ophthalmol.* **1994**, *112*, 17–18.
88. Aydin, E.; Kazi, A.A.; Peyman, G.A.; Esfahani, M.R.; Muñoz-Morales, A.; Kivilcim, M.; Caro-Magdaleno, M. Retinal toxicity of intravitreal doxycycline. A pilot study. *Arch. Soc. Espanola Oftalmol.* **2007**, *82*, 223–228.
89. Iyer, M.N.; He, F.; Wensel, T.G.; Mieler, W.F.; Benz, M.S.; Holz, E.R. Intravitreal clearance of moxifloxacin. *Trans. Am. Ophthalmol. Soc.* **2005**, *103*, 76–83. [CrossRef]
90. Oztürk, F.; Kortunay, S.; Kurt, E.; Ilker, S.S.; Basci, N.E.; Bozkurt, A. Penetration of topical and oral ciprofloxacin into the aqueous and vitreous humor in inflamed eyes. *Retina* **1999**, *19*, 218–222. [CrossRef]
91. Barza, M.; McCue, M. Pharmacokinetics of aztreonam in rabbit eyes. *Antimicrob. Agents Chemother.* **1983**, *24*, 468–473. [CrossRef] [PubMed]
92. Ay, G.M.; Akhan, S.C.; Erturk, S.; Aktas, E.S.; Ozkara, S.K.; Caglar, Y. Comparison of Intravitreal Ceftazidime and Meropenem in Treatment of Experimental Pseudomonal Posttraumatic Endophthalmitis in a Rabbit Model. *J. Appl. Res.* **2004**, *4*, 10.
93. Loewenstein, A.; Zemel, E.; Lazar, M.; Perlman, I. Drug-induced retinal toxicity in albino rabbits: The effects of imipenem and aztreonam. *Investig. Ophthalmol. Vis. Sci.* **1993**, *34*, 3466–3476. [PubMed]
94. Conway, B.P.; Campochiaro, P.A. Macular Infarction After Endophthalmitis Treated With Vitrectomy and Intravitreal Gentamicin. *Arch. Ophthalmol.* **1986**, *104*, 367–371. [CrossRef]
95. Zachary, I.G.; Forster, R.K. Experimental Intravitreal Gentamicin. *Am. J. Ophthalmol.* **1976**, *82*, 604–611. [CrossRef]
96. Bakri, S.J.; Snyder, M.R.; Reid, J.M.; Pulido, J.S.; Singh, R.J. Pharmacokinetics of Intravitreal Bevacizumab (Avastin). *Ophthalmology* **2007**, *114*, 855–859. [CrossRef]
97. Bakri, S.J.; Snyder, M.R.; Reid, J.M.; Pulido, J.S.; Ezzat, M.K.; Singh, R.J. Pharmacokinetics of Intravitreal Ranibizumab (Lucentis). *Ophthalmology* **2007**, *114*, 2179–2182. [CrossRef]
98. Drug Product Development for the Back of the Eye by Uday B. Kompella, Henry F. Edelhauser | 9781441999191 | Reviews, Description and More @ BetterWorldBooks.com. Available online: https://www.betterworldbooks.com/product/detail/drug-product-development-for-the-back-of-the-eye-1441999191 (accessed on 6 April 2018).
99. Schopf, L.R.; Popov, A.M.; Enlow, E.M.; Bourassa, J.L.; Ong, W.Z.; Nowak, P.; Chen, H. Topical Ocular Drug Delivery to the Back of the Eye by Mucus-Penetrating Particles. *Transl. Vis. Sci. Technol.* **2015**, *4*. [CrossRef]
100. Madni, A.; Rahem, M.A.; Tahir, N.; Sarfraz, M.; Jabar, A.; Rehman, M.; Kashif, P.M.; Badshah, S.F.; Khan, K.U.; Santos, H.A. Non-invasive strategies for targeting the posterior segment of eye. *Int. J. Pharm.* **2017**, *530*, 326–345. [CrossRef]

101. Ruponen, M.; Urtti, A. Undefined role of mucus as a barrier in ocular drug delivery. *Eur. J. Pharm. Biopharm.* **2015**, *96*, 442–446. [CrossRef]
102. Jünemann, A.G.M.; Choragiewicz, T.; Ozimek, M.; Grieb, P.; Rejdak, R. Drug bioavailability from topically applied ocular drops. Does drop size matter? *Ophthalmol. J.* **2016**, *1*, 29–35. [CrossRef]
103. Vadlapudi, A.D.; CholKAr, K.; Dasari, S.R.; Mitra, A.K. *Ocular Drug Delivery*; Jones Bartlett Learn: Burlington, MA, USA, 2015; pp. 219–263.
104. Watsky, M.A.; Jablonski, M.M.; Edelhauser, H.F. Comparison of conjunctival and corneal surface areas in rabbit and human. *Curr. Eye Res.* **1988**, *7*, 483–486. [CrossRef] [PubMed]
105. Coca-Prados, M. The blood-aqueous barrier in health and disease. *J. Glaucoma* **2014**, *23*, S36–S38. [CrossRef] [PubMed]
106. Barar, J.; Javadzadeh, A.R.; Omidi, Y. Ocular novel drug delivery: Impacts of membranes and barriers. *Expert Opin. Drug Deliv.* **2008**, *5*, 567–581. [CrossRef] [PubMed]
107. Kaur, I.P.; Kakkar, S. Nanotherapy for posterior eye diseases. *J. Control. Release* **2014**, *193*, 100–112. [CrossRef] [PubMed]
108. Boddu, S.H.S.; Gunda, S.; Earla, R.; Mitra, A.K. Ocular microdialysis: A continuous sampling technique to study pharmacokinetics and pharmacodynamics in the eye. *Bioanalysis* **2010**, *2*, 487–507. [CrossRef] [PubMed]
109. Bravo-Osuna, I.; Andrés-Guerrero, V.; Pastoriza Abal, P.; Molina-Martínez, I.T.; Herrero-Vanrell, R. Pharmaceutical microscale and nanoscale approaches for efficient treatment of ocular diseases. *Drug Deliv. Transl. Res.* **2016**, *6*, 686–707. [CrossRef]
110. Quantitative and Qualitative Prediction of Corneal Permeability for Drug-Like Compounds—ScienceDirect. Available online: https://www.sciencedirect.com/science/article/pii/S003991401100779X?via%3Dihub (accessed on 18 April 2018).
111. Shen, J.; Deng, Y.; Jin, X.; Ping, Q.; Su, Z.; Li, L. Thiolated nanostructured lipid carriers as a potential ocular drug delivery system for cyclosporine A: Improving in vivo ocular distribution. *Int. J. Pharm.* **2010**, *402*, 248–253. [CrossRef]
112. Sociedad Española de Oftalmología. Available online: http://www.oftalmo.com/seo/archivos/articulo.php?idSolicitud=905&numR=9&mesR=9&anioR=2001&idR=50 (accessed on 20 April 2018).
113. Ramsay, E.; Del Amo, E.M.; Toropainen, E.; Tengvall-Unadike, U.; Ranta, V.-P.; Urtti, A.; Ruponen, M. Corneal and conjunctival drug permeability: Systematic comparison and pharmacokinetic impact in the eye. *Eur. J. Pharm. Sci.* **2018**, *119*, 83–89. [CrossRef]
114. Stjernschantz, J.; Selén, G.; Astin, M.; Karlsson, M.; Resul, B. Effect of latanoprost on regional blood flow and capillary permeability in the monkey eye. *Arch. Ophthalmol.* **1999**, *117*, 1363–1367. [CrossRef]
115. Utility of Transporter/Receptor(s) in Drug Delivery to the Eye. Available online: https://www.researchgate.net/publication/236974311_Utility_of_transporterreceptors_in_drug_delivery_to_the_eye (accessed on 6 April 2018).
116. Thrimawithana, T.R.; Young, S.; Bunt, C.R.; Green, C.; Alany, R.G. Drug delivery to the posterior segment of the eye. *Drug Discov. Today* **2011**, *16*, 270–277. [CrossRef] [PubMed]
117. Kent, A.R.; Nussdorf, J.D.; David, R.; Tyson, F.; Small, D.; Fellows, D. Vitreous concentration of topically applied brimonidine tartrate 0.2%. *Ophthalmology* **2001**, *108*, 784–787. [CrossRef]
118. Balguri, S.P.; Adelli, G.R.; Majumdar, S. Topical ophthalmic lipid nanoparticle formulations (SLN, NLC) of indomethacin for delivery to the posterior segment ocular tissues. *Eur. J. Pharm. Biopharm.* **2016**, *109*, 224–235. [CrossRef] [PubMed]
119. Ying, L.; Tahara, K.; Takeuchi, H. Drug delivery to the ocular posterior segment using lipid emulsion via eye drop administration: Effect of emulsion formulations and surface modification. *Int. J. Pharm.* **2013**, *453*, 329–335. [CrossRef] [PubMed]
120. Gan, L.; Wang, J.; Jiang, M.; Bartlett, H.; Ouyang, D.; Eperjesi, F.; Liu, J.; Gan, Y. Recent advances in topical ophthalmic drug delivery with lipid-based nanocarriers. *Drug Discov. Today* **2013**, *18*, 290–297. [CrossRef] [PubMed]
121. Davis, B.M.; Normando, E.M.; Guo, L.; Turner, L.A.; Nizari, S.; O'Shea, P.; Moss, S.E.; Somavarapu, S.; Cordeiro, M.F. Topical delivery of Avastin to the posterior segment of the eye in vivo using annexin A5-associated liposomes. *Small Weinh. Bergstr. Ger.* **2014**, *10*, 1575–1584. [CrossRef]

122. Wang, Y.; Zheng, Y.; Zhang, L.; Wang, Q.; Zhang, D. Stability of nanosuspensions in drug delivery. *J. Control. Release* **2013**, *172*, 1126–1141. [CrossRef]
123. Koeberle, M.J.; Hughes, P.M.; Skellern, G.G.; Wilson, C.G. Pharmacokinetics and disposition of memantine in the arterially perfused bovine eye. *Pharm. Res.* **2006**, *23*, 2781–2798. [CrossRef]
124. Acheampong, A.A.; Shackleton, M.; John, B.; Burke, J.; Wheeler, L.; Tang-Liu, D. Distribution of brimonidine into anterior and posterior tissues of monkey, rabbit, and rat eyes. *Drug Metab. Dispos. Biol. Fate Chem.* **2002**, *30*, 421–429. [CrossRef]
125. Loftsson, T.; Hreinsdóttir, D.; Stefánsson, E. Cyclodextrin microparticles for drug delivery to the posterior segment of the eye: Aqueous dexamethasone eye drops. *J. Pharm. Pharmacol.* **2007**, *59*, 629–635. [CrossRef]
126. Sigurdsson, H.H.; Konráethsdóttir, F.; Loftsson, T.; Stefánsson, E. Topical and systemic absorption in delivery of dexamethasone to the anterior and posterior segments of the eye. *Acta Ophthalmol. Scand.* **2007**, *85*, 598–602. [CrossRef] [PubMed]
127. Díez, J.E.B.; Pujol, M.M. *Farmacología Ocular*; Univ. Politèc. de Catalunya: Catalunya, Spain, 2002; ISBN 978-84-8301-647-3.
128. Del Amo Páez, E.M. Ocular and Systemic Pharmacokinetic Models for Drug Discovery and Development. Ph.D. Dissertation, University of Helsinki, Helsinki, Finland, 2015.
129. Mitra, A.K.; Anand, B.S.; Duvvuri, S. Drug delivery to the eye. In *The Biology of the Eye*; Fischbarg, J., Ed.; Academic Press: New York, NY, USA, 2006; Volume 10, pp. 307–351.
130. Janoria, K.G.; Gunda, S.; Boddu, S.H.S.; Mitra, A.K. Novel approaches to retinal drug delivery. *Expert Opin. Drug Deliv.* **2007**, *4*, 371–388. [CrossRef] [PubMed]
131. Hughes, P.; Olejnik, O.; Changlin, J.; Wilson, C. Topical and systemic drug delivery to the posterior segments. *Adv. Drug Deliv. Rev.* **2005**, *57*, 2010–2032. [CrossRef] [PubMed]
132. Kwan, A.S.L.; Barry, C.; McAllister, I.L.; Constable, I. Fluorescein angiography and adverse drug reactions revisited: The Lions Eye experience. *Clin. Exp. Ophthalmol.* **2006**, *34*, 33–38. [CrossRef]
133. Vellonen, K.-S.; Soini, E.-M.; del Amo, E.M.; Urtti, A. Prediction of Ocular Drug Distribution from Systemic Blood Circulation. *Mol. Pharm.* **2016**, *13*, 2906–2911. [CrossRef]
134. Hosoya, K.; Tomi, M. Advances in the cell biology of transport via the inner blood-retinal barrier: Establishment of cell lines and transport functions. *Biol. Pharm. Bull.* **2005**, *28*, 1–8. [CrossRef]
135. Routes of Administration for Ocular Medications—Pharmacology. Available online: https://www.msdvetmanual.com/pharmacology/systemic-pharmacotherapeutics-of-the-eye/routes-of-administration-for-ocular-medications (accessed on 14 May 2018).
136. Gkretsi, V.; Zacharia, L.C.; Stylianopoulos, T. Targeting inflammation to improve tumor drug delivery. *Trends Cancer* **2017**, *3*, 621–630. [CrossRef]
137. Urtti, A. Challenges and obstacles of ocular pharmacokinetics and drug delivery. *Adv. Drug Deliv. Rev.* **2006**, *58*, 1131–1135. [CrossRef]
138. Toda, R.; Kawazu, K.; Oyabu, M.; Miyazaki, T.; Kiuchi, Y. Comparison of Drug Permeabilities across the Blood–Retinal Barrier, Blood–Aqueous Humor Barrier, and Blood–Brain Barrier. *J. Pharm. Sci.* **2011**, *100*, 3904–3911. [CrossRef]
139. Gaudana, R.; Jwala, J.; Boddu, S.H.S.; Mitra, A.K. Recent Perspectives in Ocular Drug Delivery. *Pharm. Res.* **2009**, *26*, 1197–1216. [CrossRef] [PubMed]
140. Jiye, Y.; Jianting, Z. Multidrug resistance-associated protein 1 (MRP1/ABCC1) polymorphism: From discovery to clinical application. *Zhong Nan Da Xue Xue Bao Yi Xue Ban* **2011**, *36*, 927–938.
141. ABCC1 Gene—GeneCards | MRP1 Protein | MRP1 Antibody. Available online: https://www.genecards.org/cgi-bin/carddisp.pl?gene=ABCC1 (accessed on 16 May 2018).
142. Pitkänen, L.; Ranta, V.-P.; Moilanen, H.; Urtti, A. Binding of Betaxolol, Metoprolol and Oligonucleotides to Synthetic and Bovine Ocular Melanin, and Prediction of Drug Binding to Melanin in Human Choroid-Retinal Pigment Epithelium. *Pharm. Res.* **2007**, *24*, 2063–2070. [CrossRef] [PubMed]
143. Demetriades, A.M.; Deering, T.; Liu, H.; Lu, L.; Gehlbach, P.; Packer, J.D.; Gabhann, F.M.; Popel, A.S.; Wei, L.L.; Campochiaro, P.A. Trans-scleral Delivery of Antiangiogenic Proteins. *J. Ocul. Pharmacol. Ther.* **2008**, *24*, 70–79. [CrossRef]
144. Menon, I.A.; Wakeham, D.C.; Persad, S.D.; Avaria, M.; Trope, G.E.; Basu, P.K. Quantitative determination of the melanin contents in ocular tissues from human blue and brown eyes. *J. Ocul. Pharmacol. Ther.* **1992**, *8*, 35–42. [CrossRef]

145. Schoenwald, R.D.; Tandon, V.; Wurster, D.E.; Barfknecht, C.F. Significance of melanin binding and metabolism in the activity of 5-acetoxyacetylimino-4-methyl-Δ2-1, 3, 4,-thiadiazoline-2-sulfonamide1. *Eur. J. Pharm. Biopharm.* **1998**, *46*, 39–50. [CrossRef]
146. Leblanc, B.; Jezequel, S.; Davies, T.; Hanton, G.; Taradach, C. Binding of drugs to eye melanin is not predictive of ocular toxicity. *Regul. Toxicol. Pharmacol.* **1998**, *28*, 124–132. [CrossRef]
147. Larsson, B.S. Interaction between chemicals and melanin. *Pigment Cell Res.* **1993**, *6*, 127–133. [CrossRef]
148. Bill, A.; Törnquist, P.; Alm, A. Permeability of the intraocular blood vessels. *Trans. Ophthalmol. Soc.* **1980**, *100*, 332–336.
149. Guymer, R.H.; Bird, A.C.; Hageman, G.S. Cytoarchitecture of Choroidal Capillary Endothelial Cells. *Investig. Opthalmol. Vis. Sci.* **2004**, *45*, 1660. [CrossRef]
150. Ranta, V.-P.; Mannermaa, E.; Lummepuro, K.; Subrizi, A.; Laukkanen, A.; Antopolsky, M.; Murtomäki, L.; Hornof, M.; Urtti, A. Barrier analysis of periocular drug delivery to the posterior segment. *J. Control. Release* **2010**, *148*, 42–48. [CrossRef] [PubMed]
151. Patel, A. Ocular drug delivery systems: An overview. *World J. Pharmacol.* **2013**, *2*, 47. [CrossRef] [PubMed]
152. Constable, P.A.; Lawrenson, J.G.; Dolman, D.E.M.; Arden, G.B.; Abbott, N.J. P-Glycoprotein expression in human retinal pigment epithelium cell lines. *Exp. Eye Res.* **2006**, *83*, 24–30. [CrossRef]
153. Eye Drugs—Prescribing and Administering. Patient. Available online: https://patient.info/doctor/eye-drugs-prescribing-and-administering (accessed on 14 May 2018).
154. Samtani, S.; Amaral, J.; Campos, M.M.; Fariss, R.N.; Becerra, S.P. Doxycycline-Mediated Inhibition of Choroidal Neovascularization. *Investig. Opthalmol. Vis. Sci.* **2009**, *50*, 5098. [CrossRef] [PubMed]
155. Kampougeris, G. Penetration of moxifloxacin into the human aqueous humour after oral administration. *Br. J. Ophthalmol.* **2005**, *89*, 628–631. [CrossRef] [PubMed]
156. García, D.A.R. Chapter 5 Quimioterapia inmunosupresora en uveítis. In *Oftalmología en la Opinión de los Expertos*; Temas Selectos en Uveítis; Santos Garcia, A., Ed.; Publisher Garaitia Editores S.A. de C.V.: México D.F., México, 2011; Volume 7.
157. Kaur, I.P.; Smitha, R.; Aggarwal, D.; Kapil, M. Acetazolamide: Future perspective in topical glaucoma therapeutics. *Int. J. Pharm.* **2002**, *248*, 1–14. [CrossRef]
158. Shirasaki, Y. Molecular Design for Enhancement of Ocular Penetration. *J. Pharm. Sci.* **2008**, *97*, 2462–2496. [CrossRef]
159. Pérez-Blázquez, E.; Redondo, M.I.; Gracia, T. Sida y oftalmología: Una visión actual. *An. Sist. Sanit. Navar.* **2008**, *31*, 69–81. [CrossRef]
160. Benatar-Haserfaty, J.; Flores, J.A.P. Anestesia locorregional en oftalmología: Una puesta al día. *Oculoplastia* **2003**, *50*, 11.
161. García, E.; Mensa, J.; Martínez, J.A. Diffusion and pharmacokinetics of antibiotics in the ocular globus. Therapeutic implications. *Rev. Esp. Quim.* **2001**, *14*, 331–339.
162. Lin, P.; Suhler, E.B.; Rosenbaum, J.T. The Future of Uveitis Treatment. *Ophthalmology* **2014**, *121*, 365–376. [CrossRef] [PubMed]
163. Duica, I.; Voinea, L.-M.; Mitulescu, C.; Istrate, S.; Coman, I.-C.; Ciuluvica, R. The use of biologic therapies in uveitis. *Rom. J. Ophthalmol.* **2018**, *62*, 105–113. [CrossRef] [PubMed]
164. Kahn, M. Bioavailability of vitamin B using a small-volume nebulizer ophthalmic drug delivery system. *Clin. Exp. Ophthalmol.* **2005**, *33*, 402–407. [CrossRef]
165. Yoo, W.S.; Kim, C.R.; Kim, B.J.; Ahn, S.K.; Seo, S.W.; Yoo, J.M.; Kim, S.J. Successful Treatment of Infectious Scleritis by Pseudomonas aeruginosa with Autologous Perichondrium Graft of Conchal Cartilage. *Yonsei Med. J.* **2015**, *56*, 1738–1741. [CrossRef] [PubMed]
166. Schwartz, S.G.; Flynn, H.W. Update on the prevention and treatment of endophthalmitis. *Expert Rev. Ophthalmol.* **2014**, *9*, 425–430. [CrossRef] [PubMed]
167. Sallam, A.B.; Kirkland, K.A.; Barry, R.; Soliman, M.K.; Ali, T.K.; Lightman, S. A Review of Antimicrobial Therapy for Infectious Uveitis of the Posterior Segment. *Med. Hypothesis Discov. Innov. Ophthalmol.* **2018**, *7*, 140–155. [PubMed]
168. Unidad de Enfermedades Vitreorretinianas—FISABIO. Available online: http://fisabio.san.gva.es/unidad-de-enfermedades-vitreorretinianas1 (accessed on 14 May 2018).

169. Andrés, S.; Higueras, M.I.; Mozaz, T. Efectos Adversos Oculares Asociados a Medicamentos y Productos Oftálmicos. Colegio Oficial de Farmacéuticos de Zaragoza. Vocalía de Optica. 2008. Available online: https://www.academiadefarmaciadearagon.es/docs/Documentos/Documento24.pdf (accessed on 14 March 2020).
170. Kim, H.; Robinson, M.R.; Lizak, M.J.; Tansey, G.; Lutz, R.J.; Yuan, P.; Wang, N.S.; Csaky, K.G. Controlled Drug Release from an Ocular Implant: An Evaluation Using Dynamic Three-Dimensional Magnetic Resonance Imaging. *Investig. Opthalmology Vis. Sci.* **2004**, *45*, 2722. [CrossRef]
171. Geroski, D.H.; Edelhauser, H.F. Drug delivery for posterior segment eye disease. *Investig. Ophthalmol. Vis. Sci.* **2000**, *41*, 961–964.
172. Prausnitz, M.R.; Noonan, J.S. Permeability of cornea, sclera, and conjunctiva: A literature analysis for drug delivery to the eye. *J. Pharm. Sci.* **1998**, *87*, 1479–1488. [CrossRef]
173. Conrad, J.M.; Robinson, J.R. Mechanisms of anterior segment absorption of pilocarpine following subconjunctival injection in albino rabbits. *J. Pharm. Sci.* **1980**, *69*, 875–884. [CrossRef]
174. Kaiser, P.K.; Goldberg, M.F.; Davis, A.A. Posterior Juxtascleral Depot Administration of Anecortave Acetate. *Surv. Ophthalmol.* **2007**, *52*, S62–S69. [CrossRef] [PubMed]
175. Ambati, J.; Adamis, A.P. Transscleral drug delivery to the retina and choroid. *Prog. Retin. Eye Res.* **2002**, *21*, 145–151. [CrossRef]
176. Ghate, D.; Edelhauser, H.F. Ocular drug delivery. *Expert Opin. Drug Deliv.* **2006**, *3*, 275–287. [CrossRef] [PubMed]
177. Lee, S.-B.; Geroski, D.H.; Prausnitz, M.R.; Edelhauser, H.F. Drug delivery through the sclera: Effects of thickness, hydration, and sustained release systems. *Exp. Eye Res.* **2004**, *78*, 599–607. [CrossRef]
178. Bourges, J.L.; Bloquel, C.; Thomas, A.; Froussart, F.; Bochot, A.; Azan, F.; Gurny, R.; BenEzra, D.; Behar-Cohen, F. Intraocular implants for extended drug delivery: Therapeutic applications. *Adv. Drug Deliv. Rev.* **2006**, *58*, 1182–1202. [CrossRef] [PubMed]
179. Raghava, S.; Hammond, M.; Kompella, U.B. Periocular routes for retinal drug delivery. *Expert Opin. Drug Deliv.* **2004**, *1*, 99–114. [CrossRef] [PubMed]
180. Olsen, T.W.; Edelhauser, H.F.; Lim, J.I.; Geroski, D.H. Human scleral permeability. Effects of age, cryotherapy, transscleral diode laser, and surgical thinning. *Investig. Ophthalmol. Vis. Sci.* **1995**, *36*, 1893–1903.
181. Ambati, J.; Gragoudas, E.S.; Miller, J.W.; You, T.T.; Miyamoto, K.; Delori, F.C.; Adamis, A.P. Transscleral delivery of bioactive protein to the choroid and retina. *Investig. Ophthalmol. Vis. Sci.* **2000**, *41*, 1186–1191.
182. Marmor, M.F.; Negi, A.; Maurice, D.M. Kinetics of macromolecules injected into the subretinal space. *Exp. Eye Res.* **1985**, *40*, 687–696. [CrossRef]
183. Geroski, D.H.; Edelhauser, H.F. Transscleral drug delivery for posterior segment disease. *Adv. Drug Deliv. Rev.* **2001**, *52*, 37–48. [CrossRef]
184. Kim, S.H.; Csaky, K.G.; Wang, N.S.; Lutz, R.J. Drug elimination kinetics following subconjunctival injection using dynamic contrast-enhanced magnetic resonance imaging. *Pharm. Res.* **2008**, *25*, 512–520. [CrossRef] [PubMed]
185. Guo, W.; Zhu, Y.; Yu, P.K.; Yu, X.; Sun, X.; Cringle, S.J.; Su, E.-N.; Yu, D.-Y. Quantitative study of the topographic distribution of conjunctival lymphatic vessels in the monkey. *Exp. Eye Res.* **2012**, *94*, 90–97. [CrossRef] [PubMed]
186. Myles, M.E.; Neumann, D.M.; Hill, J.M. Recent progress in ocular drug delivery for posterior segment disease: Emphasis on transscleral iontophoresis. *Adv. Drug Deliv. Rev.* **2005**, *57*, 2063–2079. [CrossRef]
187. Shah, S.S.; Denham, L.V.; Elison, J.R.; Bhattacharjee, P.S.; Clement, C.; Huq, T.; Hill, J.M. Drug delivery to the posterior segment of the eye for pharmacologic therapy. *Expert Rev. Ophthalmol.* **2010**, *5*, 75–93. [CrossRef] [PubMed]
188. Kompella, U.B.; Bandi, N.; Ayalasomayajula, S.P. Subconjunctival nano- and microparticles sustain retinal delivery of budesonide, a corticosteroid capable of inhibiting VEGF expression. *Investig. Ophthalmol. Vis. Sci.* **2003**, *44*, 1192–1201. [CrossRef] [PubMed]
189. Ayalasomayajula, S.P.; Kompella, U.B. Celecoxib, a selective cyclooxygenase-2 inhibitor, inhibits retinal vascular endothelial growth factor expression and vascular leakage in a streptozotocin-induced diabetic rat model. *Eur. J. Pharmacol.* **2003**, *458*, 283–289. [CrossRef]
190. Ayalasomayajula, S.P.; Kompella, U.B. Retinal delivery of celecoxib is several-fold higher following subconjunctival administration compared to systemic administration. *Pharm. Res.* **2004**, *21*, 1797–1804. [CrossRef]

191. Ayalasomayajula, S.P.; Kompella, U.B. Subconjunctivally administered celecoxib-PLGA microparticles sustain retinal drug levels and alleviate diabetes-induced oxidative stress in a rat model. *Eur. J. Pharmacol.* **2005**, *511*, 191–198. [CrossRef]
192. Amrite, A.C.; Ayalasomayajula, S.P.; Cheruvu, N.P.S.; Kompella, U.B. Single periocular injection of celecoxib-PLGA microparticles inhibits diabetes-induced elevations in retinal PGE2, VEGF, and vascular leakage. *Investig. Ophthalmol. Vis. Sci.* **2006**, *47*, 1149–1160. [CrossRef]
193. Misra, G.P.; Singh, R.S.J.; Aleman, T.S.; Jacobson, S.G.; Gardner, T.W.; Lowe, T.L. Subconjunctivally implantable hydrogels with degradable and thermoresponsive properties for sustained release of insulin to the retina. *Biomaterials* **2009**, *30*, 6541–6547. [CrossRef]
194. Tsui, J.Y.; Dalgard, C.; Van Quill, K.R.; Lee, L.; Grossniklaus, H.E.; Edelhauser, H.F.; O'Brien, J.M. Subconjunctival topotecan in fibrin sealant in the treatment of transgenic murine retinoblastoma. *Investig. Ophthalmol. Vis. Sci.* **2008**, *49*, 490–496. [CrossRef] [PubMed]
195. Gangaputra, S.; Newcomb, C.W.; Liesegang, T.L.; Kaçmaz, R.O.; Jabs, D.A.; Levy-Clarke, G.A.; Nussenblatt, R.B.; Rosenbaum, J.T.; Suhler, E.B.; Thorne, J.E.; et al. Methotrexate for Ocular Inflammatory Diseases. *Ophthalmology* **2009**, *116*, 2188–2198.e1. [CrossRef] [PubMed]
196. Wong, C.W.; Czarny, B.; Metselaar, J.M.; Ho, C.; Ng, S.R.; Barathi, A.V.; Storm, G.; Wong, T.T. Evaluation of subconjunctival liposomal steroids for the treatment of experimental uveitis. *Sci. Rep.* **2018**, *8*, 1–11. [CrossRef] [PubMed]
197. Rowe-Rendleman, C.L.; Durazo, S.A.; Kompella, U.B.; Rittenhouse, K.D.; Di Polo, A.; Weiner, A.L.; Grossniklaus, H.E.; Naash, M.I.; Lewin, A.S.; Horsager, A.; et al. Drug and Gene Delivery to the Back of the Eye: From Bench to Bedside. *Investig. Ophthalmol. Vis. Sci.* **2014**, *55*, 2714–2730. [CrossRef]
198. Imai, H.; Misra, G.P.; Wu, L.; Janagam, D.R.; Gardner, T.W.; Lowe, T.L. Subconjunctivally Implanted Hydrogels for Sustained Insulin Release to Reduce Retinal Cell Apoptosis in Diabetic Rats. *Investig. Ophthalmol. Vis. Sci.* **2015**, *56*, 7839–7846. [CrossRef]
199. Ghate, D.; Brooks, W.; McCarey, B.E.; Edelhauser, H.F. Pharmacokinetics of intraocular drug delivery by periocular injections using ocular fluorophotometry. *Investig. Ophthalmol. Vis. Sci.* **2007**, *48*, 2230–2237. [CrossRef]
200. Roper-Hall, M.J. *Anesthesia and Akinesia for Eye Operations*; Wright & Sons Ltd.: Bristol, UK, 1989.
201. Canavan, K.S.; Dark, A.; Garrioch, M.A. Sub-Tenon's administration of local anaesthetic: A review of the technique. *Br. J. Anaesth.* **2003**, *90*, 787–793. [CrossRef]
202. JJ, K.; Bowling, B. *Clinical Ophthalmology: A Systematic Approach*, 7th ed.; Saunders/Elsevier: Philadelphia, PA, USA, 2011.
203. Ehlers, J.P.; Gregory, L.F. *The Wills Eye Manual: Office and Emergency Room Diagnosis and Treatment of Eye Disease*, 5th ed.; Lippincott Williams & Wilkins: Philadelphia, PA, USA, 2008.
204. Lafranco Dafflon, M.; Tran, V.T.; Guex-Crosier, Y.; Herbort, C.P. Posterior sub-Tenon's steroid injections for the treatment of posterior ocular inflammation: Indications, efficacy and side effects. *Graefes Arch. Clin. Exp. Ophthalmol.* **1999**, *237*, 289–295. [CrossRef]
205. Tanner, V.; Kanski, J.J.; Frith, P.A. Posterior sub-Tenon's triamcinolone injections in the treatment of uveitis. *Eye Lond. Engl.* **1998**, *12 Pt 4*, 679–685. [CrossRef]
206. Choi, Y.J.; Oh, I.K.; Oh, J.R.; Huh, K. Intravitreal versus posterior subtenon injection of triamcinolone acetonide for diabetic macular edema. *Korean J. Ophthalmol. KJO* **2006**, *20*, 205–209. [CrossRef]
207. Cardillo, J.A.; Melo, L.A.S.; Costa, R.A.; Skaf, M.; Belfort, R.; Souza-Filho, A.A.; Farah, M.E.; Kuppermann, B.D. Comparison of intravitreal versus posterior sub-Tenon's capsule injection of triamcinolone acetonide for diffuse diabetic macular edema. *Ophthalmology* **2005**, *112*, 1557–1563. [CrossRef] [PubMed]
208. Ozkiriş, A.; Erkiliç, K. Complications of intravitreal injection of triamcinolone acetonide. *Can. J. Ophthalmol.* **2005**, *40*, 63–68. [CrossRef]
209. Shen, L.; You, Y.; Sun, S.; Chen, Y.; Qu, J.; Cheng, L. Intraocular and systemic pharmacokinetics of triamcinolone acetonide after a single 40-mg posterior subtenon application. *Ophthalmology* **2010**, *117*, 2365–2371. [CrossRef] [PubMed]
210. Accola, P.J.; Bentley, E.; Smith, L.J.; Forrest, L.J.; Baumel, C.A.; Murphy, C.J. Development of a retrobulbar injection technique for ocular surgery and analgesia in dogs. *J. Am. Vet. Med. Assoc.* **2006**, *229*, 220–225. [CrossRef] [PubMed]

211. Kazancioglu, L.; Batcik, S.; Kazdal, H.; Sen, A.; Sekeryapan Gediz, B.; Erdivanli, B. Complication of Peribulbar Block: Brainstem Anaesthesia. *Turk. J. Anesth. Reanim.* **2017**, *45*, 231–233. [CrossRef] [PubMed]
212. Mehta, S.; Laird, P.; Debiec, M.; Hwang, C.; Zhang, R.; Yan, J.; Hendrick, A.; Hubbard, G.B.; Bergstrom, C.S.; Yeh, S.; et al. Formulation of a Peribulbar Block for Prolonged Postoperative Pain Management in Vitreoretinal Surgery. *Ophthalmol. Retina* **2018**, *2*, 268–275. [CrossRef]
213. Iriyama, A.; Obata, R.; Inoue, Y.; Takahashi, H.; Tamaki, Y.; Yanagi, Y. Effect of posterior juxtascleral triamcinolone acetonide on the efficacy and choriocapillaris hypoperfusion of photodynamic therapy. *Graefes Arch. Clin. Exp. Ophthalmol.* **2008**, *246*, 339–344. [CrossRef]
214. Hayek, S.; Scherrer, M.; Barthelmes, D.; Fleischhauer, J.; Kurz-Levin, M.; Menghini, M.; Helbig, H.; Sutter, F. First Clinical Experience with Anecortave Acetate (Retaane®). *Klin. Monatsblätter Für Augenheilkd.* **2007**, *224*, 279–281. [CrossRef]
215. Patel, S.R.; Lin, A.S.P.; Edelhauser, H.F.; Prausnitz, M.R. Suprachoroidal Drug Delivery to the Back of the Eye Using Hollow Microneedles. *Pharm. Res.* **2011**, *28*, 166–176. [CrossRef]
216. Krohn, J.; Bertelsen, T. Corrosion casts of the suprachoroidal space and uveoscleral drainage routes in the human eye. *Acta Ophthalmol. Scand.* **2009**, *75*, 32–35. [CrossRef]
217. Krohn, J.; Bertelsen, T. Light microscopy of uveoscleral drainage routes after gelatine injections into the suprachoroidal space. *Acta Ophthalmol. Scand.* **1998**, *76*, 521–527. [CrossRef] [PubMed]
218. Einmahl, S.; Savoldelli, M.; D'Hermies, F.; Tabatabay, C.; Gurny, R.; Behar-Cohen, F. Evaluation of a Novel Biomaterial in the Suprachoroidal Space of the Rabbit Eye. *Retina* **2002**, *43*, 7.
219. Olsen, T.W.; Feng, X.; Wabner, K.; Conston, S.R.; Sierra, D.H.; Folden, D.V.; Smith, M.E.; Cameron, J.D. Cannulation of the Suprachoroidal Space: A Novel Drug Delivery Methodology to the Posterior Segment. *Am. J. Ophthalmol.* **2006**, *142*, 777–787.e2. [CrossRef] [PubMed]
220. Kompella, U.B.; Edelhauser, H.F. *Drug Product Development for the Back of the Eye*; American Association of Pharmaceutical Scientists, Ed.; AAPS advances in the pharmaceutical sciences series; AAPS Press: New York, NY, USA, 2011; ISBN 978-1-4419-9919-1.
221. Liu Suprachoroidal Injection of Ketorolac Tromethamine Does Not Cause Retinal Damage. Available online: http://www.nrronline.org/article.asp?issn=1673-5374;year=2012;volume=7;issue=35;spage=2770;epage=2777;aulast=Liu (accessed on 21 July 2018).
222. Patel, S.R.; Berezovsky, D.E.; McCarey, B.E.; Zarnitsyn, V.; Edelhauser, H.F.; Prausnitz, M.R. Targeted Administration into the Suprachoroidal Space Using a Microneedle for Drug Delivery to the Posterior Segment of the Eye. *Investig. Opthalmol. Vis. Sci.* **2012**, *53*, 4433. [CrossRef]
223. Falavarjani, K.G.; Nguyen, Q.D. Adverse events and complications associated with intravitreal injection of anti-VEGF agents: A review of literature. *Eye* **2013**, *27*, 787. [CrossRef]
224. Peng, Y.; Tang, L.; Zhou, Y. Subretinal Injection: A Review on the Novel Route of Therapeutic Delivery for Vitreoretinal Diseases. *Ophthalmic Res.* **2017**, *58*, 217–226. [CrossRef]
225. Johnson, C.J.; Berglin, L.; Chrenek, M.A.; Redmond, T.M.; Boatright, J.H.; Nickerson, J.M. Technical brief: Subretinal injection and electroporation into adult mouse eyes. *Mol. Vis.* **2008**, *14*, 2211.
226. Timmers, A.M.; Zhang, H.; Squitieri, A.; Gonzalez-Pola, C. Subretinal injections in rodent eyes: Effects on electrophysiology and histology of rat retina. *Mol. Vis.* **2001**, *7*, 131–137.
227. Qi, Y.; Dai, X.; Zhang, H.; He, Y.; Zhang, Y.; Han, J.; Zhu, P.; Zhang, Y.; Zheng, Q.; Li, X.; et al. Trans-Corneal Subretinal Injection in Mice and Its Effect on the Function and Morphology of the Retina. *PLoS ONE* **2015**, *10*, e0136523. [CrossRef]

pharmaceutics

Article

Novel Sustained-Release Drug Delivery System for Dry Eye Therapy by Rebamipide Nanoparticles

Noriaki Nagai [1,*], Miyu Ishii [1], Ryotaro Seiriki [1], Fumihiko Ogata [1], Hiroko Otake [1], Yosuke Nakazawa [2], Norio Okamoto [3], Kazutaka Kanai [4] and Naohito Kawasaki [1]

[1] Faculty of Pharmacy, Kindai University, 3-4-1 Kowakae, Higashi-Osaka, Osaka 577-8502, Japan; 1833420012r@kindai.ac.jp (M.I.); 1611610157u@kindai.ac.jp (R.S.); ogata@phar.kindai.ac.jp (F.O.); hotake@phar.kindai.ac.jp (H.O.); kawasaki@phar.kindai.ac.jp (N.K.)

[2] Faculty of Pharmacy, Keio University, 1-5-30 Shibakoen, Minato-ku, Tokyo 105-8512, Japan; nakazawa-ys@pha.keio.ac.jp

[3] Okamoto Eye Clinic, 5-11-12-312 Izumicho, Suita, Osaka 564-0041, Japan; eyedoctor9@msn.com

[4] Department of Small Animal Internal Medicine, School of Veterinary Medicine, University of Kitasato, Towada, Aomori 034-8628, Japan; kanai@vmas.kitasato-u.ac.jp

* Correspondence: nagai_n@phar.kindai.ac.jp; Tel.: +81-6-4307-3638

Received: 17 January 2020; Accepted: 13 February 2020; Published: 14 February 2020

Abstract: The commercially available rebamipide ophthalmic suspension (CA-REB) was approved for clinical use in patients with dry eye; however, the residence time on the ocular surface for the traditional formulations is short, since the drug is removed from the ocular surface through the nasolacrimal duct. In this study, we designed a novel sustained-release drug delivery system (DDS) for dry eye therapy by rebamipide nanoparticles. The rebamipide solid nanoparticle-based ophthalmic formulation (REB-NPs) was prepared by a bead mill using additives (2-hydroxypropyl-β-cyclodextrin and methylcellulose) and a gel base (carbopol). The rebamipide particles formed are ellipsoid, with a particle size in the range of 40–200 nm. The rebamipide in the REB-NPs applied to eyelids was delivered into the lacrimal fluid through the meibomian glands, and sustained drug release was observed in comparison with CA-REB. Moreover, the REB-NPs increased the mucin levels in the lacrimal fluid and healed tear film breakup levels in an *N*-acetylcysteine-treated rabbit model. The information about this novel DDS route and creation of a nano-formulation can be used to design further studies aimed at therapy for dry eye.

Keywords: rebamipide; sustained delivery system; dry eye; eyelid; mucin

1. Introduction

Dry eye is a multifactorial disease of the tears and the ocular surface that results in symptoms of discomfort, visual disturbance, and tear film instability with potential damage to the ocular surface. It is accompanied by increased osmolarity of the tear film and inflammation of the ocular surface [1]. In addition, the negative effects that dry eye have on visual function, quality of life, and economic burden are well recognized [2,3]. In many patients, the condition is chronic and requires long-term treatment, and potentially more effective ophthalmic pharmacological drugs targeting various distinct pathophysiological pathways of dry eye have been investigated. In Japan, the formulation to enhance the aqueous humor and mucin secretion are mainly used in the therapy of dry eye.

Rebamipide has followed a unique course in drug discovery and has long been used as a treatment for gastric ulcers. The logP and pK of rebamioide are 2.9 and 3.3, respectively, and the Biopharmaceutical Classification System (BCS) lists rebamipide as a class IV drug. In recent years, its mucosal-protective effect has also been applied to protection of the keratoconjunctival epithelium [4,5] after the development of ophthalmic rebamipide products for the treatment of dry eye [4–7]. With regard to the pharmacological mechanisms of rebamipide in dry eye, the majority of studies have focused on mucin production. The commercially available rebamipide ophthalmic suspension (CA-REB, Mucosta Ophthalmic Suspension UD 2%, Otsuka Pharmaceutical, Co., Ltd., Tokyo, Japan) was approved for the treatment of dry eye at the end of 2011 and was launched in Japan in 2012. In the clinical trial, the instillation of rebamipide was performed four times/day for the patient with dry eye, and in clinical studies, rebamipide has been demonstrated to be effective in improving the symptoms and signs of dry eye [6–8]. The use of rebamipide has been extended to dry eye treatment due to the discovery of its ocular surface mucin-increasing action. Previous studies showed that topical rebamipide may increase the number of goblet cells and promote the secretion of mucin-like substances in the bulbar conjunctiva and lacrimal caruncle of humans [9,10], and rebamipide has been found to improve both vital staining and tear film breakup time.

The ophthalmic application of drugs is the primary route of administration for the treatment of various eye diseases and is well-accepted by patients. However, in traditional formulations, only small amounts of the administered drug reach their target due to dilution caused by lacrimation and evacuation through the nasolacrimal duct [11]. Consequently, frequent instillation is needed to obtain a sufficient therapeutic effect. Eye ointment formulations are also used in the clinic. However, there are problems of convenience with the application of an eye ointment. Therefore, it is very important to design a sustained drug delivery system (DDS) in the ophthalmic field.

Solid drug nanoparticles come with the added benefits of possible cellular targeting and improvement in cellular uptake and have been used widely as nanotechnology-based delivery systems. We previously designed solid nanoparticles created by a breakdown method (bead mill), and reported on their low toxicity and high transdermal penetration via endocytosis when used in nano-formulations [12–16]. It is expected that the application of solid nanoparticles to the eyelid may be a possible route to sustained drug supplementation to the ocular surface and provide a novel strategy for ophthalmic DDS. In this study, we attempted to design a rebamipide nano-DDS through the eyelid and evaluate its usefulness for dry eye treatment.

2. Materials and Methods

2.1. Animals

Adult rabbits (male, weight 2.71 ± 0.43 kg, $n = 26$) were used in experiments performed according to the guidelines for The Association for Research in Vision and Ophthalmology (ARVO) and the protocol approved by the Pharmacy Committee Guidelines for the Care and Use of Laboratory Animals in Kindai University (KAPS-25-003, 1 April 2013). The rabbit model of dry eye was obtained by the instillation of 10% *N*-acetylcysteine (dry eye model), and 1.5% REB formulations (0.3 g) were applied to the shaved eyelid skin in single or repetitive applications at 14:00. For the repetitive applications, 1.5% rebamipide formulations (0.3 g) were applied once a day (14:00) for six days, and the measurements of lacrimal fluid volume, mucin levels, tear film breakup time (TBUT), ocular surface, and tea film breakup levels were started at 18:00.

2.2. Preparation of Rebamipide Solid Nanoparticle-Based Ophthalmic Formulations (REB-NPs)

Ophthalmic dispersions containing rebamipide nanoparticles were prepared following the previous reports [12–16]. Briefly, rebamipide powder (particle size 741 ± 12.7 nm) purchased from Wako Pure Chemical Industries, Ltd. (Osaka, Japan) was mixed with 2-hydroxypropyl-β-cyclodextrin (HPβCD, Nihon Shokuhin Kako Co., Ltd., Tokyo, Japan) and type SM-4 methylcellulose (MC, Shin-Etsu Chemical Co., Ltd., Tokyo, Japan) in distilled water, and the dispersions were milled at 5500 rpm for 1 min × 30 times using 0.1 mm zirconia beads and a Micro Smash MS-100R (TOMY SEIKO Co. Ltd., Tokyo, Japan). The milled mixtures were gelled with carboxypolymethylene (Carbopol® 934, carbopol, Serva, Heidelberg, Germany) and used as REB-NPs. The preparation of the rebamipide powder (solid microparticle)-based ophthalmic formulation was performed according to same protocol without the bead mill treatment (REB-MPs). The compositions of REB-MPs and REB-NPs were as follows: 1.5% rebamipide, 5% HPβCD, 0.5% MC, carbopol, in distilled water.

2.3. Measurement of Rebamipide Levels

The rebamipide in samples was extracted with *N*,*N*-dimethylformamide on ice and measured on an HPLC LC-20AT system (Shimadzu Corp. Kyoto, Japan). The HPLC conditions were as follows: wavelength, 287 nm; temperature, 35 °C; internal standard, 1 μg/mL methyl p-hydroxybenzoate; mobile phase, 50 mM phosphate buffer/acetonitrile (75/25, *v*/*v*); flow rate, 0.25 mL/min; column, 2.1 × 50 mm Inertsil® ODS-3 column (GL Science Co., Inc., Tokyo, Japan). The detection limit of HPLC was 70.4 ng/mL, and the R value was 0.9992 in the calibration curve.

2.4. Evaluation of Rebamipide Particles in REB Formulations

A nanoparticle size analyzer laser diffraction SALD-7100 (Shimadzu Corp.) with the refractive index set to 1.60–0.10i was used to measure the size distribution of rebamipide particles in REB-MPs and REB-NPs. The size distribution and number of nanoparticles in REB-NPs were analyzed by a dynamic light scattering NANOSIGHT LM10 (QuantumDesign Japan, Tokyo, Japan). The measurement time was as 60 s, and wavelength and viscosity of the suspension were set to 405 nm (blue) and 1.27 mPa·s, respectively. A scanning probe microscope SPM-9700 (Shimadzu Corp.) was used to obtain an atomic force microscopic (AFM) image in this study.

2.5. Dispersity and Stability in REB Formulations

REB-MPs and REB-NPs, 0.3 g each, were divided into 10 parts, and the rebamipide content in each part was measured to investigate dispersity. In addition, the REB-MPs and REB-NPs preparations were kept at 25 °C for one month under dark conditions to measure stability. The size distribution and concentration for demonstrating dispersity and stability were determined by the SALD-7100, NANOSIGHT, and HPLC methods described above.

2.6. Rebamipide Release from REB Formulations

A membrane filter and Franz diffusion cell were used to evaluate the release of rebamipide from REB formulations [13]. The reservation chamber of the diffusion cell was filled with 12.2 mL of 10 mM phosphate, and a 25 nm- or 450 nm-pore size MF™-MEMBRANE FILTER (Merck Millipore, Tokyo, Japan) was set into Franz diffusion cell to which 0.3 g of the 1.5% REB formulations was applied gently. The area under the rebamipide concentration-time curve (AUC_{Release}) was analyzed by the trapezoidal rule for the data for 0–24 h, and the size distribution of nanoparticles and concentration in the reservoir chamber were determined by the NANOSIGHT and HPLC methods described above.

2.7. Rebamipide Levels in Lacrimal Fluid and Meibum of Rabbits Applied with REB Formulations

REB-MPs or REB-NPs formulations (1.5%; 0.3 g) were applied to the shaved eyelid of rabbits, and the meibum and lacrimal fluid without meibum were collected with Schirmer tear test strips. The lacrimal fluid without meibum was harvested as follows: space was made between the eyelid and the ocular surface of a rabbit, and the Schirmer tear test strips were attached to the eyelid side (conjunctival sac). The Schirmer tear test strips containing samples were homogenized in *N*,*N*-dimethylformamide, and the rebamipide was extracted. The rebamipide concentrations were determined by HPLC as described above, and the *AUC* for rebamipide levels in lacrimal fluid (AUC_{LF}) were analyzed by the trapezoidal rule up to 180 min.

2.8. Monitoring the Ocular Surface of Rabbits Applied with REB Formulations

Schirmer tear test strips were used to measure the volume of lacrimal fluid in rabbits applied with REB-MPs and REB-NPs. The TBUT and changes in the ocular surface were measured 6 h after the application of REB formulation (18:00). A rabbit treated with a fluorescein strip was allowed to blink several times to distribute the fluorescein. The time from opening of the eyes to the appearance of the first dry spot in the central cornea was analyzed, and the time was presented as TBUT. The measurement was performed three times, and the mean was used as the value. The changes in tear film after winkling were monitored, and tear film breakup levels were evaluated by dry eye monitor DR-1 (KOWA Co., LTD., Aichi, Japan).

2.9. Mucin Levels in Rabbits Applied with REB Formulations

The lacrimal fluid was collected by Schirmer tear test strips and homogenized in *N*,*N*-dimethylformamide. The mucin in the supernatants was measured using a tear mucin assay ELISA kit (Cosmo Bio Co., Ltd., Tokyo, Japan) according to the manufacturer's instructions. A fluorescence microplate reader was used to measure the mucin levels (Absorption/Emission = 336 nm/383 nm), which are expressed as the ratios to the mucin levels at the start of the experiment (normal rabbit, 0.69 ± 0.06 mg/mL, $n = 24$; rabbit model with dry eye, 0.42 ± 0.03 mg/mL, $n = 27$).

2.10. Statistical Analysis

Statistical data from the SALD-7100 are expressed as the mean ± S.D., and other data are expressed as the mean ± S.E. Differences between mean values were analyzed with ANOVA followed by the Student's *t*-test and Dunnett's multiple comparisons. P-values less than 0.05 were considered significant.

3. Results

3.1. Design of a Rebamipide Solid Nanoparticle-Based Ophthalmic Formulation

Our previous study showed that bead mill treatment with MC allows a decreased particle size to the nano level, and that the addition of HPβCD prevents aggregation of the nanoparticles [12–16]. In addition, we also reported that carbopol is suitable as a base for dermal formulations [13]. Taken together, we attempted to prepare rebamipide nanoparticles based on our previous studies using additives (HPβCD and MC) and a gel base (carbopol). Rebamipide particles (approximately 100 nm–25 μm) were crushed by mill treatment. The milled rebamipide nanoparticles had a size of approximately 40–200 nm in the carbopol gel (Figure 1A,B, Figure S1) and were ellipsoid in form (Figure 1C). The rebamipide solubility increased by approximately 3.4-fold with the decrease in particle size, although the solubility remained low, and 99.92% still existed as solid particles (Figure 1D). On the other hand, the solubility of REB-MPs and REB-NPs without HPβCD were 0.003 fM, 0.011 fM, respectively, and it was suggested that the both of nano crystallization and enhanced inclusion complexes with HPβCD were related the increase of drug solubility in the REB-NPs.

Figure 2 shows the changes in REB-NPs one month after preparation. No differences were observed in the size or form of the rebamipide nanoparticles in REB-NPs (Figure 2A–C), and the ratio of solid to solution in REB-NPs was similar one month after preparation as it had been immediately (day 0) after preparation (Figure 2D). In addition, the rebamipide particles were distributed more evenly in the REB-NPs than in REB-MPs (S.D., REB-MPs 0.0571%, REB-NPs, 0.0034%, $n = 6$). No degradation was observed one month after preparation (rebamipide content of 1 month/0 month = 99.9%).

Figure 3 shows the release of rebamipide particles from the REB formulation in the in vitro study. Dissolved rebamipide was detected in both the REB-MPs and REB-NPs formulations, but no nanoparticles were detectable in the reservoir chamber when it was separated from the sample chamber by a 25 nm membrane filter (Figure 3A and Figure S2-A). On the other hand, when the chambers were separated by a 450 nm membrane filter, rebamipide nanoparticles were released from REB-NPs (Figure 3B, Figure S2-B), and both dissolved rabamipide and solid nanoparticles were detected after the application of REB-NPs. The reservoir chamber was found to contain 3.36×10^{11} particles (Figure 3C,D), and the plateau showed that all rebamipide in the REB-NPs sifted to reservoir side. Otherwise, the drug release from REB-NPs was slow in comparison with formulation containing dissolved rebamipide (Figure S3).

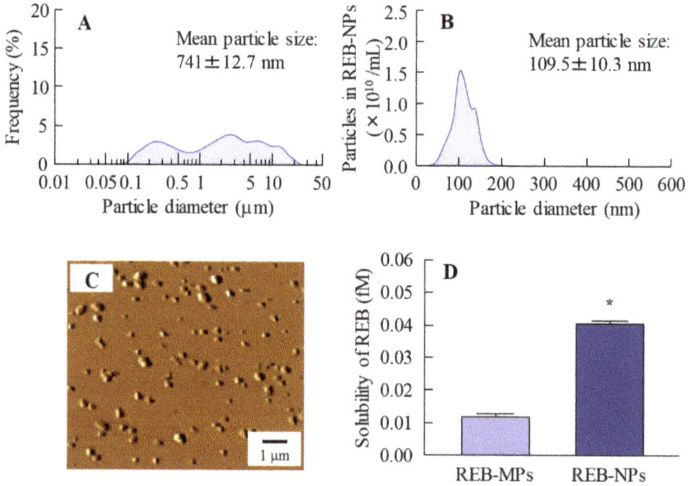

Figure 1. Characterization of the particle size, shape and solubility of rebamipide solid microparticles (REB-MPs) and nanoparticle (REB-NPs)-based ophthalmic formulation. (**A**) REB-MPs size by laser diffraction measurement. (**B**) REB-NPs size by dynamic light scattering measurement. (**C**) AFM image of REB-NPs. (**D**) Drug solubility in REB-MPs and REB-NPs. $n = 6$. $^*P < 0.05$, vs. REB-MPs. 99.92% of the rebamipide existed in the solid form in REB-NPs, and the mean particle size was 109.5 nm.

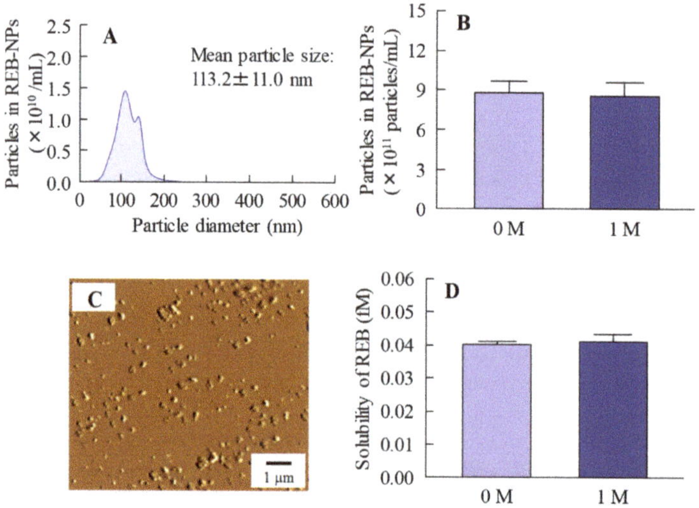

Figure 2. Stability of rebamipide solid in REB-NPs one month after preparation. (**A**) REB-NPs size by dynamic light scattering measurement. (**B**) Number of rebamipide nanoparticles in REB-NPs. (**C**) AFM image of REB-NPs. (**D**) Drug solubility in REB-MPs and REB-NPs. $n = 6$. The rebamipide solid in REB-NPs remained in the nano-size range, and no difference was observed in either the shape or solubility after one month.

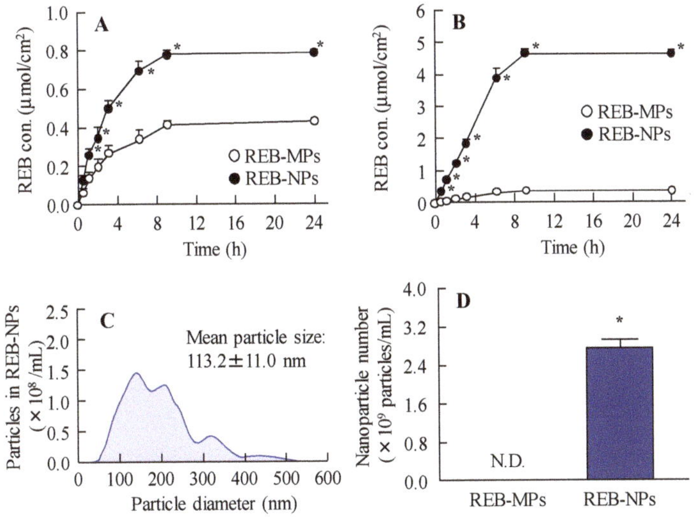

Figure 3. Rebamipide release from REB-MPs and REB-NPs through 25 nm and 450 nm pore membranes. Drug release from REB-MPs and REB-NPs through (**A**) 25 nm and (**B**) 450 nm pore membranes. (**C**) Particle size and (**D**) number of rebamipide nanoparticles that passed through the 450 nm pore membrane 24 h after the application of REB-NPs. Data show the size distribution and number of nanoparticles in the reservoir chamber. n = 5–6. N.D., not detectable. *$P < 0.05$, vs. REB-MPs. The rebamipide solid was released as nanoparticles from REB-NPs.

3.2. Drug Delivery of REB-NPs through the Eyelid

It is important to investigate the drug delivery route for the novel rebamipide solid nanoparticle-based ophthalmic formulations. Figure 4 shows the trans-eyelid penetration of rebamipide in rabbits to which REB-NPs was applied. Although no residual rebamipide can be detected 60 min after the instillation of commercially available eye drops, the rebamipide shifted from the eyelid to the lacrimal fluid of rabbits treated with REB-NPs (Figure 4A) with an AUC_{LF} that was 28.8-fold higher than that in rabbits to which REB-MPs was applied (Figure 4B). On the other hand, little penetrated rebamipide was present in the lacrimal fluid without meibum, and almost all of the penetrated rebamipide was detected in the meibum (Figure 4C). In addition, no solid nanoparticles were detected in meibum or lacrimal fluid with meibum by the dynamic light scattering measurement. These results suggested that the rebamipide was dissolved in the meibum, and meibum may show a high binding affinity to hydrophobic drugs.

3.3. Therapeutic Potential of the REB-NPs for Dry Eye

Next, we demonstrated the usefulness of REB-NPs as therapy for dry eye. Figure 5A,B show the lacrimal fluid volume (Figure 5A) and mucin levels (Figure 5B) after the application of REB-NPs to the eyelid (Figure S4-A,B). The lacrimal fluid volume and mucin levels were significantly increased by the application of REB-NPs, and at 6 h after application, the lacrimal fluid volume and mucin levels were 2.0-fold and 2.1-fold greater in comparison with the non-treatment group, respectively. Moreover, the TBUT was increased 1.3-fold by the application of REB-NPs as compared with the non-treatment group (Figure 5C and Figure S4-C). Figure 5D shows the condition of the ocular surface under a Noncontact Specular Microscope (DR-1). Although the Grade level based on the tear oil zone was Grade 4 30 min after eyelid opening in the non-treatment group, the Grade level in rabbits treated with REB-NPs remained Grade 2 at the corresponding time (Figure 5D). Figure 6 shows the changes in the lacrimal fluid volume, mucin level, and tear film breakup levels in the *N*-acetylcysteine-treated dry eye model rabbits treated with or without REB-NPs. A decrease in mucin level and strong tear film breakup levels were caused by treatment with acetylcysteine, and this damage to the ocular surface still persisted 6 days later. On the other hand, the repetitive application of REB-NPs enhanced the repair rate of the ocular surface damage: mucin levels normalized, and the lacrimal fluid volume increased (Figure 6A,B). Moreover, the tear film breakup levels were decreased 6 days after treatment (Figure 6D).

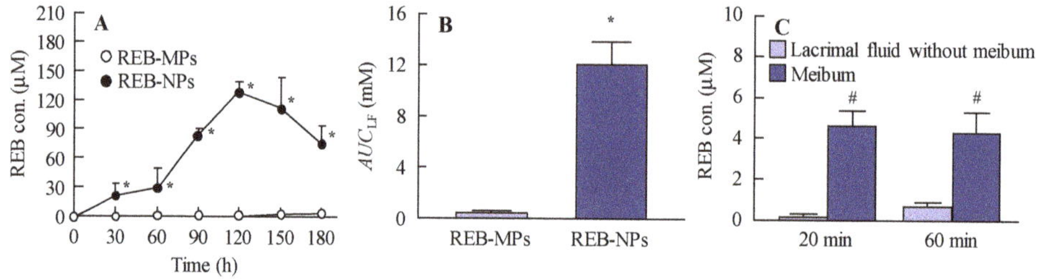

Figure 4. Changes in rebamipide levels in the lacrimal fluid and meibum of rabbits receiving a single treatment of REB-NPs or REB-MPs. (**A**) Rebamipide profile and (**B**) AUC_{LF} in the lacrimal fluid after the application of REB-MPs or REB-NPs. (**C**) Rebamipide levels in the meibum and lacrimal fluid without meibum after the application of REB-MPs or REB-NPs. Here, 20 min and 60 min after the application of REB-NPs, the lacrimal fluid without meibum was collected from the eyelid side using Schirmer tear test strips. n = 5–7. $^{*}P < 0.05$, vs. REB-MPs for each group. $^{\#}P < 0.05$, vs. lacrimal fluid without meibum for each group. The rebamipide in the REB-NPs penetrated the eyelid, and was delivered to the lacrimal fluid through the meibomian glands.

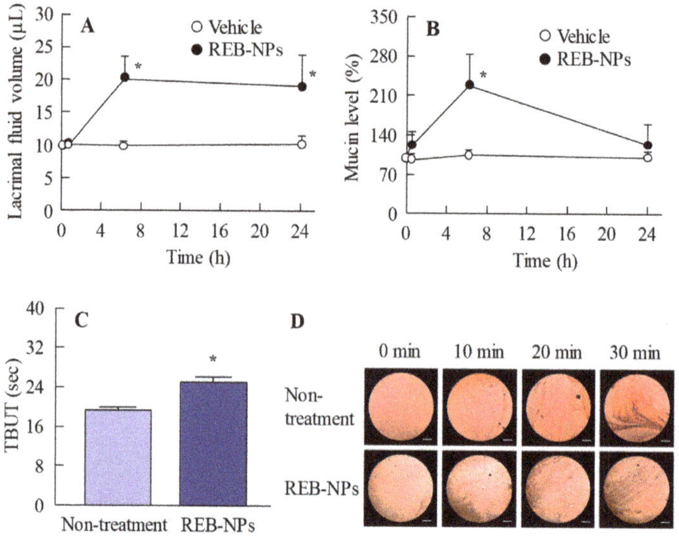

Figure 5. Effect of a single application of REB-NPs on lacrimal fluid volume, mucin levels, and TBUT in rabbits. (**A**) Changes in lacrimal fluid volume and (**B**) mucin levels after the application of REB-MPs or REB-NPs. (**C**) Changes in TBUT in rabbits treated with or without REB-NPs. (**D**) Images of the ocular surface over the range of 0-30 min after eyelid opening in rabbits treated with or without REB-NPs. The bar indicates 1 mm. In Figure 5C,D, REB-NPs measurements were begun 6 h after the application of the formulation to the eyelid. n = 6. $^{*}P < 0.05$, vs. REB-MPs for each group. The application of REB-NPs induced an increase in lacrimal fluid volume, mucin levels, and TBUT in the rabbit eye and led to the stabilization of the ocular surface.

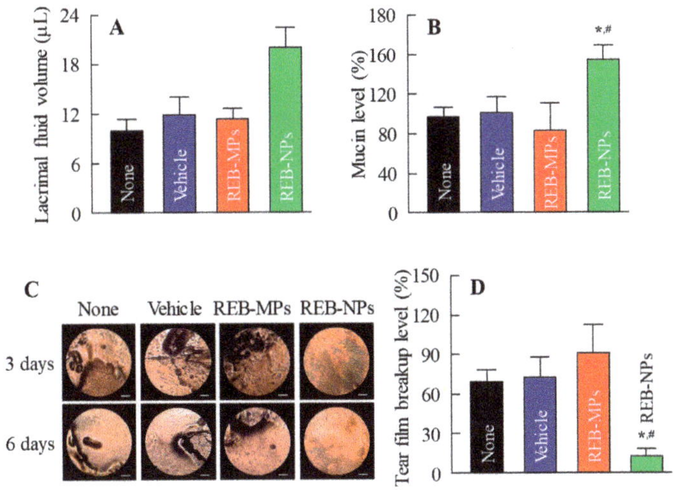

Figure 6. Therapeutic effect of the repetitive application of REB-NPs on dry eye in the *N*-acetylcysteine-treated rabbit model (dry eye model). Effect of REB-NPs on (**A**) the lacrimal fluid volume and (**B**) mucin levels in the dry eye model. (**C**) Images of the ocular surface in the dry eye model after repetitive applications of REB-NPs. The bar indicates 1 mm. (**D**) Effect of REB-NPs on tear film breakup levels in the dry eye model. Rabbits were treated repetitively with REB formulations at 14:00, and the experiments were performed at 18:00. $n = 5$–8. $^{*}P < 0.05$, vs. none for each group. $^{\#}P < 0.05$, vs. Vehicle for each group. In the dry eye model, the application of REB-NPs enhanced the lacrimal fluid volume, and normalized the decreased mucin levels. In addition, the tear film breakup levels decreased by the application of REB-NPs.

4. Discussion

CA-REB was approved for clinical use in dry eye patients [17] even though the residence time is short since the drug is diluted by lacrimation after instillation of the traditional ophthalmic formulation and removed from the ocular surface through the nasolacrimal duct [11]. Therefore, it is expected that the design of a novel ophthalmic DDS will make possible sustained drug supplementation onto the ocular surface. In this study, we developed a novel rebamipide solid nanoparticle-based ophthalmic formulation (REB-NPs), and clarified its penetration route to the ocular surface: rebamipide applied to the eyelid shifts to the ocular surface through the meibomian glands. Moreover, we found that drug supplementation from REB-NPs is sustained and that REB-NPs appears to provide a useful therapy for dry eye (Figure 7).

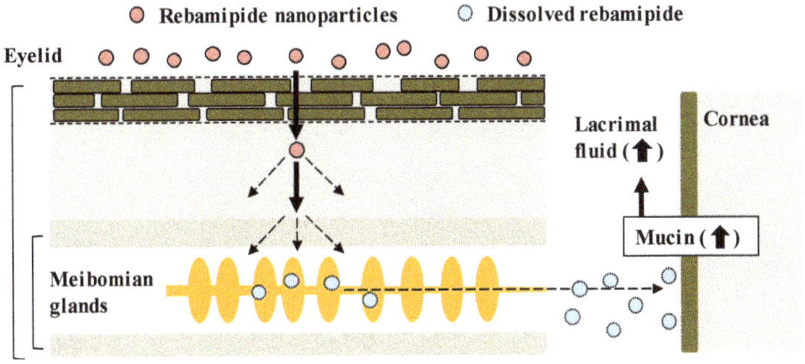

Figure 7. Drug delivery routes of rebamipide in REB-NPs, and the therapeutic mechanism for dry eye.

There are many methods for preparing solid drug nanoparticles by break down and build up, and we also previously reported a break down-based method using special additives [12–16]. The selection of additives is important for preparing REB-NPs, and MC and HPβCD lead to an enhancement in the crushing force and dispersion stability, respectively [12–16]. According to these findings, MC and HPβCD were used to prepare rebamipide nanoparticles, and the rebamipide nanoparticles were gelled by carbopol. The particle size of the rebamipide solid nanoparticles in the REB-NPs formulation was in the range of 40–200 nm (Figure 1B,C), and almost all of it was present in the solid form (Figure 1D). In addition, the rebamipide solid in the REB-NPs remained nano-size, with no differences observed in shape, solubility, dispersity, or content for 1 month after preparation (Figure 2). We demonstrated the release of rebamipide particles from the rebamipide formulation using membrane filters and a Franz diffusion cell (Figure 3). There was more drug released from the REB-NPs than from the REB-MPs (Figure 3A,B), and solid nanoparticles were detected in the reservoir chamber (Figure 3C,D). These results show that REB-NPs is stable, and that rebamipide solid is released as nanoparticles from the gel base.

Next, the drug delivery route was investigated in rabbits to which REB-NPs was applied to the eyelid. The rebamipide in REB-NPs penetrated to the lacrimal fluid side, and sustained release was observed in comparison with traditional rebamipide eye drops. No residual rebamipide can be detected 60 min after the instillation of commercially available eye drops, but when the REB-NPs was applied it the eyelid, rebamipide was still detected for more than 180 min after application (Figure 4A,B). Moreover, the high rebamipide levels were detected in the meibum (lipid), and the penetrated rebamipide dissolved in the meibum and lacrimal fluid without meibum. The meibomian glands are large sebaceous glands located in the eyelid that secrete meibum into the tear film in order to prevent excessive evaporation of lacrimal fluid [18]. Meibum shows a high binding affinity to hydrophobic drugs, such as rebamipide, since meibum is lipid, and we showed that the rebamipide was dissolved in the meibum in this study. From these results, it is hypothesized that the rebamipide in the REB-NPs penetrates into the eyelid, and shifts to the meibomian glands with high affinity. After that, the dissolved rebamipide in the meibum is delivered to the lacrimal fluid. On the other hand, we previously reported that some forms of endocytosis, such as caveolae-dependent endocytosis, clathrin-dependent endocytosis and micropinocytosis, are related to the transdermal penetration mechanism of solid nanoparticles in the epidermis layer of skin [13]. In addition, rabbits have a lot of hair follicles that provide openings in the skin. Therefore, nanoparticle permeation in that case may be much higher than in the human skin. Further studies are needed to evaluate the delivery mechanism of REB-NPs in the human eyelid.

It is important to demonstrate the therapeutic effect of REB-NPs for dry eye. Dry eye is caused by decreases in mucin secretion and lacrimal fluid volume on the ocular surface. Mucin has many important roles on the ocular surface (i.e., lacrimal fluid maintenance, lubrication of the ocular surface to facilitate smooth blinking, formation of a smooth spherical surface for good vision, provision of a barrier for the ocular surface, and the trapping and removal of pathogens and debris) [17–19]. Thus, dry eye is defined as a multifactorial disease of the tears and ocular surface. I was previously demonstrated that the topical administration of rebamipide increases mucin levels in the tear film and improves the condition of the ocular surface in dry eye [6]. Therefore, the volume of lacrimal fluid and mucin levels after the application of REB-NPs were measured in this study. REB-NPs enhanced both the lacrimal fluid volume and mucin levels on the ocular surface (Figure 5A,B), and the TBUT was also increased (Figure 5C). These results support previous reports about rebamipide and the drug behavior data (Figure 4) in this study.

It is necessary to investigate the therapeutic effect in a dry eye model. *N*-acetylcysteine is generally recognized to cause a shift to low-molecular-weight mucin molecules by breaking mucoprotein disulfide bonds. The instillation of *N*-acetylcysteine leads to histologic reductions in the mucin layer covering the cornea and conjunctiva, elimination of microvilli, and desquamation of corneal and conjunctival epithelial cells [20], and the thickness of the tear fluid layer is reduced [21]. In addition, it has been reported that the instillation of rebamipide increases the number of conjunctival goblet cells in normal rabbits [22], and the mucin-like substance content on the ocular surface in the *N*-acetylcysteine-treated rabbit model [4]. These findings suggest that the *N*-acetylcysteine-treated rabbit model is suitable for evaluating the therapeutic effect of rebamipide. The repetitive application of REB-NPs attenuated the decrease in mucin levels and the lacrimal fluid volume was increased in the eyes of the *N*-acetylcysteine model rabbits (Figure 6A,B). Moreover, the ocular surface normalized in the model rabbits (Figure 6C), and the tear film breakup levels were enhanced after six days of repetitive application of REB-NPs (Figure 6D). These results show that the REB-NPs are useful as therapy for dry eye. Further studies are needed to develop a rebamipide nano-delivery system through the eyelid, and it is important to clarify the mechanism of the transeyelid penetration of REB-NPs. Therefore, we will investigate the relationships of endocytosis pathways with the transeyelid penetration of REB-NPs using endocytosis-specific inhibitors such as nystatin, dynasore, rottlerin and cytochalasin D.

5. Conclusions

We designed a rebamipide solid nanoparticle-based ophthalmic formulation (REB-NPs) and showed that it provides sustained rebamipide supplementation to the ocular surface through the meibomian glands. In addition, REB-NPs provided a highly therapeutic treatment for dry eye, probably caused by an enhancement in mucin levels. Significant information about the novel route of transport through the meibomian glands, and the highly effective therapy for dry eye can be used to design further studies aimed at discovering new therapies for dry eye.

Supplementary Materials: The following are available online at http://www.mdpi.com/1999-4923/12/2/155/s1. Figure S1. Particle size distribution of rebamipide solid in REB-NPs on day 0 (A) and 1 month (B) after its preparation by laser diffraction measurement.; Figure S2. $AUC_{release}$ of rebamipide from REB-MPs and REB-NPs through 25 nm (A) and 450 nm (B) pore membranes.; Figure S3. Drug release from REB formulations containing dissolved rebamipide through 450 nm pore membranes; Figure S4. Lacrimal fluid volume (A), mucin levels (B), and TBUT (C) in normal rabbits applied with of a single dose of REB formulations.

Author Contributions: Conceptualization, N.N.; Data curation, M.I., R.S., F.O., and H.O.; Formal analysis, M.I., R.S., F.O., H.O., N.O., K.K., and N.K.; Funding acquisition, N.N.; Investigation, M.I., R.S., F.O., H.O., Y.N. and N.O.; Methodology, N.N., F.O., Y.N., K.K., and N.K.; Supervision, N.N., K.K., and N.K.; Visualization, N.N.; Writing—original draft, N.N.; Writing—review and editing, N.N. All authors have read and agreed to the published version of the manuscript.

Funding: This work was supported in part by a grant, 18K06769, from the Ministry of Education, Culture, Sports, Science, and Technology of Japan.

Conflicts of Interest: The authors declare no conflicts of interest. The founding sponsors had no role in the design of the study; in the collection, analyses, or interpretation of data; in the writing of the manuscript, and in the decision to publish the results.

References

1. Lemp, M.A.; Foulks, G.N. The definition and classification of dry eye disease: Report of the Definition and Classification Subcommittee of the International Dry Eye WorkShop. *Ocul. Surf.* **2007**, *5*, 75–92.
2. Li, M.; Gong, L.; Chapin, W.J.; Zhu, M. Assessment of vision-related quality of life in dry eye patients. *Investig. Ophthalmol. Vis. Sci.* **2012**, *53*, 5722–5727. [CrossRef] [PubMed]
3. McDonald, M.; Patel, D.A.; Keith, M.S.; Snedecor, S.J. Economic and Humanistic Burden of Dry Eye Disease in Europe, North America, and Asia: A Systematic Literature Review. *Ocul. Surf.* **2016**, *14*, 144–167. [CrossRef] [PubMed]
4. Urashima, H.; Okamoto, T.; Takeji, Y.; Shinohara, H.; Fujisawa, S. Rebamipide increases the amount of mucin-like substances on the conjunctiva and cornea in the N-acetylcysteine-treated in vivo model. *Cornea* **2004**, *23*, 613–619. [CrossRef] [PubMed]
5. Ríos, J.D.; Shatos, M.; Urashima, H.; Tran, H.; Dartt, D.A. OPC-12759 increases proliferation of cultured rat conjunctival goblet cells. *Cornea* **2006**, *25*, 573–581. [CrossRef] [PubMed]

6. Kinoshita, S.; Awamura, S.; Oshiden, K.; Nakamichi, N.; Suzuki, H.; Yokoi, N. Rebamipide Ophthalmic Suspension Phase II Study Group. Rebamipide (OPC-12759) in the treatment of dry eye: A randomized, double-masked, multicenter, placebo-controlled phase II study. *Ophthalmology* **2012**, *119*, 2471–2478. [CrossRef] [PubMed]
7. Kinoshita, S.; Oshiden, K.; Awamura, S.; Suzuki, H.; Nakamichi, N.; Yokoi, N. Rebamipide Ophthalmic Suspension Phase 3 Study Group. A randomized, multicenter phase 3 study comparing 2% rebamipide (OPC-12759) with 0.1% sodium hyaluronate in the treatment of dry eye. *Ophthalmology* **2013**, *120*, 1158–1165. [CrossRef] [PubMed]
8. Koh, S.; Inoue, Y.; Sugmimoto, T.; Maeda, N.; Nishida, K. Effect of rebamipide ophthalmic suspension on optical quality in the short break-up time type of dry eye. *Cornea* **2013**, *32*, 1219–1223. [CrossRef] [PubMed]
9. Kase, S.; Shinohara, T.; Kase, M. Effect of topical rebamipide on human conjunctival goblet cells. *JAMA Ophthalmol.* **2014**, *132*, 1021–1022. [CrossRef] [PubMed]
10. Kase, S.; Shinohara, T.; Kase, M. Histological observation of goblet cells following topical rebamipide treatment of the human ocular surface: A case report. *Exp. Ther. Med.* **2015**, *9*, 456–458. [CrossRef] [PubMed]
11. Goto, H.; Yamada, M.; Yoshikawa, K.; Iino, M. *Ganka-Kaigyoui Notameno Gimon·Nanmon Kaiketusaku*; Shindan to Chiryosha Co.: Tokyo, Japan, 2006; pp. 216–217. (In Japanese)
12. Nagai, N.; Ogata, F.; Otake, H.; Nakazawa, Y.; Kawasaki, N. Energy-dependent endocytosis is responsible for drug transcorneal penetration following the instillation of ophthalmic formulations containing indomethacin nanoparticles. *Int. J. Nanomed.* **2019**, *14*, 1213–1227. [CrossRef] [PubMed]
13. Nagai, N.; Ogata, F.; Otake, H.; Nakazawa, Y.; Kawasaki, N. Design of a transdermal formulation containing raloxifene nanoparticles for osteoporosis treatment. *Int. J. Nanomed.* **2018**, *13*, 5215–5229. [CrossRef] [PubMed]
14. Ishii, M.; Fukuoka, Y.; Deguchi, S.; Otake, H.; Tanino, T.; Nagai, N. Energy-Dependent Endocytosis is Involved in the Absorption of Indomethacin Nanoparticles in the Small Intestine. *Int. J. Mol. Sci.* **2019**, *20*, 476. [CrossRef] [PubMed]
15. Nagai, N.; Ono, H.; Hashino, M.; Ito, Y.; Okamoto, N.; Shimomura, Y. Improved corneal toxicity and permeability of tranilast by the preparation of ophthalmic formulations containing its nanoparticles. *J. Oleo Sci.* **2014**, *63*, 177–186. [CrossRef] [PubMed]
16. Nagai, N.; Yoshioka, C.; Ito, Y.; Funakami, Y.; Nishikawa, H.; Kawabata, A. Intravenous Administration of Cilostazol Nanoparticles Ameliorates Acute Ischemic Stroke in a Cerebral Ischemia/Reperfusion-Induced Injury Model. *Int. J. Mol. Sci.* **2015**, *16*, 29329–29344. [CrossRef] [PubMed]
17. Gipson, I.K.; Argueso, P. Role of mucins in the function of the corneal and conjunctival epithelia. *Int. Rev. Cytol.* **2003**, *231*, 1–49. [PubMed]
18. Mishima, S.; Maurice, D.M. The oily layer of the tear film and evaporation from the corneal surface. *Exp. Eye Res.* **1961**, *1*, 39–45. [CrossRef]
19. Gipson, I.K.; Hori, Y.; Argueso, P. Character of ocular surface mucins and their alteration in dry eye disease. *Ocul. Surf.* **2004**, *2*, 131–148. [CrossRef]
20. Thermes, F.; Molon-Noblot, S.; Grove, J. Effects of acetylcysteine on rabbit conjunctival and corneal surfaces. *Investig. Ophthalmol. Vis. Sci.* **1991**, *32*, 2958–2963.
21. Anderton, P.; Tragoulias, S. Mucous contribution to rat tear-film thickness measured with a microelectrode technique. In *Lacrimal Gland, Tear Film, and Dry Eye Syndrome 2*; Plenum Press: New York, NY, USA, 1998; pp. 247–252.
22. Urashima, H.; Takeji, Y.; Okamoto, T.; Fujisawa, S.; Shinohara, H. Rebamipide increases mucin-like substance contents and periodic acid Schiff reagent-positive cells density in normal rabbits. *J. Ocul. Pharmacol. Ther.* **2012**, *28*, 264–270. [CrossRef] [PubMed]

pharmaceutics

Review

Retinal Cell Protection in Ocular Excitotoxicity Diseases. Possible Alternatives Offered by Microparticulate Drug Delivery Systems and Future Prospects

Javier Rodríguez Villanueva [1,*], Jorge Martín Esteban [2] and Laura J. Rodríguez Villanueva [2]

[1] Human resources for I+D+i Department, National Institute for Agricultural and Food Research and Technology, Ctra. de la Coruña (Autovía A6) Km. 7.5, 28040 Madrid, Spain
[2] University of Alcalá, Ctra. de Madrid-Barcelona (Autovía A2) Km. 33,600, 28805 Alcalá de Henares, Madrid, Spain; jorge.martin@edu.uah.es (J.M.E.); julia.rodriguez@edu.uah.es (L.J.R.V.)
* Correspondence: javier.rodriguez@inia.es; Tel.: +34-91-347-4158

Received: 25 December 2019; Accepted: 22 January 2020; Published: 24 January 2020

Abstract: Excitotoxicity seems to play a critical role in ocular neurodegeneration. Excess-glutamate-mediated retinal ganglion cells death is the principal cause of cell loss. Uncontrolled glutamate in the synapsis has significant implications in the pathogenesis of neurodegenerative disorders. The exploitation of various approaches of controlled release systems enhances the pharmacokinetic and pharmacodynamic activity of drugs. In particular, microparticles are secure, can maintain therapeutic drug concentrations in the eye for prolonged periods, and make intimate contact by improving drug bioavailability. According to the promising results reported, possible new investigations will focus intense attention on microparticulate formulations and can be expected to open the field to new alternatives for doctors, as currently required by patients.

Keywords: excitotoxicity; neurodegeneration; retina; microparticles; controlled drug release

1. Introduction

Glutamate plays an important function in the regulation of relevant neurophysiological processes. For example, it has been proposed as a molecular substrate for learning and memory [1]. However, long-term overactivation of excess glutamate receptors in the central nervous system is associated with neuronal cell death. In the eye, an outward extension to interact with the world around us, controlled by the autonomic and central nervous systems, this happens in exactly the same way. It is released by photoreceptors, bipolar and ganglion cells and is responsible for the transmission of the light signal [2]. Examples of the participation of glutamate in other eye functions are related with synaptic transmission and plasticity, the transcriptional control of the glutathione biosynthesis and the maintenance of the cellular redox balance [3]. Glutamate homeostasis in the eye is controlled among others by macroglial cells (such as astrocytes and Müller cells) and the microglia. Microglia phagocytes monitor the environment and are rapidly alerted by a variety of injurious signal inputs, triggered by either genetic or environmental factors, as the result of external damage from ocular infections or due to cellular malfunctions. Their activation causes the secretion of neuroactive molecules, termed "gliotransmitters" affecting neurotransmission [4]. These include, among others, neurotransmitters (ATP, glutamate), eicosanoids, lactate, and the cytokine tumor necrosis factor α, factors that modulate astrocytes and Müller cells, thus ensuring proper functioning of the healthy retina [5].

When a rapid return to normality is not achieved, uncontrolled high concentrations of glutamate in synaptic and extrasynaptic locations lead to excitotoxicity, a downstream mechanism that activates cytotoxic cascades culminating in neuronal damage and/or death [6]. This excess glutamate (and related compounds that mimics its action) induced excitotoxicity acts primarily through *N*-methyl-D-aspartate acid (NMDA) receptors (NMDARs) [7], which, with kainite receptors (KARs) and α-amino-3-hydroxy-5-methyl-4-isoxazolepropionic acid receptors (AMPARs), is one of the three-ionotropic glutamate receptor subtypes expressed abundantly in inner retinal cells, making them particularly susceptible to excitotoxicity [8]. NMDARs are usually composed of two obligatory GluN1 subunits and two regulatory GluN2 subunits (GluN2A, 2B, 2C, 2D) [9]. The mechanism of action is related with a perturbation of Na^{+}/K^{+} homeostasis and an excessive calcium influx (Ca^{2+} overload), activation of extracellular signal regulated kinases 1/2 (ERK 1/2) [10] and increased release of reactive oxygen species (ROS), oxidative stress, and cytochrome c (mitochondrial dysfunction), resulting in apoptotic cell death (Figure 1). Intravitreal injection of excess glutamate has elicited loss of retinal ganglion cells (RGC) [11], the output neurons of the retina that connect the eye to the brain [12]. RGC collect and integrate visual information from second-order neurons and then transmit electrical impulses from the retina to the brain [8]. Furthermore, it reduces thickness of the retinal nerve fiber layer and attenuates the amplitude of the a- and b-wave components in pattern electroretinogram [13]. Another value, implicit time, is also altered in a- and b-waves, and oscillatory potentials are drastically affected by glutamate disturbances, indicating a neuronal dysfunction [5].

Excitotoxicity has been linked to the pathogenesis of several serious degenerative ocular diseases and injuries [9]. Apart from glaucoma, retinitis pigmentosa [14], diabetic retinopathy [15], retinal ischemia [16], age-related macular degeneration (AMD) [17] or Leber hereditary optic neuropathy are characterized by progressive retinal neurodegeneration. These disorders include cell stress and inflammatory response, at least in part due to increased glutamate levels [18], what ends in retinal remodeling. RGC and photoreceptors death by apoptosis is the characteristic of most degenerative ocular disorders [19].

Among them, particular emphasis should be placed on glaucoma. This disease remains the main reason for irreversible visual loss worldwide and the second most common in many developed countries [20,21]. It is estimated that this disease affected approximately 70 million people in 2014 [22] and the prevalence of this disease is expected to grow as the population ages, affecting more than 80 million people worldwide by 2020, with at least 6 to 8 million of them becoming bilaterally blind. It is a neurodegenerative disease of the inner retina and optic nerve characterized by morphological change of the optic nerve head and progressive degeneration of RGC and their axons. Glaucoma is subdivided into three main groups: open-angle glaucoma, closed-angle glaucoma, and secondary glaucoma. Furthermore, open-angle glaucoma is subdivided into high-pressure glaucoma and low-pressure glaucoma [23]. In closed-angle glaucoma, the peripheral iris blocks the anterior chamber angle by apposition or synechiae, preventing the drainage of the aqueous humor. In the case of open-angle glaucoma, the anterior chamber angle is open but the aqueous humor drainage through the trabecular meshwork is almost shut (especially in the juxtacanalicular tissue regions). Primary glaucoma is not associated with pre-existing diseases whereas secondary glaucoma is a consequence of another ocular or systemic disease, trauma, or from drug adverse effects [24].

While elevated intraocular pressure (IOP) is considered the major risk factor for causing optic nerve damage, ocular ischemia and subsequent remodelation (among others by endotheline-1 release), and lowering IOP is well established as a glaucoma pharmacological or surgical treatment, the precise causal mechanisms of glaucoma are not fully understood. In some patients, IOP reduction alone is not adequate and they continue to lose vision despite well-controlled IOPs [25]. Recent research has shown that it is the death of RGC that manifests visual field deficits. For this reason, it is critical to develop treatment that actively prevents the death of RGC, which are at risk in this condition [26]. Damage initiates by uncontrolled inflammation and excitotoxicity in response to ischemic injury, with lack of visual symptoms until substantial damage has occurred to the RGC and primary symptom of glaucoma, progressive loss of the visual field, appears. NMDA receptor antagonists have been used to treat neurodegenerative diseases in clinics. However, the universality of the glutamic acid neurotransmitter system makes the glutamic acid receptor blockers inefficient and unsafe in clinical experiments [27].

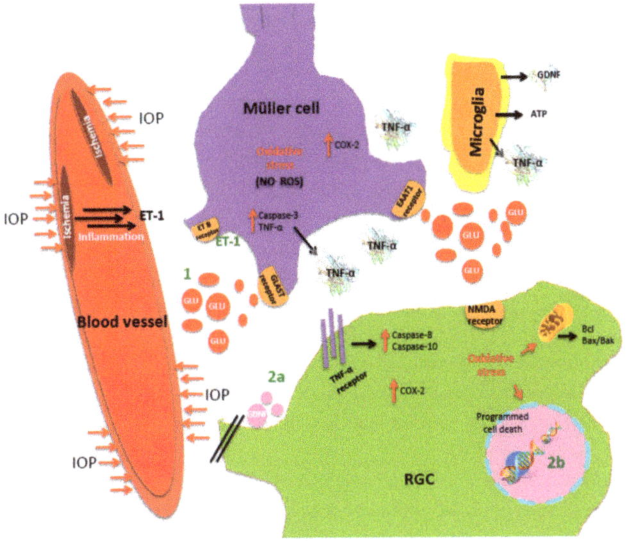

(A)

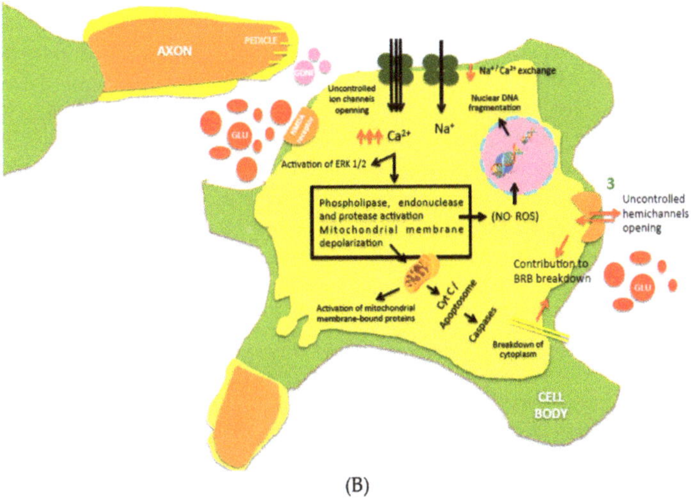

(B)

Figure 1. Schematic representation of (**A**) a synapse where intraocular pressure (IOP) and inflammation are causing optic nerve damage through excitotoxicity and the events that occur in retinal ganglion cells (RGC), Müller cells and microglia; (**B**) intracellular mechanisms activated in RGC after accumulation of excess glutamate in the synapse that lead to apoptosis. A detailed study can be found in [18] and [5]. Possible interventions to reduce excitotoxicity are indicated; 1) represents intervention over excess glutamate, 2a) administration of neurotrophic factors, 2b) administration of antiapoptotic compounds and 3) maintenance of retinal structure integrity.

Until now, there is no consensus on a clinical approach to treat glaucoma by directly targeting the neural tissue to protect them from degeneration [28]. This is partly due to the numerous numbers of different substances that have been suggested as candidates for neuroprotective therapy or neuroprotection. This is the term used for therapies that are independent of IOP lowering [21] and that protect the RGC by inhibiting various mechanisms of RGC degeneration and apoptosis, or promoting their survival [29]. The authors of [30] and [27] proposed that, among others, RGC survival can be achieved by blocking apoptosis (as, i.e., caspase and semaphorin inhibitors do), preventing glutamate induced RGC excitotoxicity (using NMDA receptor antagonists such as memantine), acting on mitochondrial injury (i.e., through the iron ion metabolism system as deferoxamine), administering various "neurotrophins" (i.e., glial cell line-derived neurotrophic factor, ciliary neurotrophic factor or brain-derived neurotrophic factor), free radical capturing elements (such as carnitine, carnosine, co-enzyme Q10, omega-3 fatty acids, flavonoids as hesperidin or vitamin B12) or calcium channel blockers (i.e., "-dipine" drugs or possibly anti-inflammatory compounds with a free carboxyl groups such as ketorolac, ibuprofen or dexamethasone [31]).

Nowadays, it is known that preservation of adequate protein folding, mitochondrial function, inflammation process and scavenging pathways directly avoids programmed cell death and irreversible damage of the neuronal cells [32]. Also, inhibition of retinal microglial and Müller glia activation via sigma-1 receptor agonism with neurosteroids (e.g., dehydroepiandrosterone, that has anti-inflammatory functions as well) has been described recently as an innovative and viable strategy [28]. However, not only should the pathway and the mechanism be effective, but also the drug should access the target site and maintain availability of the active agent for prolonged periods of time.

Solid ophthalmic devices, contact lenses, viscous liquids, gels, suspensions, colloidal systems (nanoparticles and nanosuspension), matrix system (ocular inserts, minitablets and collagen shields) liposomes, dendrimers, solid lipid nanoparticles, niosomes, and microparticles (the intraocular drug delivery systems or IODDS) have been developed with varying success. They emerge as an interesting alternative to repeated intravitreal injections of active substances in solution [33]. The administration of IODDS not only avoids serious complications related to frequent repeated injections, i.e., endophthalmitis and retinal detachment [34], but also reduces the risk of initial toxicity, due to high local drug concentrations typically occurring when they are administered in bolus [14]. Because of their micro- and nano-sized dimensions, the use of particulate systems has been explored as an appropriate alternative to conventional options in ophthalmology. They offer the possibility to enhance delivery and transport of drugs across ocular tissues [35].

However, until now, nano-sized systems have hardly been able to maintain stable drug concentration levels due to their small size they are cleared quickly through the conjunctival, sclerotic, and other periocular circulation systems [36]. Microparticles (MP), even so, are able to release an active substance for longer periods of time (up to 6 months) compared to nanoparticles. Generally, when they are elaborated for ophthalmic use, they must be extremely small-sized to avoid ocular damage due to abrasion and irritation while also providing easy injectability. Particles of a diameter less than 100 μm are considered suitable for intravitreal administration [37]. When MP are in a range between 2 to 40 μm, they can be injected through devices that include a needle (30–32 G) in a minimally invasive intervention. Among their possibilities there must be highlighted that they are good candidates to be used in personalized medicine as different amounts of particles can be administered depending on patient needs [38] and drug dosage could also be diminished to optimal, leading to a reduction of the possible side effect [39]. After administration, microparticles are not expected to move as they have the tendency to aggregate several days and remains in the vitreous cavity. Aggregation have been suggested, by some authors cited in [38], as a phenomenon that contributes to microparticles' implant behavior, what would led to some benefits as predictable kinetics. MP prepared with polylactic-co-glycolic acid (PLGA), a biodegradable polymer that is gradually converted into CO_2 and water in vivo by ocular tissues, revealed safe, stable, biocompatible, without intrinsic immunogenicity and relatively easy to produce on a large scale [40]. It fulfills the basic requirements that an ideal material for a vector should possess: compatibility with the host tissue, no immunological reaction, minimal damage at the injection site and controlled release of the drug.

In this review, we present the latest and most promising scientific communications on the field of ocular neuroprotection, focusing on those where microparticles are employed as drug controlled release systems. Emphasis, when possible, is made on their security profile and the drug release period these systems achieve as a potential advantage among intravitreal injections. This work is divided in three chapters. In the first one the intervention over excess glutamate is screened. Then, the use of neuroprotective therapies is discussed. In this case, the chapter is divided in two different parts. First, one for neurotrophic factors and then a second, where the possibility of using antiapoptotic compounds is analyzed. Finally, the approach of maintaining the retinal structure integrity as an alternative is considered.

2. Intervention over Excess Glutamate

If excitotoxicity is caused primarily by overactivation of NMDA receptors, the first idea proposed as a pharmacological approach for the treatment of degenerative diseases has been NMDA receptor antagonism where excitotoxicity is involved. However, NMDA receptors' complete blockade, as has been previously mention, implies intolerable side effects [8]. Another possibility, then, is reducing the level of glutamate in the synapsis. To this end, scientists know that one of the important functions of Müller cells is the regulation of synaptic activity through preserving low concentration of glutamate via activation of the P2 × 7 receptor [41] or upregulating high-affinity carriers such as the excitatory amino acid transporter 1 (EAAT1) or 2 (EAAT2) [42] and the glutamate/aspartate transporter (GLAST) [20]. In this last case, their activation by an α_2 agonist may contribute to the neuroprotective effects in RGC by decreasing synaptic glutamate levels. Brimonidine is a selective alpha 2-adrenergic agonist that has demonstrated the ability to lower intraocular pressure and protect retinal ganglion cells against glutamate excitotoxicity. Its mechanisms of action include inhibition of glutamate release, upregulation of brain-derived neurotrophic factor expression, regulation of cytosolic Ca^{2+} signaling, modulation of *N*-methyl-D-aspartate receptor through *N*-methyl-D-aspartate receptors 1 and 2A protein expression, reduction of aqueous humor production by the ciliary body and increased clearance through either the trabecular meshwork into the episcleral veins or the uveoscleral outflow pathway into the suprachoroidal space [43–45].

In-vivo studies carried out by [46] demonstrated that brimonidine in intravitreal application (3.6 nmol) protects retinal ganglion cells in a rabbit retinal NMDA excitotoxicity model. Ocular excitotoxicity severity correlates well with RGC disturbance. A study of viable RGC, their morphology and functionality can give yield information about ocular diseases progression and the results of therapeutical interventions. In line with [12], most of the current research investigating the pathological mechanisms underlying RGC death or evaluating novel therapeutics is conducted in genetic or experimental mouse models of glaucomatous optic neuropathies. All these models share their dependence on RGC quantification to follow the course of glaucomatous degeneration. The multiple methods that can be used to visualize RGCs in naive and experimentally manipulated rodent retinas includes basic histological [47], Nissl staining, neuronal immunostainings, retrograde tracers (such as fluorogold, dextran tetramethylrhodamine, or DiI into areas of the brain that are targeted by RGCs or by exposure of an axotomized optic nerve to these dyes [48]) or specific RGCs immunostainings (highlighting Brn3a, a POU domain class 4 transcription factor able to label their nucleus). After that, RGC counting can be done on retinal sections or in retinal flatmounts. In both methods, small frames are selected from the central, mid-peripheral and peripheral retina and RGC density is averaged and often extrapolated for the entire retina as a percentage versus control. As a result, the most common problems are related with inter- and intra-observer variation. Furthermore, if it is done manually, the technique proves to be laborious. In animal models of retinal degeneration, a- and b-wave amplitudes provide key information about disease-associated functional changes in the retina, but also about morphological alterations occurring during degenerative processes, including the progressive loss of photoreceptors and synaptic connectivity impairment [5]. In spite of this, most current animal models display rapid RGC degeneration incident, what is atypical of most human glaucomas and cannot be assumed to accurately reflect the disease process but up to date they are the most reliable preclinical models to develop pharmaceutics.

Later, [45] corroborated this observation and demonstrated that 0.2 mg brimonidine/day intravitreally injected to female Sprague-Dawley rats were enough to protect RGC specifically against mitochondrial dysfunction, the main rescue mechanism activated, induced by glutamate excitotoxicity and/or oxidative stress in ischemic retina. This small amount of drug could be maintained for almost a month by sustained release systems as proposed by [43]. These authors elaborated poly-lactic acid (RESOMER® 202H) and PLGA (75:25) microspheres (MS) using oil-in-water (O/W) emulsion solvent-evaporation method. 20 to 45 µm poly-lactic acid MS prepared exhibit good physico-chemical properties and reduced burst effect (8.0 ± 1.3%). Brimonidine was released from MS imbebed in PBS (37 °C and pH = 7.4) by roughly zero-order kinetic. After a month, only 75% of the drug content was released. Administered in-vivo in the supraciliary space (adjacent to the drug's site of action in the ciliary body using microneedles) of albino New-Zeland rabbits, these systems have demonstrated reduction of IOP for one month, but it would not be unreasonable to evaluate these systems for RGC protection. Upregulation of the glutamate transporters GLAST-1 and GLT-1 (another EAAT) has been shown to be the RGC neuroprotective mechanism behind neurturin [49]. No serious adverse effects were noticed, the eyes did not look inflamed and the animals did not show signs of pain, irritation or distress.

Finally, there must be mentioned that Ca^{2+} channel blocking has been proposed to be a mechanism that can be used to enhance RGC survival [50]. L-type Ca^{2+} channels play an important role in glutamate release from photoreceptors and bipolar cells. Dihydropyridines such as nimodipine and derivatives selectively blocks L-type Ca^{2+} channels and have demonstrated neuroprotection in cellular retinal ischemia/excitotoxicity models [51]. However, to date, results in our laboratory for RGC neuroprotection in a rat model of acute excitotoxicity has not shown positive results different from placebo. So, we agree with [52] that these statements are not reproduced in all studies, and it remains unclear whether this mechanism can exert a potential protective effect.

3. Neuroprotection

"Neuroprotective therapies" can be defined as pharmacological treatments focused on the relative preservation of neuronal survival, which is the reduction in the rate of neuronal loss over time [30]. These are plausible strategies for the treatment of various retinal dystrophies.

3.1. *Neurotrophic Factors*

The administration of neurotrophic factors is one of the most promising alternatives to enhance RGC survival. Over 2 decades ago, Faktorovitch et al. first proposed that neuro-growth factors, soluble small basic proteins for nervous system signaling, could be used to treat retinal degenerative diseases [53]. In general, a shortage of neurotrophins in the glaucomatous optic nerve has been implicated in RGC and photoreceptors loss [40]. Neurotrophic factors have the ability to promote the survival of neurons after optic nerve damage and to influence their growth [26]. Many of them (brain-derived neurotrophic factor, basic fibroblast growth factor, insulin-like growth factor 1, nerve growth factor and glial cell line-derived neurotrophic factor, to cite some of them) activate receptors that possess intrinsic tyrosine kinase activity resulting in upregulation of genes' encoding antioxidant enzymes, and proteins involved in antiapoptotic pathways, plasticity, energy metabolism and ion homeostasis [54]. For this reason the retrograde axonal transport of neurotrophic factors synthesized in target structures has been specifically associated with RGC survival [26] and a shortage with poor prognosis. Nowadays, in addition, a novel indirect strategy that involves the administration of actives, such as growth hormones, that are able to increase over-expression of neurotrophic factors has been proposed [55].

Neurotrophic factors can be administrated intravitreally. However, they have short half-life values in the vitreous, which makes necessary the use of sustained delivery systems. Particular emphasis should be made on Human Glial cell line-derived neurotrophic factor (GDNF). This factor is a 20-kDa glycosylated protean homodimer belonging to the TGF-β-superfamily [26]. It is produced and release from Müller glia [5]. GDNF signals directly through the cell surface receptor, GFR- α, and indirectly through the transmembrane Ret receptor, tyrosine kinases like. At the cellular level, exogenous GDNF has demonstrated neuroprotective effect for RGC, promoting the survival of axotomized cells [56]. When it is intravitreally injected on rats, it improves the damaged RGC survival [57]. Beneficial effects of GDNF could be related to the increased levels of glutamate transporters shown after its administration, what increase the removal of glutamate from the synapse by GLAST-1 and protects the RGC against excitotoxicity [49,58]) and with the Müller cell proliferation observed in a pig model [59]. Because of the GDNF potency and mechanism of action, the concentration needed to provide neuroprotection is low; in vitro, the EC_{50} of GDNF that enhances dopaminergic neuron survival is 40 pg/mL [60].

Based on these observations, [61] elaborated by spontaneous emulsification method GDNF MP with an average diameter of approximately 10 mm that released in PBS at 37 °C on a labquake rotating shaker the drug over a total of 71 days with three stages. These authors observed a first release phase in the first day immediately following immersion of the spheres (20 ng or 59% of total release). This burst was followed by a 30-day plateau stage (1–2 ng/mg MP). During the final 40 days, 15 ng/mg was released (total cumulative release 35.4 ng/mg/71 days). MP were administered to an animal model suffering "early degeneration" of RGC (30% lost in the first 8 months) and "late degeneration (80% or RGC lost at 10 months). During the "early degeneration" after 8 months, RGC survival was 18.6%. After continuous delivery through 13 months, RGC densities were 2.9 times greater in treated eyes. However, the best part of their findings appears when the same GDNF MP were administered to what can be considered a "chronic" model of glaucoma. Hypertonic saline (1.9 M) was injected into the episcleral vein of the left eye in adult male Brown Norway rats while the right eye served as a normal control. Two weeks later, the injection procedure was repeated on a second episcleral vein on the opposite side of the same eye. The IOP elevation seen in this study was sustained up until the end of the experiment at the 10th week time point, eight weeks beyond the second hypertonic saline injection, that can be similar to the progression of glaucoma in human eye almost for what concerns IOP. Results were very satisfactory. The administration of 5 μl of a 10% GDNF microspheres suspension significantly increased RGC survival compared with either the administration of 5 μl of the 2% GDNF microspheres suspension, although this suspension resulted in significant preservation of RGCs compared with PBS treatment after seven weeks (total theorical amount 35.4 ng GDNF (obtained from [61])).

In an attempt to take it a step further, [62] proposed one of the most feasible therapeutic approaches. They elaborated PLGA microspheres (MS) using a novel S/O/W emulsion solvent evaporation technique including GDNF and vitamin E as an oily additive. The combination of several active substances with additives has been seen to be of optimal therapeutic strategy to achieve synergistic effects. Not only does vitamin E modulate release from microparticles allowing better-controlled release, but it also exerts a positive effect over RGC survival and optic nerve functionality. Protein was incorporated maintaining integrity into MS on solid state, protected from cavitation stress, in a high production yield. MS characterization results in spherical particles ranging from 19 to 26 μm (mean particle size 19.1 ± 9.4 μm) with a high number of pores in their surface. Particles in this range are suitable for administration as suspension through standard injection needles (27–34 G). The loading data obtained was 25.4 ± 2.9 ng GDNF/mg MS corresponding with an encapsulation efficiency (EE) of 27.8 ± 3.1%. The profile obtained when MS were suspended in PBS buffer alone and with different concentrations of BSA (0.1 and 1%) showed the typical triphasic shape of PLGA systems. The initial phase was characterized by a burst effect (protein release during the first 24 h of the release assay) followed by a short rapid release period, and a second long period of slow release. As injectable systems, these MS requires effective sterilization. Gamma-irradiation showed successful when MS where protected with dry ice, remaining the amount of protein release practically unchanged [63].

GDNF biological function preservation after microencapsulation and sterilization was first evaluated on retina cultures. The RGC survival percentage was higher than 70% for no sterilized MS addition in contrast to less than 28% when no sterilized blank microspheres were plated. After gamma-irradiation cell death showed similar results. In light of these good results, in vivo assays were carried out in adult male Brown Norway rats. Extremely low amounts of GDNF released from their MS (0.8 pg/day) achieved a therapeutic effect on the retina, protecting RGC in a glaucoma model (damage caused by increasing the IOP in a non-aggressive manner). RGC counting showed significant protection in animals administered MS. The average number of preserved RGC in treated rats was 51.6 ± 3.2 mm with 0.5% GDNF/Vit E microspheres (0.64 ng/eye) compared with 22.8 ± 3.2 mm using an equivalent amount of GDNF in a single dose. The percentage of axon survival was 72.68% with GDNF/Vit E microspheres compared to 28.96% with blank microspheres. No obvious side effects on the retinal integrity were noted. Recent studies confirmed this system to be safe. These MS did not show abnormalities during a six-month follow up after intravitreal administration on adult female New Zealand albino rabbits [32].

The insulin-related growth factors, proinsulin, insulin and insulin-like growth factor (IGF) I and II, regulate multiple processes in neural cells, including survival during development and in adult life [64]. In the eye, insulin and its precursor proinsulin delay photoreceptor cell death, preserves the structure and function of cones and rods, as well as their contacts with postsynaptic neurons [65]. PLGA proinsulin particles with a smooth surface and 10 to 32 μm in diameter, an adequate size for intravitreal injection, were elaborated by [53] from a $W_1/O/W_2$ emulsion using the solvent evaporation technique. Protein was not in solid state here, as in S/O/W emulsion techniques [17]. However, protein maintained enough conformation and integrity at least to exert therapeutic effects. The selected microsphere formulation, due to the needs of therapeutic concentration after 24 h, displays a high burst effect as well as continuous in vitro release of pronsulin for at least 45 days (release profile obtained in PBS, pH 7.4 and 37 °C). Notice that the authors find values on vitreous from undetectable to 203 pmol/g of total protein, with most values in the range of 16 to 32 pmol/g with undetectable levels in control eye and serum. This gives an idea of the low but sustained concentration that must be achieved in posterior segment of the eye and the possibilities that MP systems offer [35]. The neuroprotective effect was evaluated by ERG in mice in dark- and light-adapted conditions. ERG lines were better defined and greater in amplitude on treated eyes in comparison with control. The average b-mixed, b-cone, and oscillatory potential amplitudes were significantly higher in proinsuline-treated eyes versus control. While these authors did not specifically investigate the mechanism of action of proinsulin as a prosurvival molecule, it has been shown also to involve the activation of the PI3K pathway.

3.2. *Antiapoptotic Compounds*

An antiapoptotic compound is a substance for which biosynthesis and secretion do not occur in the mature nervous system and with an intrinsic ability of action in apoptosis pathways preventing their progress and promoting neuronal survival.

Tauroursodeoxycholic acid (TUDCA), the most important component of bear bile (*Ursus thibetanus* or *Selenarctos thibetanus*, also known as the Moon bear due to its coat markings [66]) has been shown to display cytoprotective and antiapoptotic effects in rodent models of retinal degeneration [14]. The mechanism of action is not fully understood though it seems to block apoptosis at various levels, including the alleviation of endoplasmic reticulum stress, the stimulation of the PI3K and MAPK (p38, ERK1/2) survival pathways and the blockade of Bax translocation to the mitochondria impeding subsequent cytochrome c release. These effects in the retina means less oxidative stress and inflammation overactivation what prevents microglia cascade pathway triggering and photoreceptor degeneration [8].

The authors of [14] developed, using an oil-in-water emulsion solvent evaporation method, novel 20 to 40 μm PLGA TUDCA MS (mean particle size 22.89 ± 0.04 μm), spherical in shape with a smooth surface in a high production yield (78.2 ± 2.1%). MS burst effect (drug released in the first 24 h) was low and represented only 4.45 ± 0.62% (0.55 ± 0.04 μg TUDCA/mg MSs) of the encapsulated drug. After that, two phases can be clearly distinguished. The first one had a slower release rate of 0.0368 μg TUDCA/mg MSs/day from day 1 to day 14, increasing to 0.2873 μg TUDCA/mg MSs/day from day 14 to day 28. After 28 days, at the end of the study, MS had released 40% of the content. After intravitreal MS administration (4 μL of a suspension of 5 mg TUDCA MS on 1.5 mL of PBS, pH = 7,4) in the right eye of homozygous P23H line albino rats (commonly accepted as a model of retinitis pigmentosa [67]) and age-matched Sprague-Dawley rats, on both groups, electrorretinograms responses were less deteriorated compared to left eyes responses where blank PLGA MS were injected as a control. As a result of the neuroprotection, higher a- and b-wave amplitudes were shown in the TUDCA-PLGA MS groups. Immunostaining with combinations of antibodies (anti-guinea pig IgG, anti-rabbit IgG and/or donkey anti-mouse IgG secondary antibodies at different dilutions, nuclear marker TO-PRO-3 iodide was also added) were used to evaluate the protective effect of the controlled delivery of TUDCA. To evaluate TUDCA controlled release ability to preserve retina, the degree of photoreceptor cells neurodegeneration was assessed. Few photoreceptors were found in the right P23H rat retinas compared to those observed in the right retinas of age-matched TUDCA-PLGA-MSs-treated animals. Apoptosis distribution was not homogenous throughout the retina and the number of preserved cells was higher in central areas of the retina with the maximum protection at the optic nerve level in the central retina. Protected photoreceptors maintain typical morphology and structure, with long axons, well-defined outer segments and typical pedicles containing numerous synaptic vesicles that surround well-structured synaptic ribbons. Cone photorreceptors in the negative control groups degenerate and cells were practically undistinguished. Finally, these authors demonstrate the preservation of synaptic contact between photoreceptor cells and second order neurons within the outer plexiform layer. A double immunostaining for α-PKC and Bassoon (a component of synaptic ribbons of both cone pedicles and rod spherules) evidenced the contact between the axon terminals of photoreceptor and bipolar cell dendrites. Not only was the dendritic arbor better conserved on PH23H rats, but also the contacts between photoreceptors and bipolar cells are similar to those observed in normal Sprague-Dawley retinas.

Other compounds have shown antiapoptotic effects in several animal models of ocular excitotoxicity. Between them, it is necessary to highlight I) apelin-36 and apelin- 17 involved on the activation of Akt and ERK1/2 signaling pathways required for neuronal survival and inhibition of apoptosis in the retina [68], II) cannabinoids via a mechanism involving the CB1 receptors, the PI3K/Akt and MEK/ERK1/2 signaling pathways [69], III) capsaicin, a transient receptor potential vanilloid type1 agonist that activates opioid receptors, calcitonin gene-related peptide receptor and the tachykinin NK1 receptor involved in the protective effect against the NMDA receptor induced neuronal death [70], IV) pituitary adenylate cyclase-activating polypeptide through phosphatidylcholine-specific PLC pathway and cAMP production [71], V) compounds acting on adenosine A_3 receptor that attenuates the rise in calcium in RGC after activation of glutamate and P2X receptors protecting retinal cells, particularly RGC [72], VI) geranylgeranylacetone involved on the reduction in the activities of caspase-9 and -3, achieving protective results using a normal tension glaucoma mouse model which lacks GLAST [73], VII) CYM-5442 a known sphingosine 1-phosphate receptor agonist that administrated systemically in rats protected RGC from apoptotic death and preserve neuronal function after ET-1 induced RGC loss [19], VIII) adamantane derivatives such as memantine that blocks excessive activation of NMDARs without disrupting normal activity and has recently demonstrated significant preservation of RGCs density in a rodent ocular model of ocular hypertension when administrated in PLGA-polyethylene glycol (commonly PLGA-PEGylated) biodegradable nanoparticles [25], IX) tetramethylpyrazines, commonly known as TMPs, compounds able to block L-type voltage-gated calcium channels [7], X) tranylcypromine, a major lysine-specific demethylase 1 (LSD-1) and monoamine oxidase (MAO) inhibitor, that enhances expression of p38 MAPK and KEGG pathway genes [74], XI) melatonin, an autocrine or paracrine neuromodulator that regulates the local circadian physiology, that can be an effective antioxidant and antiapoptotic compound in the retina, acting as a direct and indirect free radical scavenger [75], XII) serotonin receptor (5-HT1A) agonists via the inhibition of cAMP-PKA signaling pathway that modulates GABAergic presynaptic activity [76], XIII) mTOR pathway stimulating APIs such as ciliary neurotrophic factors, lipopeptide N-fragment osteopontin mimic or lipopeptide phosphatase tension homologue inhibitors [77] or XIV) curcumin that modulates NMDA receptor subunit composition [78]. Finally, compounds with dual mechanism of action could be of special interest in multifactorial diseases as those related with RGC loss. In this sense, Mg acetyltaurate combines NMDARs' inhibition and antioxidant effects [79] (Table 1).

Table 1. Compounds evaluated in retina cells for their antiapoptotic activities. The pathway and/or mechanism involved/proposed is included.

Compounds	Pathway/Mechanism Involved	Bibliography
Apelin-36 and apelin- 17	Akt and ERK1/2 signaling pathways.	[68]
Cannabinoids	CB1 receptors, PI3K/Akt and MEK/ERK1/2 signaling pathways.	[69]
Capsaicin	Opioid, calcitonin gene-related peptide and tachykinin NK1 receptor.	[70]
Pituitary adenylate cyclase-activating polypeptide	Phosphatidylcholine-specific PLC pathway and cAMP production.	[71]
Adenosine A_3 receptor agonists	Attenuates the rise in calcium in RGC.	[72]
Geranylgeranylacetone	Reduction in the activities of caspase-9 and caspase-3.	[73]
CYM-5442	Sphingosine 1-phosphate receptor agonism.	[19]
Adamantane derivatives	Blockage of NMDARs excessive overactivation	[25]
Tetramethylpyrazines	Blockage of L-type voltaje-gated Ca^{2+} channels.	[7]
Tranylcypromine	P38 MAPK and KEGG pathway genes expression.	[74]
Dual compounds (e.g., Mg acetyltaurate)	NMDAR inhibition + antioxidant effect.	[79]
Melatonin	Direct and indirect free radical scavenger.	[75]
5-HT1A agonists	Inhibition of cAMP-PKA signaling pathway.	[76]
Ciliary neurotrophic factors, lipopeptide *N*-fragment osteopontin mimic, lipopeptide phosphatase tension homologue inhibitors	mTOR pathway stimulation.	[77]
Curcumin	Modulation of NMDA receptor subunits composition.	[78]

Recently, in an interesting approach [80] prepared PLGA 50:50 MS by the Oil/Water emulsion solvent extraction-evaporation technique including dexamethasone, melatonin and CoQ10, three recognized neuroprotective agents that were able to provide simultaneous controlled co-delivery and maintain drug concentrations above the minimum effective level and the maximum safe concentration for, at least, more than a month. When multiloaded MSs formulation were administered and the in vivo neuroprotective effect over glaucoma induction in rats (by Morrison's ocular hypertension model) evaluated, a significantly promotion of RGCs survival was found compared to administration of empty MSs. Special interest shows the fact that the administration of MSs loaded with a combination of the three drugs significantly promote RGCs survival compared to administration of empty MSs, what reveals that a combined therapy of some of those APIs could achieve synergistic results. The co-incorporation of different drugs into a single microcarrier can also reduce the amount of biomaterial (in this case PLGA) required for intraocular administration compared to equivalent dosing of single drug loaded formulations (here more than a half), which reduce the risk of PLGA associated retinal stress. Although several fixed combination therapies of antihypertensive drugs are currently in clinical practice, an equivalent neuroprotective combination therapy has not yet been clinically translated and that strategy may result in promising neuroprotective results for the treatment of multifactorial retinal diseases.

4. Retinal Structure Integrity

The structural complexity of the retina makes this tissue vulnerable to alterations from any sort of pathological injury. During retinal degeneration, retinal neurons are rewired while extracellular matrix (ECM) structural properties are changed. These changes alter matrix metalloproteinase (MMP) activity levels and influence cell-cell and cell-ECM interactions [81]. The authors of [82] demonstrated that

MMP-2 and MMP-9 contribute to pathological remodeling of the inner limiting membrane and induce cell death. Their efforts to reduce MMP-mediated retinal damage with broad-spectrum inhibitors, such as GM6001, have produced encouraging results.

Recently, fragments of αβ crystalline released in a controlled way when fused with elastin like polypeptides have demonstrated prevention of retinal layers disruption, maintenance of transepithelial resistance and less disruption of tight junctions morphology in $NaIO_3$ challenged mice [83]. The peptide construct generates spontaneous multivalent nanoparticles at physiological temperature. In spite of this, preclinical explorations of elastin like polypeptides support that their use in higher structures could enhance half-life of peptides or small proteins and achieve proper controlled release. Microparticles' elaboration could be a good strategy here.

Also, connexins, transmembrane proteins serving as subunits of gap junction channels that forms two connexons, which allow rapid transport of ions or secondary messengers and small metabolites (up to 1 kDa) between connected cells within all tissues, play an important role in homeostasis too. Among all connexins, connexin43 is extensively located in the retina and its dysregulation has been observed in multiple neurodegenerative diseases. In fact, inside the retinal capillaries, endothelial cells are arranged very tightly between adjacent cells. Inferior up-regulation that results in excessive gap junction communication or uncontrolled opening of hemichannels that contribute to "center-surround" antagonism allow pro-inflammatory mediators activation, vascular permeability or interferences between intercellular transfer of ions and metabolites, ending in loss of RGC. Furthermore, it enables the release of apoptotic and necrotic signals from injured cells to the extracellular matrix where death signals can be passed to adjacent cells [37,84,85].

Thus, blocking the hemichannel opening but still keeping gap junction coupling should be explored as a potential neuroprotective tool. For this purpose, [37] try to demonstrate that hemichannel block could be potentially useful to limit blood retinal barrier disruption, inflammation, and lesion spread as well as RGC loss under retinal inflammatory and excitotoxic conditions. Based on previous studies that corroborate that structural mimetic connexin peptides, which are small peptides mimicking the sequence of connexin hemichannels, reduced cell death, optic nerve oedema, activation of astrocytes and microglia, and preserved vascular integrity, they elaborate connexin43 mimetic peptide PLGA micro (9.13 ± 0.37 μm, narrow size distribution) and nanoparticles (113.38 ± 0.74 nm) containing native connexin43 (drug loading 1.78 ± 0.05) using the double emulsion solvent evaporation method. Particles exhibited spherical structures and a relatively smooth surface. Zeta potential was neutral for MP and negative for nanoparticles at pH = 7.4. MP's free diffusion through the vitreous via electrostatic repulsion between the particles and the negatively charged vitreous meshwork may be difficult, but it is much easier for nanoparticles. However, nanoparticles were almost completely eroded with all drug content release after 30 days in the usual release media (PBS, pH = 7.4 and 37 °C) while MP showed a slight pore formation on the particle surface and drug release up to 3 months in the classical profile, polymer degradation and drug diffusion through water-filled channels created during the erosion process. MP release was 28.6% of connexin43 following immersion (burst effect), 43.6% up to the 97th day and 27.8% during the final 14 days. Immediately following rats ischaemia–reperfusion, connexin43 MP diluted in 0.9% saline was intravitreally injected. The authors intended that MO administration reach a final peptide concentration of 20 μM assuming a vitreous volume of 50 μL. This system failed to rescue RGC. The most plausible explanation is the insufficient initial connexin43 release from MP during the immediate acute stage after injury. In this case, the results suggest that the RGC rescue effect may be more attributable to the initial burst of connexin43 than the continuous slow release, suggesting that the sooner connexin43 hemichannels are blocked after ischaemia the better. Despite nanoparticles showing the most promising results in the acute model employed by these authors, it must be taken into account that neurodegenerative diseases characterized by slow and chronic progression and death of RGC significantly increases with time [38]. The biological study evaluated here suited to rapid RGC degeneration and treatments were tested in the short term. This fact, linked with the reduced injection frequency required due to the sustained release effect that renders the MP formulation vs. the bolus administration and the reduced drug concentration needed in vitreous, but expected to be high that the dose administered somelike insignificant, spotlight that MP formulations has significant potential in the treatment of chronic retinal excitotoxicity and may still provide long-term RGC protection.

5. Conclusions

Excitotoxicity seems to play a critical role in ocular neurodegeneration. Excess glutamate mediated RGC death is the principal cause of cell loss. Uncontrolled glutamate in the synapsis have significant implications in the pathogenesis of neurodegenerative disorders. At present, there are at least four mechanisms that have provided enough evidence of ocular protection where drugs could act. Acting over excess glutamate and/or its impacts, avoid the induced apoptosis underlying NMDA over-activation or the loss of retinal integrity and the use of neuroprotectants (Figure 2). The exploitation of approaches of controlled release systems enhance the pharmacokinetic and pharmacodynamic activity of drugs. Furthermore, these systems are even more interesting when, as here, sustained but minimal drug concentrations are required. In particular, microparticles are secure, can maintain therapeutic drug concentrations in the eye for prolonged periods and make intimate contact improving drug biodisponibility. These are numerous and good enough reasons to further study this ophthalmic systems to design formulations that have, in animal models, demonstrated no toxicity but a statistical reduction of RGC degeneration, loss of functionality and morphology changes. According to the promising results reported (Table 2), new investigations will focus possibly much attention on microparticulate formulations which can be expected to open the field to new alternatives for doctors, as required by patients.

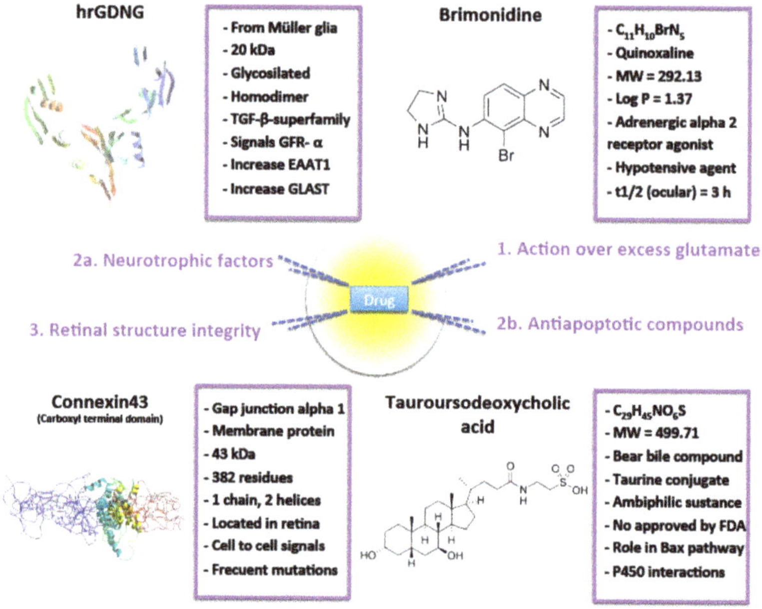

Figure 2. Drugs incorporated into microparticles to treat excitotoxicity. For each compounds the principal characteristics are highlighted.

Table 2. Alternatives for ocular neuroprotection where microparticles (MP) have been evaluated. The compound tested and its properties as well as the most relevant results obtained are shown.

Neuroprotection based on	Compound	Properties	Encapsulation	Observations	Bibliography
Intervention over excess glutamate	Brimonidine	See Figure 2	Poly-lactic acid (RESOMER® 202H) MS	Particle size between 20 to 45 µm. Reduced burst effect. After a month, only 75% of the drug was released. Reduction of IOP after a month. No serious adverse effects noticed and eyes did not look inflamed and the animals did not show signs of pain, irritation or distress. RGC protective activity was evaluated.	[43]
Neuroprotective therapies					
Neurotrophic factors	GDNF	See Figure 2	PLGA (50:50) MS	Particle size ≈ 20 µm. Drug loading ≈ 25 ng/mg. EE ≈ 28%. RGC survival in-vitro > 70%. 50% higher preservation of RGC in vivo compared to the same dose of GDNF administered in bolus. No side effects observed on retina.	[32,62,63]
Antiapoptotic compounds	TUDCA	See Figure 2	PLGA (50:50) MS	Particle size ≈ 20 µm. Spherical MS. High production yield. Low burst effect. Significant photoreceptor's survival. Well-preserved contact between photoreceptor cells and second order neurons.	[14]
	Dexamethasone (DX) Melatonin (Mel) Coenzyme Q10 (CoQ10)	Antiapoptotic Antioxidant Anti-inflammatory	PLGA (50:50) MS	Particle size ≈ 24 µm. Spherical MS. Production yield ≈ 72% EE ≈ 78% DX; 62% Mel; 96% CoQ10 Low burst effect and triphasic release. Neuroprotection—high RGC density—in the Morrison's model of ocular hypertension; whole retina density measures demonstrated that MS administration preserved RGC to a comparable extent as naïve retinas. Multidrug MS demonstrated less side effects than the same amount of drug administered in single-drug loaded MS.	[80]
Retinal structure intregrity	Connexin43 mimetic peptide	See Figure 2	PLGA (50:50) MP	Particle size ≈ 9 µm and narrow distribution. Spherical morphology. Smooth surface. Neutral zeta potential. MP release drug in sustained release more than 3 months. No enough drug released after a day to exert effective protection maybe due to rapid RGC death after ischemia lesion.	[37]

Author Contributions: All authors have read and agreed to the published version of the manuscript.

Funding: This research received no external funding.

Conflicts of Interest: The authors declare no conflict of interest.

References

1. Platt, S.R. The role of glutamate in central nervous system health and disease—A review. *Vet. J.* **2007**, *173*, 278–286. [CrossRef] [PubMed]
2. Russo, R.; Cavaliere, F.; Varano, G.P.; Milanese, M.; Adornetto, A.; Nucci, C.; Bonanno, G.; Morrone, L.A.; Corasaniti, M.T.; Bagetta, G. Impairment of Neuronal Glutamate Uptake and Modulation of the Glutamate Transporter GLT-1 Induced by Retinal Ischemia. *PLoS ONE* **2013**, *8*, e69250. [CrossRef] [PubMed]
3. Baxter, P.S.; Bell, K.F.; Hasel, P.; Kaindl, A.M.; Fricker, M.; Thomson, D.; Cregan, S.P.; Gillingwater, T.H.; Hardingham, G.E. Synaptic NMDA receptor activity is coupled to the transcriptional control of the glutathione system. *Nat. Commun.* **2015**, *6*, 6761. [CrossRef] [PubMed]
4. Meunier, C.; Wang, N.; Yi, C.; Dallerac, G.; Ezan, P.; Koulakoff, A.; Leybaert, L.; Giaume, C. Contribution of Astroglial Cx43 Hemichannels to the Modulation of Glutamatergic Currents by D-Serine in the Mouse Prefrontal Cortex. *J. Neurosci. Off. J. Soc. Neurosci.* **2017**, *37*, 9064–9075. [CrossRef]
5. Cuenca, N.; Fernandez-Sanchez, L.; Campello, L.; Maneu, V.; De la Villa, P.; Lax, P.; Pinilla, I. Cellular responses following retinal injuries and therapeutic approaches for neurodegenerative diseases. *Prog. Retin. Eye Res.* **2014**, *43*, 17–75. [CrossRef]
6. Opere, C.A.; Heruye, S.; Njie-Mbye, Y.F.; Ohia, S.E.; Sharif, N.A. Regulation of Excitatory Amino Acid Transmission in the Retina: Studies on Neuroprotection. *J. Ocul. Pharmacol. Ther.* **2018**, *34*, 107–118. [CrossRef]
7. Luo, X.; Yu, Y.; Xiang, Z.; Wu, H.; Ramakrishna, S.; Wang, Y.; So, K.F.; Zhang, Z.; Xu, Y. Tetramethylpyrazine nitrone protects retinal ganglion cells against N-methyl-d-aspartate-induced excitotoxicity. *J. Neurochem.* **2017**, *141*, 373–386. [CrossRef]
8. Gomez-Vicente, V.; Lax, P.; Fernandez-Sanchez, L.; Rondon, N.; Esquiva, G.; Germain, F.; de la Villa, P.; Cuenca, N. Neuroprotective Effect of Tauroursodeoxycholic Acid on N-Methyl-D-Aspartate-Induced Retinal Ganglion Cell Degeneration. *PLoS ONE* **2015**, *10*, e0137826. [CrossRef]
9. Vyklicky, V.; Korinek, M.; Smejkalova, T.; Balik, A.; Krausova, B.; Kaniakova, M.; Lichnerova, K.; Cerny, J.; Krusek, J.; Dittert, I.; et al. Structure, function, and pharmacology of NMDA receptor channels. *Physiol. Res.* **2014**, *63*, S191–S203.
10. Daruich, A.; Parcq, J.; Delaunay, K.; Naud, M.C.; Le Rouzic, Q.; Picard, E.; Crisanti, P.; Vivien, D.; Berdugo, M.; Behar-Cohen, F. Retinal safety of intravitreal rtPA in healthy rats and under excitotoxic conditions. *Mol. Vis.* **2016**, *22*, 1332–1341.
11. Lam, T.T.; Abler, A.S.; Kwong, J.M.; Tso, M.O. N-methyl-D-aspartate (NMDA)–induced apoptosis in rat retina. *Investig. Ophthalmol. Vis. Sci.* **1999**, *40*, 2391–2397.
12. Geeraerts, E.; Dekeyster, E.; Gaublomme, D.; Salinas-Navarro, M.; De Groef, L.; Moons, L. A freely available semi-automated method for quantifying retinal ganglion cells in entire retinal flatmounts. *Exp. Eye Res.* **2016**, *147*, 105–113. [CrossRef]
13. Gao, L.; Chen, X.; Tang, Y.; Zhao, J.; Li, Q.; Fan, X.; Xu, H.; Yin, Z.Q. Neuroprotective effect of memantine on the retinal ganglion cells of APPswe/PS1DeltaE9 mice and its immunomodulatory mechanisms. *Exp. Eye Res.* **2015**, *135*, 47–58. [CrossRef] [PubMed]
14. Fernandez-Sanchez, L.; Bravo-Osuna, I.; Lax, P.; Arranz-Romera, A.; Maneu, V.; Esteban-Perez, S.; Pinilla, I.; Puebla-Gonzalez, M.D.M.; Herrero-Vanrell, R.; Cuenca, N. Controlled delivery of tauroursodeoxycholic acid from biodegradable microspheres slows retinal degeneration and vision loss in P23H rats. *PLoS ONE* **2017**, *12*, e0177998. [CrossRef] [PubMed]
15. Xia, T.; Rizzolo, L.J. Effects of diabetic retinopathy on the barrier functions of the retinal pigment epithelium. *Vis. Res.* **2017**. [CrossRef] [PubMed]
16. Gupta, P.C.; Sood, S.; Narang, S.; Ichhpujani, P. Role of brimonidine in the treatment of clinically significant macular edema with ischemic changes in diabetic maculopathy. *Int. Ophthalmol.* **2014**, *34*, 787–792. [CrossRef]
17. Rodriguez Villanueva, J.; Bravo-Osuna, I.; Herrero-Vanrell, R.; Molina Martinez, I.T.; Guzman Navarro, M. Optimising the controlled release of dexamethasone from a new generation of PLGA-based microspheres intended for intravitreal administration. *Eur. J. Pharm. Sci.* **2016**, *92*, 287–297. [CrossRef]

18. Bringmann, A.; Grosche, A.; Pannicke, T.; Reichenbach, A. GABA and Glutamate Uptake and Metabolism in Retinal Glial (Müller) Cells. *Front Endocrinol (Lausanne)* **2013**, *4*, 48. [CrossRef]
19. Blanco, R.; Martinez-Navarrete, G.; Valiente-Soriano, F.J.; Aviles-Trigueros, M.; Perez-Rico, C.; Serrano-Puebla, A.; Boya, P.; Fernandez, E.; Vidal-Sanz, M.; de la Villa, P. The S1P1 receptor-selective agonist CYM-5442 protects retinal ganglion cells in endothelin-1 induced retinal ganglion cell loss. *Exp. Eye Res.* **2017**, *164*, 37–45. [CrossRef]
20. Jung, K.I.; Kim, J.H.; Park, C.K. alpha2-Adrenergic modulation of the glutamate receptor and transporter function in a chronic ocular hypertension model. *Eur. J. Pharmacol.* **2015**, *765*, 274–283. [CrossRef]
21. Almasieh, M.; Levin, L.A. Neuroprotection in Glaucoma: Animal Models and Clinical Trials. *Annu. Rev. Vis. Sci.* **2017**, *3*, 91–120. [CrossRef]
22. Omodaka, K.; Nishiguchi, K.M.; Yasuda, M.; Tanaka, Y.; Sato, K.; Nakamura, O.; Maruyama, K.; Nakazawa, T. Neuroprotective effect against axonal damage-induced retinal ganglion cell death in apolipoprotein E-deficient mice through the suppression of kainate receptor signaling. *Brain Res.* **2014**, *1586*, 203–212. [CrossRef] [PubMed]
23. Vohra, R.; Tsai, J.C.; Kolko, M. The role of inflammation in the pathogenesis of glaucoma. *Surv. Ophthalmol.* **2013**, *58*, 311–320. [CrossRef] [PubMed]
24. Colligris, B.; Crooke, A.; Gasull, X.; Escribano, J.; Herrero-Vanrell, R.; Benitez-del-Castillo, J.M.; Garcia-Feijoo, J.; Pintor, J. Recent patents and developments in glaucoma biomarkers. *Recent Pat. Endocr. Metab. Immune Drug Discov.* **2012**, *6*, 224–234. [CrossRef] [PubMed]
25. Sanchez-Lopez, E.; Egea, M.A.; Davis, B.M.; Guo, L.; Espina, M.; Silva, A.M.; Calpena, A.C.; Souto, E.M.B.; Ravindran, N.; Ettcheto, M.; et al. Memantine-Loaded PEGylated Biodegradable Nanoparticles for the Treatment of Glaucoma. *Small (Weinh. Der Bergstr. Ger.)* **2018**, *14*. [CrossRef] [PubMed]
26. Jiang, C.; Moore, M.J.; Zhang, X.; Klassen, H.; Langer, R.; Young, M. Intravitreal injections of GDNF-loaded biodegradable microspheres are neuroprotective in a rat model of glaucoma. *Mol. Vis.* **2007**, *13*, 1783–1792.
27. Tian, Y.; He, Y.; Song, W.; Zhang, E.; Xia, X. Neuroprotective effect of deferoxamine on N-methyl-d-aspartate-induced excitotoxicity in RGC-5 cells. *Acta Biochim. Et Biophys. Sin.* **2017**, *49*, 827–834. [CrossRef]
28. Zhao, L.; Chen, G.; Li, J.; Fu, Y.; Mavlyutov, T.A.; Yao, A.; Nickells, R.W.; Gong, S.; Guo, L.W. An intraocular drug delivery system using targeted nanocarriers attenuates retinal ganglion cell degeneration. *J. Control Release* **2017**, *247*, 153–166. [CrossRef]
29. Sandalon, S.; Konnecke, B.; Levkovitch-Verbin, H.; Simons, M.; Hein, K.; Sattler, M.B.; Bahr, M.; Ofri, R. Functional and structural evaluation of lamotrigine treatment in rat models of acute and chronic ocular hypertension. *Exp. Eye Res.* **2013**, *115*, 47–56. [CrossRef]
30. Andres-Guerrero, V.; Perucho-Gonzalez, L.; Garcia-Feijoo, J.; Morales-Fernandez, L.; Saenz-Frances, F.; Herrero-Vanrell, R.; Julvez, L.P.; Llorens, V.P.; Martinez-de-la-Casa, J.M.; Konstas, A.G. Current Perspectives on the Use of Anti-VEGF Drugs as Adjuvant Therapy in Glaucoma. *Adv. Ther.* **2017**, *34*, 378–395. [CrossRef]
31. Calvo, M.; Sanz-Blasco, S.; Caballero, E.; Villalobos, C.; Nunez, L. Susceptibility to excitotoxicity in aged hippocampal cultures and neuroprotection by non-steroidal anti-inflammatory drugs: Role of mitochondrial calcium. *J. Neurochem.* **2015**, *132*, 403–417. [CrossRef] [PubMed]
32. Garcia-Caballero, C.; Prieto-Calvo, E.; Checa-Casalengua, P.; Garcia-Martin, E.; Polo-Llorens, V.; Garcia-Feijoo, J.; Molina-Martinez, I.T.; Bravo-Osuna, I.; Herrero-Vanrell, R. Six month delivery of GDNF from PLGA/vitamin E biodegradable microspheres after intravitreal injection in rabbits. *Eur. J. Pharm. Sci.* **2017**, *103*, 19–26. [CrossRef] [PubMed]
33. Bravo-Osuna, I.; Andres-Guerrero, V.; Pastoriza Abal, P.; Molina-Martinez, I.T.; Herrero-Vanrell, R. Pharmaceutical microscale and nanoscale approaches for efficient treatment of ocular diseases. *Drug Deliv. Transl. Res.* **2016**, *6*, 686–707. [CrossRef] [PubMed]
34. Barcia, E.; Herrero-Vanrell, R.; Diez, A.; Alvarez-Santiago, C.; Lopez, I.; Calonge, M. Downregulation of endotoxin-induced uveitis by intravitreal injection of polylactic-glycolic acid (PLGA) microspheres loaded with dexamethasone. *Exp. Eye Res.* **2009**, *89*, 238–245. [CrossRef] [PubMed]
35. Rodriguez Villanueva, J.; Rodriguez Villanueva, L. Turning the screw even further to increase microparticle retention and ocular bioavailability of associated drugs: The bioadhesion goal. *Int. J. Pharm.* **2017**, *531*, 167–178. [CrossRef] [PubMed]
36. Bansal, P.; Garg, S.; Sharma, Y.; Venkatesh, P. Posterior Segment Drug Delivery Devices: Current and Novel Therapies in Development. *J. Ocul. Pharmacol. Ther.* **2016**, *32*, 135–144. [CrossRef] [PubMed]

37. Chen, Y.S.; Green, C.R.; Wang, K.; Danesh-Meyer, H.V.; Rupenthal, I.D. Sustained intravitreal delivery of connexin43 mimetic peptide by poly(D,L-lactide-co-glycolide) acid micro- and nanoparticles–Closing the gap in retinal ischaemia. *Eur. J. Pharm. Biopharm.* **2015**, *95*, 378–386. [CrossRef]
38. Herrero-Vanrell, R.; Bravo-Osuna, I.; Andres-Guerrero, V.; Vicario-de-la-Torre, M.; Molina-Martinez, I.T. The potential of using biodegradable microspheres in retinal diseases and other intraocular pathologies. *Prog. Retin. Eye Res.* **2014**, *42*, 27–43. [CrossRef]
39. Garbayo, E.; Montero-Menei, C.N.; Ansorena, E.; Lanciego, J.L.; Aymerich, M.S.; Blanco-Prieto, M.J. Effective GDNF brain delivery using microspheres–a promising strategy for Parkinson's disease. *J. Control Release* **2009**, *135*, 119–126. [CrossRef]
40. Chen, L.; Feng, W.; Zhou, X.; Yin, Z.; He, C. Thermo-and pH dual-responsive mesoporous silica nanoparticles for controlled drug release. *J. Control. Release* **2015**, *213*, e69–e70. [CrossRef]
41. Pannicke, T.; Fischer, W.; Biedermann, B.; Schadlich, H.; Grosche, J.; Faude, F.; Wiedemann, P.; Allgaier, C.; Illes, P.; Burnstock, G.; et al. P2X7 receptors in Muller glial cells from the human retina. *J. Neurosci.* **2000**, *20*, 5965–5972. [CrossRef]
42. Zhou, X.; Li, G.; Zhang, S.; Wu, J. 5-HT1A Receptor Agonist Promotes Retinal Ganglion Cell Function by Inhibiting OFF-Type Presynaptic Glutamatergic Activity in a Chronic Glaucoma Model. *Front. Cell Neurosci.* **2019**, *13*, 167. [CrossRef] [PubMed]
43. Chiang, B.; Venugopal, N.; Edelhauser, H.F.; Prausnitz, M.R. Distribution of particles, small molecules and polymeric formulation excipients in the suprachoroidal space after microneedle injection. *Exp. Eye Res.* **2016**, *153*, 101–109. [CrossRef] [PubMed]
44. Wheeler, L.A.; Woldemussie, E. Alpha-2 adrenergic receptor agonists are neuroprotective in experimental models of glaucoma. *Eur. J. Ophthalmol.* **2001**, *11* (Suppl. 2), S30–S35. [CrossRef]
45. Lee, D.; Kim, K.Y.; Noh, Y.H.; Chai, S.; Lindsey, J.D.; Ellisman, M.H.; Weinreb, R.N.; Ju, W.K. Brimonidine blocks glutamate excitotoxicity-induced oxidative stress and preserves mitochondrial transcription factor a in ischemic retinal injury. *PLoS ONE* **2012**, *7*, e47098. [CrossRef] [PubMed]
46. Dong, C.J.; Guo, Y.; Agey, P.; Wheeler, L.; Hare, W.A. Alpha2 adrenergic modulation of NMDA receptor function as a major mechanism of RGC protection in experimental glaucoma and retinal excitotoxicity. *Investig. Ophthalmol. Vis. Sci.* **2008**, *49*, 4515–4522. [CrossRef]
47. Zanoni, D.S.; Da Silva, G.A.; Ezra-Elia, R.; Carvalho, M.; Quitzan, J.G.; Ofri, R.; Laus, J.L.; Laufer-Amorim, R. Histological, morphometric, protein and gene expression analyses of rat retinas with ischaemia-reperfusion injury model treated with sildenafil citrate. *Int. J. Exp. Pathol.* **2017**, *98*, 147–157. [CrossRef]
48. Kwong, J.M.; Quan, A.; Kyung, H.; Piri, N.; Caprioli, J. Quantitative analysis of retinal ganglion cell survival with Rbpms immunolabeling in animal models of optic neuropathies. *Investig. Ophthalmol. Vis. Sci.* **2011**, *52*, 9694–9702. [CrossRef]
49. Koeberle, P.D.; Bahr, M. The upregulation of GLAST-1 is an indirect antiapoptotic mechanism of GDNF and neurturin in the adult CNS. *Cell Death Differ.* **2008**, *15*, 471–483. [CrossRef]
50. Nakazawa, M. Effects of calcium ion, calpains, and calcium channel blockers on retinitis pigmentosa. *J. Ophthalmol.* **2011**, *2011*, 292040. [CrossRef]
51. Yamada, H.; Chen, Y.N.; Aihara, M.; Araie, M. Neuroprotective effect of calcium channel blocker against retinal ganglion cell damage under hypoxia. *Brain Res.* **2006**, *1071*, 75–80. [CrossRef]
52. Zamponi, G.W. Targeting voltage-gated calcium channels in neurological and psychiatric diseases. *Nat. Rev. Drug Discov.* **2016**, *15*, 19–34. [CrossRef] [PubMed]
53. Isiegas, C.; Marinich-Madzarevich, J.A.; Marchena, M.; Ruiz, J.M.; Cano, M.J.; de la Villa, P.; Hernandez-Sanchez, C.; de la Rosa, E.J.; de Pablo, F. Intravitreal Injection of Proinsulin-Loaded Microspheres Delays Photoreceptor Cell Death and Vision Loss in the rd10 Mouse Model of Retinitis Pigmentosa. *Investig. Ophthalmol. Vis. Sci.* **2016**, *57*, 3610–3618. [CrossRef] [PubMed]
54. Mattson, M.P. Glutamate and Neurotrophic Factors in Neuronal Plasticity and Disease. *Ann. N. Y. Acad. Sci.* **2008**, *1144*, 97–112. [CrossRef]
55. Martinez-Moreno, C.G.; Fleming, T.; Carranza, M.; Avila-Mendoza, J.; Luna, M.; Harvey, S.; Aramburo, C. Growth hormone protects against kainate excitotoxicity and induces BDNF and NT3 expression in chicken neuroretinal cells. *Exp. Eye Res.* **2018**, *166*, 1–12. [CrossRef]
56. Klocker, N.; Braunling, F.; Isenmann, S.; Bahr, M. In vivo neurotrophic effects of GDNF on axotomized retinal ganglion cells. *Neuroreport* **1997**, *8*, 3439–3442. [CrossRef] [PubMed]

57. Chen, Z.Y.; Cao, L.; Lu, C.L.; He, C.; Bao, X. [Protective effect of exogenous glial cell line derived neurotrophic factor on neurons after sciatic nerve injury in rats]. *Sheng Li Xue Bao* **2000**, *52*, 295–300.
58. Naskar, R.; Vorwerk, C.K.; Dreyer, E.B. Concurrent downregulation of a glutamate transporter and receptor in glaucoma. *Investig. Ophthalmol. Vis. Sci.* **2000**, *41*, 1940–1944.
59. Kyhn, M.V.; Warfvinge, K.; Scherfig, E.; Kiilgaard, J.F.; Prause, J.U.; Klassen, H.; Young, M.; la Cour, M. Acute retinal ischemia caused by controlled low ocular perfusion pressure in a porcine model. Electrophysiological and histological characterisation. *Exp. Eye Res.* **2009**, *88*, 1100–1106. [CrossRef]
60. Lin, L.F.; Doherty, D.H.; Lile, J.D.; Bektesh, S.; Collins, F. GDNF: A glial cell line-derived neurotrophic factor for midbrain dopaminergic neurons. *Science* **1993**, *260*, 1130–1132. [CrossRef]
61. Ward, M.S.; Khoobehi, A.; Lavik, E.B.; Langer, R.; Young, M.J. Neuroprotection of retinal ganglion cells in DBA/2J mice with GDNF-loaded biodegradable microspheres. *J. Pharm. Sci.* **2007**, *96*, 558–568. [CrossRef] [PubMed]
62. Checa-Casalengua, P.; Jiang, C.; Bravo-Osuna, I.; Tucker, B.A.; Molina-Martinez, I.T.; Young, M.J.; Herrero-Vanrell, R. Retinal ganglion cells survival in a glaucoma model by GDNF/Vit E PLGA microspheres prepared according to a novel microencapsulation procedure. *J. Control. Release* **2011**, *156*, 92–100. [CrossRef] [PubMed]
63. Checa-Casalengua, P.; Jiang, C.; Bravo-Osuna, I.; Tucker, B.A.; Molina-Martinez, I.T.; Young, M.J.; Herrero-Vanrell, R. Preservation of biological activity of glial cell line-derived neurotrophic factor (GDNF) after microencapsulation and sterilization by gamma irradiation. *Int. J. Pharm.* **2012**, *436*, 545–554. [CrossRef]
64. Valenciano, A.I.; Corrochano, S.; de Pablo, F.; de la Villa, P.; de la Rosa, E.J. Proinsulin/insulin is synthesized locally and prevents caspase- and cathepsin-mediated cell death in the embryonic mouse retina. *J. Neurochem.* **2006**, *99*, 524–536. [CrossRef]
65. Vergara, M.N.; de la Rosa, E.J.; Canto-Soler, M.V. Focus on molecules: Proinsulin in the eye: Precursor or pioneer? *Exp. Eye Res.* **2012**, *101*, 109–110. [CrossRef] [PubMed]
66. Boatright, J.H.; Nickerson, J.M.; Moring, A.G.; Pardue, M.T. Bile acids in treatment of ocular disease. *J. Ocul. Biol. Dis. Inform.* **2009**, *2*, 149–159. [CrossRef] [PubMed]
67. Bovolenta, P.; Cisneros, E. Retinitis pigmentosa: Cone photoreceptors starving to death. *Nat. Neurosci.* **2009**, *12*, 5–6. [CrossRef]
68. Ishimaru, Y.; Sumino, A.; Kajioka, D.; Shibagaki, F.; Yamamuro, A.; Yoshioka, Y.; Maeda, S. Apelin protects against NMDA-induced retinal neuronal death via an APJ receptor by activating Akt and ERK1/2, and suppressing TNF-alpha expression in mice. *J. Pharmacol. Sci.* **2017**, *133*, 34–41. [CrossRef]
69. Kokona, D.; Thermos, K. Synthetic and endogenous cannabinoids protect retinal neurons from AMPA excitotoxicity in vivo, via activation of CB1 receptors: Involvement of PI3K/Akt and MEK/ERK signaling pathways. *Exp. Eye Res.* **2015**, *136*, 45–58. [CrossRef]
70. Sakamoto, K.; Kuroki, T.; Sagawa, T.; Ito, H.; Mori, A.; Nakahara, T.; Ishii, K. Opioid receptor activation is involved in neuroprotection induced by TRPV1 channel activation against excitotoxicity in the rat retina. *Eur. J. Pharmacol.* **2017**, *812*, 57–63. [CrossRef]
71. Lakk, M.; Denes, V.; Gabriel, R. Pituitary Adenylate Cyclase-Activating Polypeptide Receptors Signal via Phospholipase C Pathway to Block Apoptosis in Newborn Rat Retina. *Neurochem. Res.* **2015**, *40*, 1402–1409. [CrossRef] [PubMed]
72. Galvao, J.; Elvas, F.; Martins, T.; Cordeiro, M.F.; Ambrosio, A.F.; Santiago, A.R. Adenosine A3 receptor activation is neuroprotective against retinal neurodegeneration. *Exp. Eye Res.* **2015**, *140*, 65–74. [CrossRef] [PubMed]
73. Dong, Z.; Shinmei, Y.; Dong, Y.; Inafuku, S.; Fukuhara, J.; Ando, R.; Kitaichi, N.; Kanda, A.; Tanaka, K.; Noda, K.; et al. Effect of geranylgeranylacetone on the protection of retinal ganglion cells in a mouse model of normal tension glaucoma. *Heliyon* **2016**, *2*, e00191. [CrossRef] [PubMed]
74. Tsutsumi, T.; Iwao, K.; Hayashi, H.; Kirihara, T.; Kawaji, T.; Inoue, T.; Hino, S.; Nakao, M.; Tanihara, H. Potential Neuroprotective Effects of an LSD1 Inhibitor in Retinal Ganglion Cells via p38 MAPK Activity. *Investig. Ophthalmol. Vis. Sci.* **2016**, *57*, 6461–6473. [CrossRef] [PubMed]
75. Del Valle Bessone, C.; Fajreldines, H.D.; de Barboza, G.E.D.; Tolosa de Talamoni, N.G.; Allemandi, D.A.; Carpentieri, A.R.; Quinteros, D.A. Protective role of melatonin on retinal ganglionar cell: In vitro an in vivo evidences. *Life Sci.* **2019**, *218*, 233–240. [CrossRef] [PubMed]

76. Zhou, X.; Zhang, R.; Zhang, S.; Wu, J.; Sun, X. Activation of 5-HT1A Receptors Promotes Retinal Ganglion Cell Function by Inhibiting the cAMP-PKA Pathway to Modulate Presynaptic GABA Release in Chronic Glaucoma. *J. Neurosci.* **2019**, *39*, 1484–1504. [CrossRef]
77. Eriksen, A.Z.; Eliasen, R.; Oswald, J.; Kempen, P.J.; Melander, F.; Andresen, T.L.; Young, M.; Baranov, P.; Urquhart, A.J. Multifarious Biologic Loaded Liposomes that Stimulate the Mammalian Target of Rapamycin Signaling Pathway Show Retina Neuroprotection after Retina Damage. *ACS Nano* **2018**, *12*, 7497–7508. [CrossRef]
78. Mallozzi, C.; Parravano, M.; Gaddini, L.; Villa, M.; Pricci, F.; Malchiodi-Albedi, F.; Matteucci, A. Curcumin Modulates the NMDA Receptor Subunit Composition Through a Mechanism Involving CaMKII and Ser/Thr Protein Phosphatases. *Cell. Mol. Neurobiol.* **2018**, *38*, 1315–1320. [CrossRef]
79. Lambuk, L.; Jafri, A.J.; Arfuzir, N.N.; Iezhitsa, I.; Agarwal, R.; Rozali, K.N.; Agarwal, P.; Bakar, N.S.; Kutty, M.K.; Yusof, A.P.; et al. Neuroprotective Effect of Magnesium Acetyltaurate Against NMDA-Induced Excitotoxicity in Rat Retina. *Neurotox. Res.* **2017**, *31*, 31–45. [CrossRef]
80. Arranz-Romera, A.; Davis, B.M.; Bravo-Osuna, I.; Esteban-Perez, S.; Molina-Martinez, I.T.; Shamsher, E.; Ravindran, N.; Guo, L.; Cordeiro, M.F.; Herrero-Vanrell, R. Simultaneous co-delivery of neuroprotective drugs from multi-loaded PLGA microspheres for the treatment of glaucoma. *J. Control. Release* **2019**, *297*, 26–38. [CrossRef]
81. Shin, J.A.; Kim, H.S.; Vargas, A.; Yu, W.Q.; Eom, Y.S.; Craft, C.M.; Lee, E.J. Inhibition of Matrix Metalloproteinase 9 Enhances Rod Survival in the S334ter-line3 Retinitis Pigmentosa Model. *PLoS ONE* **2016**, *11*, e0167102. [CrossRef] [PubMed]
82. Zhang, X.; Cheng, M.; Chintala, S.K. Kainic acid-mediated upregulation of matrix metalloproteinase-9 promotes retinal degeneration. *Investig. Ophthalmol. Vis. Sci.* **2004**, *45*, 2374–2383. [CrossRef] [PubMed]
83. Sreekumar, P.G.; Li, Z.; Wang, W.; Spee, C.; Hinton, D.R.; Kannan, R.; MacKay, J.A. Intra-vitreal alphaB crystallin fused to elastin-like polypeptide provides neuroprotection in a mouse model of age-related macular degeneration. *J. Control. Release* **2018**, *283*, 94–104. [CrossRef] [PubMed]
84. Trudeau, K.; Muto, T.; Roy, S. Downregulation of mitochondrial connexin 43 by high glucose triggers mitochondrial shape change and cytochrome C release in retinal endothelial cells. *Investig. Ophthalmol. Vis. Sci.* **2012**, *53*, 6675–6681. [CrossRef] [PubMed]
85. Roy, S.; Jiang, J.X.; Li, A.F.; Kim, D. Connexin channel and its role in diabetic retinopathy. *Prog. Retin. Eye Res.* **2017**. [CrossRef] [PubMed]

MDPI
St. Alban-Anlage 66
4052 Basel
Switzerland
www.mdpi.com

Pharmaceutics Editorial Office
E-mail: pharmaceutics@mdpi.com
www.mdpi.com/journal/pharmaceutics

www.ingramcontent.com/pod-product-compliance
Lightning Source LLC
LaVergne TN
LVHW070216100526
838202LV00015B/2051